Primary Care Nutrition

Writing the Nutrition Prescription

Primary Care Nutrition

Writing the Nutrition Prescription

David Heber
Zhaoping Li

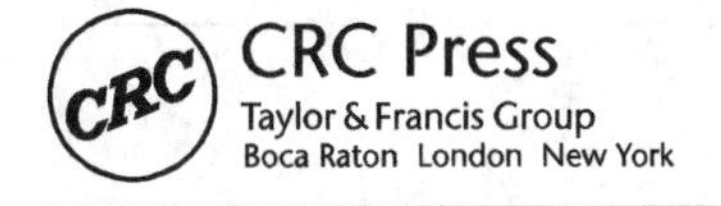

CRC Press is an imprint of the
Taylor & Francis Group, an **informa** business

CRC Press
Taylor & Francis Group
6000 Broken Sound Parkway NW, Suite 300
Boca Raton, FL 33487-2742

Printed on acid-free paper

International Standard Book Number-13: 978-1-1380-6226-9 (Paperback)
International Standard Book Number-13: 978-1-4987-4833-9 (Hardback)

Library of Congress Cataloging-in-Publication Data

Names: Heber, David, author. | Li, Zhaoping, 1962- author.
Title: Primary care nutrition : writing the nutrition prescription / David Heber, Zhaoping Li.
Description: Boca Raton : Taylor & Francis, 2017. | Includes bibliographical references and index.
Identifiers: LCCN 2016056394 | ISBN 9781498748339 (hardback : alk. paper)
Subjects: | MESH: Diet Therapy | Primary Health Care | Overweight--diet therapy |
Nutritional Physiological Phenomena | Health Promotion
Classification: LCC RA784 | NLM WB 400 | DDC 613.2--dc23
LC record available at https://lccn.loc.gov/2016056394

Visit the Taylor & Francis Web site at
http://www.taylorandfrancis.com

and the CRC Press Web site at
http://www.crcpress.com

Contents

Preface

The time is now for this textbook on primary care nutrition. Had it been written at any time during the last 30 years, it would have been thought to be totally irrelevant and an unnecessary diversion from the serious work of primary care practitioners. How could nutrition be important to a medical profession schooled in drugs and surgery for the prevention and treatment of disease?

Nutrition was an afterthought for most physicians that had nothing to do with medicine but was a supportive function delegated to dietitians. Dietitians functioned in limited ways in hospitals to help patients choose which menu items they would like to eat from the limited, cost-driven choices provided by most hospital kitchens. Some administrative dietitians came to control hospital kitchen budgets and were named directors of nutrition departments in major medical centers. Out in the world, dietitians struggled to develop private practices and were always driven by food industry–directed information that they were urged to deliver to patients. The American Dietetic Association had more members in one large state than the total number of certified by.

The creative energy in medical research funded by the National Institutes of Health in the postwar 1950s through the 1970s was directed at understanding the cellular and molecular basis of disease. This understanding revolutionized medicine into a science-based endeavor for optimal health. Subspecialties divided on the basis of organ systems sprouted in the 1970s to incorporate the large amount of special technical information that was emerging. Subspecialty divisions, including pulmonary and intensive care, nephrology, and endocrinology and metabolism, were established from what was formerly simply a division of metabolism.

As this process proceeded to become more highly specialized, the utilization of expensive and targeted treatments recommended by specialists was the main focus of patient care. The primary care physician conducted annual physical exams and analyzed routine laboratory values in an attempt to detect diseases at an early stage. Primary care doctors were called general practitioners to indicate that they really had the limited expertise of a generalist. It was much more prestigious to be a specialist during the age of expanding discoveries in the 1970s and 1980s.

Ultimately, the United States developed the most advanced and highly technical medical solutions in the world, but the distribution of that care was not cost-effective. Renal dialysis was begun to deal with the tragedy of young people dying of kidney failure due to autoimmune diseases and other rare conditions. With the advent of Medicare, dialysis expanded to include patients with type 2 diabetes, who now make up a significant portion of the hundreds of thousands of patients receiving this care in preparation for renal transplant or simply as a last resort. Cardiology has undergone a major expansion with the addition of interventional cardiologists who revascularize coronary arteries that would previously have required open-heart surgery, accompanied by cracking open the chest to reach the heart.

The advent of statins and drugs for hypertension gave patients the impression that they were protected from advanced disease solely through medication. Diet and exercise were largely not part of the medical model. Nonetheless, adherence to medications was poor. Often, this resulted from unacceptable side effects, such as muscle pain in patients taking statin drugs. In other cases, it was simply due to poor adherence that was in line with poor lifestyle habits and inattention to medical advice. In the 1970s and 1980s, the hospital was the place that care was delivered. The primary care doctor was simply a bystander and patient advocate as specialists swirled around the patient, consulting separately on each organ system. Procedures and tests that were often unnecessary were simply performed to defend against the risk of malpractice suits. Fear of omission or making a mistake drove much of this behavior without regard to costs.

Attitudes about outpatient nutrition in primary care began to change as the result of the detection of the obesity epidemic in the United States in the early 1990s. This was followed by the identification of the Global Nutrition Transition, where countries throughout the world had both malnutrition and obesity coexisting in societies that had only known malnutrition and underweight until recent years. The World Health Organization declared that for the first time in human history, there were more overweight than underweight people. While fast food and a sedentary lifestyle were identified as major factors in this global epidemic, there was little innovation in medical practice against these driving forces. Medical care continued as usual based on the molecular and cellular research engine that moved more slowly, and now more of the research was based within the drug industry, which has a vested interest in promoting their solutions over nutrition and lifestyle changes.

Over a period of 20 years, numerous hormones and peptides regulating food intake and energy expenditure were discovered in laboratories and moved to drug companies. All these drugs designed to address a bonanza of potential drug sales to the 50% of Americans who were overweight or obese failed.

The most informative example was the discovery of leptin. This was the most promising protein to emerge from the molecular revolution, whose very name is taken from the Greek root for the word that means "thinning." The full story is repeated in Chapter 5, but the point is that a basic observation in rodents that a protein could both correct a rare human genetic defect associated with obesity and prevent mice from becoming obese on a high-fat snack food-based diet called a "cafeteria diet" gained tremendous attention both at the National Institutes of Health and in the drug industry as Amgen invested $20 million to license leptin's intellectual property from the Rockefeller University in New York and many millions more to test this drug in humans. It turned out that leptin had little effect on the garden-variety obesity that was becoming increasingly common in the United States, but it worked as predicted in the genetic defect of leptin deficiency, which only occurred in a relatively small number of individuals from the Middle East and Scotland.

At the same time as these drugs were failing, many consumers were having success with meal replacements, the practice of substituting protein-rich shakes for typical cereal and milk breakfasts or high-calorie eggs, bacon, and potatoes served at restaurants and as weekend breakfasts at home. The reaction of the food industry and dietitians to this phenomenon was one of almost total rejection. In the late 1970s, extreme very low-calorie diets made from poor-quality protein and administered without medical supervision led to the deaths of about 80 women in the United States. The perception that these diets were dangerous persisted despite the development of high-quality shakes using milk protein and supplemented with vitamins and minerals. Research funded by industry demonstrated in more than 500 publications that these protein shakes were a successful modality within a healthy diet to promote weight management.

Our group at the University of California, Los Angeles (UCLA) published a multisite study in 1994 in which a minimal intervention of supplying meal replacements and paying participants to be weighed weekly in six different centers around the United States led to significant weight loss in the range of 5% of body weight. However, the weight loss required adherence to diet, and the meal replacements merely simplified the process by removing some complexity from daily nutrition plans. The next accomplishment was to show that meal replacements could be safely used in patients with type 2 diabetes, led to better weight loss than food-based diets, and were safe. While there were ongoing improvements in the taste and convenience of protein shakes, there were many people who could not accept the idea that a shake would be a meal. In our research studies, we conducted a run-in phase and often up to half of recruited subjects for a randomized study would refuse to consume shakes. The LOOK Ahead Trial was the first large multisite study funded by the National Institutes of Health to use meal replacements. There were three predictors of weight loss in participants over the first year: use of meal replacements, recording food intake, and physical activity. The more shakes an individual consumed, the greater the observed weight loss. Today, meal replacements are used around the world within a diet plan that emphasizes adequate protein and physical activity, including a healthy active lifestyle and resistance exercises.

Despite being the most easily understood variable in the obesity drug and various nutrition approaches, weight loss alone is not necessarily a good thing. Full-day symposia were held by the American Society for Nutrition differentiating unintentional weight loss, which was often associated with cancers and other chronic diseases, from the deliberate weight loss achieved by overweight and obese patients. Our group was the first to use the term *sarcopenic obesity*, which combined the idea of an increase in body fat together with a reduction in muscle mass as a clinical subtype of obesity. Incorporating resistance exercise into recommended weight management regimens for men and women to optimize body composition became the predominant philosophy of our UCLA Risk Factor Obesity Program. As described in Chapter 5, resistance exercise and protein supplementation work together to change body composition. However, the target of that supplementation was individualized optimal protein intake based on the lean body mass measured by bioelectrical impedance. The recommended amount of protein was almost twice the minimum 0.8 g/kg that was derived from a 1973 research study that identified that number as the minimum for positive nitrogen balance.

The emergence of the metabolic syndrome as a collection of risk factors for diabetes, heart disease, and even common forms of cancer led to a reassessment of body composition again. While the idea that abdominal fat was important was first proposed in the 1950s, modern research not only identified the health implications of this common condition through epidemiological observations, but also established through molecular and cellular investigations that visceral fat is an inflammatory organ releasing cytokines into the systemic circulation.

Age-related chronic diseases are not simply commonly observed conditions, but conditions with a common origin in poor diets and lifestyles. Primary care was thrown into the limelight with the development of diagnosis-related compensation from the government and private insurers. The primary care practice was invested with the function of a gatekeeper appropriately rationing inpatient care, diagnostic tests, and expensive interventions prior to the involvement of specialists. These proposed cost-cutting measures did not result in control of overall health care costs in the United States, as growth in the number of people with diabetes, heart disease, and other costly age-related chronic diseases continued to increase. As expected, ministries of health around the world have identified similar increases in poor health. Chief among these countries was Mexico, which nearly rivals the United States in the prevalence of overweight, obesity, metabolic syndrome, and type 2 diabetes. However, the largest coming wave of patients will originate in China, where 120 million people have diagnosed diabetes, and prediabetes affects about 500 million people.

Our key mission in writing this textbook is to provide primary care practices with the information and tools to address this global epidemic of obesity and nutrition-related diseases. After initial chapters on integrating nutrition into your primary care practice, there is a revealing look at the process of developing dietary guidelines and how the guidelines have slowly evolved to incorporate new findings in nutritional science and medicine. In the chapters that follow, the messages go beyond the dietary guidelines that are for healthy people and not for disease conditions. The chapters cover obesity, eating disorders and food intolerance, lipid disorders, heart disease and heart failure, renal disease, pulmonary disease, cancer prevention, and cancer survival.

We want to acknowledge the support of Dr. Jieping Yang, who assisted in editing and formatting the text, as well as setting the framework for our writing schedules over the last year. We also want to thank Randy Brehm at CRC Press, whose vision resulted in the development of the concept for this book.

David Heber, MD, PhD, FACP, FASN
Professor Emeritus of Medicine and Public Health
Founding Director, UCLA Center for Human Nutrition
David Geffen School of Medicine at UCLA

Zhaoping Li, MD, PhD
Professor of Medicine
Lynda and Stewart Resnick Chair in Human Nutrition
Chief, Division of Clinical Nutrition
and Director, UCLA Center for Human Nutrition
David Geffen School of Medicine at UCLA

Authors

David Heber, MD, PhD, FACP, FASN, is a professor emeritus of medicine and public health at the David Geffen School of Medicine at University of California, Los Angeles (UCLA) and is internationally prominent in the fields of nutrition, metabolism, and obesity and its associated complications. He is also the founding director of the UCLA Center for Human Nutrition and the founding chief of the Division of Clinical Nutrition in the UCLA Department of Medicine where he directed multiple National Institutes of Health-funded research programs, including the UCLA Clinical Nutrition Research Unit, the UCLA Dietary Supplements Research Center: Botanicals and the UCLA Nutrition and Obesity Training Grant. Dr. Heber is the founding chair of the Herbalife Nutrition Institute, and is a member of the McCormick Science Institute.

Dr. Heber is board certified in internal medicine, and endocrinology and metabolism by the American Board of Internal Medicine and is a certified physician nutrition specialist. He earned his MD at Harvard Medical School and his PhD in physiology at the UCLA. Dr. Heber served as chair of the Medical Nutrition Council of the American Society for Nutrition and, in 2014, was elected as a fellow of the American Society for Nutrition, the highest honor of the society. He has been listed multiple times since 2000 as one of the Best Doctors in America including 2015–2016 based on a survey of over 35,000 physicians in the United States. In 2014, according to Reuters News Agency, he was in the top 1% of cited authors in the field of agricultural sciences and was listed as one of the most influential scientific minds of 2014.

Dr. Heber's primary areas of research are obesity treatment and prevention, and the role of nutrition, phytonutrients, and botanical dietary supplements in the prevention and treatment of common forms of cancer and cardiovascular disease. He has published seminal research articles on the causes of obesity, weight loss strategies, and the relationship of obesity to cancer and cardiovascular disease, and is the author of over 250 peer-reviewed scientific articles, over 50 book chapters, several professional texts, and four books for the public including "What Color Is Your Diet?" and "The LA Shape Diet."

Zhaoping Li, MD, PhD, FACP, FACN is the director of the Center for Human Nutrition, chief of the Division of Clinical Nutrition, and the Lynda and Stewart Resnick Endowed Chair in Human Nutrition at David Geffen School of Medicine at the University of California, Los Angeles (UCLA). Currently, she is the vice president of the National Board of Physician Nutrition Specialists, the president of the World Association of Chinese Doctors in Clinical Nutrition, and a member of the American Society for Nutrition Medical Nutrition Council.

Dr. Li is board certified in internal medicine and a physician nutrition specialist. She completed her MD and PhD in physiology at Beijing University, China and has been a faculty member at UCLA. She is leading the Center for Human Nutrition to have vigorous research programs in nutrition, microbiome, and metabolism; providing mentorship and didactic and informal training for young scientists, premed, medical students, medical residents, fellows, and clinicians; and directing clinical programs that specialize in metabolic diseases, bariatric medicine, gastrointestinal diseases, and cancer prevention/treatment.

For nearly three decades, Dr Li's research interest has focused on translational research in the role of macronutrients and phytochemicals in the prevention and treatment of obesity-related chronic diseases. She has been a principal investigator for over 50 investigator-initiated National Institutes of Health- and industry-sponsored clinical trials and published over 150 peer-reviewed papers in journals such as *JAMA, Annals of Internal Medicine, American Journal of Clinical Nutrition,* and *Journal of American Dietetic Association.*

1 Incorporating Nutrition into the Primary Care Practice

1.1 INTRODUCTION

You can make a significant difference through your efforts in a world challenged by an international epidemic of chronic diseases fueled by rapidly spreading unbalanced nutrition and sedentary lifestyles. Primary care has typically presided over the relentless progress of common chronic diseases while providing palliative drugs that control blood sugar, blood pressure, and blood lipids. In this book, you will learn how to prescribe nutrition and lifestyle change for the prevention and palliation of such common diseases as type 2 diabetes mellitus, heart disease, and common forms of cancer.

It is very clear that physicians do not have the time or training to sit with patients and discuss the details of their breakfast, lunch, and dinner, or the details of their exercise program. Moreover, they do not have the time to follow up in adequate detail with patients to see if they are complying with their nutrition and exercise prescription. Previous efforts to make primary care physicians competent in all aspects of exercise and nutritional counseling have not been successful, as amply documented in studies of physicians in the United States and around the world. The only exception is the relatively small number of physician nutrition specialists in academic centers and in private practice who have a commitment to practice nutrition and weight management as a specialty.

This chapter and the balance of the book aim to arm you with the necessary tools to incorporate nutrition into your primary care practice, utilizing nurses, registered dietitians, psychologists, and physical therapists, whether within your practice or by referral to the community. In addition, there are commercial weight loss programs, Internet weight loss programs, and smartphone apps that are all available to help patients improve their diet and lifestyle.

Surveying your patient population, organizing the office staff, taking advantage of printed and Internet resources, obtaining proper office equipment, and becoming conversant in global nutrition issues affecting different populations will prepare you to incorporate nutrition into your practice. As a result of these efforts, you will begin the process of providing an environment where your patient's nutritional issues can be addressed.

While you are not expected to deliver the care, your knowledge base must be at a level where you feel comfortable endorsing the importance of diet and lifestyle as a legitimate component of primary care practice.

1.2 SURVEY YOUR PRACTICE POPULATION'S NUTRITION STATUS AND LIFESTYLE

Dietary patterns, physical activity, and lifestyle are inseparable, and the first step in understanding your practice population is to realize that nutrition is more than diet alone and encompasses all aspects of exercise and lifestyle that affect metabolism and age-related chronic diseases on an individual basis.

Practice populations differ in their demographic, socioeconomic, and cultural backgrounds, all of which affect their nutrition and lifestyle habits. Profiling your practice population is not something you have to do personally, but your office staff can build a database so that you can spend your time most efficiently in encouraging diet and lifestyle changes that are culturally, socially, and economically feasible with those individuals in your practice at highest risk, including those with the metabolic syndrome, hypertension, prediabetes, and type 2 diabetes.

A one-size-fits-all approach to nutrition intervention is not effective, and waiting to deliver services only to those patients who request nutrition consultation is an outdated and likely a wasted effort for your primary care practice. On the other hand, once you identify the at-risk groups in your practice, which will be a significant fraction of your patient population, you can survey and encourage readiness to change so that your efforts will have the greatest impact on the overall quality of care you can provide individually, within your practice, and within your community. By the way, this is not something that every primary care doctor will want to do. However, you can become an example to your patients and a resource to your colleagues and your community by taking on this challenge.

1.2.1 The Global Nutrition Transition and Your Practice

While poor nutritional habits and sedentary lifestyle are global problems, the world leader in establishing this unhealthy combination has been the United States over the past 40 years. It was only in the last years of the twentieth century that the U.S. Centers for Disease Control and Prevention identified sedentary lifestyle and unhealthy nutritional habits as causal factors that increase the risk of heart disease and common forms of cancer, the two leading killers of all adults in the United States (U.S. Department of Health and Human Services 1996).

On a global scale, 5 million deaths worldwide have been attributed to unhealthy nutritional habits, including sedentary lifestyle, making these habits among the 10 leading global causes of death and disability (Booth et al. 2000; Lees and Booth 2005; Lee et al. 2012). The World Health Organization has recognized that for the first time in human history, there are more overweight than underweight individuals in the world today, and this applies to your practice.

One of the most striking examples of this global shift is Mexico (Figure 1.1) (Romieu et al. 1997). Mexico has documented an increase in obesity in urban areas and continued malnutrition in some rural areas (Chávez et al. 1993). The Global Nutrition Transition is marked by the prevalence of overweight and obesity surpassing malnutrition and an increase in deaths from noncommunicable chronic diseases (NCDs) in low- and middle-income countries (Chávez et al. 1993; Popkin 2004; Caballero 2005; Doak and Popkin 2008). The nutrition transition often precedes or occurs in tandem with demographic, epidemiological, and socioeconomic changes resulting from globalization, urbanization, and development (Popkin and Gordon-Larsen 2004; Omran 2005; Satia 2010). For example, Brazil, Chile, Ecuador, Mexico, Peru, and the Dominican Republic are considered to

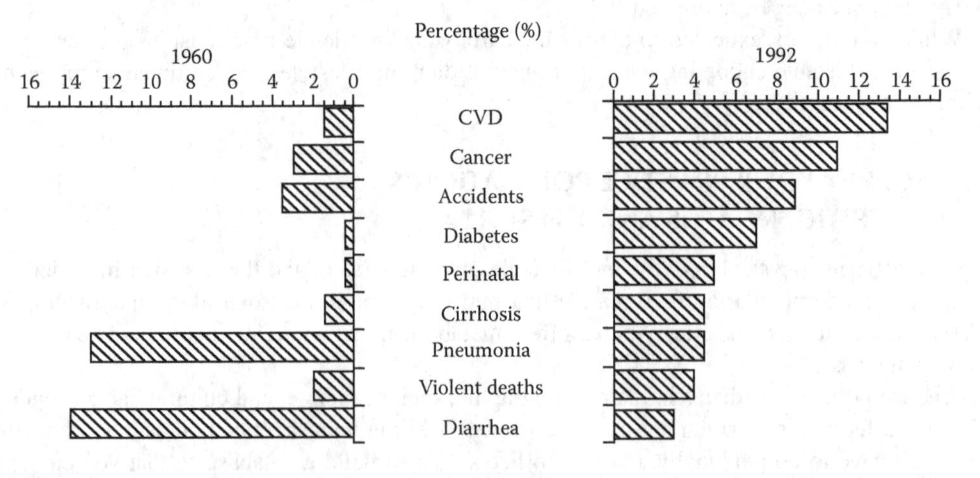

FIGURE 1.1 Principal causes of death in Mexico in 1960 and 1992. CVD, cardiovascular disease; perinatal, perinatal diseases. (Reprinted from Romieu, I. et al., *Am. J. Clin. Nutr.*, 65(4 Suppl.), 1159S–1165S, 1997.)

be advancing in the nutrition transition because, since 2000, these countries have had an increasing prevalence of obesity, increased proportion of dietary intake from fat, reduced prevalence of infant mortality and stunting, and increasing mortality from NCDs (Albala et al. 2001; Uauy et al. 2001; Ford and Mokdad 2008; Barquera et al. 2009, 2013; Bonvecchio et al. 2009; Abrahams et al. 2011; Rojas-Martínez et al. 2012).

African American and Latino adults in the United States have a higher prevalence of obesity than non-Hispanic whites (Flegal et al. 2010; Ogden et al. 2012). The relationship between acculturation to an American or Western diet pattern and overweight and obesity among Latino immigrants has been well documented in the literature (Schaffer et al. 1998; Aldrich and Variyam 2000; Bermudez et al. 2000; Edmonds 2005; Akresh 2007; Bowie et al. 2007; Ayala et al. 2008), but is clearly not restricted to that ethnic group.

1.2.2 Food Insecurity and Low Socioeconomic Status

In diverse populations in both developed and developing countries, studies have found a mild to strong relationship between food insecurity and obesity (Carlson et al. 1999; Adams et al. 2003; Hawkes 2006; Velásquez-Melendez et al. 2011). Food insecurity is a state in which the availability of nutritionally adequate foods is reduced where the ability to obtain acceptable foods is limited or uncertain.

Ethnic or racial minority status and low socioeconomic status (SES), whether conceptualized at the individual or neighborhood level, are both associated with an increased risk of morbidity and mortality for numerous age-related chronic diseases seen commonly in primary care practices (Coogan et al. 2010; Lantz and Pritchard 2010). For example, African American patients and others of lower SES are more likely than other groups to have two or more cardiovascular disease risk factors (Sharma et al. 2004), and these groups also have higher rates of hypertension (Flegal et al. 2002), poorly controlled diabetes (Romieu et al. 1997), and obesity (Chávez et al. 1993). They also exhibit low rates of meeting recommendations for fruit and vegetable intake (Popkin 2004) and, in some studies, poorer dietary profiles (Caballero 2005; Doak and Popkin 2008).

High-fat, high-salt, high-sugar foods are often the lowest-cost options available to consumers in low-income neighborhoods, as they are more affordable than healthier diet options (Omran 2005). African American neighborhood markets often have less store space devoted to fresh and frozen fruits and vegetables than markets in upper-scale neighborhoods, but similar space devoted to high-calorie energy-dense snacks with low nutrient density (Satia 2010).

Individuals with lower income and those living in ethnic minority neighborhoods have greater access to fast-food restaurants (Abrahams et al. 2011) and less access to supermarkets with fresh produce (Albala et al. 2001) than people in higher-income and majority neighborhoods. A higher frequency of fast-food consumption has been reported in African Americans (Uauy et al. 2001; Ford and Mokdad 2008) and persons of lower SES (Caballero 2005; Bonvecchio et al. 2009; Rojas-Martínez et al. 2012), and a growing body of literature shows that fast-food consumption is associated with poorer dietary habits. Studies have compared the diet composition of adults, based on dietary recalls, on days in which fast food was consumed versus days it was not. It is no surprise that overall dietary parameters on days when fast-food consumption occurs demonstrate higher total calories, total fat, saturated fat, carbohydrates, added sugar, and sugar-sweetened carbonated beverages, and lower fiber, vitamins and minerals, milk, nonstarchy vegetables, and fruit intake (Ford and Mokdad 2008; Rojas-Martínez et al. 2012). Other studies have used food frequency questionnaires or dietary screeners and more general questions about average or typical fast-food consumption with similar findings (Uauy et al. 2001; Barquera et al. 2009, 2013), including in African Americans (Uauy et al. 2001; Flegal et al. 2010). In addition to specific dietary parameters, studies have also found that more frequent fast-food consumption is associated with poorer overall dietary quality, as measured by eating indices (Uauy et al. 2001; Ogden et al. 2012), as well as weight gain and poor metabolic health outcomes (Aldrich and Variyam 2000; Uauy et al. 2001; Akresh 2007; Ayala et al. 2008).

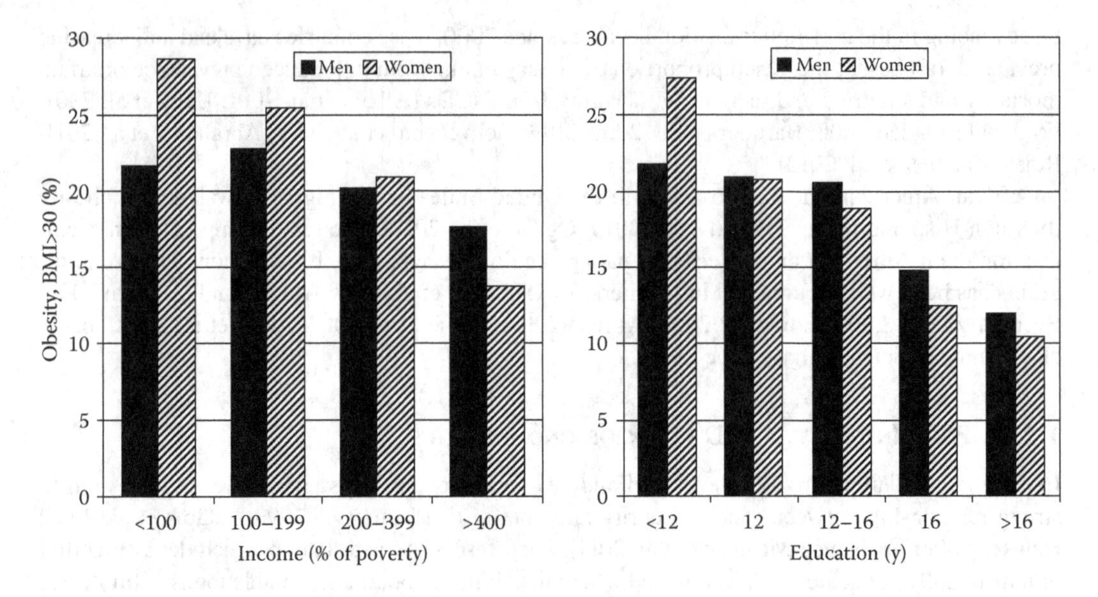

FIGURE 1.2 Obesity as a function of income and education. (Reprinted from Drewnowski, A., and Specter, S. E., *Am. J. Clin. Nutr.*, 79(1), 6–16, 2004.)

The global nutrition transition also occurs as the result of acculturation to American dietary habits with immigrants from multiple cultural and ethnic backgrounds (Schaffer et al. 1998; Carlson et al. 1999; Bermudez et al. 2000; Adams et al. 2003; Sharma et al. 2004; Edmonds 2005; Hawkes 2006; Bowie et al. 2007; Coogan et al. 2010; Lantz and Pritchard 2010; Velásquez-Melendez et al. 2011).

Among women, higher obesity rates tend to be associated with low incomes and low education levels (Kumanyika 1999; Flegal et al. 2002; Paeratakul et al. 2002; Wardle et al. 2002). The association of obesity with low SES has been less consistent among men (Flegal et al. 2002; Paeratakul et al. 2002). Minority populations, other than Asian Americans, exhibit higher rates of obesity and overweight than do U.S. whites based on body mass index (BMI) (Flegal et al. 2002). Studies of body composition have not been done in Asian American populations, but our own studies in Asian college students show a high incidence of sarcopenic obesity, where there is increased body fat despite normal BMI. Analyses of data for 68,556 U.S. adults in the National Health Interview Survey by the Centers for Disease Control and Prevention showed that the highest obesity rates were associated with the lowest incomes and low educational levels (Schoenborn et al. 2002). The relation between obesity and education and income, based on charts published by the Centers for Disease Control and Prevention (Schoenborn et al. 2002), is shown separately for men and women in Figure 1.2.

1.2.3 Relative Food Costs and Calories per Bite

Over the past 40 years, there has been a progressive global market-driven development of food technology used to make high-fat, high-sugar, high-salt snack foods and commodities used in foods available to consumers at very low cost while retaining profit margins (Bowman 1997; Maillot et al. 2007; Townsend et al. 2009). In order to determine whether the relative low cost of processed foods and ingredients in fast foods promotes poor eating habits and the global epidemic of obesity and diabetes, a number of researchers led by Dr. Adam Drewnowski of the University of Washington School of Public Health have examined the cost of foods relative to their energy density (Figure 1.3) (Darmon and Drewnowski 2015). These studies also have an impact on understanding the relationships between SES, diet quality, and health.

Using energy density values from Rolls and Barnett (2000), Drewnowski collected the energy costs of foods from supermarkets in Seattle in the winter of 2003. The concept he demonstrated is

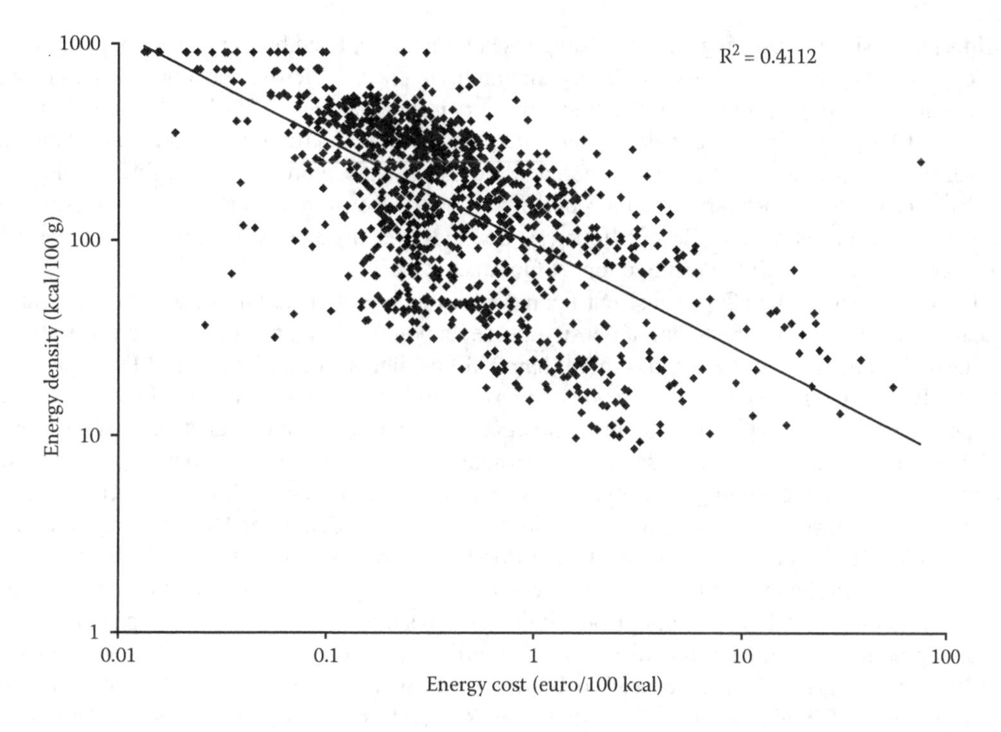

FIGURE 1.3 Energy density (kcal/100 g) and energy cost (euro/100 kcal) of foods (n = 1117) in the French food database, based on 2007 national food prices. (Reprinted from Darmon, N., and Drewnowski, A., *Nutr. Rev.*, 73(10), 643–660, 2015.)

that you get more calories per dollar with junk foods than healthy foods. The energy cost of cookies or potato chips was about 1200 kcal/dollar, whereas that of fresh carrots was only 250 kcal/dollar. The energy cost of soft drinks was 875 kcal/dollar, whereas that of orange juice from concentrate was 170 kcal/dollar. Fats and oils, sugar, refined grains, potatoes, and beans represented some of the lowest-cost options and provided dietary energy at lower cost than healthy foods. The differential in energy costs between sugar and strawberries was on the order of several thousand percent. The hierarchy of food prices is such that dry foods with a stable shelf life are generally less costly per kilocalorie than are perishable meats or fresh produce with high water content. As a rule, potato chips, chocolate, and locally bottled soft drinks provide dietary energy at a lower cost than do naturally hydrated lean meats, fish, and fresh vegetables and fruit. Energy-dense foods may contain a relatively high proportion of refined grains, added sugars, and vegetable fats.

The U.S. diet has been shown to derive close to 50% of energy from added sugars and fat (Bowman 1997; Maillot et al. 2007). Data from the Economic Research Service of the U.S. Department of Agriculture (USDA) (Townsend et al. 2009) show that the per capita availability of caloric sweeteners and fats and oils increased by 20% for each between 1977 and 1997. Retail price increases during that time were much lower for sweets and fats than for vegetables and fruit. Other studies have shown that foods identified as accounting for the greatest increase in energy intake by Americans during that time were salty snacks, desserts, soft drinks, fruit drinks, hamburgers, and cheeseburgers. For the most part, many such foods are composed of refined grains, added sugars, and fats.

1.3 IDENTIFYING MEDICAL, NUTRITIONAL, BEHAVIORAL, AND EXERCISE RESOURCES AVAILABLE

The American Society for Nutrition (ASN), with more than 4100 members, is the premier research society dedicated to improving the quality of life through the science of nutrition. The society fulfills its mission by fostering and enhancing research in animal and human nutrition, and providing opportunities for sharing, disseminating, and archiving peer-reviewed nutrition research results at its annual meeting and in its publications, the *American Journal of Clinical Nutrition* and the *Journal of Nutrition*. The society also fosters quality education and training in nutrition through its annual continuing medical education conference, Advances and Controversies in Clinical Nutrition. The society welcomes primary care physicians with an interest in nutrition. Its Medical Nutrition Council sponsors a number of Research Interest Sections, the largest of which, with more than 500 members, is the Research Interest Section on Obesity.

The Obesity Society (TOS) is a scientific and educational organization dedicated to expanding research, prevention, and treatment of obesity and reduction in stigma and discrimination affecting persons with obesity. The society has more than 2500 members. About 39% are PhDs, 35% MDs, and 2% RDs. Physician specialties include endocrinology, internal medicine, psychology, psychiatry, pediatrics bariatric surgery, and family practice. Members work in universities, hospitals, individual or group practices, medical schools, government, and other fields. The society publishes two journals, including the leading peer-reviewed scientific journal in the field, *Obesity*. The society's annual meeting, Obesity Week, is cohosted with the American Society for Metabolic and Bariatric Surgery (ASMBS) and brings in more than 5000 obesity professionals. Obesity Week is the premier annual scientific and educational conference bringing together the world's experts in obesity research, treatment, and prevention—from clinicians and surgeons to educators and policy makers. TOS members are organized into various interest groups by specialty, known as sections, including Bariatric Surgery, Basic Science, Bio-Behavioral Research, Clinical Management, Diversity, eHealth/mHealth, Epidemiology, Health Services Research, Latin American Affairs, Obesity & Cancer, and Pediatric Obesity.

The Academy of Nutrition and Dietetics is the world's largest organization of food and nutrition professionals, founded in Cleveland, Ohio, in 1917, by a visionary group of women dedicated to helping the government conserve food and improve the public's health and nutrition during World War I. Today, the academy has more than 75,000 members—registered dietitian nutritionists, dietetic technicians, registered and other dietetics professionals holding undergraduate and advanced degrees in nutrition and dietetics, and students—and is committed to improving the nation's health and advancing the profession of dietetics through research, education, and advocacy. This is an excellent resource for nutritional publications and information for dietitians. There are sections for dietitians interested in sports nutrition, research, or other areas of dietetics.

With more than 50,000 members and certified professionals, the American College of Sports Medicine (ACSM) is the largest sports medicine and exercise science organization in the world. For more than 60 years, the ACSM has advanced and translated scientific research to provide educational and practical applications of exercise science and sports medicine. ACSM and its members are dedicated to promoting well-being, sport safety, fitness, and physical activity through research, education, and public health efforts that positively impact quality of life for athletes. Primary care physicians interested in sports nutrition and medicine can obtain scientific information through position papers and attending meetings of this society.

This is not an exhaustive list, but these organizations provide well-vetted information that is accurate. Many popular authors and websites advertising nutritional products contain information that is not reliable.

1.4 OBTAINING THE EQUIPMENT NEEDED FOR PRIMARY CARE NUTRITION PRACTICE

In order to be able to classify patients by body weight for height, it is vital to have a stadiometer, as well as an accurate scale in your practice. The scales should be certified within 0.1 kg, and I prefer the electronic scales that automatically register weight, as opposed to the traditional doctor's scale, which requires balancing a counterweight. This takes more time and is often not as accurate. It is important to weigh patients consistently, with or without shoes, and ask them to remove heavy clothing as well.

Pamphlets with nutritional information and DVD presentations on televisions in the waiting room can be an excellent source of nutrition education for patients.

1.5 OUTFITTING YOUR OFFICE TO ACCOMMODATE OBESE PATIENTS

It is helpful to have industrial-capacity electronic scales that are able to accurately weigh patients up to 400 pounds if you intend to see obese patients in your practice. It is also important to have armless chairs in the waiting room and corridors able to accommodate obese patients. A number of pieces of hospital equipment have been redesigned, including MRI machines, to be able to accommodate obese patients up to 650 pounds. The need for this redesign of equipment is a sad comment on the extent of the obesity epidemic and its growth in this country over the last 40 years. TOS is a good source for specific recommendations on equipment manufacturers for a primary care practice that plans to accommodate severely obese patients.

1.6 TRAINING YOUR STAFF TO BE EMPATHETIC AND HAVE SUPPORTIVE INTERACTIONS

It is vital to identify staff members with an interest in nutrition and an empathetic attitude to the obese. Staff who believe that obesity is a moral failing are likely to mistreat obese patients or make them feel uncomfortable. Office staff without special training that dietitians or nurses typically have can welcome and encounter patients with nutritional issues, including obesity. Medical assistants and even receptionists who have a strong personal interest in nutrition can be encouraged to obtain valid information on the nutrition status of patients and record it appropriately in a practice record.

Questionnaires can be placed in the waiting room to help you determine the nutritional status and interests of your patients. These can be collected by the office staff and utilized to profile the concerns and habits of your patients. The Society for Behavioral Medicine has recommended the questionnaires listed in Table 1.1 for use in primary care practices. It also recommends including these in the electronic health record (Glasgow and Emmons 2011).

Note that many of the scales in Table 1.1 survey behavioral issues and physical activity, which are part of the nutrition landscape. Isolating food environment information alone often misses the real motivation for existing poor nutritional and lifestyle habits. Which of the above scales and questionnaires you incorporate into your practice will depend on your particular interests and the focus of your practice. In Chapters 2 and 5, on optimum nutrition and the assessment of overweight and obese patients, further suggestions for analytical tools are given. However, it is not likely you will choose to use all these. Instead, select those that make the most sense for your practice population.

Despite the epidemic of overweight and obesity in the United States today, there are still some groups at risk for nutritional deficiencies. These groups include (1) pregnant women, (2) the elderly, and (3) individuals who smoke, drink excess amounts of alcohol, or abuse drugs. While the nutritional supplementation of pregnant women is well established, including the use of prenatal vitamins, in lower socioeconomic groups, there are still many women who fail to get prenatal nutritional counseling. In clinics seeing a large number of alcoholics and drug abusers, nutrition is given little attention. Similarly, in primary care practices seeing geriatric patients, most attention is directed at chronic diseases such as diabetes, dementia, and cardiovascular diseases.

The assessment of risk of nutritional deficiency is straightforward and can be used to determine which patients require consideration for nutritional support, as described in Box 1.1.

TABLE 1.1
Recommended Domains and Example Measures

Domain	Example Measures
Smoking/tobacco use	SRNT items; one Fagerstrom item for smokers
Physical activity	BRFSS, IPAQ, or pedometer readings
Eating patterns	Starting the conversation or NCI fat and fruit/vegetable screeners
Risky drinking	2 items from AUDIT or BRFSS
Medication taking	Hill–Bone Adherence Scale
Optional items	Customized to site priorities—e.g., salt intake, sleep patterns
Psychosocial and Patient/Environmental Characteristics	
Depression/anxiety	PHQ 2 or 4
Quality of life	PROMIS questions
Stress/distress	Distress scale or distress thermometer
Health literacy/numeracy	Chin and Fagerlin health literacy and numeracy items
Patient goals	Free text on specific measurable goal and goal attainment
Demographic characteristics	Race, ethnicity, zip code for GIS coding
Optional characteristics	Customized to setting: patient priorities and preferences (e.g., preferred level of participation in medical decision making, mode of contact—e-mail vs. phone)
Issue patient most wants to discuss during next contact	

Source: Reprinted from Glasgow, R., and Emmons, K. M., *Transl. Behav. Med.*, 1(1), 108–109, 2011.

Note: AUDIT: Alcohol Use Disorder Identification Test; BRFSS: Behavioral Risk Factor Surveillance System; GIS: Geographic Information Systems; IPAQ: International Physical Activity Questionnaire; NCI: National Cancer Institute; PHQ: Patient Health Questionnaire; PROMIS: Patient-Reported Outcomes Measurement Information System; SRNT: Society for Research on Nicotine and Tobacco.

BOX 1.1 SIGNS AND SYMPTOMS OF MALNUTRITION

The presence of any of the following criteria should motivate the primary care physician to conduct a complete nutritional assessment with consideration of appropriate forms of nutritional therapy:

- Recent involuntary weight loss of greater than 5% in 1 month or more than 10% in 6 months, especially when associated with anorexia, fatigue, or weakness
- History of recent significant physiological stresses, such as organ dysfunction, major surgery, infection, or illness within the last 3 months
- Absolute lymphocyte count of <1200 cells/mm^3 or serum albumin of <3.2 g/dL.

While the above criteria are simple, it is important that these signs and symptoms are taught to your office staff, as often the vital signs of weight, blood pressure, and temperature are taken with no regard for nutrition status.

While classic vitamin deficiency diseases are rare today in the United States, except in certain high-risk groups (e.g., alcoholics, pregnant teenagers, and institutionalized elderly), there are a variety of individuals whose dietary intake is inadequate to maintain optimal health. For instance, it is recommended that Americans eat 25 g of fiber/day, but the average intake is only about 10 g. In California, only about one in five people consume five servings a day of fruits and vegetables, as recommended by the USDA. As a result, there are a number of micronutrient vitamins and minerals that are deficient, but not at levels that would cause disease. Examples include carotenoids, vitamin E, vitamin C, folate, and selenium. While the nutrient levels that constitute deficiency are established, there is little information on what is suboptimal or what types of responses can be expected following nutritional intervention. It is also unclear why there are individual variations in the absorption of a beta-carotene oral load, the effects of dietary fiber eaten at the same time, or the effects of various fats in the diet on absorption of micronutrients.

While patients look to the physician for advice, this is the point where a practice should employ a well-trained dietitian or refer to an affiliated dietitian with a modern perspective and open mind to follow the practices that you establish in your practice for nutritional counseling beyond simple nutrition deficiencies.

1.7 MODIFYING ROUTINES TO MAINTAIN EFFICIENT PATIENT FLOW

In today's environment of high patient volumes, especially in capitated care practices, it is essential to design efficient patient flow while obtaining nutritional information. There are a number of strategies available to accomplish this.

It goes without saying that there must be a carefully designed appointment schedule so that follow-up visits do not turn into lengthy encounters in an unplanned fashion. Being able to refer patients with nutrition questions to a practice-based resource can help to reduce this problem.

One of the most efficient and least costly strategies is to establish group education classes when the office space is not being used in the evenings or weekends. Groups of up to 20 people can attend education and behavior modification sessions. Professionals can be paid an hourly wage to conduct these sessions, and patients can be charged a nominal fee. It is important to ask patients to pay in advance for a set number of sessions. This puts the burden on the patient and not the practice when a patient decides to drop out of the program. Setting up a careful budget can create a win–win for the patients, the professionals conducting the groups, and the practice itself as it obtains a reputation in the medical community of providing nutrition and behavior education for nutrition-related issues.

Making e-mail contact available for questions on nutrition can be a real time saver as well. Similar questions are often asked repeatedly, and a library of frequently asked questions can be established for patients in the practice.

1.8 PROVIDING INTERNET RESOURCES FOR SELF-MONITORING AND REPORTING PROGRESS TO YOUR PRACTICE

There are a number of free apps available that can help maintain compliance.

MyFitnessPal is a free smartphone app and website that tracks diet and exercise to determine optimal calorie intake and nutrients set to the users' goals and provides e-mail and website messages to motivate users. The user may enter the name of the food or scan the barcode to find the item in a large database of more than 5 million foods or may select foods from a list of most frequently eaten foods. In 2015, the company had 80 million users.

Another popular one is Lose It. This app is a way to record both nutrition and exercise information. The food library is extensive and includes name brands plus generic categories, like fruit, coffee, and chicken. Each food type includes accurate calorie, carbohydrate, fat, and protein values, which you can track on a separate page. Daily exercises can be added, including the intensity and hours spent. The app then calculates how many calories are eaten and burned. During the day, it keeps track of how much has been eaten and how much more can be eaten within the targeted protein or calories for the day. A graph based on data over time displays the weight lost. These records can be brought to routine visits and shared with your practice. This review provides an opportunity to applaud progress or solve problems around obstacles to compliance. Apps require a lot of data entry. Smartphones are passively collecting numbers of steps taken each day, and Fitbit counts steps and interacts with a home computer each night to record progress and provide encouragement.

It is wise to discourage your patients from trying to learn about nutrition on the general Internet. Most of the information available distorts the science or makes outright false claims for various nutritional approaches and supplements. Your practice should be the ultimate resource for information that is endorsed by you once you have the background you need.

1.9 ESTABLISH METHODS TO OBTAIN REIMBURSEMENT FOR YOUR SERVICES

In the course of treating common diseases influenced by nutrition and obesity, it is your prerogative as a primary care physician to use nutrition alone or in combination with medication to treat common diseases, including hypertension, hyperlipidemia, hyperglycemia, and obesity.

By law, Medicare covers specified, medically necessary services for illness and injury. The prior legal language, because it stated that obesity was not an illness, prevented Medicare from covering treatments for diseases related to obesity.

As of August 2015, according to Medicare coverage, the question is no longer whether obesity is a disease or a risk factor. What matters is whether there is scientific evidence that an obesity-related medical treatment improves health. Essential to this process is the submission of published, clinical trial data that demonstrate that obesity-related treatments improve the health of Medicare beneficiaries.

In addition to billing for comorbid diseases where obesity or nutrition is addressed, Medicare provides coverage for intensive behavioral therapy. There is a limit of 22 individual and/or group visits (any combination) in the initial 12-month period, counted from the date of the first claim. This can be repeated annually. Face-to-face weekly visits are reimbursed in the first month. In months 2–6, visits are reimbursed twice per month, and then in months 7–12, monthly visits are reimbursed. However, in order to qualify, the patient must lose more than 3 kg (6.6 pounds) in months 2–6, and this must be documented in the medical record. As of January 2015, Medicare covers group intensive behavioral counseling using a new group code, G0473. Face-to-face behavioral counseling for groups of 2–10 individuals lasting 30 minutes is approved.

Another approach is to simply create behavioral group programs for a reasonable charge, for which patients are responsible. They can be given a master bill to submit to their insurance, or in other cases, where they use a health savings account, a brief letter to their accountant will suffice.

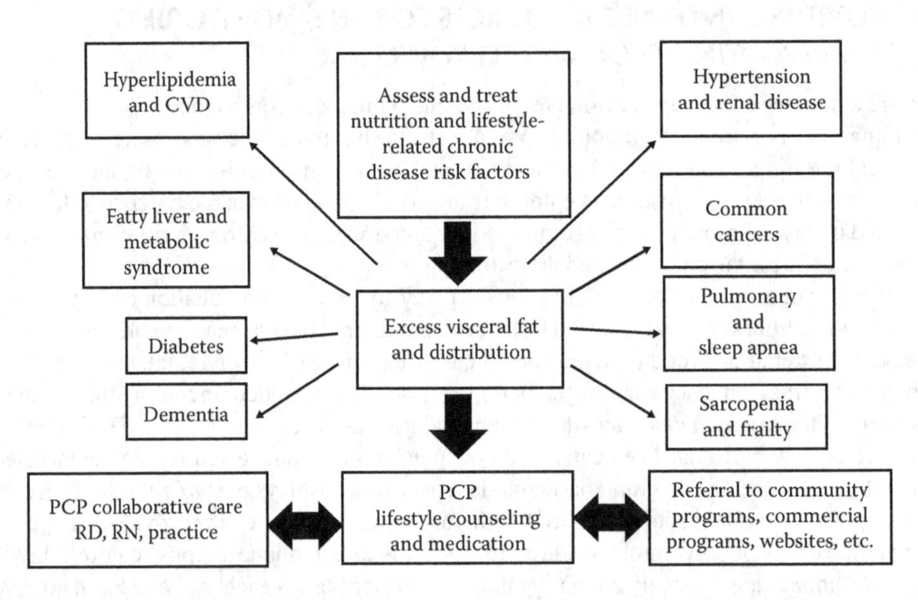

FIGURE 1.4 This algorithm describes the interaction of primary care practice and chronic age-related diseases where nutrition and lifestyle play a major role (see text). CVD, cardiovascular disease; PCP, primary care physician; RD, registered dietitian; RN, registered nurse.

1.10 PRIMARY CARE ALGORITHM

To conclude this chapter, an overview of the primary care practice paradigm is presented in Figure 1.4.

The integration of nutrition into primary care practice begins with the assessment and treatment of the nutrition- and lifestyle-related risk factors associated with common chronic diseases. The primary care physician has the primary responsibility for endorsing the nutrition and lifestyle prescription. Of equal importance are the primary care practice health care providers, including registered dietitians, nurses, exercise physiologists, psychologists, nurse practitioners, and physician assistants, as well as the referral to community resources, websites, and commercial programs, as described in this chapter. The chronic diseases included in the algorithm in Figure 1.4 are among the most common encountered in primary care practice. Excess visceral fat and obesity are primary factors in most of these conditions.

REFERENCES

Abrahams, Z., Z. McHiza, and N. P. Steyn. 2011. Diet and mortality rates in sub-Saharan Africa: Stages in the nutrition transition. *BMC Public Health* 11:801.

Adams, E. J., L. Grummer-Strawn, and G. Chavez. 2003. Food insecurity is associated with increased risk of obesity in California women. *J Nutr* 133:1070–1074.

Akresh, H. R. 2007. Dietary acculturation and health among Hispanic immigrants to the United States. *J Health Soc Behav* 48:404–417.

Albala, C., F. Vio, J. Kain, and R. Uauy. 2001. Nutrition transition in Latin America: The case of Chile. *Nutr Rev* 59 (6):170–176.

Aldrich, L., and J. N. Variyam. 2000. Acculturation erodes the diet quality of US Hispanics/Latinos. *ERS-USDA Diet Qual Food Rural Econ Div* 23 (1):51–55.

Ayala, G., B. Baquero, and S. Klinger. 2008. A systematic review of acculturation and diet among Latino immigrants in the US. *J Am Diet Assoc* 108:1330–1344.

Barquera, S., I. Campos, and J. A. Rivera. 2013. Mexico attempts to tackle obesity: The process, results, push backs and future challenges. *Obes Rev* 14 (Suppl 2):69–78.

Barquera, S., L. Hernandez-Barrera, I. Campos-Nonato, J. Espinosa, M. Flores, A. B. J, and J. A. Rivera. 2009. Energy and nutrient consumption in adults: Analysis of the Mexican National Health and Nutrition Survey 2006. *Salud Publica Mex* 51 (Suppl 4):S562–S573.

Bermudez, O. I., L. M. Falcon, and K. L. Tucker. 2000. Intake and food sources of macronutrients among older Hispanic adults: Association with ethnicity, acculturation, and length of residence in the United States. *J Am Diet Assoc* 100:665–673.

Bonvecchio, A., M. Safdie, E. A. Monterrubio, T. Gust, S. Villalpando, and J. A. Rivera. 2009. Overweight and obesity trends in Mexican children 2 to 18 years of age from 1988 to 2006. *Salud Publica Mex* 51 (Suppl 4):S586–S594.

Booth, F. W., S. E. Gordon, C. J. Carlson, and M. T. Hamilton. 2000. Waging war on modern chronic diseases: Primary prevention through exercise biology. *J Appl Physiol (1985)* 88 (2):774–787.

Bowie, J. V., H. S. Juon, J. Cho, and E. M. Rodriguez. 2007. Factors associated with overweight and obesity among Mexican Americans and Central Americans: Results from the 2001 California health interview survey. *Prev Chronic Dis* 4:8.

Bowman, S. A. 1997. A methodology to price food consumed: Development of a food price database. *Fam Econ Nutr Rev* 10:26–33.

Caballero, B. 2005. A nutrition paradox—Underweight and obesity in developing countries. *N Engl J Med* 352 (15):1514–1516.

Carlson, S. J., M. S. Andrews, and G. W. Bickel. 1999. Measuring food insecurity and hunger in the United States: Development of a national benchmark measure and prevalence estimates. *J Nutr* 129 (2S Suppl):510S–516S.

Chávez, A., M. de Chávez, and J. Roldán. 1993. La nutrición en México y la transición epidemiológica. Mexico: División de Nutrición en Comunidad, Instituto Nacional de Ciencias Médicas y Nutrición Salvador Zubirán.

Coogan, P. F., Y. C. Cozier, S. Krishnan, L. A. Wise, L. L. Adams-Campbell, L. Rosenberg, and J. R. Palmer. 2010. Neighborhood socioeconomic status in relation to 10-year weight gain in the Black Women's Health Study. *Obesity (Silver Spring)* 18 (10):2064–2065.

Darmon, N., and A. Drewnowski. 2015. Contribution of food prices and diet cost to socioeconomic disparities in diet quality and health: A systematic review and analysis. *Nutr Rev* 73 (10):643–660.

Doak, C. M., and B. Popkin. 2008. The rapid emergence of obesity in developing countries. In *Nutrition and Health in Developing Countries*, ed. R. D. Semba and M. W. Bloem, 617–638. 2nd ed. New York: Humana Press.

Drewnowski, A., and S. E. Specter. 2004. Poverty and obesity: The role of energy density and energy costs. *Am J Clin Nutr* 79 (1):6–16.

Edmonds, V. M. 2005. The nutritional patterns of recently immigrated Honduran women. *J Transcult Nurs* 16 (3):226–235.

Flegal, K. M., M. D. Carroll, C. L. Ogden, and L. R. Curtin. 2010. Prevalence and trends in obesity among US adults, 1999–2008. *JAMA* 303:235–241.

Flegal, K. M., M. D. Carroll, C. L. Ogden, and C. I. Johnson. 2002. Prevalence and trends in obesity among US adults 1999–2000. *JAMA* 288:1723–1727.

Ford, E. S., and A. H. Mokdad. 2008. Epidemiology of obesity in the Western hemisphere. *J Clin Endocrinol Metab* 93 (11 Suppl 1):S1–S8.

Glasgow, R., and K. M. Emmons. 2011. The public health need for patient-reported measures and health behaviors in electronic health records: A policy statement of the Society of Behavioral Medicine. *Transl Behav Med* 1 (1):108–109.

Hawkes, C. 2006. Uneven dietary development: Linking the policies and processes of globalization with the nutrition transition, obesity and diet-related chronic diseases. *Global Health* 2:4.

Kumanyika, S. K. 1999. Understanding ethnic differences in energy balance: Can we get there from here? *Am J Clin Nutr* 70 (1):1–2.

Lantz, P. M., and A. Pritchard. 2010. Socioeconomic indicators that matter for population health. *Prev Chronic Dis* 7:A74.

Lee, I. M., E. J. Shiroma, F. Lobelo, P. Puska, S. N. Blair, and P. T. Katzmarzyk. 2012. Effect of physical inactivity on major non-communicable diseases worldwide: An analysis of burden of disease and life expectancy. *Lancet* 380 (9838):219–229.

Lees, S. J., and F. W. Booth. 2005. Physical inactivity is a disease. *World Rev Nutr Diet* 95:73–79.

Maillot, M., N. Darmon, F. Vieux, and A. Drewnowski. 2007. Low energy density and high nutritional quality are each associated with higher diet costs in French adults. *Am J Clin Nutr* 86 (3):690–696.

Ogden, C. L., M. D. Carroll, B. K. Kit, and K. M. Flegal. 2012. Prevalence of obesity and trends in body mass index among US children and adolescents, 1999–2010. *JAMA* 307:482–490.

Omran, A. R. 2005. The epidemiologic transition: A theory of the epidemiology of population change. *Milbank Q* 83 (4):731–757.

Paeratakul, S., J. C. Lovejoy, D. H. Ryan, and G. A. Bray. 2002. The relation of gender, race and socioeconomic status to obesity and obesity comorbidities in a sample of US adults. *Int J Obes Relat Metab Disord* 26 (9):1205–1210.

Popkin, B. M. 2004. The nutrition transition: An overview of world patterns of change. *Nutr Rev* 62 (7 Pt 2):S140–S143.

Popkin, B. M., and P. Gordon-Larsen. 2004. The nutrition transition: Worldwide obesity dynamics and their determinants. *Intl J Obes* 28:S2–S9.

Rojas-Martínez, R., C. A. Aguilar-Salinas, A. Jimenez-Corona, F. J. Gómez-Pérez, S. Barquera, and E. Lazcano-Ponce. 2012. Prevalence of obesity and metabolic syndrome components in Mexican adults without type II diabetes or hypertension. *Salud Publica Mex* 54 (1):7–12.

Rolls, B., and R. A. Barnett. 2000. *The Volumetrics Weight-Control Plan: Feel Full on Fewer Calories.* New York: HarperCollins.

Romieu, I., M. Hernandez-Avila, J. A. Rivera, M. T. Ruel, and S. Parra. 1997. Dietary studies in countries experiencing a health transition: Mexico and Central America. *Am J Clin Nutr* 65 (4 Suppl):1159S–1165S.

Satia, J. A. 2010. Dietary acculturation and the nutrition transition: An overview. *Appl Physiol Nutr Metab* 35 (2):219–223.

Schaffer, D. M., E. M. Velie, G. M. Shaw, and K. P. Todoroff. 1998. Energy and nutrient intakes and health practices of Latinas and white non-Latinas in the 3 months before pregnancy. *J Am Diet Assoc* 98 (8):876–884.

Schoenborn, C. A., P. F. Adams, and P. M. Barnes. 2002. Body weight status of adults: United States, 1997–98. *Adv Data* (330):1–15.

Sharma, S., A. M. Malarcher, W. H. Giles, and G. Myers. 2004. Racial, ethnic and socioeconomic disparities in the clustering of cardiovascular disease risk factors. *Ethn Dis* 14 (1):43–48.

Townsend, M. S., G. J. Aaron, P. Monsivais, N. L. Keim, and A. Drewnowski. 2009. Less-energy-dense diets of low-income women in California are associated with higher energy-adjusted diet costs. *Am J Clin Nutr* 89 (4):1220–1226.

Uauy, R., C. Albala, and J. Kain. 2001. Obesity trends in Latin America: Transiting from under- to overweight. *J Nutr* 131 (3):893S–899S.

U.S. Department of Health and Human Services. 1996. *Physical Activity and Health: A Report of the Surgeon General*. Atlanta, GA: U.S. Department of Health and Human Services.

Velásquez-Melendez, G., M. M. Schlussel, A. S. Brito, A. A. M. Silva, J. D. Lopes-Filho, and G. Kac. 2011. Mild but not light or severe food insecurity is associated with obesity among Brazilian women. *J Nutr* 141:898–902.

Wardle, J., J. Waller, and M. J. Jarvis. 2002. Sex differences in the association of socioeconomic status with obesity. *Am J Public Health* 92 (8):1299–1304.

2 Personalization of Nutrition Advice

2.1 INTRODUCTION

The interest of the public in nutrition, health, and longevity is something you will encounter frequently in your primary care practice. Often, this information is presented as strong opinions and preconceived misconceptions. Much of the misinformation about nutrition in the public arena is found on the Internet, and your patients will bring this misinformation to your attention. In addition to information that makes no physiological sense, there is a great deal of information that your patients will find confusing or conflicting, such as the controversy around dietary fats and sugars. Official governmental and nongovernmental advisory groups, in an effort to reach a political consensus meeting the needs of various vested interests, often issue generalized guidelines that are of little practical value to you in responding to a patient's specific questions.

Government guidelines are based on established but incomplete nutrition science. They fail to account for the many aspects of the emerging science of nutrition, including phytonutrients, antioxidants, the microbiome, and the wealth of information emerging on the role of the microbiome in intermediary metabolism. Humans evolved on a plant-based diet eating animals that were also plant eaters on land and at sea. Processing and food production has made food plentiful and enabled the feeding of the world's hungry in unprecedented ways.

There is also "hidden hunger," a term popularized by Dr. Hans Biesalski of the University of Hohenheim in Germany. This is the intracellular and sometimes localized deficiency of vitamins and minerals that is not easily diagnosed using the usual clinical methods.

A key example of hidden hunger is the well-known need for vitamin C or ascorbic acid, an important dietary antioxidant and stimulant of collagen synthesis. The amounts of vitamin C needed to prevent scurvy are minimal, but the optimum intake of vitamin C for antioxidant protection in the body is much higher. Humans do not synthesize vitamin C, so it must come from the diet. Ironically, it is believed that the genetic machinery for making vitamin C evolved due to the vitamin C-rich environment in the ancient plant-based diet in Africa. A single fruit contains more vitamin C than the amount needed to prevent scurvy. Nonetheless, scurvy was common among sailors until the middle of the eighteenth century.

The fictional captain of a Portuguese ship sailing to Japan in the novel *Shogun*, set in the 1700s, would take a tiny slice of apple each day and squeeze its juice onto a spoon and drink it to prevent scurvy. Today, while scurvy is uncommon, the intakes of vitamin C are still too low in many population groups in the United States and globally.

While, along with scurvy, beriberi, pellagra, and the other classical vitamin deficiencies are no longer common, suboptimal intakes of vitamins, minerals, and phytonutrients from fruits and vegetables have been associated with increased incidences of heart disease and common forms of cancer.

Often, the information in dietary guidelines that set the basis for healthy nutrition is ignored by the public, but these guidelines are used by industry and government to modify the food supply. The many assumptions underlying dietary guidelines and government advice are that they are meant for healthy people. Unfortunately, we live in an era where two-thirds of all Americans are overweight or obese, and many more have excess body fat due to a sedentary lifestyle and an unhealthy diet. Fat-soluble vitamins such as vitamin D and phytonutrients such as lutein, which are fat soluble, distribute into fat tissue, lowering circulating and cellular levels of these substances and other lipid-soluble vitamins and phytonutrients.

The information and recommendations in this book will remain within the dietary guidelines, but focus them to go beyond what can be observed in an epidemiology study to what can be prescribed to an individual patient to achieve healthy results. As a primary care physician, you may be called upon for an instant consensus decision on a nutritional issue that is controversial. Partnering with dietitians, nurses, and other health care personnel will be a vital way to make your nutrition endorsement and prescription of balanced nutrition and healthy active lifestyles effective. However, it will be important that you and your dietitians and health care personnel are aligned on the advice being given. Even minor inconsistencies in advice can undermine the confidence of patients in the validity of the information you are providing. Education of the staff in your practice, along with discussions of any disagreements on approach, is critical to establishing a viable nutrition focus in your practice.

Federal regulations in the United States, as part of the Dietary Supplements Health Education Act, mandate that a dietary supplement may not "prevent, cure, treat, or mitigate" any disease. It also cleverly excludes tobacco, which contains nicotine and could in the broadest sense be considered a drug or botanical. Clearly, humans should meet their needs from the hundreds of thousands of substances found in plant-based foods, spices, and herbs, as ancient man defined the genetics of our metabolism. Eating a variety of foods, spices, and herbs can approximate what we need for optimal health, but no diet is perfect, and reasonable supplementation has demonstrated benefits. Many benefits cannot be demonstrated in clinical trials since they are an integral part of combined effects that we cannot study with presently available methods. However, individuals with certain genetic polymorphisms demonstrate the need for supplementation in terms of reduced risks of chronic diseases, such as heart disease and cancer. These examples are discussed in greater detail in this chapter. The risks of dietary supplements have been overemphasized by those sectors of the medical and scientific communities that prefer drugs and surgery over nutrition for the treatment and prevention of disease.

It is important to realize that nutrition is both an applied science and a political science. The advice emerging from government advisory committees in many countries reflects the concerns of individual food lobbying groups and many other stakeholders. Once the Dietary Guidelines Advisory Committee summarized the science in the 2015–2020 guidelines and submitted them to the U.S. Department of Agriculture (USDA) and the Department of Health and Human Services, the guidelines underwent congressional review, where the inputs of commodity groups were considered.

At the level of congressional review, one of the recommendations of the Scientific Advisory Committee on eating less meat protein, which they based on extensive review of the scientific literature, was removed following complaints from the beef industry interests. In addition, recommendations on developing sustainable food sources reflecting environmental concerns were removed during congressional review. Nonetheless, the content of the guidelines is constantly improving decade by decade, and the next set of guidelines, after 2020, may well overcome some or all of the objections raised in the 2015–2020 guidelines. This process is a progressive one that ultimately leads the nation and the world to a better understanding of healthy diet and lifestyle. However, the slow rate of evolution is a strong rationale for providing nutrition advice that is both within and in some aspects beyond the current dietary guidelines.

2.2 UNDERSTANDING THE DIETARY GUIDELINES AND GOVERNMENT ADVICE

Many in the food industry and the dietetic community view the dietary guidelines issued by the government as laws that must not be violated. Clearly, they behave like laws for the marketing and regulatory departments of food companies and public agencies. However, these guidelines are not unchanging laws, but have evolved over many decades, largely based on data derived from the field of nutritional epidemiology (Willett 1998). This field depends on self-reported dietary intake, and measurement of a limited number of biomarkers, such as height and weight. Nutritional epidemiology has resulted in some of the most influential publications in nutrition science in humans. While there is a large nutrition science literature in animal nutrition, the data on human intervention studies are usually conducted on small numbers of people, with the exceptions of a few large studies, such as the Women's Health Initiative (WHI) and the Dietary Approaches to Stop Hypertension (DASH) (Sacks et al. 1995; Howard et al. 2006; Prentice et al. 2006).

Today, the guidelines are still a work in progress, as combinations of foods eaten together in dietary patterns have evolved from the epidemiological data, including the Healthy Eating Index (Kennedy et al. 1995) and the Mediterranean diet (Trichopoulou et al. 2003). Nutritional scientists, physicians, and dietitians who volunteer to do the hard work of examining large epidemiological evidence bases for the development of nutrition advice are often faced with too little information or even conflicting information. Further analysis of the same data sets led to the expected conclusion that those who adhered to the dietary guidelines had a reduced risk of chronic disease compared with those who did not (McCullough et al. 2000a,b, 2002).

As a result, many dietary guidelines are meant to be broad in nature and not too far out in front of the science. Others are compromises that do not reflect the science that is known. There is also a natural bias toward foods and against dietary supplements, which does not reflect the knowledge, attitudes, and behaviors of the public or the extensive body of data on micronutrient supplementation.

Dietary supplements are meant to be an addition to the diet, and they do not substitute for a poor dietary pattern. It is also true that obtaining all the micronutrients that have been implicated in a healthy lifestyle by simply eating a healthy dietary pattern (formerly the four or five basic food groups) is no longer possible given the explosion of nutrition knowledge. Supplements can be a useful way to adhere to the dietary guidelines, even though they are only beginning to receive minimal mention in the guidelines. Fears of toxicity are overblown, and safe levels of supplements are discussed further in this chapter.

2.2.1 Personalization of Dietary Guidelines

As stated above, government advice on diet and physical activity is well meaning, but it is too general to be very useful in advising individual patients. In this chapter, we describe not only the guidelines and how to stay within them broadly, but also how to personalize them to help your patients achieve a better diet and lifestyle that meets their individual goals for health and quality of life. Once again, it is important to remember there has been a positive evolution of the dietary guidelines over the last few decades, and this chapter is not an attack on the dietary guidelines or a criticism of the dedicated professionals who developed recommendations.

The process of evolution of dietary guidelines will continue, always following and not leading science, but you do not need to wait for approval from these government bodies before instituting the advice that you think is best for your patients. Since nutrition advice does not participate in the costly aspects of the health care system and may help prevent age-related chronic diseases, physician-led teams should retain the liberty to give individualized advice for many years to come. Arrayed against this freedom are several powerful stakeholders, including the food industry and the regimenting systems of primary care that threaten to control physician behavior, through direct regulation or indirectly by controlling government reimbursement for services rendered.

In the United States, the American Dietetic Association has changed its name to the Academy for Nutrition and Dietetics. Beginning in 2017, dietitians will be required to have a master's degree in nutrition to be registered dietitians. These changes will enhance the communication and cooperation between physicians and dietitians to ideally form a functioning nutrition expert team within primary care medical practices.

2.2.2 Recommended Dietary Allowances: A Brief History

The National Research Council issued the first recommended dietary allowances (RDAs) for vitamins, minerals, protein, and energy in 1941. These recommendations were intended to serve as a guide for good nutrition. In early 1977, after years of discussion, scientific review, and debate, the U.S. Senate Select Committee on Nutrition and Human Needs, led by Senator George McGovern, recommended dietary goals for the American people (U.S. Congress 1977). The goals consisted of complementary nutrient-based and food-based recommendations. The first goal focused on energy balance and recommended that, to avoid overweight, Americans should consume only as much energy as they expended. Overweight Americans should consume less energy and expend more energy. For the nutrient-based goals, the Senate committee recommended that Americans make the following modifications:

1. Increase consumption of complex carbohydrates and naturally occurring sugars
2. Reduce consumption of refined and processed sugars, total fat, saturated fat, cholesterol, and sodium
3. Increase consumption of fruits, vegetables, and whole grains
4. Decrease the consumption of refined and processed sugars and foods high in such sugars
5. Decrease the consumption of foods high in total fat and animal fat, while partially replacing saturated fats with polyunsaturated fats
6. Decrease intake of eggs, butter fat, and other high-cholesterol foods
7. Decrease salt and foods high in salt
8. Choose low-fat and nonfat dairy products instead of high-fat dairy products (except for young children)

While this also sounds reasonable by modern standards, with a few exceptions, the issuance of the dietary goals was met with considerable debate and controversy, as industry groups and the scientific community expressed doubt that the science available at the time supported the specificity of the numbers provided in the dietary goals.

To support the credibility of the science used by the committee, the USDA and U.S. Department of Health and Human Services (then called the Department of Health, Education, and Welfare) selected scientists from the two departments and obtained additional expertise from the scientific community throughout the country to address the public's need for authoritative and consistent guidance on diet and health.

In the 1980s, there were controversies over the RDA recommendations. In a celebrated case, there was an argument over whether the RDA for vitamin C should be 45 or 60 mg/day, with the hard scientists citing biochemical data, while public health-oriented nutritionists cited the need for increased intake of fruits and vegetables as a way to reduce the risk of common forms of cancer and other age-related chronic diseases (Levine et al. 1999).

When issued in 1989, the RDA had expanded from a coverage of 8 original nutrients to 27 nutrients. The RDA generally reflected changes resulting from the emergence of new concepts in the field of nutrition science. The RDAs have served as the basis for federal and state food and nutrition programs and policies.

By the 1990s, a number of developments had occurred that dramatically altered the nutrition science landscape and ultimately challenged the RDA. Prominent among these were the significant gains made in scientific knowledge regarding epidemiological associations between diet, health, and chronic disease, and the availability of advanced technologies that could measure the variations in nutrition metabolism among individuals (van Ommen and Stierum 2002; Goodman et al. 2003). Additionally, the use of fortified or enriched foods and the increased consumption of nutrients in pure form, either singly or in combination with others, as dietary supplements outside of the context of food, prompted examination of the potential effects of excess nutrient intake (Greenwald and McDonald 2001; Honein et al. 2001).

2.2.3 Dietary Reference Intakes

The Food and Nutrition Board of the National Academy of Sciences Institute of Medicine began in 1994 to work to develop a new, broader set of dietary reference values, known as the Dietary Reference Intakes (DRIs) (Otten et al. 2006). The DRIs expanded on and replaced the RDAs with four categories of values intended to help individuals optimize their health, prevent disease, and avoid consuming too much of a nutrient.

The DRIs include five nutrient-based reference values that are used to assess and plan the diets of healthy people. The reference values include the acceptable macronutrient range, estimated average requirement (EAR), RDA, adequate intake (AI), and tolerable upper intake level (UL) (Figure 2.1 and Box 2.1).

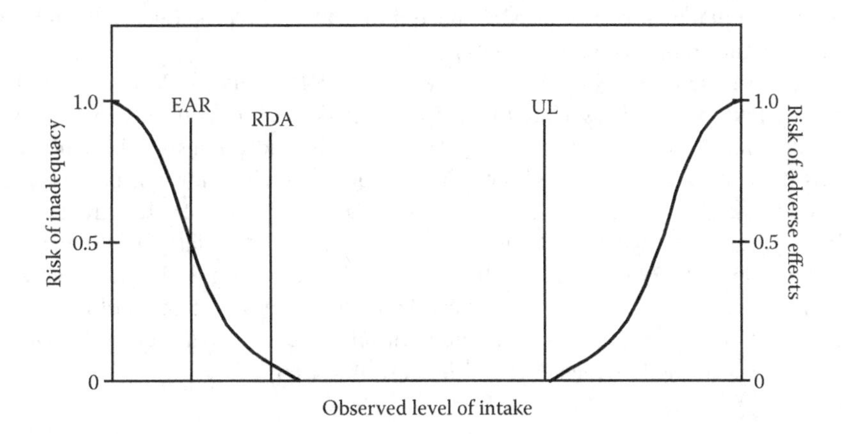

FIGURE 2.1 The EAR is the intake at which the risk of inadequacy is 0.5 (50%) to an individual. The RDA is the intake at which the risk of inadequacy is very small—only 0.02–0.03 (2–3%). The AI does not bear a consistent relationship to the EAR or the RDA because it is set without the estimate of the requirement. At intakes between the RDA and UL, the risks of inadequacy and excess are both close to 0. At intakes above the UL, the risk of adverse effects may increase. (Reprinted from Institute of Medicine (U.S.), Panel on Dietary Reference Intakes for Electrolytes and Water, *DRI, Dietary Reference Intakes for Water, Potassium, Sodium, Chloride, and Sulfate*, National Academies Press, Washington, DC, 2005.)

BOX 2.1 Definition of the DRI Components

Acceptable macronutrient distribution ranges (AMDRs): Ranges of macronutrient intakes that are associated with reduced risk of chronic disease, while providing recommended intakes of other essential nutrients.

Adequate intake (AI): The recommended average daily intake level based on observed or experimentally determined approximations or estimates of nutrient intake by a group (or groups) of apparently healthy people that are assumed to be adequate; used when an RDA cannot be determined.

Estimated average requirement (EAR): The average daily nutrient intake level that is estimated to meet the requirements of half of the healthy individuals in a particular life stage and gender group.

Recommended dietary allowance (RDA): The average daily dietary nutrient intake level that is sufficient to meet the nutrient requirements of nearly all (97–98%) healthy individuals in a particular life stage and gender group.

Tolerable upper intake level (UL): The highest average daily nutrient intake level that is likely to pose no risk of adverse health effects to almost all individuals in the general population. As intake increases above the UL, the potential risk of adverse effects may increase.

The DRI process included several principles that differed from the isolated nutrient approach of the RDAs. The concepts of probability and risk were used in the determination of the DRIs and in their application in assessment and nutritional planning. Greater emphasis was placed on the distribution of nutrient requirements within a population, rather than on a single value, as was the case in the RDAs. Where data existed, upper levels of intake were established regarding the risk of adverse health effects. Compounds found naturally in foods that may not meet the traditional concept of a nutrient, but have a potential risk or possible benefit to health, could be reviewed, and if sufficient data existed, reference intakes could be established.

Among the most useful innovations introduced by the RDA was the development of ranges of macronutrient intakes that are associated with reduced risk of chronic disease, which were called acceptable macronutrient distribution ranges (AMDRs). This innovation solved one of the most vexing problems in the area of popular high-protein diets by lifting the allowable protein intake above 0.8 g/kg of body weight. At the time, evidence was mounting that protein requirements should be higher. The requirements for essential fats in the diet are so low that fatty acid deficiency disease does not occur unless individuals have gastrointestinal disorders. Similarly, carbohydrates are not essential nutrients, and refined carbohydrates can be reduced. As sweet and fat foods in excess are a significant driver of the obesity epidemic and chronic disease, flexibility in designing healthy dietary patterns was enabled by the advent of the AMDRs (Zello 2006).

2.2.4 The 2015–2020 Dietary Guidelines

A greater focus on the importance of healthy eating patterns as a whole, and how foods and beverages act synergistically to affect health, has developed and is reflected in the 2015–2020 dietary guidelines (U.S. Department of Health and Human Services and U.S. Department of Agriculture 2015).

The 2015–2020 dietary guidelines provided five overarching guidelines that encourage healthy eating patterns. The guidelines also embody the idea that a healthy eating pattern is not a rigid prescription, but rather an adaptable framework in which individuals can enjoy foods that meet their personal, cultural, and traditional preferences and fit within their budget. Several examples of healthy eating patterns that translate and integrate the recommendations in overall healthy ways to eat are provided.

The overarching guidelines can easily be met while individualizing your patient's nutrition prescription. The guidelines are as follows:

1. Follow a healthy eating pattern across the life span. All food and beverage choices matter. Choose a healthy eating pattern at an appropriate calorie level to help achieve and maintain a healthy body weight, support nutrient adequacy, and reduce the risk of chronic disease.
2. Focus on variety, nutrient density (high content of nutrients per calorie), and amount. To meet nutrient needs within calorie limits, choose a variety of nutrient-dense foods across and within all food groups in recommended amounts.
3. Limit calories from added sugars and saturated fats and reduce sodium intake. Consume an eating pattern low in added sugars, saturated fats, and sodium. Cut back on foods and beverages higher in these components to amounts that fit within healthy eating patterns.

4. Shift to healthier food and beverage choices. Choose nutrient-dense foods and beverages across and within all food groups in place of less healthy choices. Consider cultural and personal preferences to make these shifts easier to accomplish and maintain.
5. Support healthy eating patterns for all. Everyone has a role in helping to create and support healthy eating patterns in multiple settings nationwide, from home to school to work to communities.

Key recommendations on healthy eating patterns include (1) a variety of vegetables from all the subgroups, including dark green, red and orange, and legumes (beans and peas); (2) fruits, especially whole fruits; (3) grains, at least half of which are whole grains; (4) fat-free or low-fat dairy, including milk, yogurt, cheese, and/or fortified soy beverages; and (5) a variety of protein foods, including seafood, lean meats, poultry, eggs, legumes (beans and peas), nuts, seeds, and soy products, and healthy oils. It also limits saturated fats and *trans* fats, added sugars, and sodium.

Key recommendations that are quantitative are provided for several components of the diet that should be limited. These components are of particular public health concern in the United States, and the specified limits can help individuals achieve healthy eating patterns within calorie limits, as follows: (1) consume less than 10% of calories per day from added sugars; (2) consume less than 10% of calories per day from saturated fats; (3) consume less than 2300 mg/day of sodium; (4) if alcohol is consumed, it should be consumed in moderation—up to one drink per day for women and up to two drinks per day for men—and only by adults of legal drinking age.

2.2.5 Dietary Patterns Recommended by the 2015–2020 U.S. Dietary Guidelines

To get away from individual nutrients such as fats, carbohydrates, and proteins, the dietary guidelines shifted to recommending dietary patterns. There are many different healthy eating patterns. The healthy Mediterranean-style eating pattern and healthy vegetarian eating pattern, which were developed by modifying the healthy U.S.-style eating pattern, are two examples of healthy eating patterns individuals are provided in the guidelines. Similar to the healthy U.S.-style eating pattern, these patterns were designed to consider the types and proportions of foods Americans typically consume, but in nutrient-dense forms and appropriate amounts, which result in eating patterns that are attainable and relevant in the U.S. population. Additionally, healthy eating patterns can be flexible with respect to the intake of carbohydrates, protein, and fats within the context of the AMDR.

2.2.6 Physical Activity Guidelines

The Department of Health and Human Services issued the federal government's first-ever physical activity guidelines for Americans in 2008 to help Americans understand the types and amounts of physical activity that offer important health benefits (Tucker et al. 2011). Physical activity is any form of exercise or movement of the body that uses energy. Some of your daily life activities, including doing active chores around the house, yard work, and walking the dog, are provided as examples of physical activity. The physical activity guidelines for Americans recommend 60 minutes of physical aerobic activity daily for children ages 6–17 and 30 minutes daily for adults ages 18–64. Only 21% of Americans follow these guidelines in recent surveys, again demonstrating that simply issuing guidelines does not accomplish behavior change when it comes to exercise.

Dietary guidelines and physical activity guidelines by their nature are too generalized to be directly used in writing the nutrition prescription for individual patients. The guidelines have recognized the increased prevalence of obesity, but are still largely based on data developed considering nutritional deficiency rather than optimum nutrition. In the next section, the commonality of overfatness even in individuals with normal body mass index (BMI) and waist circumference is a striking indicator of how common nutritional issues are in the general primary care practice community.

2.2.7 Daily Values and Label Reading

Since the DRIs report recommendations according to age, sex, and life stage, they contain too much information to include on the Nutrition Facts label on packages of foods. To solve this problem, the Food and Drug Administration (FDA) uses information from the DRIs to create one number that represents the daily requirement for each nutrient.

This number, called the daily value (DV), is based on the amount of each nutrient needed for a diet of 2000 calories/day. You will not find the DV on the Nutrition Facts label. Instead, it is used to calculate the information you will find on the label: the percent DV. The percent DV tells you what percentage of your daily requirement you will get from one serving of the product.

Since it is based on eating 2000 calories daily, your actual percentage will certainly vary according to the calories in your diet, but it is still a good frame of reference and an easy way to track your daily intake. It is also a helpful tool for identifying whether the food is a high or low source of nutrients. A percent DV of 5% or less is considered low, while 20% or more indicates a high source, according to the FDA. I find this percent DV to be misleading to many consumers and teach my patients to read food labels as follows: proteins and carbohydrates each provide about 4 calories/g. Fat provides 9 calories/g. It takes a little math, but multiplying fat grams by 9 and the protein and carbohydrate grams by 4 will provide your patients with a better assessment of the percent fat in a food. The amounts of sugars are also listed on the food label. The only other tricky part is determining what a serving size should be. Sometimes, the serving size is not realistic in terms of what they will be eating (e.g., one-quarter package of corn chips). While many people read the food labels mandated by the Nutrition Labeling and Education Act enacted under the administration of President George H. W. Bush, many consumers are baffled by the information they find there.

About half of all American adults have one or more preventable chronic diseases, many of which are related to poor-quality eating patterns and physical inactivity. These include cardiovascular disease, high blood pressure, type 2 diabetes, some cancers, and poor bone health. More than two-thirds of adults and nearly one-third of children and youth are overweight or obese. These high rates of overweight and obesity and chronic disease have persisted for more than two decades and come not only with increased health risks, but also at a high cost to the economy.

2.3 BODY COMPOSITION AND PERSONALIZATION OF THE NUTRITION PRESCRIPTION

In this section, the basis of a nutrition prescription individualized on the basis of lean body mass and used to determine protein and calorie requirements is described. From that basis, it is possible to build a personalized diet incorporating fruits, vegetables, whole grains, and healthy fats. Colorful fruits and vegetables and spices provide antioxidant phytonutrients with little impact on overall calorie intake. Many of the phytonutrients we have identified have established cellular actions, but for others, there is much more to learn. For those who wish to begin with the end in mind, Box 2.2 describes how to build a diet based on these principles, while the following subsections provide the rationale. Variations in this diet are useful for weight management in obese patients, but the general guidelines given in what follows will aid healthy individuals in maintaining optimal body composition when combined with a regular exercise program.

BOX 2.2 BUILDING A PERSONALIZED DIET BASED ON LEAN BODY MASS

Between what we know about nutrition and what our patients do about nutrition, there is an implementation gap. When meeting with patients, a simple plan that a primary care doctor can endorse and a dietitian or nurse can reinforce will change eating behaviors more readily than generalized dietary guidelines, which by nature must be a compromise among several different commodity-driven economically influenced arguments.

It is possible to build a balanced diet based on lean body mass determined using bioelectrical impedance. First, determine the protein foods that will result in providing personalized protein at 1 g/pound of lean body mass per day. This can be accomplished by prescribing 25 g units of protein providing about 140 calories/portion in units of 4–8 providing between 100 and 200 g/day.

Food Item	1 Unit	Calories	Protein (g)
	Breakfast		
Egg whites	7 whites	115	25
Greek yogurt (0% fat) *without* fruit added	1 cup	130	23
Nonfat cottage cheese	1 cup	140	28
	Vegetarian		
Soy Canadian bacon	4 slices	80	21 (varies)
Soy protein powder	1 ounce	110	20–25
Soy cereal	½ cup	140	25 (varies)
	Lunch and Dinner		
Poultry breast	3 ounces, cooked weight	115–140	25
Ocean-caught fish	4 ounces, cooked weight	130–170	25–31
Shrimp, crab, lobster	4 ounces, cooked weight	120	22–24
Tuna	4 ounces, water pack	145	27
Scallops	4 ounces, cooked weight	135	25
Egg whites	7 whites	115	25
Nonfat cottage cheese	1 cup	140	28
	Vegetarian		
Soy protein powder	1 ounce	110	20–25
Soy hot dog	2 links	110	22 (varies)
Soy ground round	¾ cup	120	24
Morningstar Farms Better'n Burgers	2 patties	160	26
Tofu, firm	½ cup	180	20 (varies)
Boca Burgers (all varieties)	2 patties	180–220	26–28

Carbohydrates and fiber can come from seven servings per day of colorful fruits and vegetables, with a typical 100 g serving of vegetable providing about 50 calories and a 100 g serving of fruit providing about 70 calories. Listed next are the calories and fiber content of fruits and vegetables organized according to the color grouping used in my clinic.

Food Item	Portion	Calories	Fiber
	Red		
Tomato juice	1 cup	40	1
Tomato sauce/puree	1 cup	100	5
Tomato soup, made with water	1 cup	85	0
Tomato vegetable juice	1 cup	45	2
Tomatoes, cooked	1 cup	70	3
Tomatoes, raw	1 large	40	2
Watermelon	1 cup of balls	50	1

(*Continued*)

Food Item	Portion	Calories	Fiber
	Red/Purple		
Beets, cooked	1 cup	75	3
Blackberries	1 cup	75	8
Blueberries	1 cup	110	5
Cranberries	1 cup raw	60	5
Cranberry sauce	¼ cup	100	1
Eggplant, cooked	2 cups	60	5
Peppers, red	1 large	45	3
Plums	3 small	100	3
Red apple	1 medium	100	4
Red cabbage, cooked	2 cups	60	6
Red pear	1 medium	100	4
Red wine	4-ounce glass	80	0
Strawberries	1½ cups, sliced	75	6
	Orange		
Acorn squash, baked	1 cup	85	6
Apricot	5 whole	85	4
Cantaloupe	½ medium	80	2
Carrots, cooked	1 cup	70	5
Carrots, raw	3 medium	75	6
Mango	½ large	80	3
Pumpkin, cooked	1 cup	50	3
Winter squash, baked	1 cup	70	7
	Orange/Yellow		
Nectarine	1 large	70	2
Orange	1 large	85	4
Papaya	½ large	75	3
Peach	1 large	70	3
Peach nectar	⅔ cup	90	1
Pineapple	1 cup, diced	75	2
Tangerine	2 medium	85	5
Yellow grapefruit	1 fruit	75	2
	Yellow/Green		
Avocado	¼ average fruit	80	2
Banana	1 average	90	2
Collard greens, cooked (ckd)	2 cups	100	10
Corn	½ cup kernels or 1 ear	75	2
Cucumber	1 average	40	2
Green beans, ckd	2 cups	85	8
Green peas	½ cup	70	4
Green peppers	1 large	45	3
Honeydew	¼ large melon	100	2
Kiwi	1 large	55	3
Mustard greens, ckd	2 cups	40	6
Romaine lettuce	4 cups	30	4
Spinach, cooked	2 cups	80	8
Spinach, raw	4 cups	30	4
Turnip greens, ckd	2 cups	60	10
Yellow peppers	1 large	50	2
Zucchini with skin, ckd	2 cups	60	5

(*Continued*)

Food Item	Portion	Calories	Fiber
	Green		
Broccoli, cooked	2 cups	85	9
Brussels sprouts	1 cup	60	4
Cabbage, cooked	2 cups	70	8
Cabbage, raw	2 cups	40	4
Cauliflower, ckd	2 cups	55	6
Chinese cabbage, ckd	2 cups	40	5
Kale, cooked	2 cups	70	5
Swiss chard	2 cups	70	7
	White/Green		
Artichoke	1 medium	60	6
Asparagus	18 spears	60	4
Celery	3 large stalks	30	3
Chives	2 tablespoons	2	0
Endive, raw	½ head	45	8
Garlic	1 clove	5	0
Leeks, cooked	1 medium	40	1
Mushrooms, cooked	1 cup	40	3
Onion	1 large	60	3

Whole grain and refined grain foods provide about 250 calories/100 g, so breads, cakes, pastries, and cookies should be minimized in the diet. Two slices of whole grain sprouted bread will have 140–200 calories while providing 4–8 g of protein. Instead of suggesting breads and cereals as the base of the diet with six to eight servings per day, recommend having more fruits and vegetables and fewer refined grains. This will both increase fiber intake and provide more vitamins, minerals, and phytonutrients to the diet.

Grain/Starch	Serving Size	Calories	Fiber (g)	Protein (g)
Cooked beans	1 cup, cooked	230–280	10–14	14
Brown rice	1 cup, cooked	220	4	6
Lentils	1 cup, cooked	230	16	18
Potato, baked	1 medium	220	8	4
Sweet potato	1 small	100	2	2
Whole grain pasta	1 cup, cooked		2	6
Plain instant oatmeal	1 packet	100	3	4
Shredded Wheat, bite size	¾ cup	85	3	4
Fiber One cereal	¾ cup	90	21	4
All-Bran with extra fiber cereal	¾ cup	75	18	5
Kashi GOLEAN cereal	¾ cup	120	10	8
Kashi Good Friends cereal	¾ cup	90	8	3
Kellogg's All-Bran cereal	¾ cup	120	15	6
Bran Chex cereal	¾ cup	120	5	4
Kellogg All-Bran Buds cereal	⅓ cup	85	12	2
Bread, Vogel	1 slice	100	3	5
Bread, Ezekiel sprouted wheat	1 slice	80	3	4

Then, you consider balancing the omega-6 and omega-3 fatty acids by reducing total fat, which includes hidden *trans* fats and omega-6 fats, while consuming about 2 g of fish oils from fish oil supplements or ocean-caught fish.

This is not a low-fat or high-fat diet. A practical reduction in hidden fats results in a diet containing between 20% and 25% of total calories from fat. If a higher-fat diet is desired with reduced carbohydrates, then omega-9 fats should be used from olive oil or avocados, since these are neutral fats that do not upset the balance of omega-3 and omega-6.

This method is simple enough to enable personal choices of foods to obtain a diet that will help maintain healthy body composition when combined with physical activity daily. It begins from the assumption that most Americans are struggling to keep from storing excess body fat due to a sedentary lifestyle and omnipresent high-fat, high-sugar foods.

The above foods can be used as building blocks incorporated into recipes using spices and various cooking techniques, which are becoming increasingly popular. Recipes are outside the scope of this book, but your partnering dietitians can develop recipes to provide to your patients using widely available cookbooks and Internet recipe sites.

2.3.1 Rationale for a Balanced Diet Based on Supplemented Personalized Protein

Protein is the macronutrient that is most satiating and, in combination with exercise, can maintain or build muscle mass. Increasing muscle mass has significant positive effects on metabolism and joint health. Muscle cells take up glucose independent of insulin, reducing stress on the pancreas even while glucose levels are normal in individuals with prediabetes or metabolic syndrome. Nutritional assessment using bioelectrical impedance to estimate lean body mass is central to developing diets to maintain optimal body composition, especially internal abdominal or visceral fat, which rapidly accumulates when individuals are sedentary and in a positive calorie balance.

Dr. Jimmy Bell and colleagues at Hammersmith Hospital and Imperial College in London found that 40% of apparently healthy individuals with a normal BMI and normal waist circumference had excess intra-abdominal fat based on MRI studies (Thomas et al. 2012).

Dr. Bell originated the term *TOFI* (thin outside, fat inside), which is used to describe lean individuals with a disproportionate amount of fat stored within their abdomen. Figure 2.2 illustrates this by showing two men, both aged 35 years, with a BMI of 25 kg/m^2. Despite their similar size, the TOFI man had 5.86 L of internal fat, while the healthy control had only 1.65 L.

To classify an individual as TOFI, it is essential to measure his or her internal fat content. The only way that this is possible is by using MRI or computed tomography (CT) scanning. The parameters of the MRI scanner are manipulated to show fat as bright (white) and lean tissue as dark. Indirect methods, such as waist circumference, are not suitable, as individuals with an identical waist circumference can have vastly different levels of internal fat. Figure 2.3 clearly shows that despite having an identical waist circumference (in this example, all men had a waist of 84 cm), there is considerable variation in the amount of visceral fat (volumes shown on the image in liters) present.

While the exact incidence of TOFI globally has not been established, the existence of this syndrome suggests a much wider distribution of excess body fat among those with reduced lean body mass and increased body fat at normal body weight.

The amount of lean body mass is critical in estimating the resting energy expenditure, as each pound of lean body mass burns about 14 (13.8 is the original number) calories/pound/day, while each pound of fat burns only about 3 calories/pound/day (Cunningham 1980).

Using bioelectrical impedance analysis (BIA) is a practical and cost-effective way to assess body composition in the office (Kyle et al. 2004). BIA depends on the fact that muscle is about 70% water and conducts electricity, while fat is an insulator. The most commonly used machines are modified scales with four contact points. By placing two contact points on the hands and two on the feet and separating these by a wide distance, it is possible to pass an alternating microcurrent at 50 cycles/second (50 Hz) through the body and assess impedance. The computer in the machine using proprietary algorithms then estimates both lean body mass and fat mass. The lean body mass measurement is accurate, within 5–10%, while the body fat measurement is an estimate and does not specify the location of the fat, as was done with MRI.

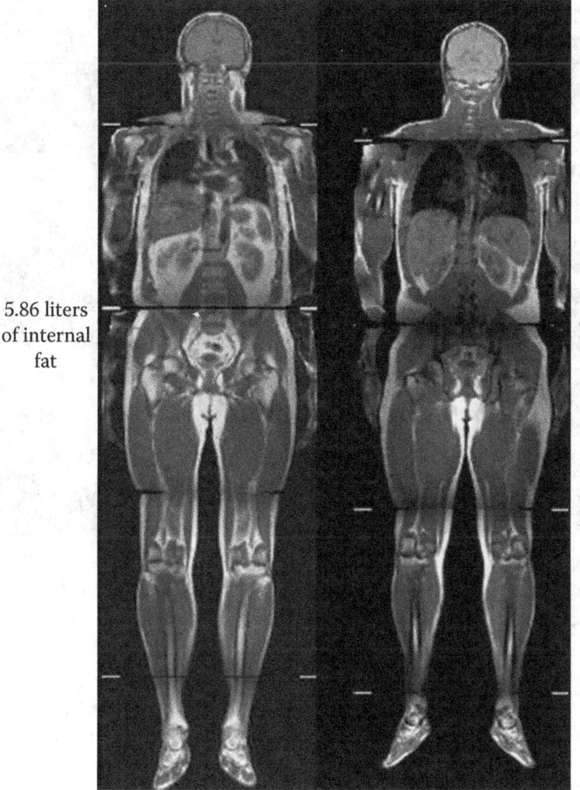

FIGURE 2.2 Coronal image of a TOFI and a normal control. Subjects defined as TOFI with a BMI of <25 kg/m^2 have increased levels of many of the risk factors associated with the metabolic syndrome. This phenotype is a further refinement of "metabolically obese but normal weight" (MONW). (Reprinted from Imaging fat—MRI images of subjects we have scanned, CC BY-SA 3.0, https://commons.wikimedia.org/w/index.php?curid=20135561.)

While the dietary guidelines suggest that Americans get enough protein in their diet, the evidence suggests that the pattern of intake at each meal leads to insufficient intake over the whole day (Schaafsma 2005). As shown in Figure 2.4, many individuals eat little protein at breakfast, a little more for lunch, and a large amount at dinner, much of which is not utilized by the muscles for protein synthesis. A balanced distribution of protein throughout the day provides support of muscle protein synthesis.

The amount of lean body mass can be used to prescribe an AI of lean protein to both control hunger and maintain lean body mass. In the University of California, Los Angeles (UCLA) Risk Factor Obesity Program, we utilize a nutrition prescription of 1 g/pound of lean body mass determined by BIA. The variations in body composition can be significant and affect resting energy expenditure, and this is does not correlate with BMI. It has been established that lean body mass (also called fat free mass) is the strongest correlate of resting energy expenditure (Jew et al. 2009) (Figure 2.5).

While resting energy expenditure is not the same as total energy expenditure, it does accurately describe the greatest personal differences in the ability to lose or gain weight among individuals. A loss of 10 pounds of fat-free mass due to sedentary lifestyle and inadequate protein intake leads to a reduction in resting energy expenditure of 140 calories/day. This can be significant for a small woman who burns 1500 calories/day at age 25 but loses 20 pounds of lean body mass by age 40 and

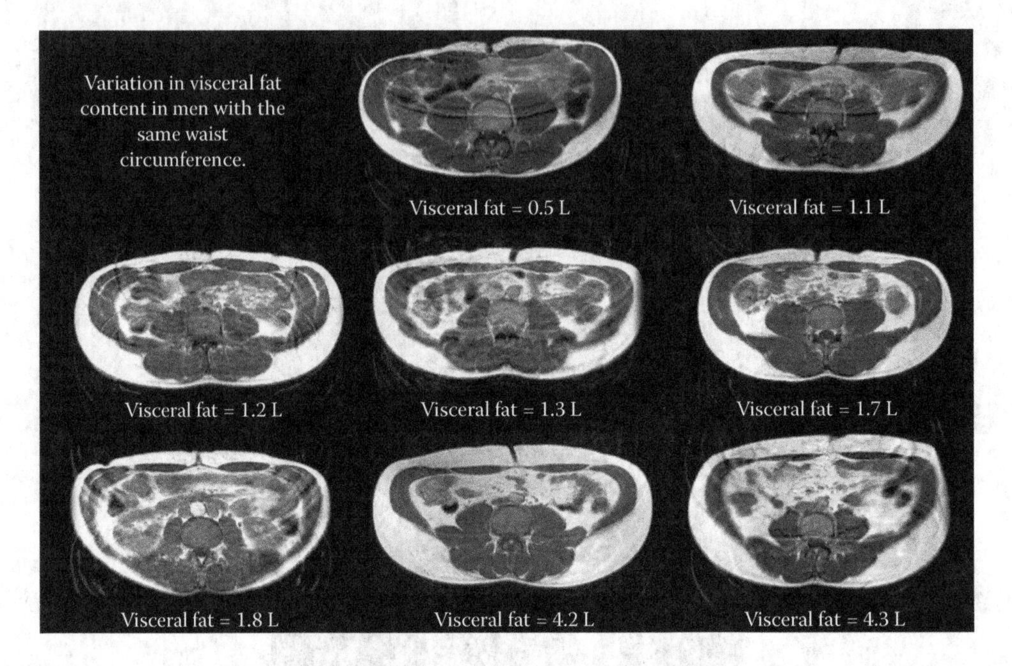

FIGURE 2.3 Variation in visceral fat in men with the same waist circumference. (Reprinted from Imaging fat—Images from cohort of volunteers, CC BY-SA 3.0, https://commons.wikimedia.org/w/index.php?curid=20139540.)

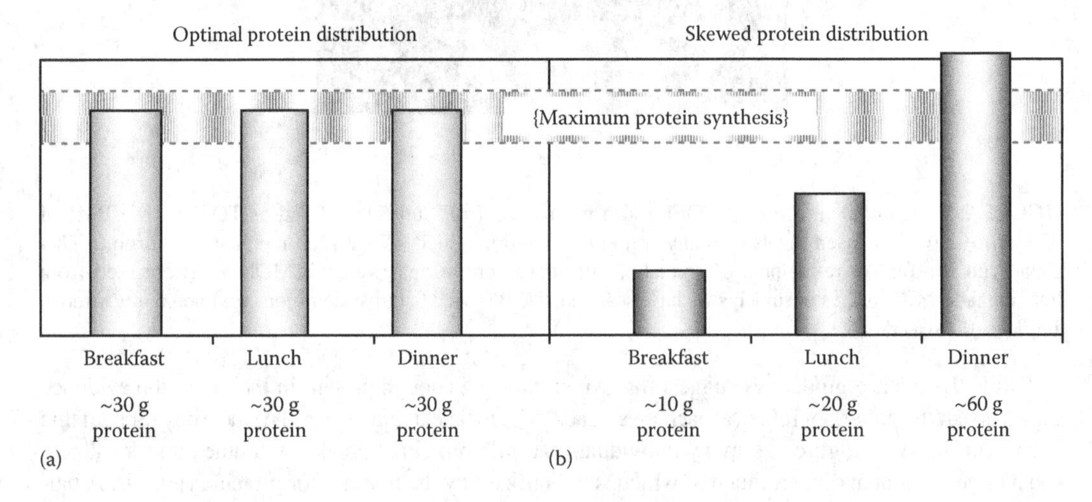

FIGURE 2.4 Protein distribution at meals. (a) Ingestion of 90 g of protein, distributed evenly at three meals. (b) Ingestion of 90 g of protein unevenly distributed throughout the day. Stimulating muscle protein synthesis to a maximal extent during the meals (a) is more likely to provide a greater 24-hour protein anabolic response than the unequal protein distribution in B. (Reprinted from Paddon-Jones, D., and Rasmussen, B. B., *Curr. Opin. Clin. Nutr. Metab. Care*, 12(1), 86–90, 2009.)

then burns only 1250 calories at rest. This results in the common clinical paradigm of a middle-aged women stating that she is gaining weight while still eating the same number of calories.

The RDA for protein was determined using a method called nitrogen balance. In this method, the average protein is considered to have 1 g of nitrogen/6.25 g of protein in the diet. This is an obvious approximation since there are 21 different amino acids, some having two nitrogen atoms, while most have only one. Urinary urea excretion is the primary method of nitrogen exit from the body.

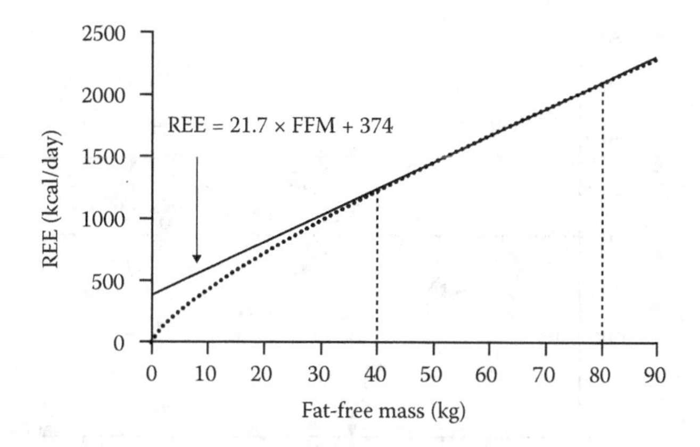

FIGURE 2.5 Resting energy expenditure (REE) and fat-free mass (FFM) are related in a curvilinear fashion. However, for FFM between 40 and 80 kg, the REE-FFM relation is linear. (Reprinted from Wang, Z. et al., *Am. J. Physiol. Endocrinol. Metab.*, 279(3), E539–E545, 2000.)

While some exists as ammonia and some in cells in stool, urinary urea nitrogen is an acceptable clinical method to test for the adequacy of protein intake.

In 1973, Dr. Vernon Young at the Massachusetts Institute of Technology (MIT) studied young healthy men eating egg whites and found that they achieved positive nitrogen balance at an intake of 0.8 g/kg of body weight/day (Young et al. 1973). Young healthy men eating 0.8 g/kg of body weight went into positive nitrogen balance (Figure 2.6). This was assumed to hold for all men, leading to a recommendation of 56 g/day for men and 46 g/day for women as the RDA.

However, studies in 1989 found that in endurance athletes, more than 1.2 g/kg/day was needed to achieve positive nitrogen balance (Figure 2.7). In weight lifters, a higher amount of more than 2 g/kg of body weight was needed (Figure 2.8).

Taken together, these observations led us to conclude that the RDA was too low and too general. The protein in the diet must be increased when lean body mass is increased. While the body tends to conserve lean body mass during starvation, optimal lean body mass can only be achieved with resistance exercise and surplus protein intake, as evidenced by elimination of excess urinary urea nitrogen.

It turns out that a reasonable recommendation to implement is 1 g/pound of lean body mass per day. Lean body mass can be estimated with BIA, which is widely available. The math works out that this level of protein intake represents 29% of resting energy expenditure. Therefore, as a percent of

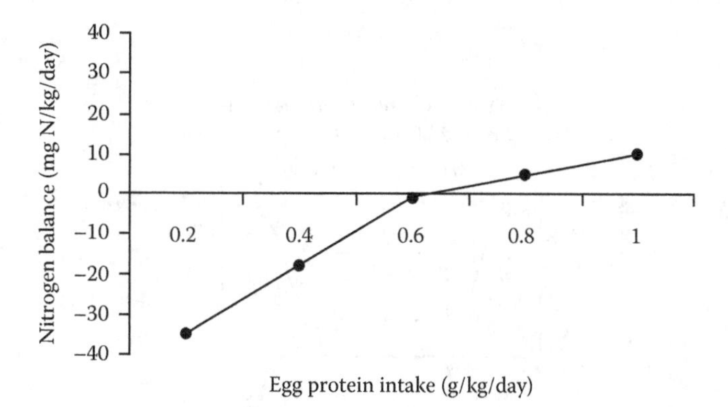

FIGURE 2.6 Studies in normal volunteers in 1973 demonstrated positive nitrogen balance when fed egg white protein at a dose of 0.8 gm/kg/day. These data are still the basis of RDA values in many countries. (Adapted from Young, V. R. et al., *J. Nutr.*, 103(8), 1164–1174, 1973.)

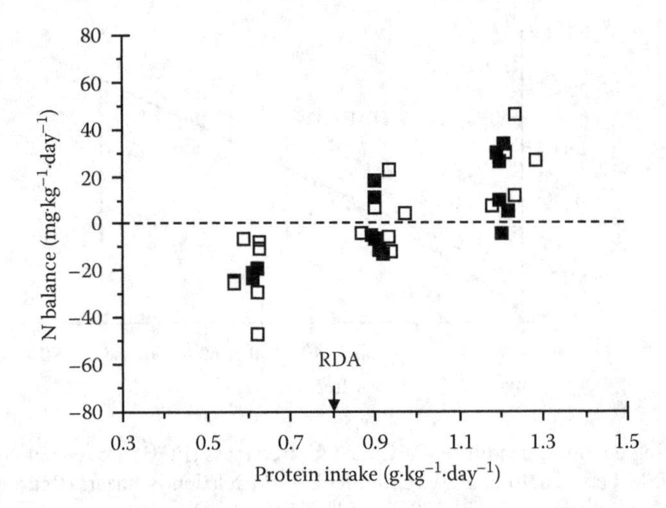

FIGURE 2.7 More than 1.2 g/kg/day is needed to achieve positive nitrogen balance. (Reprinted from Meredith, C. N. et al., *J. Appl. Physiol. (1985)*, 66(6), 2850–2856, 1989.)

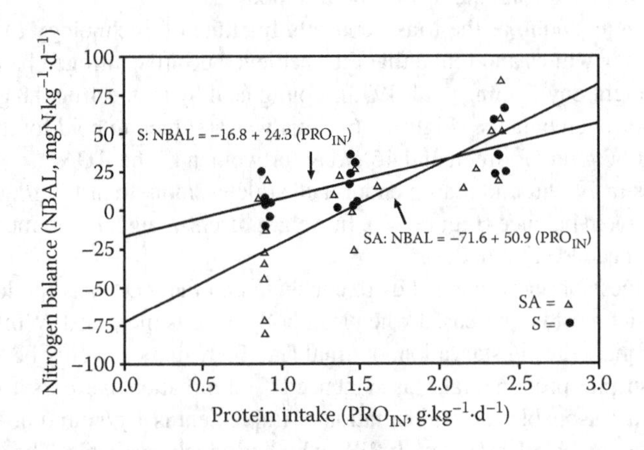

FIGURE 2.8 More than 2 g/kg of body weight/day is needed to achieve positive nitrogen balance in weight lifters with a large lean body mass. (Reprinted from Tarnopolsky, M. A. et al., *J. Appl. Physiol. (1985)*, 73(5), 1986–1995, 1992.)

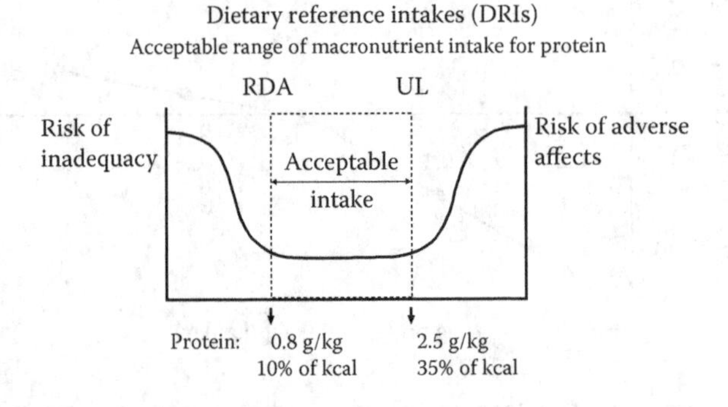

FIGURE 2.9 Acceptable range of protein intake within the DRI for protein. (Adapted from Fulgoni, V. L., 3rd, *Am. J. Clin. Nutr.*, 87(5), 1554S–1557S, 2008.)

total energy expenditure, this amounts to somewhere around 25% of the total, including exercise, dietary thermogenesis, and fidgeting.

As shown in Figure 2.9, this recommended amount of protein intake per day is well within the acceptable macronutrient range of 10–35% established by the Institute of Medicine of the National Academy of Sciences.

2.3.2 Protein Quantity and Quality

There are 21 common amino acids, and while some amino acids can be made from other amino acids in the liver through a chemical exchange called transamination, other amino acids are essential (Box 2.3) and must be obtained from the diet. Some amino acids are called conditionally essential because they must be consumed in the diet during growth to provide adequate growth rates, but become nonessential in adults who are not growing. One such amino acid is histidine, which is essential for growing rats but not adult rats. Much of the data on the essentiality of amino acids are obtained from rats, where single amino acid elimination is a way of determining whether a given amino acid is essential. For example, lysine and threonine cannot be made from other amino acids by transamination and must be included in the diet.

BOX 2.3 AMINO ACIDS

Essential Amino Acids	
Histidine	Phenylalanine
Isoleucine	Threonine
Leucine	Tryptophan
Lysine	Valine
Methionine	
Nonessential Amino Acids	
Alanine	Glycine
Arginine	Proline
Asparagine	Serine
Aspartic acid	Taurine
Cysteine	Tyrosine
Glutamic acid	Glutamine

Proteins containing all the essential amino acids and nonessential amino acids in proper amounts are called complete, while proteins missing some essential amino acids are called incomplete. Two incomplete proteins, such as those found in corn and beans or rice and beans, can be combined to produce a mixed protein with higher protein quality. The original biological value tables found in many nutrition textbooks were assessed in animals and did not evaluate digestibility, leading to the impression that soy protein, the highest-quality protein in the plant world, had a biological value of 73 compared with egg white, which has a value of 100. The protein digestibility-corrected amino acid score (PDCAAS) has been adopted by the Food and Agriculture Organization (FAO) and World Health Organization (WHO) as the preferred method for the measurement of the protein value in human nutrition. The method is based on comparison of the concentration of the first limiting essential amino acid in the test protein with the concentration of that amino acid in a reference scoring pattern. This scoring pattern is derived from the essential amino acid requirements of the preschool-aged child. The chemical score obtained in this way is corrected for true digestibility of the test protein. PDCAAS values higher than 100% are not accepted as such but are truncated to 100%. Using this method, soy protein, whey protein, and egg white all have a biological value of 100% (Schaafsma 2005).

2.3.3 Carbohydrates and Fibers

Carbohydrates contain carbon, hydrogen, and oxygen but no nitrogen, and are broken down into sugars, such as glucose and fructose, or excreted from the body in undigested form. The term *carbohydrate*, while useful for classifying macronutrients, includes both the carbohydrates that have been industrially processed to a refined form and the indigestible carbohydrates found in fruits, vegetables, and whole grains. Refined carbohydrates are often free of vitamins, minerals, and phytonutrients unless they are fortified. Moreover, fruits and vegetables, as noted in the above diet plan have, much lower-calorie density, such that a 100 g serving of a vegetable provides only 50 calories and fruit provides 70 calories, while a 100 g serving of a refined carbohydrate such as white rice provides 250 calories.

Those carbohydrates excreted in undigested form or those partially or completely digested by colonic bacteria are referred to as dietary fibers. Since they are not digested, dietary fibers do not contribute directly to the nutritive value of foods in terms of calories, but they have many effects on human physiology. Ancient humans ate a great deal of fiber, and this fiber resulted in numerous large bulky stools that filled the colon and caused it to contract against a large-volume load. Modern man eats a small amount of fiber, approximately 10–15 g/day, compared with 35 g/day in a healthy plant-based diet and well over 50 g/day in ancient diets.

One consequence of eating a low-fiber diet is that the colonic muscles contract against a smaller volume of stool and so exert higher pressures. It is generally believed that these higher pressures account for the common occurrence of diverticulosis (outpouching of mucosa between strands of muscle) in the colons of elderly individuals. Constipation is also very common in modern society, since a low-fiber diet does not stimulate intestinal motility as well as a higher-fiber diet does.

This slowing of transit time—the time it takes foods to get through the gastrointestinal tract—also permits greater reabsorption of substances normally excreted through the intestines. For example, estrogen (the female hormone) is excreted in the bile from the liver into the intestine. In the intestine, it is bound to fibers and excreted in the stool. Women with low-fiber diets and constipation reabsorb this estrogen in the distal small intestine, called the ileum, rather than excreting the estrogen. This is not a minor effect, and results in 20% higher blood estrogen levels in women on a low-fiber diet than in those consuming a high-fiber diet (Rose et al. 1991).

Total dietary fiber is classified as either soluble or insoluble dietary fiber. Insoluble dietary fibers, such as cellulose (a structural carbohydrate making up plant cell walls), are not digested in the intestine and pass out in the stool, where they can be found intact. Soluble carbohydrates, such as pectin, guar, and starches, are digested by bacteria in the colon. Stool mass is determined by the mass of fibers and the mass of bacteria in stool. A significant portion of stool mass is bacteria. Soluble fibers contribute to stool mass by promoting the growth of the bacteria that digest the soluble fiber and use it as fuel.

2.3.4 Simple Sugars and Complex Carbohydrates

Simple sugars include glucose, fructose, lactose, and sucrose. These are listed as sugars on food labels, while the so-called "complex carbohydrates" are not included in this list, despite the similarity discussed above. Lactose and sucrose are disaccharides made up of galactose or glucose and glucose or fructose, respectively. The tastes of corn sugar, sucrose or table sugar, and fructose are different. Fructose is the sweetest-tasting sugar and is the one found in fruits such as oranges. Corn sugar tastes like pancake syrup and is the primary sweetener in colas in the United States. In some countries, such as Mexico, sucrose is used to sweeten colas, and they taste distinctly different from their U.S. counterparts.

The term *complex carbohydrate* usually means a long-chain carbohydrate made up of many glucose or carbohydrate molecules linked together. According to the FDA, maltodextrin, or corn sugar, made up of 15 glucose molecules linked together, is a complex carbohydrate. In fact, as soon as corn sugar is dissolved in stomach acid, it breaks up, giving exactly the same glucose release into the blood as table sugars.

From the standpoint of dental health, corn sugar can promote tooth decay (Ma et al. 2013). The original patent on maltodextrin claimed that it would enable infants to get more calories with less diarrhea, since each maltodextrin molecule had 15 times the calories of an equivalent caloric load of glucose with much less osmolality (the physical chemical property of dissolved chemicals that draws fluid into the colon). In fact, this does help, but many infants still have colicky diarrhea as the infant expression of stress and food intolerance. Declaration of the different types of carbohydrates, especially of maltodextrin or corn syrup, is insufficient in some products, and consequently, the consumer is not alerted to their cariogenic potential when used in older children. Complex carbohydrates by the FDA definition help neither dental health nor the development of diabetes.

2.3.5 Glycemic Index, Glycemic Load, and Calories

Years ago, we simply talked about refined and complex carbohydrates. The refined were called bad, because they caused a rapid rise in blood sugar, which could trigger snacking through effects on brain chemistry. Then in 1981, Dr. David Jenkins of the University of Toronto developed the glycemic index (GI) (Jenkins et al. 1981). To determine GI, compare how much the blood sugar rises over a several-hour period with a fixed dose of pure corn sugar (or dextrose). In practice, a plot is made of the values of blood sugar over a 2-hour period, and the dots are connected, creating a curve. The area under the curve of blood sugars after the administration of a fixed portion of carbohydrate (usually 50 g) of the test food is calculated and compared with the area under the curve following the administration of the same number of grams of carbohydrate from glucose, which is given an arbitrary score of 100. The higher the number, the greater the blood sugar response and the resulting emotional impact on sugar craving. So, a low-GI food will cause a small rise, while a high-GI food will trigger a dramatic spike in blood sugar. Table 2.1 lists common foods with their GI.

One problem with the GI is that it only detects carbohydrate quality, not quantity. A GI value tells you only how rapidly a particular carbohydrate turns into sugar. It does not tell you how much of that carbohydrate is in a usual serving of a particular food. You need to know both things to understand a food's effect on blood sugar. The best example of this is the carrot. The form of sugar in the carrot has a high GI, but the total carbohydrate content of the carrot in a usual serving is low, so it does not have much effect on blood sugar. This is where glycemic load (GL) comes in: it takes into consideration a food's GI, as well as the amount of carbohydrates per serving. A carrot has only 4 g of carbohydrate. To get 50 g, you would have to eat about a pound and a half of them. GL takes the GI value and multiplies it by the actual number of carbohydrates in a typical serving. While this number is useful for research studies, especially epidemiological studies, for the purpose of educating patients in primary care practice, it is enough to encourage the intake of healthy carbohydrates from low-GI foods, such as fruits, vegetables, and whole grains, while advising reductions in foods with refined carbohydrates, such as cookies, candy bars, cakes, and pastries. These foods typically have hidden fats as well. Reducing the intake of sugar-sweetened drinks, such as colas, which have a high GI, is also vital, as about one-third of all sugar in the diets of Americans come from this one source. Substituting water and unsweetened teas when not exercising is an important piece of advice. During prolonged exercise that is vigorous, sports drinks with added sugar are needed to maintain muscle glycogen, but for most minimal exercise, simply drinking water to maintain hydration is adequate.

The studies of the effects and potential benefits of eating foods with a low GI require taking into account GL. A food with a low GL is defined by consensus as one with a value of less than 16. GL has been found to be an important variable in epidemiological studies of diet and the risk of chronic disease. Populations eating a diet that has a high GL, such as the U.S. diet of processed grains and few fruits and vegetables, have a higher risk of diabetes and heart disease than those in some Asian

TABLE 2.1
GIs of Food

Food	GI
Cornflakes	92
Potatoes	85
Jelly beans	80
Cream of wheat	74
French bread	73
Watermelon	72
White bread	70
Life Savers	70
Rye bread	65
Mars bar	65
Rice, white	64
Pineapple	59
Banana	52
Whole wheat bread	51
Orange	48
All-Bran	42
Peach	42
Apple	40
Ice cream, full fat	38
Milk, skim	32
Yogurt, low fat, fruit	31
Lentils	29
Milk, full fat	27
Soybeans	18

Source: Heber, D., and S. Bowerman, *The L.A. Shape Diet: The 14-Day Total Weight Loss Plan*, 1st ed., Regan Books, New York, 2004.

countries where they eat lots of fruits and vegetables with few processed foods. This has been documented both in population studies, such as those conducted by the Harvard School of Public Health (Bhupathiraju et al. 2014), and in weight loss studies in children conducted at Children's Hospital in Boston, where a low-GL diet was more effective in promoting weight loss than a high-GL diet (Ebbeling et al. 2012).

Researchers at Harvard University also examined the relationship between diet and risk of non-insulin-dependent diabetes mellitus (NIDDM) in a cohort of 42,759 men without NIDDM or cardiovascular disease, who were 40–75 years of age in 1986 (Bhupathiraju et al. 2014). Diet was assessed at baseline by a validated semiquantitative food frequency questionnaire. During 6 years of follow-up, 523 incident cases of NIDDM were documented. The dietary GL (an indicator of carbohydrate's ability to raise blood glucose levels multiplied by the number of grams of carbohydrate per serving) was positively associated with risk of NIDDM after adjustment for age, BMI, smoking, physical activity, family history of diabetes, alcohol consumption, cereal fiber, and total energy intake.

The above findings support the hypothesis that diets with a high GL and a low cereal fiber content increase the risk of NIDDM in men, as recently reviewed by an international group of nutrition experts (Augustin et al. 2015). Further, they suggest that grains should be consumed in a minimally refined form to reduce the incidence of NIDDM. So once again, we are back to whole foods. Those foods with more dietary fiber, such as natural fruits and vegetables, are less likely to lead to obesity and diabetes than modern refined and processed carbohydrates with the fiber removed.

Poor gastrointestinal health is common in Americans, with up to 40% suffering from diarrhea or constipation at any time. At the same time, diets that are high in refined grains are more calorie dense, with refined grains having 20–30 times the calorie density (calories per bite) as fruits, vegetables, and whole grains.

The GI, GL, and total calories of foods are listed here (Foster-Powell et al. 2002). The GI of foods is based on the GI—where glucose is set to equal 100. The other is the GL, which is the GI divided by 100 multiplied by its available carbohydrate content (i.e., carbohydrates minus fiber) in grams per serving (Tables 2.2 through 2.7).

TABLE 2.2
Low GI (<55) and Low GL (<16) Foods (Lowest Calorie, 110 Calories/Serving or Less)

	GI	GL	Serving Size	Calories
Most vegetables	<20	<5	1 cup, cooked	40
Apple	40	6	1 average	75
Banana	52	12	1 average	90
Cherries	22	3	15 cherries	85
Grapefruit	25	5	1 average fruit	75
Kiwi	53	6	1 average fruit	45
Mango	51	14	1 small fruit	110
Orange	48	5	1 average fruit	65
Peach	42	7	1 average fruit	70
Plums	39	5	2 medium	70
Strawberries	40	1	1 cup	50
Tomato juice	38	4	1 cup	40

Source: Heber, D., and S. Bowerman, *The L.A. Shape Diet: The 14-Day Total Weight Loss Plan*, 1st ed., Regan Books, New York, 2004.

TABLE 2.3
High GI (>55) but Low GL (<16) Foods (All Low Calorie, 110 or Less per Serving)

	GI	GL	Serving Size	Calories
Apricots	57	6	4 medium	70
Orange juice	57	15	1 cup	110
Papaya	60	9	1 cup of cubes	55
Pineapple	59	7	1 cup of cubes	75
Pumpkin	75	3	1 cup, mashed	85
Shredded wheat	75	15	1 cup of mini-squares	110
Toasted oats	74	15	1 cup	110
Watermelon	72	7	1 cup of cubes	50

Source: Heber, D., and S. Bowerman, *The L.A. Shape Diet: The 14-Day Total Weight Loss Plan*, 1st ed., Regan Books, New York, 2004.

TABLE 2.4
Moderate Calorie, Low GI, Low GL (110–135 Calories/Serving or Less)

	GI	GL	Serving Size	Calories
Apple juice	40	12	1 cup	135
Grapefruit juice	48	9	1 cup	115
Pear	33	10	1 medium	125
Peas	48	3	1 cup	135
Pineapple juice	46	15	1 cup	130
Whole grain bread	51	14	1 slice	80–120

Source: Heber, D., and S. Bowerman, *The L.A. Shape Diet: The 14-Day Total Weight Loss Plan*, 1st ed., Regan Books, New York, 2004.

TABLE 2.5
Higher Calorie, Low GI, Low GL (160–300 Calories/Serving)

	GI	GL	Serving Size	Calories
Barley	25	11	1 cup, cooked	190
Black beans	20	8	1 cup, cooked	235
Brown rice	50	16	1 cup	215
Garbanzo beans	28	13	1 cup, cooked	285
Grapes	46	13	40 grapes	160
Kidney beans	23	10	1 cup, cooked	210
Lentils	29	7	1 cup, cooked	230
Soybeans	18	1	1 cup, cooked	300
Yam	37	13	1 cup, cooked	160

Source: Heber, D., and S. Bowerman, *The L.A. Shape Diet: The 14-Day Total Weight Loss Plan*, 1st ed., Regan Books, New York, 2004.

TABLE 2.6
Low GI and Low GL, but High Fat and High Calorie

	GI	GL	Serving Size	Calories
Cashews	22	4	½ cup	395
Premium ice cream	38	10	1 cup	360
Low-fat ice cream	37–50	13	1 cup	220
Peanuts	14	1	½ cup	330
Potato chips	54	15	2 ounces	345
Whole milk	27	3	1 cup	150
Vanilla pudding	44	16	1 cup	250
Fruit yogurt	31	9	1 cup	200+
Soy yogurt	50	13	1 cup	200+

Source: Heber, D., and S. Bowerman, *The L.A. Shape Diet: The 14-Day Total Weight Loss Plan*, 1st ed., Regan Books, New York, 2004.

TABLE 2.7
High GI (>55) and High GL (>16) (Many Trigger Foods, Many Higher Calorie)

	GI	GL	Serving Size	Calories
Baked potato	85	34	1 small	220
Cola	63	33	16-ounce bottle	200
Corn	60	20	1 ear, 1 cup kernels	130
Corn chips	63	21	2 ounces	350
Cornflakes	92	24	1 cup	100
Cream of wheat	74	22	1 cup, cooked	130
Croissant	67	17	1 average	275
French fries	75	25	1 large order	515
Macaroni and cheese	64	46	1 cup	285
Oatmeal	75	17	1 cup, cooked	140
Pizza	60	20	1 large slice	300
Pretzels	83	33	1 ounce	115
Raisin Bran	61	29	1 cup	185
Raisins	66	42	½ cup	250
Soda crackers	74	18	12 crackers	155
Waffles	76	18	1 average	150
White bread	73	20	2 small slices	160
White rice	64	23	1 cup, cooked	210

Source: Heber, D., and S. Bowerman, *The L.A. Shape Diet: The 14-Day Total Weight Loss Plan*, 1st ed., Regan Books, New York, 2004.

2.3.6 Fats and Oils

Fats and oils provide the most concentrated source of calories of any foodstuffs. Fats provide essential fatty acids (linoleic and linolenic acids), which are precursors for prostaglandins. They are called essential because they must be consumed similar to vitamins. Animals can be demonstrated to die within weeks on a fat-free diet, but humans with intact gastrointestinal tracts do not clinically demonstrate fat deficiency since only 5–10% of calories from essential fats are needed to avoid fatty acid deficiency. Fats also require prolonged digestion and contribute to satiety, carry fat-soluble vitamins, and concentrate the tastes of foods to make them more palatable. The key problem for most people eating a Western diet is an excess of fat from processed foods, and these fats are rich in pro-inflammatory omega-6 fatty acids.

Ninety-five percent or more of the fats you eat and store are triglycerides. These fats have a 3-carbon backbone and three fatty acids esterified at each of the three positions (Figure 2.10). When all the fatty acids on a triglyceride are the same, they are called simple; otherwise, they are called mixed triglycerides, which are more common. Excess calories, regardless of source, are stored as triglycerides (Figure 2.11).

The principal dietary sources of fat are meats, dairy products, poultry, fish, nuts, and vegetable oils and fats used in processed foods. Vegetables and fruits contain only small amounts of fat, so that vegetable oils are only sources of fat due to the processing of vegetables. The most commonly used oils and fats for salad oils, cooking oils, shortenings, and margarines in the United States include soybean, corn, cottonseed, palm, peanut, olive, canola (low erucic acid rapeseed oil), safflower, sunflower, coconut, palm kernel, tallow, and lard. These fats and oils contain varying compositions of fatty acids, which have particular physiological properties (Table 2.8).

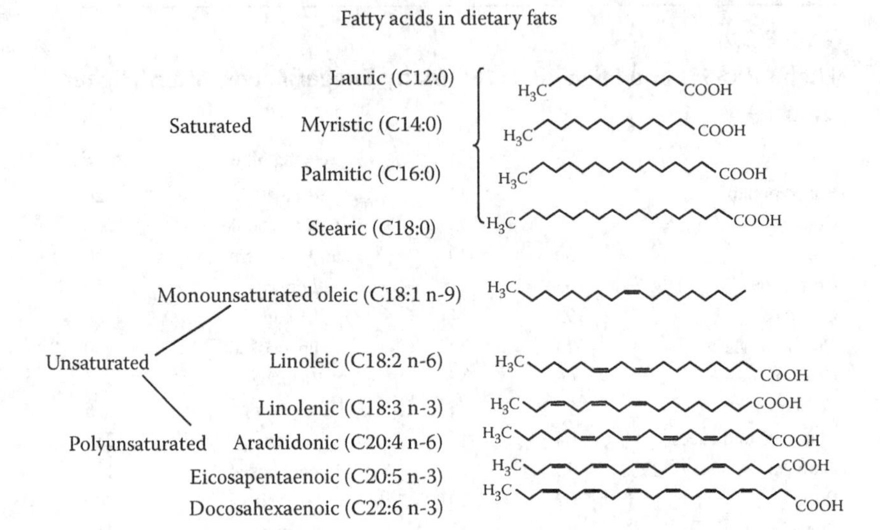

FIGURE 2.10 Chemical structure of the most common dietary fatty acids. These fatty acids are found in triglycerides with a 3-carbon backbone, so that three fatty acids occur together. In the body, triglycerides are digested and the fatty acids incorporated into body fat, where over a period of time the chemical composition of the fat correlates with dietary fat structures to a certain extent. The cellular balance between the 20- and 22-carbon omega-6 (also called n-6) and omega-3 (also called n-3) polyunsaturated fatty acids can affect immune function. Humans are very inefficient in converting the 18-carbon fatty acids to 20- and 22-carbon-length n-3 fatty acids, so these must be consumed from the diet as ocean-caught fish or from fish oil supplements. The n-3 and n-6 designations for polyunsaturated fats are based on the first double bond being three or six carbons from one end. The monounsaturated fats, such as olive oil or avocado oil, have the first double bond nine carbons from one end and are called n-9.

If a fat contains among the three fatty acids predominantly saturated, monounsaturated, or saturated fats (Table 2.8), then we use the shorthand of calling these saturated, monounsaturated, or saturated fats. Commonly eaten fats all have varying mixtures of the fatty acids shown in Table 2.8 in their triglyceride lipids, the primary dietary source of fatty acids (USDA 2003).

Table 2.9 lists the comparative ratios of omega-6 to omega-3 fatty acids in Paleolithic, Mediterranean, US, UK, and northern European diets. The differences in omega-6 to omega-3 ratios are due to both increases in animal fat intake and the intake of vegetable oils rich in omega-6 fatty acids. Humans are inefficient at converting 18-carbon to 20- and 22-carbon fatty acids, especially in face of the high refined carbohydrate and fat intake of the modern diet. Fish are efficient at this conversion and also obtain some fish oils from algae. Their contribution of omega-3 fatty acids is discussed below.

BOX 2.4 WHICH IS BETTER: CHICKEN OR BEEF?

There are some surprising differences in the ratios of omega-6 to omega-3 between grass-fed and corn-fed beef and chicken in the ratios of omega-6 to omega-3 fatty acids they contain.

Ratio of Omega-6 to Omega-3	
Grass-fed beef	1.95
Grain-fed beef	6.38
Grain-fed chicken breast	185

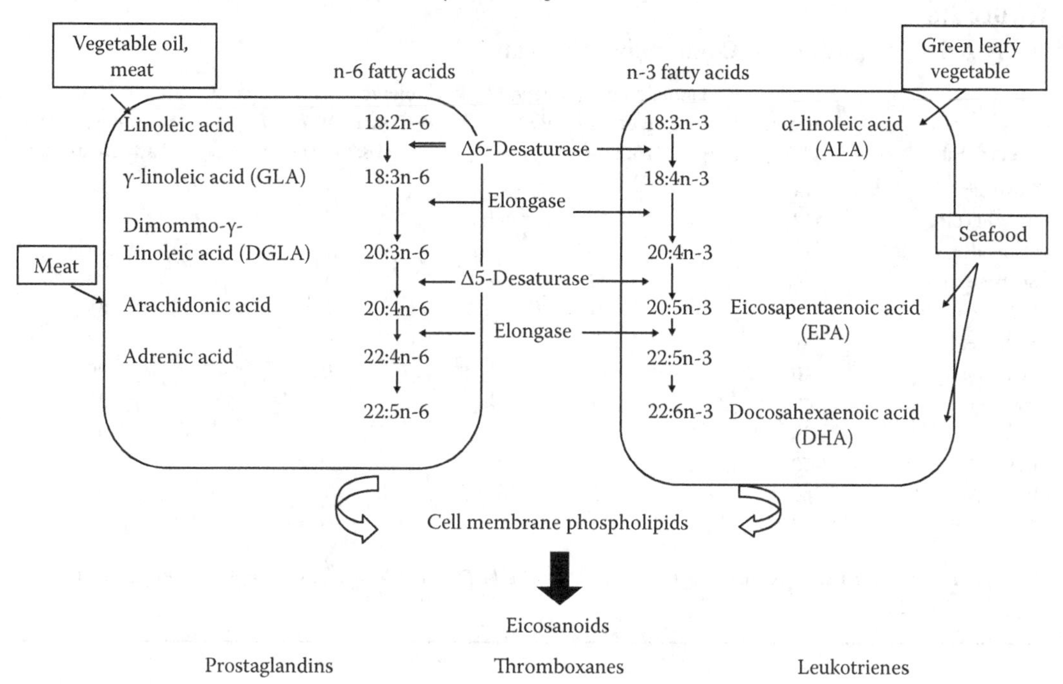

FIGURE 2.11 Within the cell, the long-chain omega-6 and omega-3 fatty acids compete for the same enzymes, leading to potentially different compositions of the cell membrane phospholipids. In turn, the phospholipids used to synthesize eicosanoids are a group of signaling compounds, including prostaglandins, thromboxanes, and leukotrienes, which affect cellular function in numerous ways. The balance of omega-6 and omega-3 promotes the synthesis of pro-inflammatory (2 and 4 series from omega-6) or anti-inflammatory (3 series from omega-3) eicosanoids. In this sense, the fatty acids are signal molecules involved in inflammation, as well as serving as building blocks for stored triglycerides in fat cells.

These ratios can be misleading, because the total fat in chicken breast is far less than the total fat in grain-fed beef or grass-fed beef. Therefore, chicken breast is still a better choice overall than beef. The flesh of wild game is typically only 2–4% fat by weight compared with domestic meats, which are 20–25% fat by weight, much of it in the form of saturated fat. Wild meat has its gamey taste due to both omega-3 fatty acids and aromatic oils from the plant foods eaten by these animals.

Note: You will not find this type of information in the dietary guidelines.

Another interesting comparison is that between farmed salmon and ocean-caught salmon. The fat in farmed salmon contains less of the healthy omega-3 fatty acids than the fat in wild salmon. Salmon fat is rich in omega-3 fatty acids, essential nutrients important to fetal brain development and linked to reductions in the occurrence or symptoms of autoimmune disease, headaches, cramps, arthritis, other inflammatory diseases, hardening of the arteries, Alzheimer's disease, and heart attacks. But USDA testing data show that the fat of farmed salmon contains an average of 35% fewer omega-3 fatty acids (USDA 2003). Because farmed salmon contains 52% more total fat than wild salmon, the total omega-3 fatty acid content of farmed and wild fish is similar. However, in the case of farmed salmon, the fat is contaminated with polychlorinated biphenyls (PCBs) and more than 100 other pollutants and pesticides. Frequent farmed salmon eaters may exceed government health limits for these pollutants.

TABLE 2.8
Fatty Acid Composition in Commonly Eaten Fats

Dietary Fat	Total Saturated (%)	Linoleic Acid (Omega-6) Polyunsaturated) (18:2 n-6) (%)	Linolenic Acid (Omega-3) Polyunsaturated) (18:3 n-3) (%)	Total Monounsaturated Fatty Acids (%)
Olive oil	14	9	1	74
Avocado oil	12	13	1	71
Corn oil	13	58	1	24
Soybean oil	14	51	7	23
Peanut oil	17	32	0	46
Safflower oil	6	75	0	14
Sunflower oil	10	66	0	20
Palm oil	49	9	0	37
Lard	39	10	1	45
Beef tallow	50	3	1	42
Butter fat	62	2	1	29
Coconut oil	87	2	0	6

Source: Heber, D., and S. Bowerman, *The L.A. Shape Diet: The 14-Day Total Weight Loss Plan*, 1st ed., Regan Books, New York, 2004.

TABLE 2.9
Comparative Ratios of Omega-6 to Omega-3 Fats in Different Diets

Population	Ratio of Omega-6 to Omega-3
Paleolithic	0.79
Mediterranean (Greece prior to 1960)	1.0–2.0
Current United States	16.74
Current United Kingdom and northern Europe	15.0
Current Japan	4.0

Source: Adapted from Simopoulos, A. P., *Biol. Res.*, 37(2), 263–277, 2004.

The simple solution for modern times is to select low-fat fish, white meat of poultry, and occasionally very lean meat, preferably grass fed. The ratio of omega-6 to omega-3 for fish is not comparable to those shown in Box 2.4. Wild salmon has a ratio of 0.08, and farmed salmon has a ratio of 0.29. Addition of just 3 ounces of ocean-caught fish (e.g., herring) or 3 g of fish oil capsules to a low-fat diet will reduce the proportion of predicted omega-6 fatty acids in tissues from 80% to 40%. This amazing impact of fish oils is a potent argument for including fish and fish oil supplements in a healthy diet.

2.3.7 Dietary Pattern That Prevents Weight Gain

Since the major nutrition problem in the world of primary care is no longer malnutrition but overweight and obesity, the major preventive challenge is to find a dietary pattern that helps to maintain body weight and prevent the weight gain that occurs so commonly with aging in a sedentary population.

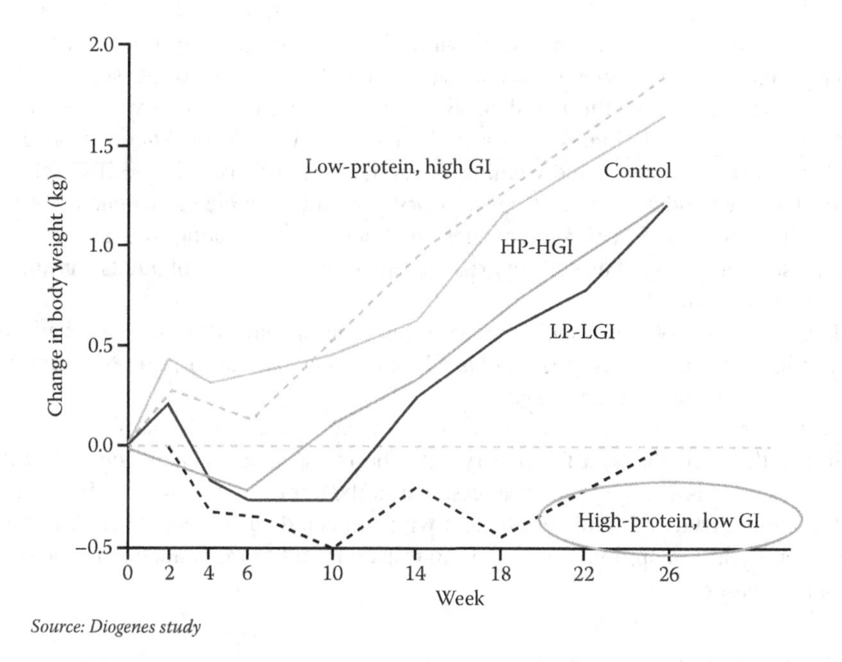

FIGURE 2.12 **(See color insert.)** Science backs protein: change in body weight during the DIOGENES study. As the chart shows, the high-protein, low-GI diet produced the best weight loss results. HP, high protein; LP, low protein; HGI, high GI; LGI, low GI. (Reprinted from Larsen, T. M., *N. Engl. J. Med.*, 363(22), 2102–2113, 2010.)

The Pan-European Weight Loss Study (DIOGENES) was conducted in eight European countries, and after an 8-week weight loss phase, those who lost weight on a very low-calorie diet were randomized to one of five different diets for the next 6 months (Figure 2.12) (Aller et al. 2014). All the combinations of high and low protein and high and low GI with constant fat intake were tested. Only those subjects consuming the high-protein diet at 30% of calories combined with low-GI fruits, vegetables, and grains maintained their weight over the next 6 months. Subjects eating all the other possible diet combinations gained between 2 and 4 pounds over the next 6 months. In these studies, the percent of fat calories was held constant. While every effort to reduce the intake of high-fat foods with hidden fats is desirable, as discussed, efforts to reduce fat intake below 25% of calories have not been successful in intervention trials. Nonetheless, there are societies where lower amounts of fat are eaten. Given the many advantages that fat provides to food taste and the transport of fat-soluble phytonutrients, substitution of healthy fats, such as olive oil, is a more practical alternative than restricting total fat intake below 25%.

This dietary pattern was not mentioned in the dietary guidelines but is within the AMDR and, as indicated, can be individualized for weight maintenance or weight management, discussed in Chapters 2 and 5. This is a dietary pattern that can provide simple instruction to your primary care patients quickly, and your dietitians and nurses can participate in the instruction. It can even be accomplished in small groups of patients.

2.4 OPTIMIZING VITAMIN, MINERAL, AND MICRONUTRIENT INTAKE FROM FOODS AND SUPPLEMENTS

Vitamin and mineral deficiency diseases in the United States were relatively common prior to World War II. Today, with the fortification of the food supply, classical vitamin deficiency diseases such as scurvy and rickets are rare outside the setting of specific disease states, drug–nutrient interactions, or extreme malnutrition due to poverty.

The 2007–2010 National Health and Nutrition Examination Survey (NHANES) study found that the large majority of Americans, despite having a high prevalence of obesity, failed to get adequate levels of micronutrients through their diet. Vitamin D and E intakes were below the EAR in 94% and 88% of the population, respectively. In addition, 33–50% of Americans had inadequate intakes of magnesium, calcium, and vitamins A and C. This was noted in the 2015 scientific report of the 2015 Dietary Guidelines Scientific Advisory Committee, which also stated that vitamins A, C, D, and E, as well as folate, calcium, magnesium, fiber, and potassium, were nutrients of concern. While all these data are based on self-report, it is remarkable that 90% of adults consumed an inadequate amount of vitamin D.

Significant portions of the population with common chronic diseases also have inadequate intakes of micronutrients. Obesity is associated with inadequate absorption of vitamins A, C, D, and E, as well as calcium and magnesium.

Despite the uncommon occurrence of classical vitamin deficiencies sufficient to cause acute disease in healthy individuals, a familiarity with the roles of the various common vitamins and minerals, and some knowledge of their assessment in the clinical laboratory, will aid in the assessment of the hospitalized or ambulatory patient with suspected nutritional deficiency. It will also be helpful in identifying suboptimal intakes of vitamins relevant to the reduction of the risk for common chronic diseases.

2.4.1 Fat-Soluble Vitamins: A, D, E, and K

2.4.1.1 Vitamin A

Night blindness was well recognized in ancient Egypt, where it was treated with juice from cooked liver or by including liver in the diet. The active agent, vitamin A, was discovered as a fat-soluble growth factor necessary for the rat in 1914 and structurally analyzed in 1930 (Moore 1957). The parent compound of the vitamin A family is all-*trans*-retinol. Its aldehyde and acid forms are retinal and retinoic acid (RA).

The active form of vitamin A for vision is 11-*cis*-retinal, which is converted to *trans*-retinal following the absorption of the energy of a light photon. Called photoisomerization, this light-mediated change in conformation from the *cis*- to the *trans*- form results in the dissociation of the protein rhodopsin, which results in nerve impulses through the optic nerve to regions in the visual cortex where sight is formed from the integration of these impulses.

A second active function for vitamin A is cellular differentiation. RA is a morphogen derived from retinol (vitamin A) that plays important roles in cell growth, differentiation, and organogenesis. The production of RA from retinol requires two consecutive enzymatic reactions catalyzed by different sets of dehydrogenases. The retinol is first oxidized into retinal, which is then oxidized into RA. The RA interacts with the retinoic acid receptor (RAR) and retinoic acid X receptor (RXR), which then regulate the target gene expression within the nucleus of cells where they promote differentiation. Vitamin A deficiency accounts for 500,000 cases of blindness in children in the developing world. Vitamin A deficiency results in a thickening of the conjunctiva of the eye called xerophthalmia. The latter is due to the second function of vitamin A in maintaining the epithelial integrity of the cornea. In young children, Bitot's spots, foamy white accumulations of sloughed cells on the conjunctiva, can be useful in diagnosing vitamin A deficiency.

The recent discovery of four RA receptors (termed RAR-alpha through RAR-gamma) in the nucleus of cells has begun to elucidate the molecular mechanisms by which vitamin A induces differentiation of many types of cells (Anon 1987). A number of retinoids or synthetic vitamin A analogs (the best known is 13-*cis*-RA, or Accutane) are used to treat acne and have been studied for their differentiating activities in the prevention and treatment of premalignant lesions of the mouth, trachea, and cervix (Petkovich et al. 1987). Given the importance of vitamin A, it is fortunate that it can be formed from provitamin A carotenoids found in carrots, yellow squash, dark green leafy

TABLE 2.10
Blood Levels of Vitamin A and Laboratory Diagnosis

Deficient	Marginal	Satisfactory	Excessive	Toxic
<0.35 μmol/L	0.35–0.70	0.70–1.75	1.75–3.5	>3.5

Source: Adapted from Olson, J. A., *Vitamin A: In Present Knowledge in Nutrition*, ILSI Press, Washington, DC, 1990.

vegetables, corn, tomatoes, papaya, and oranges. Preformed vitamin A is found as retinyl palmitate in liver; various dairy products, including milk, cheese, butter, and ice cream; and fish, such as herring, sardines, and tuna. In the United States, about 75% of vitamin A is obtained from preformed dietary sources and 25% from provitamin A carotenoids (Olson 1987).

The term *vitamin A* applies to all compounds with biological activity similar to that of vitamin A. The interconversion and pharmacology of these various vitamin A's is controversial and still under study. The international units (IU) apply only to animal experiments under standardized conditions. In the IU system, 0.3 μg of retinol or 0.34 μg of retinyl acetate or 0.6 μg of beta-carotene corresponds to 1 IU. Diet can provide numerous vitamin A-like substances. Requirements and intakes are listed as retinal activity equivalents (RAE): 1 mg RAE = 1 mg of retinal, 1.15 mg of retinal acetate, 6 mg of beta-carotene, and 3000 IU of vitamin A.

Low plasma concentrations of retinol (<0.35 μmol/L) are associated with clinical symptoms of vitamin A deficiency (Control of vitamin A deficiency and xerophthalmia 1982). The RDA for vitamin A is 5000 IU (800–1000 μg retinol equivalents [RE]) per day, and toxicity has been reported at intakes of 25,000 IU/day. This makes vitamin A one of the most toxic vitamins known. The plasma levels of vitamin A can be used to assess status as shown in Table 2.10 (Olson 1990).

2.4.1.2 Vitamin D

There are two forms of vitamin D: vitamin D3 and vitamin D2. Vitamin D3 (cholecalciferol) occurs in some foods but is primarily produced in the skin on exposure to sunlight (Baggerly et al. 2015; Holick 2016). Vitamin D2 (ergocalciferol) does not occur naturally but is manufactured by the ultraviolet irradiation of ergosterol, which occurs in molds, yeasts, and plants. Vitamin D3 differs from vitamin D2 in that D2 has a double bond between carbon 22 and carbon 23 and a methyl group on carbon 24.

Only a few foods (cod liver oil, fatty fish, and egg yolks) contain substantial amounts of naturally occurring vitamin D3. The amount of vitamin D typically obtained from food sources other than fortified foods and skin synthesis often is insufficient. For this reason, food is supplemented with vitamin D in most developed countries. In North America, food is supplemented with both vitamin D2 and vitamin D3, with milk being the principal fortified dietary component. Since dairy products have been fortified with vitamins A and D, dietary rickets has become rare in the United States. Vitamin D acts to enhance calcium absorption from the intestine and has been shown to have differentiating effects on a number of different cell types, including white blood cells and prostate cancer cells. The active form of vitamin D is 1,25-dihydroxyvitamin D3 formed from 25-hydroxyvitamin D (25(OH)D) in the kidneys. 25(OH)D is a large inactive pool formed and stored in the liver. The kidney also has an inactivation enzyme (24-hydroxylase), which converts 25(OH)D to inactive 24,25-dihydroxyvitamin D. When 1,25-dihydroxyvitamin D acts at the nucleus, it turns on the genes necessary to produce the 24-hydroxylase enzyme. Whenever there is such a branch point in the body, there is additional protection from toxicity, and it indicates a substance with important metabolic roles (e.g., apolipoprotein B and thyroid hormones).

As people age, the skin becomes less effective in forming vitamin D and people are advised to use sunscreens and avoid sun exposure to prevent skin cancer (Kockott et al. 2016). Vitamin D3 as a supplement is preferable to D2 (found in plants) since D2 is more rapidly cleared and is less biologically active than D3. Taking a dose of 2000 IU/day is not toxic since it translates into an increase in 25(OH)D levels of only 24 ng/mL (Table 2.11). The Institute of Medicine has only recognized the benefits of vitamin D for bone and has set the requirements accordingly.

However, toxicity is only noted at doses greater than 20,000 units/day, and many consumers take 1000–5000 units daily to take advantage of emerging science on the actions of vitamin D beyond its role in calcium absorption. Vitamin D is not just a vitamin, but a hormone that, like the retinoids, travels to the nucleus to program the transcription of specific proteins. Research over the last three decades has brought to light many additional functions of vitamin D and redefined what is considered optimal vitamin D nutrition. It is now estimated that approximately 1 billion people worldwide have blood concentrations of vitamin D that are considered suboptimal. Low vitamin D serum concentrations are linked to several types of cancers, cardiovascular disease, diabetes, upper respiratory tract infections, and all-cause mortality.

Immune effects of vitamin D have been recognized for more than a century, and are now appreciated as having had a role in the use of sunlight in the therapy of tuberculosis in the preantibiotic era. Topical application of vitamin D cutaneous tuberculosis resulted in disappearance of lesions. In the last few years, the significance of these observations to normal human physiology has become apparent (Hewison 2012). There are increasing data linking vitamin insufficiency with prevalent immune disorders. Improved awareness of low circulating levels of precursor 25(OH)D in populations across the globe has prompted epidemiological investigations of health problems associated with vitamin D insufficiency. Prominent among these are autoimmune diseases such as multiple sclerosis, type 1 diabetes, and Crohn's disease, but more recent studies indicate that infections such as tuberculosis may also be linked to low 25(OH)D levels. Moreover, it is now clear that cells from the immune system contain all the machinery needed to convert 25(OH)D to active 1,25-dihydroxyvitamin D, and for subsequent responses to 1,25-dihydroxyvitamin D. Mechanisms such as this are important for promoting antimicrobial responses to pathogens in macrophages, and for regulating the maturation of antigen-presenting dendritic cells. The latter may be a key pathway by which vitamin D controls T-lymphocyte (T-cell) function. However, T-cells also exhibit direct responses to 1,25-dihydroxyvitamin D, notably the development of suppressor regulatory T-cells. Collectively, these observations suggest that vitamin D is a key factor linking innate and adaptive immunity, and both of these functions may be compromised under conditions of vitamin D insufficiency.

These actions of vitamin D were excluded from the dietary guidelines or the Institute of Medicine report. Yet many of your patients may be taking 1000–5000 units of vitamin D supplements with no ill effects due to the natural deactivation of excess vitamin D.

TABLE 2.11
Serum 25-Hydroxyvitamin D Concentrations by Category

Category	25(OH)D Concentrations, ng/mL (nmol/L)
Deficiency	<20 (<50)
Insufficiency	20–32 (50–80)
Sufficiency	32–100 (80–250)
Excess	>100 (>250)
Intoxication	>150 (>325)

Source: Adapted from Hossein-nezhad, A., and M. F. Holick, *Mayo Clin. Proc.*, 88(7), 720–755, 2013.

Vitamin D is not just a vitamin, but a hormone that, like the retinoids, travels to the nucleus to program the transcription of specific proteins. Research over the last three decades has brought to light many additional functions of vitamin D and redefined what is considered optimal vitamin D nutrition. It is now estimated that approximately 1 billion people worldwide have blood concentrations of vitamin D that are considered suboptimal. Low vitamin D serum concentrations are linked to several types of cancers, cardiovascular disease, diabetes, upper respiratory tract infections, and all-cause mortality.

Several observational studies and a few prospectively randomized controlled trials have demonstrated that adequate levels of vitamin D can decrease the risk and improve survival rates for several types of cancers, including breast, rectum, ovary, prostate, stomach, bladder, esophagus, kidney, lung, pancreas, uterus, non-Hodgkin lymphoma, and multiple myeloma (John et al. 2007; Davis and Milner 2011). Individuals with serum vitamin D concentrations of less than 20 ng/mL are considered most at risk, whereas those who achieve levels of 32–100 ng/mL are considered to have sufficient serum vitamin D concentrations, as in Table 2.11 (Hossein-nezhad and Holick 2013).

Vitamin D can be obtained from exposure to the sun, through dietary intake, and via supplementation. Obtaining a total of approximately 4000 IU/day of vitamin D3 from all sources has been shown to achieve serum concentrations considered to be in the sufficient range. Most individuals will require a dietary supplement of 2000 IU/day of vitamin D3 to achieve sufficient levels, as up to 20,000 IU/day is considered safe. The Endocrine Society has issued clinical guidelines recommending 1000 IU/day as a safe dose (Rosen et al. 2012). Vitamin D3 is available as an over-the-counter product at most pharmacies and is relatively inexpensive, especially when compared with potential and demonstrated benefits. Since vitamin D is fat soluble, it disperses into adipose tissue, and overfat individuals are known to have decreased levels compared with lean individuals and to require higher doses to normalize blood levels of vitamin D.

2.4.1.3 Vitamin E

A group of fat-soluble substances, the tocopherols are referred to as vitamin E. One of these substances, alpha-D-tocopherol, is biologically active in rodents, where a deficiency can cause infertility. Tocopherols have antioxidant properties protecting tissues and substances from the effects of oxygen. For example, these compounds can prevent oxidation of cholesterol, polyunsaturated fats, and other membrane lipids and proteins. The antioxidant effects of vitamin E have been demonstrated only at doses that cannot be derived from usual diets, but can only be achieved by using supplement capsules.

In humans, severe vitamin E deficiency occurs as a result of genetic defects in the a-tocopherol transfer protein (a-TTP), causing ataxia (Di Donato et al. 2010). The lack of functional a-TTP results in the rapid depletion of plasma a-tocopherol (Traber et al. 1990; Morley et al. 2008), thereby demonstrating that a-TTP is needed to maintain plasma a-tocopherol concentrations. Fat malabsorption also leads to vitamin E deficiency, including patients with cholestatic liver disease or cystic fibrosis (Traber and Manor 2012). In humans, when there is a vitamin E deficiency, in addition to spinocerebellar ataxia, which gets worse over time, there is also muscle deterioration, including cardiomyopathy, ultimately resulting in death.

The use of vitamin E supplements has been associated with lower cardiovascular disease risk in males, and has also been used effectively to retard oxygen-induced damage to the eye in infants given 100% oxygen, known as retrolental fibroplasia. There is increased interest in using vitamin E as an antioxidant for the prevention of cardiovascular disease and common forms of cancer. The RDA for vitamin E is between 8 and 12 μg equivalents per day to prevent vitamin E deficiency (infertility seen only in animals), but many individuals take 400–800 IU supplements without ill effects.

A recent analysis of multiple studies found that above 330 IU/day was associated with a 5% increase in overall mortality from cardiovascular disease. These results have been discounted by many nutrition scientists and remain controversial. Studies have shown evidence of benefits of tocotrienols, as well as tocopherols, but most supplements and multivitamins provide only synthetic alpha-D-tocopherol.

2.4.1.4 Vitamin K

Vitamin K is a fat-soluble vitamin. The *K* is derived from the German word *koagulation*. Coagulation refers to blood clotting, because vitamin K is essential for the functioning of several proteins involved in blood clotting. Vitamin K acts on target proteins in the clotting cascade BY, adding a gamma-carboxyl group to activate clotting proteins.

Half of vitamin K comes from the diet, and the other half is synthesized from precursors by intestinal bacteria. Spinach, green leafy vegetables, cabbage, potatoes, cereals, and liver are good sources (Booth 2012).

Since vitamin K is found in so many foods and is also formed by intestinal bacteria, deficiency is rare. Individuals receiving prolonged antibiotic therapy destroying intestinal bacteria and individuals with fat malabsorption are at risk for vitamin K deficiency. The RDA for adults ranges from 45 to 80 μg/day. Because warfarin antagonizes the action of vitamin K, rich dietary sources of vitamin K are restricted in patients on warfarin, also known as coumadin. For patients whose blood tests, called the international normalized ratio (INR), vary greatly, it is an art to adjust the warfarin dose, as dose adjustments often require 36 hours to manifest.

Vitamin K2 acts in bone as a cofactor for gamma-carboxylase, which converts the glutamic acid in osteocalcin molecules to gamma-carboxyglutamic acid (Kidd 2010). It is also a transcriptional regulator of bone-specific genes that act through steroid and xenobiotic receptors to favor the expression of osteoblastic markers. Vitamin K deficiency has been shown to be a risk factor for hip fractures in the elderly, and vitamin K2 supplementation increases serum levels of osteocalcin and has a modest effect on bone mineral density.

A deficiency of this vitamin in newborn babies results in hemorrhagic disease, as well as postoperative bleeding and hematuria, while muscle hematomas and intercranial hemorrhages have been reported. A shortage of this vitamin may manifest itself in nosebleeds or internal hemorrhaging.

There are two naturally occurring forms of vitamin K (Figure 2.13). Plants synthesize phylloquinone, also known as vitamin K1. Bacteria synthesize a range of vitamin K forms, using

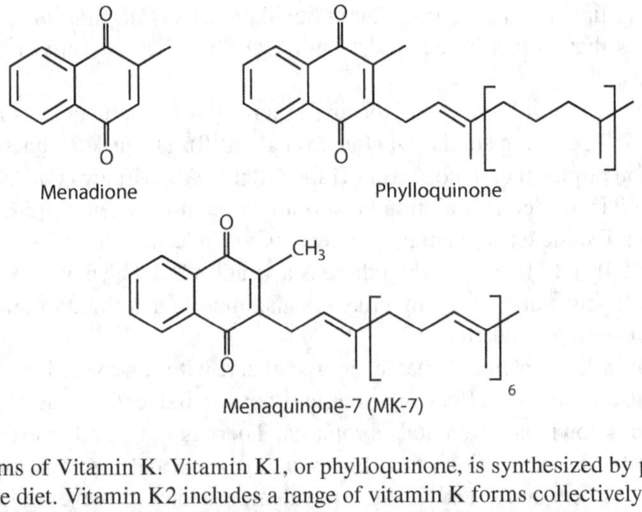

Menadione

Phylloquinone

Menaquinone-7 (MK-7)

FIGURE 2.13 Forms of Vitamin K. Vitamin K1, or phylloquinone, is synthesized by plants and is the predominant form in the diet. Vitamin K2 includes a range of vitamin K forms collectively referred to as menaquinones. Most menaquinones are synthesized by human intestinal microbiota and found in fermented foods and in animal products. Menaquinones differ in length from 1 to 14 repeats of 5-carbon units in the side chain of the molecules. These forms of vitamin K are designated MK-n, where n stands for the number of 5-carbon units (MK-2 to MK-14).

repeating 5-carbon units in the side chain of the molecule. These forms of vitamin K are designated menaquinone-n (MK-n), where n stands for the number of 5-carbon units. MK-n are collectively referred to as vitamin K2. The synthetic compound known as menadione (vitamin K3) is a provitamin that needs to be converted to MK-4 to be active. MK-4 is not produced in significant amounts by bacteria, but appears to be synthesized by animals (including humans) from phylloquinone, which is found in plants (Nakagawa et al. 2010). MK-4 is found in a number of organs other than the liver at higher concentrations than phylloquinone. This fact, along with the existence of a unique pathway for its synthesis, suggests that there is some unique function of MK-4 that is yet to be discovered.

2.4.2 Water-Soluble Vitamins

2.4.2.1 Vitamin B1 (Thiamin)

Thiamin deficiency disease, still seen today in alcoholics, is known as beriberi (McCullough et al. 2000a). This disease, which damages the nervous and cardiovascular systems, is found in two forms, wet beriberi with edema and congestive heart failure, and dry beriberi characterized by muscle atrophy due to nerve damage. In alcoholics, Wernicke–Korsakoff syndrome, characterized by mental confusion, memory disturbances, ataxia, opthalmoplegia, and nystagmus, can be fatal if not treated with intravenous thiamin (Haas 1988).

The dietary vitamin is phosphorylated by transfer of a high-energy phosphate from ATP to form thiamin pyrophosphate in the intestine. Its primary function is to act as a coenzyme for the oxidative decarboxylation of alpha-keto acids to carboxylic acids (e.g., pyruvate to acetyl-CoA) and the transketolase reaction of the pentose phosphate shunt. The latter pathway is important for nucleic acid synthesis and the formation of NADPH for fatty acid synthesis and other reactions. Decreased transketolase activity in red cells can be detected early in the course of thiamin deficiency. The RDA of thiamin is 0.5 mg/1000 kcal, and this is four times the intake at which deficiency signs are observed.

2.4.2.2 Vitamin B2 (Riboflavin)

Riboflavin is a yellow fluorescent compound found throughout the animal and plant kingdoms. Humans and other mammals cannot synthesize these compounds, which function in numerous enzyme complexes (including flavin mononucleotide and flavin adenine dinucleotide) involved in electron transport oxidation–reduction reactions. It is the central component of the cofactors FAD and FMN and, as such, is required for a variety of flavoproteoin enzyme reactions, including the activation of other vitamins (Merrill et al. 1981).

Flavins are transported in the blood by albumin and immunoglobulins. Uncomplicated riboflavin deficiency is uncommon, but dietary lack of the vitamin can lead to a deficit, not only in flavin coenzyme functions, but also in the conversion of vitamin B6 to pyridoxal phosphate. The RDA for riboflavin ranges between 1.2 and 1.8 mg/day for adults.

2.4.2.3 Vitamin B6 (Pyridoxine)

The active form of vitamin B6 is pyridoxal 5′-phosphate (PLP), and this coenzyme is involved in more than 60 different enzymatic reactions in the body, including such common reactions as decarboxylation and aminotransferase reactions (Mooney et al. 2009).

Isolated deficiencies of vitamin B6 are rare, and it is most common to see deficiencies of multiple B vitamins. The best measure of vitamin B6 status is plasma PLP, which can be measured by high-performance liquid chromatography (HPLC). An intake of 2 mg/day is recommended as the RDA, and doses greater than 1 mg must be given to change PLP levels. At intakes of greater than 25 mg, PLP levels do not change further, with the excess vitamin B6 excreted in the urine as pyridoxal and pyridoxic acid. Very large doses (e.g., 500 mg/day) can cause peripheral neuropathy by inducing a conditioned deficiency of other B vitamins catabolized in a manner similar to that of the excess vitamin B6 ingested.

2.4.2.4 Niacin

Vitamin B3, also known as niacin or nicotinic acid, can be synthesized by the body from tryptophan. The nickname *niacin* came from linking several letters in the words *nicotinic*, *acid*, and *vitamin*. When the properties of nicotinic acid, made by oxidation of nicotine, were first discovered, it was decided that vitamin B3, or nicotinic acid, should be named in such a way as to dissociate it from nicotine and not create the impression that either smoking provided this vitamin or wholesome food contained a poison.

Once again, niacin refers to both nicotinic acid and nicotinamide, although sometimes it is used just to indicate niacin. Nicotinamide is converted to the nicotinamide adenine dinucleotide cofactors (NAD and NADH) essential for a number of enzymatic reactions and electron transport. Niacin causes flushing and can reduce triglyceride levels in individuals with dyslipidemia at high doses of 500 mg three times a day, usually taken with aspirin to reduce the flushing reaction (Brown et al. 2001). Nicotinamide does not have these lipid-lowering effects.

The deficiency disease, pellagra, was observed to occur in populations consuming a maize-based diet deficient in the amino acid tryptophan, which is the precursor for endogenous niacin formation. Large doses of nicotinic acid (1.5–3 g/day), but not nicotinamide, will lower cholesterol and triglyceride levels and raise HDL levels in subgroups of hypercholesterolemic individuals. However, long-acting forms of niacin in large doses have been associated with liver damage, facial flushing, and worsening of hyperglycemia in diabetics. The RDA for niacin ranges between 13 and 20 mg/day for adults.

2.4.2.5 Folic Acid

Folate is a micronutrient, once called vitamin M, which frequently is deficient in American diets since it is derived from dark green, leafy vegetables. The root of the name folic comes from the Latin word for *leaf*. Folic acid acts in cell maturation and differentiates epithelial tissues. In the lung and the cervical epithelium, pro-differentiation effects have been demonstrated. Folic acid has also been associated with the prevention of neural tube defects, such as spina bifida, through its effects in epigenetic methylation in utero. It is included in all prenatal vitamins at an enhanced level.

Folate supplementation is restricted to 400 μg/tablet in over-the-counter vitamins given the fear that someone with excessive folate and B12 deficiency (see Section 2.4.2.6) will develop subacute combined spinal degeneration and paralysis (Drazkowski et al. 2002). Patients with pernicious anemia are among those susceptible to subacute combined spinal degeneration from excess folate intake, as are those who have had a gastric bypass operation or gastrectomy. *Folate* and *folic acid* are *not* interchangeable terms. Folic acid is the oxidized form found in fortified foods and supplements, while folate is the reduced form found naturally in foods as polyglutamates, which must be cleaved and converted in a series of steps to 5-methyltetrahydrofolate, which plays a key role in methyl donor reactions.

Food sources of folate include mushrooms and green vegetables. Raw foods have higher amounts than cooked foods. Enrichment of white flour began in 1998 and is now the major source of folate in the American diet. The bioavailability of dietary folate is about 50%.

One dietary folate equivalent (DFE) is equal to 1 μg of food folate, 0.6 μg of folic acid from a supplement or fortified food consumed with a meal, or 0.5 μg of folic acid from a supplement taken without food (empty stomach). Stated alternately, DFE = 1 μg of food folate + (1.7 × 1 μg of folic acid).

2.4.2.6 Vitamin B12

Vitamin B12, also called cyanocobalamin, is needed to make red blood cells and is necessary for the synthesis of nerve sheaths, fatty acids, and DNA. Since this vitamin is stored in the liver, nutritional deficiency usually takes years to develop. It is much more common to see metabolic deficiencies. Most commonly, an anemia due to B12 deficiency results from an autoimmune disease called pernicious anemia, in which the parietal cells in the stomach that make a binding protein (intrinsic factor) necessary for B12 absorption are destroyed (Seetharam and Alpers 1982). The healthy individuals most at risk of a dietary vitamin B12 deficiency are vegetarians, since there is no B12 in any plant product. There is also a decreased capability for absorption of vitamin B12 in the elderly due to decreased gastric acid secretion (Carmel 1997).

Vitamin B12 levels need to be measured in individuals at risk, since folate administered to an individual with B12 deficiency will result in subacute combined degeneration of the spine and paralysis. The RDA for adults is only 2–2.6 µg/day.

Vitamin B12 consists of a class of chemically related compounds, all of which have vitamin activity. It contains the biochemically rare element cobalt sitting in the center of a planar tetrapyrrole ring called a corrin ring. More recently, hydroxocobalamin, methylcobalamin, and adenosylcobalamin can be found in more expensive pharmacological products and food supplements. Their extra utility is currently controversial.

2.4.2.7 Choline

Choline is not considered a B vitamin since a portion of the choline requirement can be met via endogenous de novo synthesis of phosphatidylcholine catalyzed by phosphatidylethanolamine N-methyltransferase (PEMT) in the liver. A recommended dietary intake for choline of 550 mg/day in humans was set in 1998, and although many foods contain choline, 90% of Americans do not get enough in their diets (Zeisel 2011).

When deprived of dietary choline, most adult men and postmenopausal women develop signs of organ dysfunction, such as fatty liver, liver or muscle cell damage, and reduced capacity to handle a methionine load, resulting in elevated homocysteine levels in the blood.

Only some premenopausal women with a genetic polymorphism develop problems, because estrogen induces expression of the PEMT gene and allows premenopausal women to make more of their needed choline endogenously. The dietary requirement for choline can vary based on common polymorphisms in genes of choline and folate metabolism, including the methylenetetrahydrofolate reductase (MTHFR) gene. The CC polymorphism is the most common and protects individuals from choline deficiency. The less common TT polymorphism in about 10% of individuals does not protect individuals from choline deficiency.

Choline is critical during fetal development, when it alters DNA methylation and thereby influences neural precursor cell proliferation and apoptosis. This results in long-term alterations in brain structure and function, specifically memory function. Along with folate and B12 deficiency, inadequate consumption of choline can lead to high homocysteine and all the risks associated with that, including cardiovascular disease, neuropsychiatric illness (Alzheimer's disease and schizophrenia), and osteoporosis. Inadequate choline intake can also lead to fatty liver or nonalcoholic fatty liver disease (NAFLD). The issues around homocysteine are an excellent example of the impact of nutrigenetics, the differences among individuals impacting risk of age-related chronic diseases.

DNA methylation is dependent on a methyl donor. and S-adenosyl-L-methionine (SAM) is the primary methyl group donor for most biological methylation reactions (Chiang et al. 1996). SAM is generated by the methionine cycle, in which 5-methyltetrahydrofolate transfers single methyl groups to homocysteine in a reaction catalyzed by methionine synthase to produce methionine. After donating the methyl group, 5-methyltetrahydrofolate is converted to tetrahydrofolate and then to 5,10-methylenetetrahydrofolate by serine hydroxymethyltransferase. 5,10-Methylenetetrahydrofolate is a key substrate that can be directed toward nucleotide biosynthesis or methionine regeneration. MTHFR catalyzes the irreversible conversion of 5,10-methylenetetrahydrofolate to 5-methyltetrahydrofolate, which can be used in the methionine cycle to generate SAM (Schwahn and Rozen 2001).

The *MTHFR* C677T polymorphism leads to the amino acid alanine being replaced by valine (p.Ala222Val) and the production of a thermolabile variant of MTHFR with 30% less enzyme activity (Sharp and Little 2004). The *MTHFR* C677T polymorphism has been suspected to induce hypomethylation and then activate proto-oncogenes, which could explain the association between this polymorphism and some types of cancer, including oral cancer (Sailasree et al. 2011).

2.4.2.8 Pantothenic Acid and Coenzyme A

Pantothenic acid is also called pantothenate or vitamin B5. Pantothenic acid is required to synthesize coenzyme A (CoA), which is intrinsic to the synthesis of proteins, carbohydrates, and fats (Robishaw and Neely 1985). The structure of pantothenic acid is made up of an amide linkage between pantoic acid and alanine. Its name derives from a Greek root meaning "from everywhere," since small quantities of pantothenic acid are found in nearly every food, with high amounts in avocado, whole grains, legumes, eggs, and meats. It commonly occurs in its alcohol form, pantothenol, and as calcium pantothenate. Pantothenic acid is used as an ingredient in some hair and skin care products, since it is reputed with no proof to prevent graying of the hair. It was discovered in 1933 by Dr. Roger Williams.

Within cells, pyruvate produced from the breakdown of glucose via the glycolytic pathway is transported into mitochondria for the production of ATP via oxidative phosphorylation, as discussed earlier. When oxygen is available, pyruvate is converted into a 2-carbon acetyl group (acetyl-CoA), which is then picked up by CoA. Acetyl-CoA can be used in a variety of ways by the cell, but its major function is to deliver the acetyl group derived from pyruvate to the Krebs cycle of glucose catabolism to produce ATP energy for the cell. In all living organisms, CoA is synthesized in a five-step process that requires four molecules of ATP, from pantothenate and cysteine. The structure of CoA was identified in the early 1950s at the Lister Institute in London, together with workers at the Massachusetts General Hospital and Harvard Medical School (Theodoulou et al. 2014).

Since CoA contains a sulfhydryl group (SH), it can react with a carboxylic acid group to form a thioester, which can be used to help transfer fatty acids with more than 10 carbons from the cytoplasm to the mitochondria. A molecule of CoA carrying an acetyl group is also referred to as acetyl-CoA. Examples of uses of CoA include fatty acyl-CoAs (proprionyl-CoA, butyryl-CoA, myristoyl-CoA, crotonyl-CoA, acetoacetyl-CoA, benzoyl-CoA, and phenylacetyl-CoA), malonyl-CoA, succinyl-CoA, and hydroxymethylglutaryl (HMG)-CoA. The last compound is involved in the rate-limiting step in cholesterol biosynthesis, which is HMG-CoA reductase.

2.4.2.9 Biotin

Biotin, also known as vitamin B7, vitamin H, or coenzyme R, is a coenzyme for carboxylase enzymes, involved in the synthesis of fatty acids, isoleucine, and valine, and in gluconeogenesis. Biotin exists in food as protein-bound form or biocytin. Proteolysis by protease is required prior to absorption. This process assists free biotin release from biocytin and protein-bound biotin. The biotin present in corn is readily available; however, most grains have about a 20–40% bioavailability of biotin. Biotin is found in a wide variety of foods, with high biotin content in peanuts, Swiss chard, liver, Saskatoon berries, and leafy green vegetables.

Biotin deficiency can be caused by inborn metabolic errors affecting biotin-related enzymes. In animals fed raw egg whites, biotin deficiency occurs due to a protein called avidin, which binds biotin. Avidin is denatured with cooking, so cooked egg white does not affect biotin availability. Patients with gastric bypass or gastrectomy can develop biotin deficiency in the absence of supplementation since proteolysis is required in the stomach to release protein-bound biotin found in foods. Symptoms include hair loss, dermatitis, and conjunctivitis (Mock and Said 2009). The reason it is called vitamin H is from the German for *hair* and *skin* (*hair* and *haut*), since these are characteristic of biotin deficiency. Neurological and psychological symptoms can occur with only mild deficiencies. Dermatitis, conjunctivitis, and hair loss will generally occur only when deficiency becomes more severe. Pregnant women tend to have a high risk of biotin deficiency. Nearly half of pregnant women have abnormal increases of 3-hydroxyisovaleric acid, which reflects a reduced status of biotin.

2.5 WRITING THE EXERCISE PRESCRIPTION AND EVALUATING FITNESS

A great deal of evidence indicates that regular physical activity is one of the most powerful influences on patient health that physicians and other health care professionals can have (Kraus et al. 2015). The lack of physical activity counseling in the primary care setting represents a lost opportunity to improve the health and well-being of patients with minimal cost. Among adults with prediabetes, only 40% report receiving counseling on physical activity.

While time constraints, lack of tools, and skeptical attitudes are cited as reasons for the lack of physical activity counseling, in the Activity and Counseling Trial clinicians in primary care were taught to deliver a brief intervention over 3–4 minutes during routine office visits (Writing Group for the Activity Counseling Trial Research Group 2001). At 2 years of follow-up, there were improvements in cardiorespiratory fitness, as determined by measurement of maximum oxygen consumption. Most clinicians reported that the counseling did not disrupt or increase the length of the visit and that the counseling was an asset to their practice.

There are a number of practical steps that can be taken in order to incorporate physical activity counseling into your primary care practice (Berra et al. 2015).

1. Make physical activity a vital sign at every visit.
2. Ask if the patient exercises regularly or engages in a physical activity.
   a. If yes, ask what type, for how many minutes, and how often.
   b. If no, ask if the patient is willing to start.
3. Associate physical activity with reduced risks of common diseases.
4. Write a prescription for agreed-upon daily physical activity, working up to at least 30 minutes of walking or other moderate-intensity activity daily.
5. Encourage use of a pedometer or the free health app on some smartphones and advise record keeping of daily activity.
6. Recognize success and encourage reluctant adopters.

Physicians and other health care professionals can help set priorities for patients with regard to physical activity by personalizing the exercise prescription.

The first step in encouraging personalized exercise is to recommend walking 10,000 steps/day. However, this is just a beginning for most patients. Thirty minutes per day of aerobic exercise at one time or two bouts of exercise lasting 15 minutes each is the next level. For these sessions, it is simple to calculate a personal target heart rate for aerobic activities, such as walking on a treadmill or elliptical or riding an exercise bike. Simply subtract the patient's age from 220 and multiply by 0.7. At this heart rate, fat burning is optimized.

The next level of exercise prescription may require the help of a knowledgeable physical therapist with experience in biomechanics. An assessment of muscle strength through various muscle groups will make it possible to design a personalized exercise regimen with specific endpoints in mind. This type of program requires the highest level of commitment from your patients. For patients who are working, it is important to consider ways to link the exercise in time and geography either before or after work.

In order to adapt patients to exercising regularly, encourage a routine that includes special fitness clothing, a low-calorie sports drink, and fitness music with a rapid beat, which tends to reduce feelings of fatigue and add some fun to the workout.

The next level of fitness awareness requires the involvement of a physical therapist and trainer knowledgeable in muscle biomechanics. The concept is to educate and rehabilitate muscles that have atrophied due to disuse. When muscles atrophy, they do so in an asymmetrical way, putting increased strain on joints.

An important example is the atrophy of the hamstring muscles due to a sedentary lifestyle. With lack of use, the hamstring muscles foreshorten, and this puts a strain on the hip joints. Atrophy of the gluteal muscles and poor abdominal tone put a strain on the lower back.

In the upper body, round shoulders are due to atrophy of the scapula muscles and maintenance of poor posture. Exercising the upper back muscles, abdominal muscles, and gluteus posture muscles can help correct poor posture.

The main message is to recommend exercises that have a goal and a measurable or visible result. Reduced joint pain is a benefit, as is correction of poor posture. While walking and aerobic exercise are good places to begin the exercise prescription, they are not the end of an exercise prescription.

2.6 LEVERAGING DIETETIC AND NURSING SUPPORT

It is critical to realize that you cannot do this yourself. You must build a team within your practice and communicate sufficiently to align your messages. A system for communication can be established if you are not already using the electronic health record. You will find that you and your dietitians and nurses have complementary skills that can be combined to improve the nutrition and fitness programs prescribed in your practice.

Since the education of many dietitians has centered around philosophies generated by the food industry, it is important that the dietitians in your practice align with your philosophy. Take what you like from this chapter and create your own messaging that is reinforced by your dietitians and nurses.

2.7 ISSUES AROUND BOTANICAL DIETARY SUPPLEMENTS

Only very small clinical trials have been conducted with certain preparations of botanical dietary supplements. The FDA has established good manufacturing practices and inspects manufacturing sites to ensure compliance. Few companies have established the necessary, preclinical, clinical, and postmarketing resources to responsibly monitor botanical dietary supplements. Raw materials should be chemically characterized using chromatography or mass spectrometry to fully identify the amounts of marker ingredients. This is an expensive effort and should be followed by careful analysis of the finished products at the factory and during shipping. A full discussion of the positive and negative aspects of botanical dietary supplements is outside the scope of this book. Your primary role will be to screen out any supplements known to be toxic. In addition, the FDA conducts postmarket surveillance for side effects, so you should use this reporting system whenever you encounter a side effect that you attribute to a botanical dietary supplement.

2.8 ENABLING PATIENT CHOICE IN NUTRITION FOR DIETS AND SUPPLEMENTS

The most practical basic micronutrient supplementation program includes a daily multivitamin or multimineral, calcium and magnesium, a vitamin D supplement, and a fish oil supplement. When combined with dietary counseling, there is a good rationale for this simple approach.

A number of medical and government advisory groups have argued against the use of a daily multivitamin supplement, but the overwhelming evidence is that this is only the first step in a supplementation program. A Canadian study of men and women over 50 years of age found that less than 5% of those who used a daily multivitamin or multimineral supplement had a deficiency of vitamins A, C, B6, and B12, and folate (Shakur et al. 2012). Between one-third and one-half of all Americans take multivitamin or multimineral supplements. By themselves, these supplements do not make up for an unhealthy diet, but they have no adverse effects. As patients learn more about nutrition, they will explore additional supplements with you and your dietitian, so it is important to keep up on the latest trends in dietary supplements as they develop.

Here are just a few examples of supplements you may be asked about:

Coenzyme Q10 or ubiquinone: This is an antioxidant for which there is some evidence of benefit in heart failure. Many heart patients will ask about this supplement. There are no adverse effects associated with consuming this supplement.

SAMe: This is S-Adenosyl methionine, and there are some studies showing benefit for osteoarthritis and depression.

Glucosamine or chondroitin sulfate: Glucosamine has been shown to slow the loss of knee cartilage in patients with osteoarthritis. There is less evidence for additional ingredients in many supplements in this category. There are no adverse effects.

Phytosterols: Plants do not make cholesterol, but they synthesize phytosterols, which compete with cholesterol for intestinal uptake. Their use is associated with about a 5% decrease in cholesterol levels. There are no adverse effects.

Cranberry extracts for urinary tract prevention: There are specific compounds in cranberry, called proanthocyanidins, with a unique structure that inhibits the adhesion of bacteria to the bladder wall.

None of the above supplements have toxic effects. Rather than condemn all supplements, consider allowing patients to consume those they think are helpful. Very few dietary supplements have the scientific evidence from placebo-controlled trials that are typical of prescription drugs. However, many patients with psychophysiological disorders benefit from taking supplements, even when the rationale is weak and not scientifically based. There are multiple sources of information, including the National Institutes of Health guide on dietary supplements, that can provide you with key information on this topic. Unless there is a safety issue, it is best to enable, rather than criticize, the use of botanical supplements as a rule.

REFERENCES

Aller, E. E., T. M. Larsen, H. Claus, A. K. Lindroos, A. Kafatos, A. Pfeiffer, J. A. Martinez et al. 2014. Weight loss maintenance in overweight subjects on ad libitum diets with high or low protein content and glycemic index: The DIOGENES trial 12-month results. *Int J Obes (Lond)* 38 (12):1511–1517.

Anonymous. 1987. Nomenclature policy: Generic descriptors and trivial names for vitamins and related compounds. *J Nutr* 117:7–14.

Augustin, L. S., C. W. Kendall, D. J. Jenkins, W. C. Willett, A. Astrup, A. W. Barclay, I. Bjorck et al. 2015. Glycemic index, glycemic load and glycemic response: An International Scientific Consensus Summit from the International Carbohydrate Quality Consortium (ICQC). *Nutr Metab Cardiovasc Dis* 25 (9):795–815.

Baggerly, C. A., R. E. Cuomo, C. B. French, C. F. Garland, E. D. Gorham, W. B. Grant, R. P. Heaney et al. 2015. Sunlight and vitamin D: Necessary for public health. *J Am Coll Nutr* 34 (4):359–365.

Berra, K., J. Rippe, and J. E. Manson. 2015. Making physical activity counseling a priority in clinical practice: The time for action is now. *JAMA* 314 (24):2617–2618.

Bhupathiraju, S. N., D. K. Tobias, V. S. Malik, A. Pan, A. Hruby, J. E. Manson, W. C. Willett, and F. B. Hu. 2014. Glycemic index, glycemic load, and risk of type 2 diabetes: Results from 3 large US cohorts and an updated meta-analysis. *Am J Clin Nutr* 100 (1):218–232.

Booth, S. L. 2012. Vitamin K: Food composition and dietary intakes. *Food Nutr Res* 56.

Brown, B. G., X. Q. Zhao, A. Chait, L. D. Fisher, M. C. Cheung, J. S. Morse, A. A. Dowdy et al. 2001. Simvastatin and niacin, antioxidant vitamins, or the combination for the prevention of coronary disease. *N Engl J Med* 345 (22):1583–1592.

Carmel, R. 1997. Cobalamin, the stomach, and aging. *Am J Clin Nutr* 66 (4):750–759.

Chiang, P. K., R. K. Gordon, J. Tal, G. C. Zeng, B. P. Doctor, K. Pardhasaradhi, and P. P. McCann. 1996. S-Adenosylmethionine and methylation. *FASEB J* 10 (4):471–80.

Control of vitamin A deficiency and xerophthalmia. 1982. *World Health Organ Tech Rep Ser* 672:1–70.
Cunningham, J. J. 1980. A reanalysis of the factors influencing basal metabolic rate in normal adults. *Am J Clin Nutr* 33 (11):2372–2374.
Davis, C. D., and J. A. Milner. 2011. Nutrigenomics, vitamin D and cancer prevention. *J Nutrigenet Nutrigenomics* 4 (1):1–11.
Di Donato, I., S. Bianchi, and A. Federico. 2010. Ataxia with vitamin E deficiency: Update of molecular diagnosis. *Neurol Sci* 31 (4):511–515.
Drazkowski, J., J. Sirven, and D. Blum. 2002. Symptoms of B12 deficiency can occur in women of child bearing age supplemented with folate. *Neurology* 58 (10):1572–1573.
Ebbeling, C. B., H. A. Feldman, V. R. Chomitz, T. A. Antonelli, S. L. Gortmaker, S. K. Osganian, and D. S. Ludwig. 2012. A randomized trial of sugar-sweetened beverages and adolescent body weight. *N Engl J Med* 367 (15):1407–1416.
Foster-Powell, K., S. H. Holt, and J. C. Brand-Miller. 2002. International table of glycemic index and glycemic load values: 2002. *Am J Clin Nutr* 76 (1):5–56.
Fulgoni, V. L., 3rd. 2008. Current protein intake in America: Analysis of the National Health and Nutrition Examination Survey, 2003–2004. *Am J Clin Nutr* 87 (5):1554S–1557S.
Goodman, G. E., S. Schaffer, G. S. Omenn, C. Chen, and I. King. 2003. The association between lung and prostate cancer risk, and serum micronutrients: Results and lessons learned from beta-carotene and retinol efficacy trial. *Cancer Epidemiol Biomarkers Prev* 12 (6):518–526.
Greenwald, P., and S. S. McDonald. 2001. The beta-carotene story. *Adv Exp Med Biol* 492:219–231.
Haas, R. H. 1988. Thiamin and the brain. *Annu Rev Nutr* 8:483–515.
Heber, D., and S. Bowerman. 2004. *The L.A. Shape Diet: The 14-Day Total Weight Loss Plan*. 1st ed. New York: Regan Books.
Hewison, M. 2012. Vitamin D and immune function: An overview. *Proc Nutr Soc* 71 (1):50–61.
Holick, M. F. 2016. Biological effects of sunlight, ultraviolet radiation, visible light, infrared radiation and vitamin D for health. *Anticancer Res* 36 (3):1345–1356.
Honein, M. A., L. J. Paulozzi, T. J. Mathews, J. D. Erickson, and L. Y. Wong. 2001. Impact of folic acid fortification of the US food supply on the occurrence of neural tube defects. *JAMA* 285 (23):2981–2986.
Hossein-nezhad, A., and M. F. Holick. 2013. Vitamin D for health: A global perspective. *Mayo Clin Proc* 88 (7):720–755.
Howard, B. V., L. Van Horn, J. Hsia, J. E. Manson, M. L. Stefanick, S. Wassertheil-Smoller, L. H. Kuller et al. 2006. Low-fat dietary pattern and risk of cardiovascular disease: The Women's Health Initiative Randomized Controlled Dietary Modification Trial. *JAMA* 295 (6):655–666.
Institute of Medicine (U.S.), Panel on Dietary Reference Intakes for Electrolytes and Water. 2005. *DRI, Dietary Reference Intakes for Water, Potassium, Sodium, Chloride, and Sulfate*. Washington, DC: National Academies Press.
Jenkins, D. J., T. M. Wolever, R. H. Taylor, H. Barker, H. Fielden, J. M. Baldwin, A. C. Bowling, H. C. Newman, A. L. Jenkins, and D. V. Goff. 1981. Glycemic index of foods: A physiological basis for carbohydrate exchange. *Am J Clin Nutr* 34 (3):362–366.
Jew, S., S. S. AbuMweis, and P. J. Jones. 2009. Evolution of the human diet: Linking our ancestral diet to modern functional foods as a means of chronic disease prevention. *J Med Food* 12 (5):925–934.
John, E. M., G. G. Schwartz, J. Koo, W. Wang, and S. A. Ingles. 2007. Sun exposure, vitamin D receptor gene polymorphisms, and breast cancer risk in a multiethnic population. *Am J Epidemiol* 166 (12):1409–1419.
Kennedy, E. T., J. Ohls, S. Carlson, and K. Fleming. 1995. The Healthy Eating Index: Design and applications. *J Am Diet Assoc* 95 (10):1103–1108.
Kidd, P. M. 2010. Vitamins D and K as pleiotropic nutrients: Clinical importance to the skeletal and cardiovascular systems and preliminary evidence for synergy. *Altern Med Rev* 15 (3):199–222.
Kockott, D., B. Herzog, J. Reichrath, K. Keane, and M. F. Holick. 2016. New approach to develop optimized sunscreens that enable cutaneous vitamin D formation with minimal erythema risk. *PLoS One* 11 (1):e0145509.
Kraus, W. E., V. Bittner, L. Appel, S. N. Blair, T. Church, J. P. Despres, B. A. Franklin et al. 2015. The national physical activity plan: A call to action from the American Heart Association: A science advisory from the American Heart Association. *Circulation* 131 (21):1932–1940.
Kyle, U. G., I. Bosaeus, A. D. De Lorenzo, P. Deurenberg, M. Elia, J. M. Gomez, B. L. Heitmann et al. 2004. Bioelectrical impedance analysis. Part I. Review of principles and methods. *Clin Nutr* 23 (5):1226–1243.
Larsen, T. M., S. M. Dalskov, M. van Baak, S. A. Jebb, A. Papadaki, A. F. Pfeiffer, J. A. Martinez et al. 2010. Diets with high or low protein content and glycemic index for weight-loss maintenance. *N Engl J Med* 363 (22):2102–2113.

Levine, M., S. C. Rumsey, R. Daruwala, J. B. Park, and Y. Wang. 1999. Criteria and recommendations for vitamin C intake. *JAMA* 281 (15):1415–1423.

Ma, R., M. Sun, S. Wang, Q. Kang, L. Huang, T. Li, and W. W. Xia. 2013. Effect of high-fructose corn syrup on the acidogenicity, adherence and biofilm formation of *Streptococcus mutans*. *Aust Dent J* 58 (2):213–218.

McCullough, M. L., D. Feskanich, E. B. Rimm, E. L. Giovannucci, A. Ascherio, J. N. Variyam, D. Spiegelman, M. J. Stampfer, and W. C. Willett. 2000a. Adherence to the dietary guidelines for Americans and risk of major chronic disease in men. *Am J Clin Nutr* 72 (5):1223–1231.

McCullough, M. L., D. Feskanich, M. J. Stampfer, E. L. Giovannucci, E. B. Rimm, F. B. Hu, D. Spiegelman, D. J. Hunter, G. A. Colditz, and W. C. Willett. 2002. Diet quality and major chronic disease risk in men and women: Moving toward improved dietary guidance. *Am J Clin Nutr* 76 (6):1261–1271.

McCullough, M. L., D. Feskanich, M. J. Stampfer, B. A. Rosner, F. B. Hu, D. J. Hunter, J. N. Variyam, G. A. Colditz, and W. C. Willett. 2000b. Adherence to the dietary guidelines for Americans and risk of major chronic disease in women. *Am J Clin Nutr* 72 (5):1214–1222.

Meredith, C. N., M. J. Zackin, W. R. Frontera, and W. J. Evans. 1989. Dietary protein requirements and body protein metabolism in endurance-trained men. *J Appl Physiol (1985)* 66 (6):2850–2856.

Merrill, A. H., Jr., J. D. Lambeth, D. E. Edmondson, and D. B. McCormick. 1981. Formation and mode of action of flavoproteins. *Annu Rev Nutr* 1:281–317.

Mock, D. M., and H. Said. 2009. Introduction to "Advances in understanding of the biological role of biotin at the clinical, biochemical, and molecular level." *J Nutr* 139 (1):152–153.

Mooney, S., J. E. Leuendorf, C. Hendrickson, and H. Hellmann. 2009. Vitamin B6: A long known compound of surprising complexity. *Molecules* 14 (1):329–351.

Moore, T. 1957. *Vitamin A*. Amsterdam: Elsevier.

Morley, S., M. Cecchini, W. Zhang, A. Virgulti, N. Noy, J. Atkinson, and D. Manor. 2008. Mechanisms of ligand transfer by the hepatic tocopherol transfer protein. *J Biol Chem* 283 (26):17797–17804.

Nakagawa, K., Y. Hirota, N. Sawada, N. Yuge, M. Watanabe, Y. Uchino, N. Okuda, Y. Shimomura, Y. Suhara, and T. Okano. 2010. Identification of UBIAD1 as a novel human menaquinone-4 biosynthetic enzyme. *Nature* 468 (7320):117–121.

Olson, J. A. 1987. Recommended dietary intakes (RDI) of vitamin A in humans. *Am J Clin Nutr* 45 (4):704–716.

Olson, J. A. 1990. *Vitamin A: In Present Knowledge in Nutrition*. Washington, DC: ILSI Press.

Otten, J. J., J. P. Hellwig, and L. D. Meyers. 2006. *DRI, Dietary Reference Intakes: The Essential Guide to Nutrient Requirements*. Washington, DC: National Academies Press.

Paddon-Jones, D., and B. B. Rasmussen. 2009. Dietary protein recommendations and the prevention of sarcopenia. *Curr Opin Clin Nutr Metab Care* 12 (1):86–90.

Petkovich, M., N. J. Brand, A. Krust, and P. Chambon. 1987. A human retinoic acid receptor which belongs to the family of nuclear receptors. *Nature* 330 (6147):444–450.

Prentice, R. L., B. Caan, R. T. Chlebowski, R. Patterson, L. H. Kuller, J. K. Ockene, K. L. Margolis et al. 2006. Low-fat dietary pattern and risk of invasive breast cancer: The Women's Health Initiative Randomized Controlled Dietary Modification Trial. *JAMA* 295 (6):629–642.

Robishaw, J. D., and J. R. Neely. 1985. Coenzyme A metabolism. *Am J Physiol* 248 (1 Pt 1):E1–E9.

Rose, D. P., M. Goldman, J. M. Connolly, and L. E. Strong. 1991. High-fiber diet reduces serum estrogen concentrations in premenopausal women. *Am J Clin Nutr* 54 (3):520–525.

Rosen, C. J., J. S. Adams, D. D. Bikle, D. M. Black, M. B. Demay, J. E. Manson, M. H. Murad, and C. S. Kovacs. 2012. The nonskeletal effects of vitamin D: An Endocrine Society scientific statement. *Endocr Rev* 33 (3):456–492.

Sacks, F. M., E. Obarzanek, M. M. Windhauser, L. P. Svetkey, W. M. Vollmer, M. McCullough, N. Karanja et al. 1995. Rationale and design of the Dietary Approaches to Stop Hypertension trial (DASH). A multicenter controlled-feeding study of dietary patterns to lower blood pressure. *Ann Epidemiol* 5 (2):108–118.

Sailasree, R., K. R. Nalinakumari, P. Sebastian, and S. Kannan. 2011. Influence of methylenetetrahydrofolate reductase polymorphisms in oral cancer patients. *J Oral Pathol Med* 40 (1):61–66.

Schaafsma, G. 2005. The protein digestibility-corrected amino acid score (PDCAAS)—A concept for describing protein quality in foods and food ingredients: A critical review. *J AOAC Int* 88 (3):988–994.

Schwahn, B., and R. Rozen. 2001. Polymorphisms in the methylenetetrahydrofolate reductase gene: Clinical consequences. *Am J Pharmacogenomics* 1 (3):189–201.

Seetharam, B., and D. H. Alpers. 1982. Absorption and transport of cobalamin (vitamin B12). *Annu Rev Nutr* 2:343–369.

Shakur, Y. A., V. Tarasuk, P. Corey, and D. L. O'Connor. 2012. A comparison of micronutrient inadequacy and risk of high micronutrient intakes among vitamin and mineral supplement users and nonusers in Canada. *J Nutr* 142 (3):534–540.

Sharp, L., and J. Little. 2004. Polymorphisms in genes involved in folate metabolism and colorectal neoplasia: A HuGE review. *Am J Epidemiol* 159 (5):423–443.

Simopoulos, A. P. 2004. Omega-3 fatty acids and antioxidants in edible wild plants. *Biol Res* 37 (2):263–277.

Tarnopolsky, M. A., S. A. Atkinson, J. D. MacDougall, A. Chesley, S. Phillips, and H. P. Schwarcz. 1992. Evaluation of protein requirements for trained strength athletes. *J Appl Physiol (1985)* 73 (5):1986–1995.

Theodoulou, F. L., O. C. Sibon, S. Jackowski, and I. Gout. 2014. Coenzyme A and its derivatives: Renaissance of a textbook classic. *Biochem Soc Trans* 42 (4):1025–1032.

Thomas, E. L., J. R. Parkinson, G. S. Frost, A. P. Goldstone, C. J. Dore, J. P. McCarthy, A. L. Collins, J. A. Fitzpatrick, G. Durighel, S. D. Taylor-Robinson, and J. D. Bell. 2012. The missing risk: MRI and MRS phenotyping of abdominal adiposity and ectopic fat. *Obesity (Silver Spring)* 20 (1):76–87.

Traber, M. G., and D. Manor. 2012. Vitamin E. *Adv Nutr* 3 (3):330–331.

Traber, M. G., R. J. Sokol, G. W. Burton, K. U. Ingold, A. M. Papas, J. E. Huffaker, and H. J. Kayden. 1990. Impaired ability of patients with familial isolated vitamin E deficiency to incorporate alpha-tocopherol into lipoproteins secreted by the liver. *J Clin Invest* 85 (2):397–407.

Trichopoulou, A., T. Costacou, C. Bamia, and D. Trichopoulos. 2003. Adherence to a Mediterranean diet and survival in a Greek population. *N Engl J Med* 348 (26):2599–2608.

Tucker, J. M., G. J. Welk, and N. K. Beyler. 2011. Physical activity in U.S.: Adults compliance with the physical activity guidelines for Americans. *Am J Prev Med* 40 (4):454–461.

U.S. Congress, Senate, Select Committee on Nutrition and Human Needs. 1977. *Dietary Goals for the United States*. Washington, DC: U.S. Government Printing Office.

U.S. Department of Health and Human Services and U.S. Department of Agriculture. 2015. *2015–2020 Dietary Guidelines for Americans*. 8th ed. http://health.gov/dietaryguidelines/2015/guidelines.

USDA (U.S. Department of Agriculture), Agricultural Research Service. 2003. USDA National Nutrient Database for Standard Reference Release 28 August 2016. https://www.ars.usda.gov/northeast-area/beltsville-md/beltsville-human-nutrition-research-center/nutrient-data-laboratory/docs/usda-national-nutrient-database-for-standard-reference/. Washington, DC: USDA.

van Ommen, B., and R. Stierum. 2002. Nutrigenomics: Exploiting systems biology in the nutrition and health arena. *Curr Opin Biotechnol* 13 (5):517–521.

Wang, Z., S. Heshka, D. Gallagher, C. N. Boozer, D. P. Kotler, and S. B. Heymsfield. 2000. Resting energy expenditure-fat-free mass relationship: New insights provided by body composition modeling. *Am J Physiol Endocrinol Metab* 279 (3):E539–E545.

Willett, W. 1998. *Nutritional Epidemiology*. 2nd ed. New York: Oxford University Press.

Writing Group for the Activity Counseling Trial Research Group. 2001. Effects of physical activity counseling in primary care: The Activity Counseling Trial: A randomized controlled trial. *JAMA* 286 (6):677–687.

Young, V. R., Y. S. Taylor, W. M. Rand, and N. S. Scrimshaw. 1973. Protein requirements of man: Efficiency of egg protein utilization at maintenance and submaintenance levels in young men. *J Nutr* 103 (8):1164–1174.

Zeisel, S. H. 2011. Nutritional genomics: Defining the dietary requirement and effects of choline. *J Nutr* 141 (3):531–534.

Zello, G. A. 2006. Dietary Reference Intakes for the macronutrients and energy: Considerations for physical activity. *Appl Physiol Nutr Metab* 31 (1):74–79.

3 Nutrition and the Immune System

3.1 INTRODUCTION

Unbalanced nutrition with too much sugar, salt, and fat; a sedentary lifestyle; and the effects of a stressful obesogenic environment can compromise the host immune responses, increasing susceptibility to a wide range of age-related chronic diseases. The new field of nutritional immunology or immunonutrition primarily focuses on the role of diet and its nutritional contents in disease prevention, while there is extensive scientific evidence for the effects of malnutrition on immune function, going back more than 60 years. In fact, the system that classically fails in advanced protein–energy malnutrition (PEM) is the immune system. Deficiencies of vitamins and minerals can also lead to immune compromise, and some effects of classic vitamins, such as vitamin D, impact the immune system, as well as bone mineral metabolism. One of the assessments used since the early 1970s in clinical research on enteral and parenteral nutrition was delayed hypersensitivity to tuberculin, mumps, and streptokinase and streptodornase (SKSD) antigens. More recently, the interactions of obesity and immune function have been recognized.

3.2 THE FAT CELL AS AN ENDOCRINE AND IMMUNE CELL

The intricate interaction between immunity and fat metabolism has been recognized and investigated extensively (Scrimshaw et al. 1968). Indeed, it has been demonstrated that adipose tissue is not merely the site of energy storage, but can be considered an "immune-related" organ producing a series of molecules named "adipocytokines." Nutritional depletion, specific deficiencies, and kwashiorkor-like malnutrition suppress immune function, while accumulation of excess body fat as a result of energy imbalance results in chronic low-grade inflammation.

The cloning of the obese gene (*ob*) and identification of its protein product, leptin, have provided fundamental insight into the hypothalamic regulation of body weight. Circulating levels of this adipocyte-derived hormone are proportional to fat mass but may be lowered rapidly by fasting or increased by inflammatory mediators. The impaired T-cell immunity of mice, now known to be defective in leptin (*ob/ob*) or its receptor (*db/db*), is related to the absence of functional leptin signaling due to the absence of a functional leptin protein (*ob/ob*) or the leptin receptor protein (*db/db*) (Faggioni et al. 2001). Impaired cell-mediated immunity and reduced levels of leptin are both features of low body weight in humans. Indeed, malnutrition predisposes to death from infectious diseases, and the impaired immune function resulting from PEM and HIV infection is well documented (Thea et al. 1996). On an evolutionary basis, the ability to fight off infection and the ability to store fat in cells were both critical to survival. While the adaptation to starvation and associated gradual weight loss do not impair immune function, rapid weight loss does (Scrimshaw et al. 1959). Moreover, the close interrelationship of immune function and nutrition has been confirmed with modern molecular nutrition tools.

The immune system during adapted starvation is a fail-safe system until it decompensates. On the other hand, staying with the theme that humans are well adapted to starvation but poorly adapted to overnutrition, there is chronic low-grade inflammation associated with overweight and obesity, mediated by intra-abdominal fat-resident immune cells that cause a systemic inflammation. In order to understand these two poles of the interaction of nutrition and immune function, it is necessary to understand the difference between innate and adaptive immune mechanisms.

3.3 MALNUTRITION AND IMMUNE FUNCTION

Nutrient deficiencies can impair immune function, and nutrient supplementation can restore normal immune capacity (Bhaskaram 2002). The association of malnutrition and infection has been recorded in ancient historical accounts. For example, an examination of church records in England in the twelfth century shows an interesting association between consecutive years of famine and epidemics of pestilence or communicable diseases. Recent epidemiologic studies in the Americas and Asia have confirmed that infection, often added on malnutrition, is a major cause of morbidity and is responsible for about two-thirds of all deaths among children under 5 years of age. In 1968, Scrimshaw summarized the human and animal data on interactions, often synergistic but occasionally antagonistic, between nutritional deficiencies and infectious illness (Scrimshaw et al. 1968).

Careful observations showed a correlation between nutritional status and morbidity and mortality largely due to infections (O'Neill et al. 2012). It was shown that the risk of death increased from ~0.1% in the well-nourished to as much as 18% in severely malnourished infants. The effect of malnutrition on different infections is variable. For some organisms, for example, measles, tuberculosis, and *Pneumocystis carinii*, there is little doubt that nutritional deficiencies enhance susceptibility and worsen prognosis. For others, such as yellow fever and poliomyelitis, nutrition does not appear to have a major influence on natural history and outcome.

PEM causes widespread atrophy of lymphoid tissues, especially in children. The thymus, spleen, tonsils, and lymph nodes are all affected, with histological evidence of atrophy being greatest in the T-lymphocyte areas of these tissues. Lymphocytes and eosinophils show lowered blood counts, natural killer cells show reduced activity (Salimonu 1992), and cultured blood lymphocytes react poorly to mitogens. Production of thymic hormones is reduced, as is a patient's ability to fend off and recover from infectious illnesses. These closely linked events can initiate a "downhill spiral" or a "vicious cycle" that leads inexorably to death. PEM causes a marked repression of cell-mediated immunity and the function of T-lymphocytes. Malnourished children show dermal anergy, with loss of delayed dermal hypersensitivity (DDH) reactions, a decrease or reversal of the T-helper/suppressor cell ratio, and loss of the ability of killer lymphocytes to recognize and destroy foreign tissues. In contrast, B-lymphocyte numbers and functions generally appear to be maintained. While existing antibody production is conserved or even increased during generalized malnutrition, new primary antibody responses to T-cell-dependent antigens and antibody affinity are impaired.

Research conducted in military personnel has shown immune dysregulation caused by stress that is similar to the immune dysregulation noted in the elderly (e.g., anergy and decreased proliferative response) (Castell et al. 2010).

3.4 IMMUNE FUNCTION IN OBESITY

As abdominal fat expands in response to positive energy balance, there is a need for new blood vessel formation. However, these new vessels can often not keep up with the metabolic needs of expanding abdominal fat, leading to the death of adipocytes. As these adipocytes die, they release cellular debris, which results in the activation of macrophages, which release cytokines resulting in insulin resistance in fat cells, as well as a systemic inflammation. The macrophages gather in circular collections and engulf the fat released from dead adipose cells in both abdominal fat and subcutaneous fat tissue (Le et al. 2011).

This systemic inflammation leads to an increase in innate immune function and defects in adaptive immunity. These defects have been identified in mice fed high-fat diets to induce obesity. Mice fed a 70% fat diet develop obesity and specific defects in the ability of dendritic cells to present antigens to the immune system, leading to defects in adaptive immunity (Smith et al. 2007).

There are a number of chronic diseases that are impacted by the enhanced innate immune function and inflammation. Since inflammation is a common mechanism across many different chronic diseases of aging, obesity-associated changes in immune function are critical in mediating the obesity-associated increased risks of heart disease, diabetes, common forms of cancer, asthma, and connective tissue diseases.

3.5 IMMUNE FUNCTION AND VITAMIN AND MINERAL BALANCE

Vitamin A deficiency has long been known to be associated with increased susceptibility to viral infections, such as mumps. While it has long been recognized that vitamin A and its metabolites have immune regulatory roles, the mechanisms of action have not been known. Recently, there has been significant progress in elucidating the functions of retinoic acid in the regulation of immune cell development (Kim 2008). Retinoic acid (all-*trans*- and 9-*cis*-retinoic acid) is produced from the cells of the intestine, such as dendritic cells, and provides an intestine-specific environmental cue to differentiating immune cells. When T-cells and B-cells are activated in the intestine and associated-lymphoid tissues, gut-homing receptors are induced on the cells in a retinoic acid and antigen-dependent manner. Retinoic acid, produced by gut dendritic cells, is also an important signal that induces immunoglobulin A (IgA)-producing B-cells. The gut-homing T-cells and B-cells play essential roles in protecting the digestive tract from pathogens. Retinoic acid is also required for the production of mature phagocytes in bone marrow. On the other hand, retinoic acid induces a subset of FoxP3+ regulatory T-cells, which is important for maintaining immune tolerance in the gut. Therefore, retinoids provide both positive and negative regulatory signals to fine-control the mucosal immune system.

Although the best-known actions of vitamin D involve its regulation of bone mineral homeostasis, vitamin D exerts its influence on many physiologic processes. One of these is the immune system. Both the adaptive and innate immune systems are impacted by the active metabolite of vitamin D, 1,25(OH)(2)D. These observations have been proposed as potential mechanisms mediating the predisposition of individuals with vitamin D deficiency to infectious diseases, such as tuberculosis, as well as to autoimmune diseases, such as type 1 diabetes mellitus and multiple sclerosis (Bikle 2011).

Selenium (Se) is an essential trace element needed for the biosynthesis of a small number of mammalian selenoproteins. Selenium intake and personal selenium status are implicated in widespread human pathologies, including cancer, cardiovascular disease, and neurodegeneration (Papp et al. 2007). Positive effects of selenium supplementation have been observed in a number of clinical trials with patients suffering from sepsis, HIV infection, or autoimmune thyroid disease (Broome et al. 2004). Most importantly, the lower the selenium status during critical illness, the more likely that the patients will not survive (Manzanares et al. 2009). Supplementation with trace elements in some individuals with nutritional deficiency to correct a selenium deficiency has been shown to enhance antibody titers to influenza vaccination, and shows a trend toward fewer subjects with respiratory tract infections. Another study reported better immune responsiveness and "fewer infection-related illnesses" with a multivitamin supplement than with a placebo in apparently healthy, independent living elderly (Chandra and Chandra 1986). Other researchers have supplemented the diets of seniors with poor eating habits and found no immunological benefit or reduction in acute respiratory tract infections. The reason for the variability of results is likely related to the adaptation to starvation, which can maintain immune function until late in the process as long as multivitamin and mineral intake is normal. Some, but not all, clinical trials have proven effective in improving the outcome of critically ill patients by selenium supplementation, but the best application regimen, the most suitable selenium compound, and the mechanisms of action have not yet been established.

A randomized, double-blind, placebo-controlled trial was carried out to investigate the effects of micronutrient supplementation on immunity and the incidence of common infections in type 2 diabetic outpatients (Liu et al. 2011). A total of 196 type 2 diabetic outpatients were randomized to receive tablets of micronutrients ($n = 97$) or placebo ($n = 99$) for 6 months. Individualized dietary energy intake and daily physical activity were recommended. Anthropometric measurements, blood biochemical variables, and the incidence of common infections were measured at baseline and at 6 months. Data on diet, exercise, and infection (upper respiratory tract infection, skin infection, urinary and genital tract infections, etc.) were recorded 1 month before the study and every month during the study. Blood concentrations of total protein, iron (Fe), folic acid, and hemoglobin increased, and unsaturated iron-binding capacity (UIBC) levels were decreased in the micronutrient supplementation group compared with the placebo group at 6 months. Moreover, at 6 months, compared with the placebo group, the blood concentrations of IgE, CD4+, CD4+/CD8+, white blood cells, lymphocyte counts, and basophilic leukocytes increased and the CD8+ count decreased in the supplementation group, and the levels of IgA, IgM, IgG, and complements C3 and C4 did not differ. The incidence of upper respiratory infection, vaginitis, urinary tract infection, gingivitis, and dental ulcer were lower, and body temperature and duration of fever greatly improved in the supplementation group compared with the placebo group. These data suggest that supplementation of micronutrients might increase immune function and reduce the incidence of common infections in type 2 diabetic outpatients.

In addition, deficiencies of vitamins B6 and folate are associated with reduced immunocompetence (Chandra and Chandra 1986). Trace elements modulate immune responses through their critical role in enzyme activity. Although dietary requirements of most of these elements are met by a balanced diet, there are certain population groups and specific disease states that are likely to be associated with deficiency of one or more of these essential elements. The role of trace elements in the maintenance of immune function and their causal role in secondary immunodeficiency is increasingly being recognized. There is growing research concerning the role of zinc, copper, selenium, and other elements in immunity, and the mechanisms that underlie such roles. The problem of interaction of trace elements and immunity is complex because of the frequently associated other nutritional deficiencies, the presence of clinical or subclinical infections, which in themselves have a significant effect on immunity, and finally, the altered metabolism due to the underlying disease (Kim 2008).

3.6 INTERACTION OF OMEGA-3 FATTY ACIDS AND MACROPHAGE

As noted above, chronic activation of inflammatory pathways plays an important role in the pathogenesis of insulin resistance, and the macrophage–adipocyte nexus provides a key mechanism underlying many common chronic diseases associated with excess body fat (Schenk et al. 2008). Migration of macrophages to adipose tissue (including intramuscular fat depots) and liver, with subsequent activation of macrophage pro-inflammatory pathways and cytokine secretion, is the critical link between overnutrition and inflammation.

Omega-3 fatty acids (n-3 FAs), docosahexaenoic acid (DHA) and eicosapentaenoic acid (EPA), exert anti-inflammatory effects, but the mechanisms are poorly understood. Recently, it was discovered that the G protein-coupled receptor 120 (GPR120) functions as an n-3 FA receptor or sensor (Oh et al. 2010). Stimulation of GPR120 with n-3 FAs or a chemical agonist caused broad anti-inflammatory effects in monocytes (RAW 264.7 cells) and in macrophages obtained from the intraperitoneal fluid. All these effects were abrogated by GPR120 knockdown, demonstrating that the GPR120 membrane protein functions as an n-3 FA receptor or sensor in pro-inflammatory macrophages and mature adipocytes. Moreover, GPR120 is highly expressed in pro-inflammatory macrophages and functions as an n-3 FA receptor, mediating the anti-inflammatory effects of this class of FAs to inhibit both the TLR2/3/4 and the tumor necrosis factor α (TNF-α) response pathways and cause systemic insulin sensitization. Therefore, the *in vivo* anti-inflammatory and insulin-sensitizing effects of n-3 FAs are dependent on the expression of GPR120, as demonstrated in studies of obese GPR120 knockout (KO) animals and wild-type (WT) littermates.

The worldwide diversity of dietary intakes of n-6 and n-3 FAs influences tissue compositions of n-3 long-chain fatty acids (LCFAs) (EPA, docosapentaenoic acid, and DHA) and risks of cardiovascular and mental illnesses (Hibbeln et al. 2006) via inflammatory mechanisms mediated by eicosanoids synthesized from arachidonic acid and other n-6 LCFAs. By increasing n-3 FA intake from fish and fish oil or algae oil supplements and decreasing n-6 FA consumption from vegetable oils and processed foods, it is possible to change tissue and plasma FA balance. More research is needed to connect changes in the ratio of n-6 to n-3 fatty acids to changes in immune function despite some supportive evidence on this relationship (Patterson et al. 2012). Polyunsaturated fatty acids (PUFAs) are associated with increases in chronic inflammatory diseases such as nonalcoholic fatty liver disease (NAFLD), cardiovascular disease, obesity, inflammatory bowel disease (IBD), rheumatoid arthritis, and Alzheimer's disease (AD). By increasing the ratio of n-6:n-3 PUFA in the Western diet, reductions may be achieved in the incidence of these chronic inflammatory diseases.

3.7 CALORIC RESTRICTION WITHOUT MALNUTRITION AND IMMUNE FUNCTION

It is well known and widely taught that marasmus, the condition of adapted starvation with significant weight loss, occurs without compromising immune function. Calorie restriction (CR) without malnutrition increases life span in simple model organisms and rodents (Fontana et al. 2010). CR decreases inflammation, which is believed to protect against age-associated diseases (Meyer et al. 2006; Franceschi and Campisi 2014). Low-grade chronic inflammation has been identified as a unifying mechanism in the pathogenesis of multiple age-associated chronic diseases and in aging itself (Howcroft et al. 2013). Serum C-reactive protein (CRP) is formed in response to phospholipid oxidation and is a systemic marker of inflammation. TNF-α is a pro-inflammatory cytokine. These cytokines and others are associated with an increased risk of developing type 2 diabetes mellitus, heart disease, and common forms of cancer (Hotamisligil et al. 1993; Matzinger 2002a,b; Serhan 2007; Lavie et al. 2009; Ingersoll et al. 2011; Taube et al. 2012; Koenig 2013). Increased adipose tissue TNF-α expression (Kern et al. 1995) and serum TNF-α levels (Zahorska-Markiewicz et al. 2000; Bhaskaram 2002) are reduced by weight loss (Kern et al. 1995; Formoso et al. 2012). Some studies in monkeys (Roecker et al. 1996) have shown suppression of immune responses with CR, and studies in mice have shown increased susceptibility to infection in mice (Gardner 2005; Ritz et al. 2008), while other studies in aging mice and monkeys show that CR can enhance immune surveillance by T-cells (Messaoudi et al. 2006; Yang et al. 2009). CR in humans, when it includes a restriction of protein and essential nutrients, impairs cell-mediated immune responses (Schaible and Kaufmann 2007) and increases susceptibility to morbidity and mortality from infectious diseases.

A form of chronic CR in which protein and micronutrients are maintained has been studied extensively in a multicenter, randomized clinical trial supported by the National Institute of Aging of the National Institutes of Health (Ravussin et al. 2015). The effects of CR on inflammation and cell-mediated immunity were determined in 218 healthy nonobese adults (20–50 years) who were assigned 25% CR (n = 143) or an *ad libitum* (AL) diet (n = 75), and outcomes tested at baseline and 12 and 24 months of CR. CR induced a 10.4% weight loss over the 2-year period. Relative to AL group, CR reduced circulating inflammatory markers, including total WBC and lymphocyte counts, intercellular adhesion molecule 1 (ICAM-1), and leptin. Serum CRP and TNF-α concentrations were about 40% and 50% lower in the CR group, respectively. CR had no effect on the delayed-type hypersensitivity skin response or antibody response to vaccines, nor did it cause a difference in clinically significant infections. In conclusion, long-term moderate CR without malnutrition induces a significant and persistent inhibition of inflammation without impairing key *in vivo* indicators of cell-mediated immunity. Given the established role of these pro-inflammatory molecules in the pathogenesis of multiple chronic diseases, these CR-induced adaptations suggest a shift toward a healthy phenotype. Clearly reducing body fat without malnutrition demonstrated beneficial effects on immune function, and the observations apply to tackling both overweight and obesity in the primary care setting.

3.8 GUT MICROBIOTA AND IMMUNE FUNCTION

While some 40–50 years ago there was interest in colonic bacteria that could produce compounds from indigestible substances that could promote colon cancer, in the last decade, there has been an explosion of interest in the metabolic and immune functions of the gut microbiota and their influence on metabolism and immune function. Anaerobic culture methods for gut bacteria have been available in specialized labs for more than 40 years, but remain challenging for some bacterial strains. The very recent introduction of technologies that can identify bacterial species based on conserved sequences of 16s rRNA has enabled large-scale analysis of the genetic and metabolic profile of gut microbiota. Some have suggested that the gut microbiota represents a forgotten organ reflecting dietary intake, metabolizing indigestible substances into absorbed phytonutrients and even providing new therapeutic interventions for challenging bacterial infections of the gut and other organs. The gut microbiota is so complex in its interactions and constituents that it may be helpful to make an analogy to the immune system, which is a collection of cells that work in unison with the host that can promote health or initiate disease, depending on nutritional inputs. Moreover, the gut-associated lymphoid tissue represents 70% of the immune system and plays a critical role through interactions of dendritic cells with foreign bacterial antigens in alerting the immune system to potential pathogens, while at the same time protecting those beneficial bacteria critical to an effective barrier, protecting the single layer of epithelial cells lining the villi of the small intestine and the colonic epithelium.

The National Institutes of Health-funded Human Microbiome Project investigated the microbiota of a variety of bodily niches, including the skin, as well as the oral, vaginal, and nasal cavities (Segata et al. 2012). Currently, the majority of research is focused on the gut microbiota, since this is where the greatest density and numbers of bacteria are found. In addition, most data have been derived from fecal samples and, to a lesser extent, mucosal biopsies. While it is relatively easy to obtain fresh fecal samples, the information obtained from them does not represent the complete picture within the gut.

From a number of studies, we know that the small intestine, where most of the immune system influences occur, contains a very different abundance and composition of bacteria, with greater variation than the colon (Zoetendal et al. 2012). The colonic microbiota populations are largely driven by the efficient degradation of complex indigestible carbohydrates and polyphenol phytonutrients. The bacterial populations of the small intestine are shaped by the intestinal microbiota capacity for the fast import and conversion of relatively small carbohydrates, and rapid adaptation to overall nutrient availability. Therefore, fecal samples, while not an ideal proxy for the gastrointestinal (GI) tract, are more practical for research and provide a glimpse into the diversity of colonic microbiota populations as they are influenced by nutrition.

Five phyla represent the majority of bacteria that comprise the gut microbiota. There are approximately 160 species in the large intestine of any individual (Rajilic-Stojanovic and de Vos 2014). The ability to synthesize short-chain fatty acids (SCFAs) is found in all humans (Louis et al. 2010), but the amounts vary due to changes in microbiota populations over time in the same individual and the nutrient bacteria metabolizing.

Fermentation of indigestible carbohydrates is one of the central functions of the human gut microbiota, driving the energy and carbon economy of the colon. Dominant and prevalent species of gut bacteria, including SCFA producers, appear to play a critical role in initial degradation of complex plant-derived polysaccharides (Flint et al. 2012), in conjunction with species that ferment oligosaccharides (e.g., *Bifidobacterium*), to liberate SCFAs and gases, which are also used as carbon and energy sources by other more specialized bacteria, including reductive acetogens, sulfate-reducing bacteria, and methanogens (which cause the blue flames when some foolish individuals light a match as they produce gas from their anus) (Ze et al. 2013). Efficient conversion of complex indigestible dietary carbohydrates into SCFAs serves microbial cross-feeding communities and the host, with 10% of our daily energy requirements coming from colonic fermentation. Butyrate and propionate can regulate intestinal physiology and immune function, while acetate acts as a substrate for lipogenesis and gluconeogenesis (Macfarlane and Macfarlane 2011). Recently, key roles for these metabolites have been identified in regulating immune function in the periphery; directing appropriate immune response, oral tolerance, and resolution of inflammation; and regulating the inflammatory output of adipose tissue (Arpaia et al. 2013). In the colon, the majority of this carbohydrate fermentation occurs in the proximal colon, at least for people following a Western-style diet. As carbohydrates are broken down and the bolus of undigested material moves distally to the transverse and descending colon, the gut microbiota switches to metabolism of proteins or amino acids. Fermentation of amino acids, besides liberating beneficial SCFAs, produces a range of potentially harmful compounds. Some of these may play a role in gut diseases, such as colon cancer or IBD. Studies in animal models and *in vitro* show that compounds like ammonia, phenols, p-cresol, certain amines, and hydrogen sulfide play important roles in the initiation or progression of a leaky gut, inflammation, DNA damage, and cancer progression (Windey et al. 2012).

Dietary fiber and the intake of a plant-based diet appear to reduce these metabolites or absorb them for excretion, supporting the importance of overall dietary balance when examining the function of the microbiota (Tang et al. 2013). Carbohydrate fermentation variation by gut microbiota also provides a scientific basis for rational design of functional foods aimed at improving gut health and for impacting microbiota activities linked to systemic host physiology through the gut–liver axis, the gut–brain axis, and the gut–skin axis (Clarke et al. 2014).

Probiotics, prebiotics, and polyphenols have been shown to affect the gut microbiota and have led to the development of supplements and functional foods intended to improve gut health or modulate immune function (Tuohy and Del Rio 2014).

Probiotics are live microorganisms that when administered in sufficient amounts can confer health benefit to their host (Khani et al. 2012). Lactobacilli and bifidobacteria are the two most common types of probiotics. The global probiotic market is in the billions of U.S. dollars despite few randomized clinical trials proving efficacy (Markets and Markets 2015). Probiotics have been studied as alternative biotherapies for respiratory infection (Shida et al. 2017), IBD (Hahm et al. 2012), antibiotic-associated diarrhea (Wong et al. 2014), and ulcerative colitis (Goldin and Gorbach 2008). In spite of the booming *in vitro* and *in vivo* probiotic studies against metabolic diseases such as diabetes mellitus and obesity, their application in primary care is not common (Carvalho and Saad 2013; Gomes et al. 2014).

The dominant phyla in healthy adults ages 18–50 are Firmicutes, Bacteroidetes, Actinobacteria, and Proteobacteria. As aging begins after about 65 years, there is a reduction in Firmicutes, especially the *Bifidobacterium* genus, and an increase in Proteobacteria, which contains several opportunistic pathogens (Duncan and Flint 2013). A cross-sectional study of the fecal microbiota of different European populations showed that higher levels of bifidobacteria were seen in the 20- to 50-year-olds in Italy and Sweden in comparison with their over-60 counterparts. However, this was comparable between age groups in France and Germany, but with those in Italy possessing an average of 10- to 100-fold greater populations than other countries. *Bacteroides* species were higher in the under-50s in Italy and the over-60s in Germany. This study demonstrated variations in the age-related changes in the microbiota that probably relate to both location and dietary habits (Mueller et al. 2006).

There are several methods of changing the human gut microbiota in order to counter digestive diseases and other conditions. One is direct transplantation of healthy microbiota into a host who suffers from a gut-related disorder, such as IBD (Eiseman et al. 1958), or *Clostridium difficile*-associated diseases (Guo et al. 2012; Kelly et al. 2012). Fecal transplant is the method of using a liquid suspension of a fecal sample from a healthy (disease-free) donor and transplanting it into an individual through a nasogastric, nasoduodenal, or rectal catheter.

The consumption of probiotics and prebiotics is a more frequently used way of modulating the gut microbiota. Prebiotics, discussed further below, are essentially substrates for the beneficial commensal bacteria that already exist within the gut microbiota. They survive stomach acid and the upper GI tract in order to be fermented by specific bacteria in the large gut (Gibson and Roberfroid 1995). Probiotics are live microbial cultures of species known to elicit beneficial effects, such as the effect on intestinal cell proliferation (Blottiere et al. 2003), production of vitamins and minerals (Hooper et al. 2002), and modulation of immune function by production of anti-inflammatory cytokines (Dong et al. 2012). As mentioned, recent studies on changes in the gut microbiota with age can vary by nationality (Mueller et al. 2006). Those that are more detrimental to gut health are the reduction of bifidobacteria and the increase in pathogenic species. Probiotic use is often limited to *Lactobacillus* and *Bifidobacterium* species, which have shown positive effects when orally administered in studies with older volunteers (Ahmed et al. 2007; Lahtinen et al. 2009; Moro-Garcia et al. 2013).

Since the vast majority of live bacteria entering the stomach from most probiotic supplements and yogurts are destroyed or inactivated by stomach acid, spore-forming bacteria that can survive stomach acid to enter the intestine have been developed. *Bacillus coagulans* GBI-30, 6086 (GanedenBC30 [BC30]) is a spore-forming lactic acid-producing bacterium. Being spore formers, they have the capacity to resist adverse conditions of stomach acid and bile in the GI tract (Hyronimus et al. 2000; Maathuis et al. 2010). *In vitro* studies using continuous culture have investigated the ability of *B. coagulans* to affect pathogen survival in the human gut microbiota. This strain could competitively exclude transient pathogens *in vitro* (Honda et al. 2011). Such bacteria are also known to excrete antimicrobial peptides (Le Marrec et al. 2000; Bizani and Brandelli 2002). Moreover, use of *B. coagulans* both *in vitro* and *in vivo* demonstrated an ability to reduce distension in adults with postprandial intestinal gas-related symptoms (Kalman et al. 2009), and the probiotic has also shown immunomodulatory effects (Jensen et al. 2010).

A prebiotic is defined as a "nondigestible food ingredient that beneficially affects the host by selectively stimulating the growth and/or activity of one or a limited number of bacteria in the colon and thus improves the host's health." A more refined definition for prebiotic is a selectively fermented ingredient that allows specific changes, in both the composition and activity in the GI microflora, that confer benefits. These definitions are attracting a great deal of interest in the field of nutrition, both in scientific research and in food applications. It is necessary to establish clear criteria for classifying a food ingredient as a prebiotic. Prebiotics require a science-based demonstration that the ingredient (1) resists gastric acidity, (2) is not hydrolyzed by GI tract enzymes, (3) is not absorbed in the upper GI tract, (4) is fermented by intestinal microorganisms, and (5) induces selective stimulation of growth and/or activity of intestinal bacteria, potentially associated with health and well-being.

The daily dose of the prebiotic is not a determinant of the prebiotic effect, which is mainly influenced by the number of bifidobacteria per gram in feces before supplementation of the diet with the prebiotic begins. The ingested prebiotic stimulates the whole indigenous population of bifidobacteria to growth, and the larger that population, the larger is the number of new bacterial cells appearing in feces. In connection with this, a new concept of "prebiotic index" is proposed and is defined as the increase in the absolute number of bifidobacteria expressed divided by the daily dose of prebiotic ingested.

Prebiotics of various types are found as natural components in milk; honey; fruits, such as banana; vegetables, such as onion, Jerusalem artichoke, chicory, leek, garlic, and artichoke; and rye and barley. In most of these sources, concentrations of prebiotics range from 0.3% to 6% of fresh weight. Asparagus, sugar beet, garlic, chicory, onion, Jerusalem artichoke, wheat, honey, banana, barley, tomato, and rye are special sources of fructooligosaccharides (FOSs). Galactooligosaccharides (GOSs) are found naturally in human and bovine milk. Seeds of legumes, lentils, peas, beans, chickpeas, and mustard are rich in raffinose oligosaccharides. Xylooligosaccharide (XOS) is also an emerging prebiotic that is found in bamboo shoots, fruits, vegetables, milk, and honey.

Prebiotics include oligosaccharides that, when fermented, mediate measurable changes within the gut microbiota composition, usually an increase in the relative abundance of bacteria thought of as beneficial, such as bifidobacteria or other SCFA producers. Prebiotic FOSs consist of fructose units linked with glycosidic bonds with a terminal D-glucose unit, and GOSs are composed of galactose units with a terminal D-glucose unit. Several studies have shown beneficial effects from prebiotic supplementation in both *in vitro* and *in vivo* situations using samples from a younger (18–50 years) cohort (Tuohy et al. 2001; Meyer et al. 2006; De Preter et al. 2010; Franceschi and Campisi 2014).

Our group at University of California, Los Angeles (UCLA) conducted the first clinical study evaluating the effects of daily treatment with 2 g of XOS derived enzymatically from corn cobs on glucose tolerance and insulin resistance in prediabetic adults (Yang et al. 2015). Eight weeks of XOS supplementation tended to increase insulin sensitivity by lowering the oral glucose tolerance test (OGTT) 2-hour insulin response ($p = 0.11$), while no significant improvement of pre-diabetes mellitus subjects' metabolic situation was observed, using the parameters of body composition, serum glucose, triglyceride, satiety hormones, and inflammation marker TNF-α. In a prior study in healthy adults, we found that a dose of 2 g/day increased bifidobacteria with no effect on lactobacilli, and it did not cause any GI side effects (Finegold et al. 2014). XOS significantly modified gut microbiota in both healthy and prediabetic subjects, and resulted in dramatic shifts of four bacterial taxa associated with prediabetes. Future studies with a larger sample size are needed to study the metabolic impact of XOS and understand the connection between XOS-mediated gut microbiota changes and the pathogenesis of type 2 diabetes mellitus.

Polyphenols are a diverse class of plant secondary metabolites, often associated with the color, taste, and defense mechanisms of fruit and vegetables. They have long been studied as the most likely class of compounds present in whole plant foods capable of affecting physiological processes that protect against chronic diet-associated diseases (Clifford 2004). The gut microbiota plays a critical role in transforming dietary polyphenols into absorbable biologically active species, acting on the estimated 95% of dietary polyphenols that reach the colon. Our group at UCLA investigated the effect of pomegranate extract containing ellagitannins on the growth of major groups of intestinal bacteria and on the formation of urolithins (Li et al. 2015). Urolithins are found in the urine after ingestion of pomegranate and walnuts and are a metabolite of ellagic acid, which recirculates after conjugation in the liver and has metabolic effects on mitochondria, with extension of life span in *Caenorhabditis elegans* and enhanced muscle function in rodents (Ryu et al. 2016).

In our human study (Li et al. 2015), 20 healthy participants consumed 1000 mg of pomegranate extract daily for 4 weeks. Based on urinary and fecal content of the pomegranate metabolite urolithin A (UA), we observed three distinct groups: (1) individuals with no baseline UA presence but induction of UA formation by pomegranate extract consumption ($n = 9$); (2) individuals with baseline UA formation, which was enhanced by pomegranate extract consumption daily for 28 days ($n = 5$); and (3) individuals with no baseline UA production, which was not inducible ($n = 6$). We have demonstrated that pomegranate extract is a prebiotic in the sense that it changed bacterial populations and is known to have beneficial health effects.

A Verrucomicrobia species (*Akkermansia muciniphila*) was 33- and 47-fold higher in stool samples of UA producers than in those of nonproducers at baseline and after 4 weeks, respectively. This bacterium also occurs in the small intestine, where it breaks down mucin and stimulates more mucin production from goblet cells to protect small intestinal epithelia. In UA producers, the genera *Butyrivibrio*, *Enterobacter*, *Escherichia*, *Lactobacillus*, *Prevotella*, *Serratia*, and *Veillonella* were increased and *Collinsella* decreased significantly at week 4 compared with baseline. Pomegranate extract consumption may induce health benefits secondary to changes in the microbiota, which amplify the production of urolithins.

3.9 PRACTICAL CONSIDERATIONS FOR MODULATING IMMUNE FUNCTION

The practical applications of the interaction of immune function and nutrition are fourfold. First, it is important to achieve and maintain optimal intra-abdominal fat depots that do not trigger chronic inflammation. The growing global epidemic of obesity and type 2 diabetes associated with the adoption of Western diets and lifestyles has significant implications for immune function, but in the opposite direction of that associated with malnutrition. Chronic inflammation is associated with numerous age-related chronic diseases. Improved immune function in these individuals is achieved through a balanced diet and a healthy active lifestyle.

It is clear that malnutrition, especially PEM associated with kwashiorkor-like findings in children in the developed world or in hospitalized patients, can impair immune function. Therefore, recognizing and treating malnutrition is a critical component of maintaining normal immune function in hospitalized patients, the elderly, and military personnel working under stressed conditions.

In addition to calorie and protein balance, micronutrients and the lipid balance of n-3 and n-6 are critical. These needs can be met through a balanced diet, but in at-risk groups, including the elderly, individuals consuming unbalanced diets, and military personnel under stress, it may be advisable to include a multivitamin or multimineral dietary supplement to support healthy immune function. For balancing n-3 and n-6 FAs in cells, it is important to both increase the intake of DHA and EPA from fish or supplements and reduce the intake of n-6 FAs from foods containing vegetable oils.

Finally, studies of the microbiome, still in their infancy, are already demonstrating that gut bacteria can play an important role in modulating immune function, as well as in the efficiency of absorption of nutrients, by adapting to key elements in the diet, including fiber and polyphenol phytonutrients. Therefore, maintaining digestive health through treatment of irritable bowel syndrome and encouragement of fiber intake at 25 g/day and a regular schedule of defecation may improve immune function through the homeostatic effects of a healthy and stable microbiome.

REFERENCES

Ahmed, M., J. Prasad, H. Gill, L. Stevenson, and P. Gopal. 2007. Impact of consumption of different levels of *Bifidobacterium lactis* HN019 on the intestinal microflora of elderly human subjects. *J Nutr Health Aging* 11 (1):26–31.

Arpaia, N., C. Campbell, X. Fan, S. Dikiy, J. van der Veeken, P. deRoos, H. Liu, J. R. Cross, K. Pfeffer, P. J. Coffer, and A. Y. Rudensky. 2013. Metabolites produced by commensal bacteria promote peripheral regulatory T-cell generation. *Nature* 504 (7480):451–455.

Bhaskaram, P. 2002. Micronutrient malnutrition, infection, and immunity: An overview. *Nutr Rev* 60 (5 Pt 2):S40–S45.

Bikle, D. D. 2011. Vitamin D regulation of immune function. *Vitam Horm* 86:1–21.

Bizani, D., and A. Brandelli. 2002. Characterization of a bacteriocin produced by a newly isolated *Bacillus* sp. Strain 8 A. *J Appl Microbiol* 93 (3):512–519.

Blottiere, H. M., B. Buecher, J. P. Galmiche, and C. Cherbut. 2003. Molecular analysis of the effect of short-chain fatty acids on intestinal cell proliferation. *Proc Nutr Soc* 62 (1):101–106.

Broome, C. S., F. McArdle, J. A. Kyle, F. Andrews, N. M. Lowe, C. A. Hart, J. R. Arthur, and M. J. Jackson. 2004. An increase in selenium intake improves immune function and poliovirus handling in adults with marginal selenium status. *Am J Clin Nutr* 80 (1):154–162.

Carvalho, B. M., and M. J. Saad. 2013. Influence of gut microbiota on subclinical inflammation and insulin resistance. *Mediators Inflamm* 2013:986734.

Castell, L. M., C. D. Thake, and W. Ensign. 2010. Biochemical markers of possible immunodepression in military training in harsh environments. *Mil Med* 175 (3):158–165.

Chandra, S., and R. K. Chandra. 1986. Nutrition, immune response, and outcome. *Prog Food Nutr Sci* 10 (1–2):1–65.

Clarke, G., R. M. Stilling, P. J. Kennedy, C. Stanton, J. F. Cryan, and T. G. Dinan. 2014. Minireview: Gut microbiota: The neglected endocrine organ. *Mol Endocrinol* 28 (8):1221–1238.

Clifford, M. N. 2004. Diet-derived phenols in plasma and tissues and their implications for health. *Planta Med* 70 (12):1103–1114.

De Preter, V., G. Falony, K. Windey, H. M. Hamer, L. De Vuyst, and K. Verbeke. 2010. The prebiotic, oligofructose-enriched inulin modulates the faecal metabolite profile: An in vitro analysis. *Mol Nutr Food Res* 54 (12):1791–1801.

Dong, H., I. Rowland, and P. Yaqoob. 2012. Comparative effects of six probiotic strains on immune function in vitro. *Br J Nutr* 108 (3):459–470.

Duncan, S. H., and H. J. Flint. 2013. Probiotics and prebiotics and health in ageing populations. *Maturitas* 75 (1):44–50.

Eiseman, B., W. Silen, G. S. Bascom, and A. J. Kauvar. 1958. Fecal enema as an adjunct in the treatment of pseudomembranous enterocolitis. *Surgery* 44 (5):854–859.

Faggioni, R., K. R. Feingold, and C. Grunfeld. 2001. Leptin regulation of the immune response and the immunodeficiency of malnutrition. *FASEB J* 15 (14):2565–2571.

Finegold, S. M., Z. Li, P. H. Summanen, J. Downes, G. Thames, K. Corbett, S. Dowd, M. Krak, and D. Heber. 2014. Xylooligosaccharide increases bifidobacteria but not lactobacilli in human gut microbiota. *Food Funct* 5 (3):436–445.

Flint, H. J., K. P. Scott, P. Louis, and S. H. Duncan. 2012. The role of the gut microbiota in nutrition and health. *Nat Rev Gastroenterol Hepatol* 9 (10):577–589.

Fontana, L., L. Partridge, and V. D. Longo. 2010. Extending healthy life span—From yeast to humans. *Science* 328 (5976):321–326.

Formoso, G., M. Taraborrelli, M. T. Guagnano, M. D'Adamo, N. Di Pietro, A. Tartaro, and A. Consoli. 2012. Magnetic resonance imaging determined visceral fat reduction associates with enhanced IL-10 plasma levels in calorie restricted obese subjects. *PLoS One* 7 (12):e52774.

Franceschi, C., and J. Campisi. 2014. Chronic inflammation (inflammaging) and its potential contribution to age-associated diseases. *J Gerontol A Biol Sci Med Sci* 69 (Suppl 1):S4–S9.

Gardner, E. M. 2005. Caloric restriction decreases survival of aged mice in response to primary influenza infection. *J Gerontol A Biol Sci Med Sci* 60 (6):688–694.

Gibson, G. R., and M. B. Roberfroid. 1995. Dietary modulation of the human colonic microbiota: Introducing the concept of prebiotics. *J Nutr* 125 (6):1401–1412.

Goldin, B. R., and S. L. Gorbach. 2008. Clinical indications for probiotics: An overview. *Clin Infect Dis* 46 (Suppl 2):S96–S100; discussion S144–S151.

Gomes, A. C., A. A. Bueno, R. G. de Souza, and J. F. Mota. 2014. Gut microbiota, probiotics and diabetes. *Nutr J* 13:60.

Guo, B., C. Harstall, T. Louie, S. Veldhuyzen van Zanten, and L. A. Dieleman. 2012. Systematic review: Faecal transplantation for the treatment of *Clostridium difficile*-associated disease. *Aliment Pharmacol Ther* 35 (8):865–875.

Hahm, E.-H. K., H. Hong, K.-S. Hong, and K. Baik. 2012. High concentrated probiotics improve inflammatory bowel diseases better than commercial concentration of probiotics. *J Food Drug Anal* 20:4.

Hibbeln, J. R., L. R. Nieminen, T. L. Blasbalg, J. A. Riggs, and W. E. Lands. 2006. Healthy intakes of n-3 and n-6 fatty acids: Estimations considering worldwide diversity. *Am J Clin Nutr* 83 (6 Suppl):1483S–1493S.

Honda, H., G. R. Gibson, S. Farmer, D. Keller, and A. L. McCartney. 2011. Use of a continuous culture fermentation system to investigate the effect of GanedenBC30 (*Bacillus coagulans* GBI-30, 6086) supplementation on pathogen survival in the human gut microbiota. *Anaerobe* 17 (1):36–42.

Hooper, L. V., T. Midtvedt, and J. I. Gordon. 2002. How host-microbial interactions shape the nutrient environment of the mammalian intestine. *Annu Rev Nutr* 22:283–307.

Hotamisligil, G. S., N. S. Shargill, and B. M. Spiegelman. 1993. Adipose expression of tumor necrosis factor-alpha: Direct role in obesity-linked insulin resistance. *Science* 259 (5091):87–91.

Howcroft, T. K., J. Campisi, G. B. Louis, M. T. Smith, B. Wise, T. Wyss-Coray, A. D. Augustine, J. E. McElhaney, R. Kohanski, and F. Sierra. 2013. The role of inflammation in age-related disease. *Aging (Albany NY)* 5 (1):84–93.

Hyronimus, B., C. Le Marrec, A. H. Sassi, and A. Deschamps. 2000. Acid and bile tolerance of spore-forming lactic acid bacteria. *Int J Food Microbiol* 61 (2–3):193–197.

Ingersoll, M. A., A. M. Platt, S. Potteaux, and G. J. Randolph. 2011. Monocyte trafficking in acute and chronic inflammation. *Trends Immunol* 32 (10):470–477.

Jensen, G. S., K. F. Benson, S. G. Carter, and J. R. Endres. 2010. GanedenBC30 cell wall and metabolites: Anti-inflammatory and immune modulating effects in vitro. *BMC Immunol* 11:15.

Kalman, D. S., H. I. Schwartz, P. Alvarez, S. Feldman, J. C. Pezzullo, and D. R. Krieger. 2009. A prospective, randomized, double-blind, placebo-controlled parallel-group dual site trial to evaluate the effects of a *Bacillus coagulans*-based product on functional intestinal gas symptoms. *BMC Gastroenterol* 9:85.

Kelly, C. R., L. de Leon, and N. Jasutkar. 2012. Fecal microbiota transplantation for relapsing *Clostridium difficile* infection in 26 patients: Methodology and results. *J Clin Gastroenterol* 46 (2):145–149.

Kern, P. A., M. Saghizadeh, J. M. Ong, R. J. Bosch, R. Deem, and R. B. Simsolo. 1995. The expression of tumor necrosis factor in human adipose tissue. Regulation by obesity, weight loss, and relationship to lipoprotein lipase. *J Clin Invest* 95 (5):2111–2119.

Khani, S., H. M. Hosseini, M. Taheri, M. R. Nourani, and A. A. Imani Fooladi. 2012. Probiotics as an alternative strategy for prevention and treatment of human diseases: A review. *Inflamm Allergy Drug Targets* 11 (2):79–89.

Kim, C. H. 2008. Roles of retinoic acid in induction of immunity and immune tolerance. *Endocr Metab Immune Disord Drug Targets* 8 (4):289–294.

Koenig, W. 2013. High-sensitivity C-reactive protein and atherosclerotic disease: From improved risk prediction to risk-guided therapy. *Int J Cardiol* 168 (6):5126–5134.

Lahtinen, S. J., L. Tammela, J. Korpela, R. Parhiala, H. Ahokoski, H. Mykkanen, and S. J. Salminen. 2009. Probiotics modulate the *Bifidobacterium* microbiota of elderly nursing home residents. *Age (Dordr)* 31 (1):59–66.

Lavie, C. J., R. V. Milani, A. Verma, and J. H. O'Keefe. 2009. C-reactive protein and cardiovascular diseases—Is it ready for primetime? *Am J Med Sci* 338 (6):486–492.

Le, K. A., S. Mahurkar, T. L. Alderete, R. E. Hasson, T. C. Adam, J. S. Kim, E. Beale, C. Xie, A. S. Greenberg, H. Allayee, and M. I. Goran. 2011. Subcutaneous adipose tissue macrophage infiltration is associated with hepatic and visceral fat deposition, hyperinsulinemia, and stimulation of NF-kappaB stress pathway. *Diabetes* 60 (11):2802–2809.

Le Marrec, C., B. Hyronimus, P. Bressollier, B. Verneuil, and M. C. Urdaci. 2000. Biochemical and genetic characterization of coagulin, a new antilisterial bacteriocin in the pediocin family of bacteriocins, produced by *Bacillus coagulans* I(4). *Appl Environ Microbiol* 66 (12):5213–5220.

Li, Z., S. M. Henning, R. P. Lee, Q. Y. Lu, P. H. Summanen, G. Thames, K. Corbett, J. Downes, C. H. Tseng, S. M. Finegold, and D. Heber. 2015. Pomegranate extract induces ellagitannin metabolite formation and changes stool microbiota in healthy volunteers. *Food Funct* 6 (8):2487–2495.

Liu, Y., H. Jing, J. Wang, R. Zhang, Y. Zhang, Y. Zhang, Q. Xu, X. Yu, and C. Xue. 2011. Micronutrients decrease incidence of common infections in type 2 diabetic outpatients. *Asia Pac J Clin Nutr* 20 (3):375–382.

Louis, P., P. Young, G. Holtrop, and H. J. Flint. 2010. Diversity of human colonic butyrate-producing bacteria revealed by analysis of the butyryl-CoA:acetate CoA-transferase gene. *Environ Microbiol* 12 (2):304–314.

Maathuis, A. J., D. Keller, and S. Farmer. 2010. Survival and metabolic activity of the GanedenBC30 strain of *Bacillus coagulans* in a dynamic in vitro model of the stomach and small intestine. *Benef Microbes* 1 (1):31–36.

Macfarlane, G. T., and S. Macfarlane. 2011. Fermentation in the human large intestine: Its physiologic consequences and the potential contribution of prebiotics. *J Clin Gastroenterol* 45 (Suppl):S120–S127.

Manzanares, W., A. Biestro, F. Galusso, M. H. Torre, N. Manay, G. Pittini, G. Facchin, and G. Hardy. 2009. Serum selenium and glutathione peroxidase-3 activity: Biomarkers of systemic inflammation in the critically ill? *Intensive Care Med* 35 (5):882–889.

Markets and Markets. 2015. Probiotic ingredients market by function (regular, preventative, therapy), application (food & beverage, dietary supplements, & animal feed), end use (human & animal probiotics), ingredient (bacteria & yeast), and by region—Global trends & forecast to 2020. http://www.marketsandmarkets.com/Market-Reports/probiotic-market-advanced-technologies-and-globalmarket-69.html (retrieved July 16, 2016).

Matzinger, P. 2002a. The danger model: A renewed sense of self. *Science* 296 (5566):301–305.

Matzinger, P. 2002b. An innate sense of danger. *Ann NY Acad Sci* 961:341–342.

Messaoudi, I., J. Warner, M. Fischer, B. Park, B. Hill, J. Mattison, M. A. Lane et al. 2006. Delay of T cell senescence by caloric restriction in aged long-lived nonhuman primates. *Proc Natl Acad Sci USA* 103 (51):19448–19453.

Meyer, T. E., S. J. Kovacs, A. A. Ehsani, S. Klein, J. O. Holloszy, and L. Fontana. 2006. Long-term caloric restriction ameliorates the decline in diastolic function in humans. *J Am Coll Cardiol* 47 (2):398–402.

Moro-Garcia, M. A., R. Alonso-Arias, M. Baltadjieva, C. Fernandez Benitez, M. A. Fernandez Barrial, E. Diaz Ruisanchez, R. Alonso Santos, M. Alvarez Sanchez, J. Saavedra Mijan, and C. Lopez-Larrea. 2013. Oral supplementation with *Lactobacillus delbrueckii* subsp. *bulgaricus* 8481 enhances systemic immunity in elderly subjects. *Age (Dordr)* 35 (4):1311–1326.

Mueller, S., K. Saunier, C. Hanisch, E. Norin, L. Alm, T. Midtvedt, A. Cresci et al. 2006. Differences in fecal microbiota in different European study populations in relation to age, gender, and country: A cross-sectional study. *Appl Environ Microbiol* 72 (2):1027–1033.

Oh, D. Y., S. Talukdar, E. J. Bae, T. Imamura, H. Morinaga, W. Fan, P. Li, W. J. Lu, S. M. Watkins, and J. M. Olefsky. 2010. GPR120 is an omega-3 fatty acid receptor mediating potent anti-inflammatory and insulin-sensitizing effects. *Cell* 142 (5):687–698.

O'Neill, S. M., A. Fitzgerald, A. Briend, and J. Van den Broeck. 2012. Child mortality as predicted by nutritional status and recent weight velocity in children under two in rural Africa. *J Nutr* 142 (3):520–525.

Papp, L. V., J. Lu, A. Holmgren, and K. K. Khanna. 2007. From selenium to selenoproteins: Synthesis, identity, and their role in human health. *Antioxid Redox Signal* 9 (7):775–806.

Patterson, E., R. Wall, G. F. Fitzgerald, R. P. Ross, and C. Stanton. 2012. Health implications of high dietary omega-6 polyunsaturated fatty acids. *J Nutr Metab* 2012:539426.

Rajilic-Stojanovic, M., and W. M. de Vos. 2014. The first 1000 cultured species of the human gastrointestinal microbiota. *FEMS Microbiol Rev* 38 (5):996–1047.

Ravussin, E., L. M. Redman, J. Rochon, S. K. Das, L. Fontana, W. E. Kraus, S. Romashkan et al. 2015. A 2-year randomized controlled trial of human caloric restriction: Feasibility and effects on predictors of health span and longevity. *J Gerontol A Biol Sci Med Sci* 70 (9):1097–1104.

Ritz, B. W., I. Aktan, S. Nogusa, and E. M. Gardner. 2008. Energy restriction impairs natural killer cell function and increases the severity of influenza infection in young adult male C57BL/6 mice. *J Nutr* 138 (11):2269–2275.

Roecker, E. B., J. W. Kemnitz, W. B. Ershler, and R. Weindruch. 1996. Reduced immune responses in rhesus monkeys subjected to dietary restriction. *J Gerontol A Biol Sci Med Sci* 51 (4):B276–B279.

Ryu, D., L. Mouchiroud, P. A. Andreux, E. Katsyuba, N. Moullan, A. A. Nicolet-Dit-Felix, E. G. Williams et al. 2016. Urolithin A induces mitophagy and prolongs lifespan in *C. elegans* and increases muscle function in rodents. *Nat Med* 22 (8):879–888.

Salimonu, L. S. 1992. Acute phase proteins in "small for dates" babies. II. Haptoglobin, transferrin, alpha-1-feto protein, alpha-1-acid glycoprotein and caeruloplasmin levels. *Afr J Med Med Sci* 21 (1):55–59.

Schaible, U. E., and S. H. Kaufmann. 2007. Malnutrition and infection: Complex mechanisms and global impacts. *PLoS Med* 4 (5):e115.

Schenk, S., M. Saberi, and J. M. Olefsky. 2008. Insulin sensitivity: Modulation by nutrients and inflammation. *J Clin Invest* 118 (9):2992–3002.

Scrimshaw, N. S., C. E. Taylor, and J. E. Gordon. 1959. Interactions of nutrition and infection. *Am J Med Sci* 237 (3):367–403.

Scrimshaw, N. S., C. E. Taylor, and J. E. Gordon. 1968. Interactions of nutrition and infection. *Monogr Ser World Health Organ* 57:3–329.

Segata, N., S. K. Haake, P. Mannon, K. P. Lemon, L. Waldron, D. Gevers, C. Huttenhower, and J. Izard. 2012. Composition of the adult digestive tract bacterial microbiome based on seven mouth surfaces, tonsils, throat and stool samples. *Genome Biol* 13 (6):R42.

Serhan, C. N. 2007. Resolution phase of inflammation: Novel endogenous anti-inflammatory and proresolving lipid mediators and pathways. *Annu Rev Immunol* 25:101–137.

Shida, K., T. Sato, R. Iizuka, R. Hoshi, O. Watanabe, T. Igarashi, K. Miyazaki, M. Nanno, and F. Ishikawa. 2017. Daily intake of fermented milk with *Lactobacillus casei* strain Shirota reduces the incidence and duration of upper respiratory tract infections in healthy middle-aged office workers. *Eur J Nutr* 56 (1):45–53.

Smith, A. G., P. A. Sheridan, J. B. Harp, and M. A. Beck. 2007. Diet-induced obese mice have increased mortality and altered immune responses when infected with influenza virus. *J Nutr* 137 (5):1236–1243.

Tang, W. H., Z. Wang, B. S. Levison, R. A. Koeth, E. B. Britt, X. Fu, Y. Wu, and S. L. Hazen. 2013. Intestinal microbial metabolism of phosphatidylcholine and cardiovascular risk. *N Engl J Med* 368 (17):1575–1584.

Taube, A., R. Schlich, H. Sell, K. Eckardt, and J. Eckel. 2012. Inflammation and metabolic dysfunction: Links to cardiovascular diseases. *Am J Physiol Heart Circ Physiol* 302 (11):H2148–H2165.

Thea, D. M., R. Porat, K. Nagimbi, M. Baangi, M. E. St. Louis, G. Kaplan, C. A. Dinarello, and G. T. Keusch. 1996. Plasma cytokines, cytokine antagonists, and disease progression in African women infected with HIV-1. *Ann Intern Med* 124 (8):757–762.

Tuohy, K., and D. Del Rio, eds. 2014. *Diet-Microbe Interactions in the Gut: Effects on Human Health and Disease*. Amsterdam: Elsevier Science.

Tuohy, K. M., S. Kolida, A. M. Lustenberger, and G. R. Gibson. 2001. The prebiotic effects of biscuits containing partially hydrolysed guar gum and fructo-oligosaccharides—A human volunteer study. *Br J Nutr* 86 (3):341–348.

Windey, K., V. De Preter, and K. Verbeke. 2012. Relevance of protein fermentation to gut health. *Mol Nutr Food Res* 56 (1):184–196.

Wong, S., A. Jamous, J. O'Driscoll, R. Sekhar, M. Weldon, C. Y. Yau, S. P. Hirani, G. Grimble, and A. Forbes. 2014. A *Lactobacillus casei* Shirota probiotic drink reduces antibiotic-associated diarrhoea in patients with spinal cord injuries: A randomised controlled trial. *Br J Nutr* 111 (4):672–678.

Yang, H., Y. H. Youm, and V. D. Dixit. 2009. Inhibition of thymic adipogenesis by caloric restriction is coupled with reduction in age-related thymic involution. *J Immunol* 183 (5):3040–3052.

Yang, J., P. H. Summanen, S. M. Henning, M. Hsu, H. Lam, J. Huang, C. H. Tseng, S. E. Dowd, S. M. Finegold, D. Heber, and Z. Li. 2015. Xylooligosaccharide supplementation alters gut bacteria in both healthy and prediabetic adults: A pilot study. *Front Physiol* 6:216.

Zahorska-Markiewicz, B., J. Janowska, M. Olszanecka-Glinianowicz, and A. Zurakowski. 2000. Serum concentrations of TNF-alpha and soluble TNF-alpha receptors in obesity. *Int J Obes Relat Metab Disord* 24 (11):1392–1395.

Ze, X., F. Le Mougen, S. H. Duncan, P. Louis, and H. J. Flint. 2013. Some are more equal than others: The role of "keystone" species in the degradation of recalcitrant substrates. *Gut Microbes* 4 (3):236–240.

Zoetendal, E. G., J. Raes, B. van den Bogert, M. Arumugam, C. C. Booijink, F. J. Troost, P. Bork, M. Wels, W. M. de Vos, and M. Kleerebezem. 2012. The human small intestinal microbiota is driven by rapid uptake and conversion of simple carbohydrates. *ISME J* 6 (7):1415–1426.

4 Nutrition and Gastrointestinal Disorders

4.1 INTRODUCTION

The gastrointestinal tract is a complex system of organs that digest and absorb nutrients, micronutrients, xenobiotics, and metabolites of gut bacteria. Through the action of the liver and gallbladder, the gastrointestinal tract also detoxifies and excretes toxic and potentially toxic substances from the body. Food is converted into energy and other substances that are used by cells throughout the entire body. Many diseases can affect the various organs of the gastrointestinal tract, and nutrition can affect the course of these disorders.

Gastrointestinal disorders can result from deficiencies or excesses of specific nutrients in normal individuals. In allergic or susceptible subjects, diseases such as food allergy, lactose intolerance, gluten "sensitivity," and gluten enteropathy may occur with intake of normal daily requirements.

Treatment of gastrointestinal disease may require dietary modifications, enteral supplements, or exclusive enteral nutrition. If the gut is not functioning adequately, nutritional support via the parenteral route may be required. In subjects with inflammatory bowel disease (IBD) and short gut syndrome, replacement of specific nutrients may be required, particularly calcium, magnesium, zinc, iron, folate, and vitamins B12, D, and A.

The process of digestion begins with the visualization of a food and the attributed hedonic value of a food. This visualization can trigger central nervous system activation of gastrointestinal physiology, including insulin secretion. Ninety percent of the nerves between the brain and gastrointestinal tract carry messages from the gastrointestinal tract to the brain. The human brain is able to learn and memorize sensory inputs, including those that accompany the consumption of food and drink. From the taste of foods to their gastrointestinal sensations and social-cultural associations, nutrition takes on many psychological attributes that in many patients overtake normal physiology, resulting in strong cravings, addictions, and food intolerances.

True food allergies are much less common and are mediated through the immune system, which is anatomically associated with the gastrointestinal tract. However, food allergies are also part of the larger association of food with systemic reactions. Moreover, some patients mistake food intolerance for true food allergy, and the ability to distinguish these entities can be helpful in counseling patients presenting with complex issues around food intake. In the extreme, food intolerance can lead to established eating disorders and anorexia nervosa.

Irritable bowel syndrome (IBS) is a complex disorder that is extremely common in primary care practice. This disorder affects a significant percentage of the general primary care patient population. IBS is associated with an interaction of psychological stress-related effects on motility and effects resulting from the ingestion of food. It is a clinical syndrome with a group of specific symptoms. Food intake, particularly high-fat and low-fiber food, may play a role in triggering or perpetuating symptoms in patients with IBS.

IBD involves chronic inflammation of all or part of the digestive tract. IBD primarily includes ulcerative colitis and Crohn's disease. While the precise mechanisms underlying the development of IBD are not known, sufficient data suggest that it results from a complex interplay of genetic, environmental, and immunologic factors. An inappropriate mucosal immune response to normal intestinal constituents is a key feature, leading to an imbalance in local pro- and anti-inflammatory cytokines. Diet and nutrition play important roles in the causation, primary treatment, and adjunctive therapy of IBD.

This chapter reviews the interactions of nutrition and gastrointestinal disorders and the psychological, as well as physiological, aspects of the interactions between nutrition and the gastrointestinal tract from the brain's hedonic centers to the colonic flora digesting the substances we do not digest.

4.2 FOOD ADDICTION OR SIMPLY CRAVING?

There are similarities between food craving and drug craving, whichs support the concept of a physiological addiction to specific foods (Gearhardt et al. 2009). There are similarities in the neuroanatomy, neurochemistry, and learning of food cravings and food addictions. The brain mechanisms for craving foods likely developed during evolution to promote seeking of nutrient-dense foods such as sweet fruits with phytonutrients, vitamins, and minerals. Alcohol addiction and drug addiction activate the same brain reward centers as junk foods.

Healthy, normal-weight individuals, by definition, do not suffer from food addiction; however, some overweight and obese individuals meet criteria for addictive behavior established by the psychiatric community, such as continuing a behavior in the face of known negative consequences. While high-sweet and high-fat foods are not in themselves responsible for the obesity problem, the marketing and availability of these foods in an obesogenic environment enables addiction in susceptible individuals. Some nonpalatable foods can also come to be desired and potentially eaten in excess. In particular, pica, which is the consumption of mud or chalk by individuals, is an example of addictive behavior not linked to what would be considered palatable food.

The evidence for food addiction as a psychophysiological entity is growing (Davis et al. 2011). Clinical and evolutionary evidence has been combined with animal research and clinical research. While classic drugs of abuse activate similar brain centers as some foods, a major difference is the lack of withdrawal symptoms when the consumption of the addictive food is stopped. Food addiction is fundamentally a behavioral disorder. There is evidence that some people lose control over their food consumption, failing to reduce their intake and continuing to eat foods in the face of known negative consequences. Other aspects of food addiction as an addiction similar to that of drugs require more research, including evidence of tolerance to high-fat sweets and time spent in buying, eating, and recovering from addictive food intake, including how overall nutrition and quality of life are affected by food addiction.

As the necessary research proceeds to prove the addictive nature of some overeating, a practical approach in weight management programs in order to reduce both food cravings and addictions is to provide education on trigger foods that may lead to addictive processes. This information can be used to inform patients that for them, particular trigger foods cannot practically be included in their weight management diet, as previously taught in the philosophy of balance, variety, and moderation. These trigger foods may present special behavioral issues that make it impossible for susceptible overweight and obese patients to restrict their intake.

The Yale Food Addiction Scale was the first tool developed to identify individuals with addictive tendencies toward food. Using a sample of obese adults (aged 25–45 years), and a case-control methodology, this instrument assesses three domains relevant to the characterization of conventional substance dependence disorders: clinical comorbidities, psychological risk factors, and abnormal motivation for the addictive substance (Rogers and Smit 2000). Among subjects surveyed with this instrument, those who met the diagnostic criteria for food addiction had significantly greater comorbidities demonstrated, including binge eating disorder, depression, and attention-deficit/hyperactivity disorder, than their age- and weight-matched counterparts. Individuals with food addiction were also more impulsive and displayed greater emotional reactivity than obese controls. They also displayed greater food cravings and the tendency to "self-soothe" with food.

These findings identify some clinically relevant behavioral obesity phenotypes with different susceptibility to environmental risk factors, and thereby could inform more personalized treatment approaches for those who struggle with overeating and weight gain.

The diagnosis of food addiction is based on psychological processes of ambivalence and attribution, operating together with normal mechanisms of appetite control, the hedonic effects of certain foods, and socially and culturally determined perceptions of appropriate intakes and uses of those foods (Rogers and Smit 2000). Ambivalence is the idea that some foods are "nice but naughty," and this has been used in the marketing of chocolate, particularly to women. There is a mixed message here that chocolate is great tasting and has physiologically positive and rewarding effects, but should be eaten with restraint. Attempts to restrict intake, however, cause the desire for chocolate to become more salient, an experience that is then labeled as a craving. The example of chocolate is not meant to minimize the potential effects of high-cocoa chocolate and flavonols, and the example could easily have been savory snacks for men, or ice cream for both genders.

Behavioral strategies such as relapse prevention come directly from the addiction medicine literature and can be successfully employed once a food addiction has been identified.

4.3 EATING DISORDERS: FROM BULIMIA TO ANOREXIA NERVOSA

Anorexia nervosa and bulimia nervosa have their common origin in an obsession with body shape and weight. While relationships, work, parenting, and sports performance form the core of a person's self-worth for most individuals, for patients with eating disorders, their self-worth stems from their body shape and weight and their ability to control them. Eating disorders are commonly considered to include only anorexia nervosa and bulimia nervosa. However, there is a third eating disorder called "atypical eating disorders" (Fairburn and Brownell 2002) or "eating disorders not otherwise specified." Atypical eating disorders are the most common diagnostic category, outnumbering patients with anorexia or bulimia, as documented in three well-executed case series (Millar 1998; Ricca et al. 2001). Atypical eating disorders primarily affect adolescents and young adult women. A further eating disorder has also been proposed, termed binge eating disorder, and it affects a significant percentage of overweight and obese patients, sometimes classified as "volume eaters."

Most atypical eating disorders resemble aspects of anorexia nervosa and bulimia nervosa (Ricca et al. 2001), and many are as severe and long lasting. Some are virtually identical to the two well-known disorders, but do not meet their precise diagnostic criteria (Andersen et al. 2001). For example, such patients may not meet the body weight criteria for anorexia nervosa, or they may still have intact reproductive function. On the other hand, features such as extreme dieting, extreme exercising, and binge eating may be present. Some patients may have a past history of anorexia nervosa or bulimia nervosa. Obsession with shape and weight is usually present, but some patients primarily focus on controlling eating behavior.

Patients with anorexia and bulimia view their low body weight as an accomplishment rather than a disease. They have little motivation to change their behavior. In bulimia nervosa, the struggle to control shape and weight is interrupted by binge eating, so that patients describe themselves as failed anorexics. Patients often identify negative physical and emotional states as feeling too fat. They sometimes focus on a single fold of fat or a shape that promotes their misinterpretation of their body size and shape.

Patients with anorexia nervosa who successfully lose weight well below what most would consider healthy do this through a well-planned strategy of avoiding fattening foods and overconsuming low-calorie, high-bulk foods, such as salads. They also typically exercise aerobically to achieve an ever-thinner body. Self-induced vomiting to control body weight and the use of laxative and diuretics are also methods used by some anorectic patients.

4.4 TREATMENT OF EATING DISORDERS

Eating disorders range from picky eating to anorexia and bulimia nervosa. There is a spectrum of severity of disordered eating, ranging from picky eating in childhood and adolescent anorexia nervosa to severe and sometimes fatal eating disorders in adulthood.

In most cases, picky eating in early childhood is a part of normal development. It is more common in preschool children and usually decreases in later childhood. However, picky eating may persist into adulthood. The term refers to a range of conditions, including eating a limited variety of food, and other specific features related to food and eating, such as eating very slowly or being satiated soon after beginning to eat. Picky eating is often a major concern for parents of young children (Cardona Cano et al. 2015). The most common approach to the management of picky eating is to start with nutrition education. These programs are directed at the parents of children with picky eating and are meant to increase nutrition knowledge while also improving feeding styles in order to reduce negative interactions, including anxiety of parents and children around efforts to force eating (Cardona Cano et al. 2015).

There are two types of anorexia nervosa—primary and secondary. The secondary form occurs in the context of an underlying psychiatric condition and responds to treatment when the underlying condition is resolved. Primary anorexia nervosa is far more complex and involves genetic predisposition and the individual's behavior in relation to the family, as well as the resulting psychodynamics.

Most clinical guidelines recommend family therapy for adolescent anorexia nervosa (National Collaborating Centre for Mental Health 2004; American Psychiatric Association 2006; Hay et al. 2014; Blessitt et al. 2015), emphasizing the role of the family in the development of the illness and its potential role as a mediator of successful treatment. While family therapy for adolescent anorexia nervosa is now generally accepted as an effective treatment, there are clearly patients that do not respond (Blessitt et al. 2015). Not just for family therapy, but more generally for anorexia nervosa, there is still a strong need for more well-designed treatment studies (Hay et al. 2014). Compulsory treatment is a last resort for anorexia nervosa, and is justified given its high mortality rate of 5% per decade (Arcelus et al. 2011). In severe cases of anorexia nervosa, where the patient refuses life-saving treatment, compulsory treatment needs to be considered (Elzakkers et al. 2014).

The treatment for bulimia nervosa and binge eating disorder in adults is based on individual psychotherapy and cognitive behavioral therapy (CBT) (Fairburn et al. 2009; Kass et al. 2013; Spielmans et al. 2013). In many countries where there are not enough therapists available to serve the population, self-help manuals and interventions by the Internet have been shown to be effective for cognitive behavioral treatment of eating disorders (Fairburn and Murphy 2015).

As with overweight and obesity, the majority of people with an eating disorder in the community never enter the health care system (Hoek 2006). Therefore, the primary care practice as the first entry point for individuals and families has a special role to play in the detection and treatment or referral of patients with eating disorders.

4.5 FOOD INTOLERANCE AND FOOD ALLERGY

Food intolerance is a common nutritional problem that is encountered in primary care. Estimates of the prevalence of this condition range from about 5% to 33% based on self-report (Bender and Matthews 1981; Strobel 1993). Children have been studied more often than adults, as food intolerance and even temporary allergies are more common (Young et al. 1994; Zeiger and Heller 1995; Sampson 1996).

It is known that food allergy in adults is often associated with hay fever, and that the spectrum of relevant food allergens is different from that in children (Hofer and Wuthrich 1985; Muhlemann and Wuthrich 1991; Ring and Vieluf 1991; Jansen et al. 1994). Double-blind, placebo-controlled food challenge results in much lower estimates of the incidence of food allergy than questionnaires used in epidemiologic surveys. There are numerous alternative medicine practices based on invalid testing of foods and their mood connections, often tested by adding drops of food extracts to the tongue. It is important to distinguish food intolerance, which is a behavioral disorder often linked with IBS, nausea, or other poorly defined symptoms, from a true food allergy, which activates an immune reaction.

There is limited research on the connection between food allergies and the actual sensitization by food challenge, as well as association with manifestations of atopy (Bjornsson et al. 1996; Chng et al. 1999; Sicherer et al. 1999). When double-blind, placebo-controlled food challenge was used, the prevalence of food allergies or intolerance was between 1.4% and 2.4% (Hofer and Wuthrich 1985; Jansen et al. 1994). These studies were carried out in relatively small numbers of subjects ranging between 73 and 93. In one such study, a standard battery of eight allergens were tested, allowing inferences only on these substances. Furthermore, some nonatopic reactions were included, such as headache and behavioral and joint symptoms.

Food allergens in adults differ from those in childhood, where milk and egg account for the majority of reactions. Reactions to nuts, fruit, milk, wine, and vegetables are most frequently reported in adults. Peanut allergies are so common that the use of peanuts in producing foods is often noted. The vast majority of reactions occur in the skin or mucosa (>70%). The given percentages of reactions in population-based studies of different organ systems add to the data derived from patient populations, and in which more severe reactions were seen (Ring and Vieluf 1991; Bjornsson et al. 1996; Sicherer et al. 1999). In a nonatopic adult population from Singapore, 11.7% were found to be sensitized to at least one of 18 food allergens in the skin prick test (SPT) (Chng et al. 1999). Specific immunoglobulin E (IgE) antibodies to at least one of six food allergens were exhibited in 8% of a Swedish adult population (Bjornsson et al. 1996).

Researchers have found a strong association of sensitization to soy and celery or hazelnut, as well as sensitization to celery or peanut and hazelnut. Clustering of food reactions suggests that there is cross-reactivity between food and pollen allergens, causing food allergy in adults as a sequel to pollen sensitization. This is supported by the finding that more than 70% of subjects with food allergy have a history of physician-diagnosed allergic rhinitis (Wuthrich et al. 1995). A strong and clinically relevant association of food and pollen sensitization is known from several patient-based studies (Dreborg 1988). From patient populations, it was estimated that 65% of those with food allergy exhibit other clinical manifestations of atopy (Muhlemann and Wuthrich 1991). Associations of food allergy or sensitization with asthma and bronchial hyperresponsiveness were also reported in a population-based study (Chng et al. 1999).

4.6 IRRITABLE BOWEL SYNDROME

IBS is characterized by chronically recurring abdominal pain or discomfort and altered bowel habits. It is one of the most common syndromes seen by primary care providers, with a worldwide prevalence between 10% and 15% (Drossman et al. 2002; Mayer 2008). IBS, while common, is a diagnosis of exclusion, which in the absence of evidence of organic disease is defined by symptom-based diagnostic criteria known as the "Rome criteria" (Longstreth et al. 2006).

In addition to the association of food intolerance with atopic reactions, IBS, including incipient diarrhea, gas pain, or irregularity, is frequently reported in conjunction with specific food intake. Some of these symptoms are physiologically based, including the well-known gas production from complex sugars found in vegetables such as beans or broccoli. However, this syndrome is far more common than even those related to specific foods and is based on behavioral factors in common with food intolerance.

Other functional gastrointestinal disorders, including functional dyspepsia, are frequently seen in patients with IBS (Halder et al. 2007). In addition, fibromyalgia, chronic pelvic pain, and interstitial cystitis (Whitehead et al. 2002; Wessely and White 2004) have been reported in association with IBS. Coexisting psychological conditions are also common, primarily anxiety, somatization, and symptom-related fears (e.g., "I am worried that I will have severe discomfort during the day if I don't empty my bowels completely in the morning"); these contribute to impairments in quality of life (Spiegel et al. 2004) and excessive use of health care associated with IBS (Levy et al. 2001).

The use of fiber in treatment of IBS is well established. At least two recent meta-analyses with published studies demonstrate that soluble fiber can improve symptoms of IBS, whereas there is no evidence for recommending insoluble fiber for IBS. There were no severe adverse events seen in any of the studies included in this meta-analysis. Minor side effects were reported, including GI disturbances, which were a result of the action of soluble and insoluble fibers (Moayyedi et al. 2014; Nagarajan et al. 2015). The mechanism by which fiber helps alleviate the symptoms of IBS is not established. Soluble fibers are digested and fermented in the distal small intestine and proximal colon by endogenous bacteria to metabolites, including short-chain fatty acids (SCFAs). The presence of these carbohydrates may produce selective changes in the composition of the microbiota, inducing different fermentation patterns. As such, carbohydrates such as inulin are regarded as prebiotics, which may stimulate or alter the preferential growth of health-promoting species already residing in the colon, including lactobacilli and bifidobacteria (Gibson et al. 1995; Roberfroid 2007). An increase in the production of SCFAs in stool can aid in the nourishment of the colonic mucosa and improve mucus production. There is some emerging evidence that SCFAs can also decrease inflammation at the cellular level, but further studies are needed to confirm this observation (Nagarajan et al. 2015).

FODMAPs is an acronym for "fermentable oligo-, di-, monosaccharides and polyols," that is, low in wheat, onions, beans, many kinds of fruit, and sorbitol. In recent years, studies supporting the low-FODMAP diet for the management of IBS symptoms have been published, including several randomized controlled trials, case-control studies, and other observational studies (Nanayakkara et al. 2016). Dietary intervention studies have demonstrated that FODMAPs reduce symptoms in up to 50% of patients with IBS (Gearry et al. 2009). In a study utilizing a placebo-controlled, crossover rechallenge design (Shepherd et al. 2008), patients had fewer symptoms on the FODMAP-reduced diet, and symptoms recurred in 70–80% of them when FODMAPs were reintroduced.

FODMAP restriction may reduce both osmotic load and gas production in the distal small bowel and the proximal colon, providing symptomatic relief in patients with IBS. The long-term health effects of a low-FODMAP diet are not known; however, stringent FODMAP restriction is not recommended, owing to risks of inadequate nutrient intake and potential adverse effects from altered gut microbiota.

4.7 GLUTEN ENTEROPATHY AND GLUTEN SENSITIVITY

Gluten is the major protein component of wheat, rye, and barley (Kumar and Wijmenga 2011). Gluten enteropathy, also called celiac disease, is an immune-mediated disease of the intestines that is triggered by the ingestion of gluten in genetically susceptible individuals. Genetic predisposition plays a key role in celiac disease. Gluten enteropathy is strongly associated with specific human leukocyte antigen (HLA) class II genes located on chromosome 6p21. Approximately 95% of celiac disease patients express *HLA-DQ2*, and the remaining patients are usually *HLA-DQ8* positive. However, the *HLA-DQ2* allele is common and is carried by approximately 30% of Caucasian individuals. Thus, *HLA-DQ2* or *HLA-DQ8* is necessary for disease development but is not sufficient for disease development; its estimated risk effect is only 36–53%. An additional 13 celiac disease risk loci have been identified, but the genetic causes of celiac disease are still not established (Trynka et al. 2011). Diagnosis is established by small intestinal biopsy.

The perception that gluten causes gastrointestinal symptoms and even central nervous system symptoms in patients who do not have celiac disease, and are not allergic to wheat, is an increasing clinical problem called gluten sensitivity (Verdu et al. 2009). There are now many more people on a gluten-free diet following a self-diagnosis of gluten intolerance than there are patients with celiac disease or gluten enteropathy confirmed by biopsy (Rubio-Tapia et al. 2012). This condition, like IBS, is a clinical diagnosis without a biomarker or characteristic intestinal biopsy findings (Ludvigsson et al. 2013).

The existence of the condition called gluten sensitivity remains controversial, and if it does exist, its cause may not be gluten. Fermentable carbohydrates, including oligosaccharides, fructans, and galactooligosaccharides (Sapone et al. 2012), have been termed FODMAPs, and they are capable of triggering symptoms of IBS. Gluten-containing diets, which are low in FODMAPs, reduce symptoms (Gibson et al. 2007; Biesiekierski et al. 2011; Shepherd et al. 2013; Molina-Infante et al. 2015), indicating that the benefits of a gluten-free diet in some patients diagnosed with gluten sensitivity may not be a consequence of the elimination of gluten, but rather may be due to their reduced intake of FODMAPs.

4.8 INFLAMMATORY BOWEL DISEASES

IBDs are comprised of ulcerative colitis and Crohn's disease. These are chronic and relapsing diseases affecting both the gastrointestinal tract and the quality of life. IBD results from the interaction of genetic susceptibility and environmental factors. Even though there is no cure for IBDs, a combined pharmacological and nutritional therapy can induce remissions.

4.8.1 Malnutrition

Malnutrition and specific nutritional deficiencies are frequent among these patients. Malnutrition is common in IBDs, and the underlying pathogenesis in these disorders is multifactorial. It is often a combination of inadequate calorie intake and increased energy expenditure associated with disease flares of inflammatory lesions (Hartman et al. 2009). In addition, both pharmacological and surgical treatment can impair digestion and absorption of nutrients because of drug–nutrient interactions and reduced absorptive area of the intestine following surgical resections (O'Sullivan and O'Morain 2006). Reduced lean body mass and sarcopenia are common in patients with IBD, and these conditions are associated with osteopenia and osteoporosis (Bryant et al. 2015).

Malabsorption is a major contributor to weight loss and malnutrition in adult Crohn's disease patients. Increased gastrointestinal nutrient losses are observed in patients after ileal resection or with bile acid malabsorption (Vitek 2015). Bile acid malabsorption is common in patients, whether the disease is localized in the ileum or not. It leads to malfunction of lipid digestion with steatorrhea, impaired intestinal motility, and significant changes in intestinal microflora. Increased fat in feces could also be a result of a deficit in pancreatic enzyme secretion. Gastric acid- and pancreatic enzyme-impaired secretion have been found in 80% of Crohn's disease patients.

4.8.2 Enteral and Parenteral Nutrition

Enteral feeding using formulas or liquids should always take precedence over parenteral feeding, unless it has been completely contraindicated. Total parenteral nutrition may be used during the acute inflammatory phase with obstruction, toxic megacolon, or active fistulas. It is also used in the preoperative period and in patients with short bowel syndrome (SBS) due to previous extensive bowel resections (Forbes et al. 2011; Mihai et al. 2013).

The idea of providing all nutrition through enteral supplements rather than foods is called exclusive enteral nutrition, and it is used for active disease. It was first used in 1973 in adults with Crohn's disease resistant to other therapies (Voitk et al. 1973). Supplemental enteral nutrition may also be used to maintain a disease remission or to achieve adequate weight gain and growth (O'Sullivan and O'Morain 2006). Although research studies have confirmed its effectiveness in therapy, outcomes of this approach, when implemented in patients, are highly variable. Exclusive enteral nutrition is the initial therapy option in active Crohn's disease. Parenteral nutrition is reserved to only being considered as an alternative method of nutrition for those who cannot tolerate enteral nutrition or during perioperative periods.

4.8.3 Breastfeeding

Breastfeeding has been associated with a lower risk of IBD. The mechanism by which breastfeeding is protective is not known. Breastfeeding in the first months of life is crucial for the development of gut microflora, as the complex carbohydrates in breast milk support the growth of a particular *Bifidobacterium* species (Garrido et al. 2015). The gut microbiome stimulates innate and acquired immunity, promotes the maturation of the mucosal immune system and the integrity of the mucosa, and develops tolerance to food antigens (Scaldaferri et al. 2013; Ananthakrishnan 2015). Some authors assign a special role in this process to lactoferrin (Frolkis et al. 2013). This peptide, which is found in human milk but not in infant formula, has anti-inflammatory, antibacterial, and antiviral properties (Brock 2002).

4.8.4 Specific Carbohydrate Diet

The specific carbohydrate diet (SCD) was introduced and initially described in the early 1920s to treat celiac disease. In the years that followed, it became very popular due to several impressive lay reports indicating the potential of SCD to treat IBDs. The underlying theory of the SCD is that disaccharide and polysaccharide carbohydrates are poorly absorbed in the human intestinal tract, resulting in bacterial and yeast overgrowth that might lead to inflammation and mucosal damage. This diet restricts carbohydrate exposure to the monosaccharides glucose, fructose, and galactose. Almonds, nuts, and coconut flours are recommended, while grain flours from wheat, rice, and corn are excluded. Most dairy products are excluded, except for fermented yogurt, and the only sugar allowed is honey. There has been no significant recent study examining the modification of carbohydrate intake and its effects on the microbiome, which may be the likely mechanism of action for both improvement and exacerbation of disease episode through an interaction of the microbiome and the gut-associated immune system.

4.8.5 FODMAP Diet

Several trials have demonstrated the effect of a FODMAP-reduced diet in the treatment of IBS, as described in Section 4.6. As a high percentage of patients with IBD experience IBS-like symptoms (Appleyard et al. 2004; Soares 2014), a FODMAP-reduced diet might also be a therapeutic option in IBD (Gibson and Shepherd 2005; Gearry et al. 2009). At least in one study, FODMAPs appear to reduce some of the symptoms in Crohn's disease (Donnellan et al. 2013). However, enthusiasm for the FODMAP diet approach is reduced by the concern that such a structured dietary regimen will have adverse effects secondary to reduced dietary diversity. It is particularly important to recognize that this very same group of excluded nutrients plays a major role in modulating the composition of gut microbiome. The majority of prebiotics are FODMAPSs (Rastall and Gibson 2015). Therefore, it is important that patients following this diet do not restrict their fruit and vegetable intakes too severely, in order to avoid vitamin and mineral deficiencies.

4.8.6 Western Diet and Obesity

The Western diet is characterized by higher intakes of red and processed meat, butter, high-fat dairy products, eggs, refined grains, white potatoes, french fries in particular, and high-sugar drinks (Hu 2002). The Western dietary pattern is associated with increased IBD risk (Ananthakrishnan 2015).

A German study of monozygotic and dizygotic twins correlated high consumption of processed meat, including sausage, with an increased risk of Crohn's disease, as well as ulcerative colitis (Spehlmann et al. 2012). Similar associations have been noted in Japan, where increased intake of dairy products and meat was associated with a rising incidence of ulcerative colitis (Ng 2014). A potential mechanism is that allergy to proteins such as cow's milk could increase the risk of these diseases. Once study demonstrated that allergy to cow's milk in infancy increased the risk of Crohn's disease and ulcerative colitis in later childhood (Virta et al. 2013).

Polyunsaturated fatty acids (PUFAs) may also play a role in the pathogenesis of IBDs. Increased consumption of omega-6 fats from beef, pork, corn, sunflower oils, and polyunsaturated margarines in place of omega-3 fats from fish has been associated with an increased incidence of IBD (Ueda et al. 2008; Bernstein 2010). In addition, increased consumption of omega-6 fats has been associated with a greater risk of developing ulcerative colitis in a dose-dependent manner (IBD in EPIC Study Investigators et al. 2009). Recently, the European Prospective Investigation into Cancer (EPIC) study, which included more than 350,000 participants with IBD, examined the association between dietary pattern and IBD risks. While there was no overall association, they found that an imbalanced diet, with high consumption of sugar and soft drinks and low consumption of vegetables, was associated with increased ulcerative colitis risk (Racine et al. 2016).

A significant proportion of patients with IBD are overweight (Kugathasan et al. 2007), which is clearly associated with Western diets. A recent study showed that obesity prevalence in IBD patients reflected the obesity index in the general population of the United States (Flores et al. 2015). Visceral fat localized around the intestine lumen is suspected to be pathogenic in IBDs (Fink et al. 2012). Fat deposited around the small or large intestine is called "fat wrapping" (Weakley and Turnbull 1971). In Crohn's disease, fat surrounding more than 50% of the bowel circumference is typical (Sheehan et al. 1992). It has been suggested that pro-inflammatory adipokines secreted by this fatty tissue play a significant role in the pathophysiology of IBD (Ponemone et al. 2010).

4.8.7 Omega-3 Polyunsaturated Fatty Acids

Omega-3 PUFAs (from fish oils and some seed oils) are potent anti-inflammatory nutraceuticals, capable of inhibiting the biosynthesis of important inflammation elicitors such as prostaglandin E2 (PGE2) and tumor necrosis factor α (TNF-α). In addition, omega-3 PUFAs also act as substrates for the synthesis of the inflammation-resolving mediators resolvins, maresins, and protectins. A diet rich in olive oil and fish, but also in vegetables, fruits, grains, and nuts, was inversely associated with Crohn's disease (D'Souza et al. 2008). The role of omega-3 PUFAs in the prevention and treatment of inflammation in IBD in humans has been enthusiastically studied. However, these reports show conflicting results. In some of them, omega-3 PUFAs had an important role in the course of Crohn's disease and ulcerative colitis, with reduced inflammation, improved clinical benefits, and lower rates of relapse (Pearl et al. 2014; Calder 2015; Barbalho et al. 2016). This may be due to differences in study design, amount and formulations of the fatty acids administered, dietary background, ratio of omega-6 to omega-3, or patient compliance (Belluzzi et al. 2000).

4.8.8 Vitamin D

Vitamin D deficiency is common among patients with IBD. The effects of low plasma 25-hydroxyvitamin D (25(OH)D) on outcomes other than bone health are understudied in patients with IBD (Mouli and Ananthakrishnan 2014). There is increasing support for the role of vitamin D in strengthening the innate immune system by acting as an immunomodulator and reducing inflammation in experimental and human IBD (Reich et al. 2014). Moreover, supplementation with vitamin D and vitamin D plasma levels correlated with quality of life in IBD patients during the winter and spring period in some central European countries (Hlavaty et al. 2014).

4.9 SUMMARY

This chapter has integrated psychological, neurological, and physiological aspects of gastrointestinal tract function to food intake. The immune system is largely located in proximity to the gastrointestinal tract, leading to interactions of the immune system with foods in the disorders of food intolerance and food allergies. With further immune involvement with foods and some genetic component, IBD may be triggered in the form of Crohn's disease or ulcerative colitis. These inflammatory conditions are associated with particular foods common in the Western diet, again emphasizing the interaction of foods and the immune system in gastrointestinal tract disorders. FODMAPs and fiber present a confusing and variable effect on both IBS and IBD, implicating possible differences in response based on different gut microflora populations.

The management of these inflammatory conditions includes pharmacological, nutritional, and surgical therapy. The main goal of the treatments is induction and maintenance of remission, correction of nutritional deficiencies, and prevention of complications (Hanauer 2006).

There is no single diet or meal plan for everyone with IBD, and dietary recommendations must be individualized. Attention must be paid to avoiding foods that worsen or trigger disease symptoms and meanwhile making healthy food choices, replacing nutritional deficiencies, and maintaining a well-balanced nutrient-rich diet.

REFERENCES

American Psychiatric Association. 2006. Treatment of patients with eating disorders, third edition. American Psychiatric Association. *Am J Psychiatry* 163 (7 Suppl):4–54.

Ananthakrishnan, A. N. 2015. Epidemiology and risk factors for IBD. *Nat Rev Gastroenterol Hepatol* 12 (4):205–217.

Andersen, A. E., W. A. Bowers, and T. Watson. 2001. A slimming program for eating disorders not otherwise specified. Reconceptualizing a confusing, residual diagnostic category. *Psychiatr Clin North Am* 24 (2):10.

Appleyard, C. B., G. Hernandez, and C. F. Rios-Bedoya. 2004. Basic epidemiology of inflammatory bowel disease in Puerto Rico. *Inflamm Bowel Dis* 10 (2):106–111.

Arcelus, J., A. J. Mitchell, J. Wales, and S. Nielsen. 2011. Mortality rates in patients with anorexia nervosa and other eating disorders. A meta-analysis of 36 studies. *Arch Gen Psychiatry* 68 (7):724–731.

Barbalho, S. M., A. Goulart Rde, K. Quesada, M. D. Bechara, and C. de Carvalho Ade. 2016. Inflammatory bowel disease: Can omega-3 fatty acids really help? *Ann Gastroenterol* 29 (1):37–43.

Belluzzi, A., S. Boschi, C. Brignola, A. Munarini, G. Cariani, and F. Miglio. 2000. Polyunsaturated fatty acids and inflammatory bowel disease. *Am J Clin Nutr* 71 (1 Suppl):339S–342S.

Bender, A. E., and D. R. Matthews. 1981. Adverse reactions to foods. *Br J Nutr* 46 (3):403–407.

Bernstein, C. N. 2010. New insights into IBD epidemiology: Are there any lessons for treatment? *Dig Dis* 28 (3):406–410.

Biesiekierski, J. R., O. Rosella, R. Rose, K. Liels, J. S. Barrett, S. J. Shepherd, P. R. Gibson, and J. G. Muir. 2011. Quantification of fructans, galacto-oligosaccharides and other short-chain carbohydrates in processed grains and cereals. *J Hum Nutr Diet* 24 (2):154–176.

Bjornsson, E., C. Janson, P. Plaschke, E. Norrman, and O. Sjoberg. 1996. Prevalence of sensitization to food allergens in adult Swedes. *Ann Allergy Asthma Immunol* 77 (4):327–332.

Blessitt, E., S. Voulgari, and I. Eisler. 2015. Family therapy for adolescent anorexia nervosa. *Curr Opin Psychiatry* 28 (6):455–460.

Brock, J. H. 2002. The physiology of lactoferrin. *Biochem Cell Biol* 80 (1):1–6.

Bryant, R. V., S. Ooi, C. G. Schultz, C. Goess, R. Grafton, J. Hughes, A. Lim, F. D. Bartholomeusz, and J. M. Andrews. 2015. Low muscle mass and sarcopenia: Common and predictive of osteopenia in inflammatory bowel disease. *Aliment Pharmacol Ther* 41 (9):895–906.

Calder, P. C. 2015. Marine omega-3 fatty acids and inflammatory processes: Effects, mechanisms and clinical relevance. *Biochim Biophys Acta* 1851 (4):469–484.

Cardona Cano, S., H. W. Hoek, and R. Bryant-Waugh. 2015. Picky eating: The current state of research. *Curr Opin Psychiatry* 28 (6):448–454.

Chng, H. H., C. Y. Tang, and K. P. Leong. 1999. Healthy adults demonstrate less skin reactivity to commercial extracts of commonly ingested food than to *D. farinae*. *Asian Pac J Allergy Immunol* 17 (3):175–178.

Davis, C., C. Curtis, R. D. Levitan, J. C. Carter, A. S. Kaplan, and J. L. Kennedy. 2011. Evidence that "food addiction" is a valid phenotype of obesity. *Appetite* 57 (3):711–717.

Donnellan, C. F., L. H. Yann, and S. Lal. 2013. Nutritional management of Crohn's disease. *Therap Adv Gastroenterol* 6 (3):231–242.

Dreborg, S. 1988. Food allergy in pollen-sensitive patients. *Ann Allergy* 61 (6 Pt 2):41–46.

Drossman, D. A., M. Camilleri, E. A. Mayer, and W. E. Whitehead. 2002. AGA technical review on irritable bowel syndrome. *Gastroenterology* 123 (6):2108–2131.

D'Souza, S., E. Levy, D. Mack, D. Israel, P. Lambrette, P. Ghadirian, C. Deslandres, K. Morgan, E. G. Seidman, and D. K. Amre. 2008. Dietary patterns and risk for Crohn's disease in children. *Inflamm Bowel Dis* 14 (3):367–373.

Elzakkers, I. F., U. N. Danner, H. W. Hoek, U. Schmidt, and A. A. van Elburg. 2014. Compulsory treatment in anorexia nervosa: A review. *Int J Eat Disord* 47 (8):845–852.

Fairburn, C. G., and K. D. Brownell. 2002. *Eating Disorders and Obesity: A Comprehensive Handbook*. 2nd ed. New York: Guilford Press.

Fairburn, C. G., Z. Cooper, H. A. Doll, M. E. O'Connor, K. Bohn, D. M. Hawker, J. A. Wales, and R. L. Palmer. 2009. Transdiagnostic cognitive-behavioral therapy for patients with eating disorders: A two-site trial with 60-week follow-up. *Am J Psychiatry* 166 (3):311–319.

Fairburn, C. G., and R. Murphy. 2015. Treating eating disorders using the Internet. *Curr Opin Psychiatry* 28 (6):461–467.

Fink, C., I. Karagiannides, K. Bakirtzi, and C. Pothoulakis. 2012. Adipose tissue and inflammatory bowel disease pathogenesis. *Inflamm Bowel Dis* 18 (8):1550–1557.

Flores, A., E. Burstein, D. J. Cipher, and L. A. Feagins. 2015. Obesity in inflammatory bowel disease: A marker of less severe disease. *Dig Dis Sci* 60 (8):2436–2445.

Forbes, A., E. Goldesgeyme, and E. Paulon. 2011. Nutrition in inflammatory bowel disease. *JPEN J Parenter Enteral Nutr* 35 (5):571–580.

Frolkis, A., L. A. Dieleman, H. W. Barkema, R. Panaccione, S. Ghosh, R. N. Fedorak, K. Madsen, G. G. Kaplan, and Alberta IBD Consortium. 2013. Environment and the inflammatory bowel diseases. *Can J Gastroenterol* 27 (3):e18–e24.

Garrido, D., S. Ruiz-Moyano, D. G. Lemay, D. A. Sela, J. B. German, and D. A. Mills. 2015. Comparative transcriptomics reveals key differences in the response to milk oligosaccharides of infant gut-associated bifidobacteria. *Sci Rep* 5:13517.

Gearhardt, A. N., W. R. Corbin, and K. D. Brownell. 2009. Food addiction: An examination of the diagnostic criteria for dependence. *J Addict Med* 3 (1):1–7.

Gearry, R. B., P. M. Irving, J. S. Barrett, D. M. Nathan, S. J. Shepherd, and P. R. Gibson. 2009. Reduction of dietary poorly absorbed short-chain carbohydrates (FODMAPs) improves abdominal symptoms in patients with inflammatory bowel disease—A pilot study. *J Crohns Colitis* 3 (1):8–14.

Gibson, G. R., E. R. Beatty, X. Wang, and J. H. Cummings. 1995. Selective stimulation of bifidobacteria in the human colon by oligofructose and inulin. *Gastroenterology* 108 (4):975–982.

Gibson, P. R., E. Newnham, J. S. Barrett, S. J. Shepherd, and J. G. Muir. 2007. Review article: Fructose malabsorption and the bigger picture. *Aliment Pharmacol Ther* 25 (4):349–363.

Gibson, P. R., and S. J. Shepherd. 2005. Personal view: Food for thought—Western lifestyle and susceptibility to Crohn's disease. The FODMAP hypothesis. *Aliment Pharmacol Ther* 21 (12):1399–1409.

Halder, S. L., G. R. Locke 3rd, C. D. Schleck, A. R. Zinsmeister, L. J. Melton 3rd, and N. J. Talley. 2007. Natural history of functional gastrointestinal disorders: A 12-year longitudinal population-based study. *Gastroenterology* 133 (3):799–807.

Hanauer, S. B. 2006. Inflammatory bowel disease: Epidemiology, pathogenesis, and therapeutic opportunities. *Inflamm Bowel Dis* 12 (Suppl 1):S3–S9.

Hartman, C., R. Eliakim, and R. Shamir. 2009. Nutritional status and nutritional therapy in inflammatory bowel diseases. *World J Gastroenterol* 15 (21):2570–2578.

Hay, P., D. Chinn, D. Forbes, S. Madden, R. Newton, L. Sugenor, S. Touyz, and W. Ward. 2014. Royal Australian and New Zealand College of Psychiatrists clinical practice guidelines for the treatment of eating disorders. *Aust NZ J Psychiatry* 48 (11):977–1008.

Hlavaty, T., A. Krajcovicova, T. Koller, J. Toth, M. Nevidanska, M. Huorka, and J. Payer. 2014. Higher vitamin D serum concentration increases health related quality of life in patients with inflammatory bowel diseases. *World J Gastroenterol* 20 (42):15787–15796.

Hoek, H. W. 2006. Incidence, prevalence and mortality of anorexia nervosa and other eating disorders. *Curr Opin Psychiatry* 19 (4):389–394.

Hofer, T., and B. Wuthrich. 1985. Food allergy. II. Prevalence of organ manifestations of allergy-inducing food. A study on the basis of 173 cases, 1978–1982 [in German]. *Schweiz Med Wochenschr* 115 (41):1437–1442.

Hu, F. B. 2002. Dietary pattern analysis: A new direction in nutritional epidemiology. *Curr Opin Lipidol* 13 (1):3–9.

IBD in EPIC Study Investigators, A. Tjonneland, K. Overvad, M. M. Bergmann, G. Nagel, J. Linseisen, G. Hallmans et al. 2009. Linoleic acid, a dietary n-6 polyunsaturated fatty acid, and the aetiology of ulcerative colitis: A nested case-control study within a European prospective cohort study. *Gut* 58 (12):1606–1611.

Jansen, J. J., A. F. Kardinaal, G. Huijbers, B. J. Vlieg-Boerstra, B. P. Martens, and T. Ockhuizen. 1994. Prevalence of food allergy and intolerance in the adult Dutch population. *J Allergy Clin Immunol* 93 (2):446–456.

Kass, A. E., R. P. Kolko, and D. E. Wilfley. 2013. Psychological treatments for eating disorders. *Curr Opin Psychiatry* 26 (6):549–555.

Kugathasan, S., J. Nebel, J. A. Skelton, J. Markowitz, D. Keljo, J. Rosh, N. LeLeiko et al. 2007. Body mass index in children with newly diagnosed inflammatory bowel disease: Observations from two multicenter North American inception cohorts. *J Pediatr* 151 (5):523–527.

Kumar, V., and C. Wijmenga. 2011. Celiac disease: Update from the 14th International Celiac Disease Symposium 2011. *Expert Rev Gastroenterol Hepatol* 5 (6):685–687.

Levy, R. L., M. Von Korff, W. E. Whitehead, P. Stang, K. Saunders, P. Jhingran, V. Barghout, and A. D. Feld. 2001. Costs of care for irritable bowel syndrome patients in a health maintenance organization. *Am J Gastroenterol* 96 (11):3122–3129.

Longstreth, G. F., W. G. Thompson, W. D. Chey, L. A. Houghton, F. Mearin, and R. C. Spiller. 2006. Functional bowel disorders. *Gastroenterology* 130 (5):1480–1491.

Ludvigsson, J. F., D. A. Leffler, J. C. Bai, F. Biagi, A. Fasano, P. H. Green, M. Hadjivassiliou et al. 2013. The Oslo definitions for coeliac disease and related terms. *Gut* 62 (1):43–52.

Mayer, E. A. 2008. Clinical practice. Irritable bowel syndrome. *N Engl J Med* 358 (16):1692–1699.

Mihai, C., C. C. Prelipcean, I. Pintilie, O. Nedelciuc, A. O. Jigaranu, M. Dranga, and B. Mihai. 2013. Nutrition in inflammatory bowel diseases. *Rev Med Chir Soc Med Nat Iasi* 117 (3):662–669.

Millar, H. R. 1998. New eating disorder service. *Psychiatr Bull* 22:4.

Moayyedi, P., E. M. Quigley, B. E. Lacy, A. J. Lembo, Y. A. Saito, L. R. Schiller, E. E. Soffer, B. M. Spiegel, and A. C. Ford. 2014. The effect of fiber supplementation on irritable bowel syndrome: A systematic review and meta-analysis. *Am J Gastroenterol* 109 (9):1367–1374.

Molina-Infante, J., S. Santolaria, D. S. Sanders, and F. Fernandez-Banares. 2015. Systematic review: Noncoeliac gluten sensitivity. *Aliment Pharmacol Ther* 41 (9):807–820.

Mouli, V. P., and A. N. Ananthakrishnan. 2014. Review article: Vitamin D and inflammatory bowel diseases. *Aliment Pharmacol Ther* 39 (2):125–136.

Muhlemann, R. J., and B. Wuthrich. 1991. Food allergies 1983–1987 [in German]. *Schweiz Med Wochenschr* 121 (46):1696–1700.

Nagarajan, N., A. Morden, D. Bischof, E. A. King, M. Kosztowski, E. C. Wick, and E. M. Stein. 2015. The role of fiber supplementation in the treatment of irritable bowel syndrome: A systematic review and meta-analysis. *Eur J Gastroenterol Hepatol* 27 (9):1002–1010.

Nanayakkara, W. S., P. M. Skidmore, L. O'Brien, T. J. Wilkinson, and R. B. Gearry. 2016. Efficacy of the low FODMAP diet for treating irritable bowel syndrome: The evidence to date. *Clin Exp Gastroenterol* 9:131–142.

National Collaborating Centre for Mental Health. 2004. *Core Interventions in the Treatment and Management of Anorexia Nervosa, Bulimia Nervosa and Related Eating Disorders*. Leicester: British Psychological Society.

Ng, S. C. 2014. Epidemiology of inflammatory bowel disease: Focus on Asia. *Best Pract Res Clin Gastroenterol* 28 (3):363–372.

O'Sullivan, M., and C. O'Morain. 2006. Nutrition in inflammatory bowel disease. *Best Pract Res Clin Gastroenterol* 20 (3):561–573.

Pearl, D. S., M. Masoodi, M. Eiden, J. Brummer, D. Gullick, T. M. McKeever, M. A. Whittaker et al. 2014. Altered colonic mucosal availability of n-3 and n-6 polyunsaturated fatty acids in ulcerative colitis and the relationship to disease activity. *J Crohns Colitis* 8 (1):70–79.

Ponemone, V., A. Keshavarzian, M. I. Brand, T. Saclarides, H. Abcarian, R. J. Cabay, E. Fletcher, B. Larsen, L. J. Durstine, G. Fantuzzi, and R. Fayad. 2010. Apoptosis and inflammation: Role of adipokines in inflammatory bowel disease. *Clin Transl Gastroenterol* 1:e1.

Racine, A., F. Carbonnel, S. S. Chan, A. R. Hart, H. B. Bueno-de-Mesquita, B. Oldenburg, F. D. van Schaik et al. 2016. Dietary patterns and risk of inflammatory bowel disease in Europe: Results from the EPIC study. *Inflamm Bowel Dis* 22 (2):345–354.

Rastall, R. A., and G. R. Gibson. 2015. Recent developments in prebiotics to selectively impact beneficial microbes and promote intestinal health. *Curr Opin Biotechnol* 32:42–46.

Reich, K. M., R. N. Fedorak, K. Madsen, and K. I. Kroeker. 2014. Vitamin D improves inflammatory bowel disease outcomes: Basic science and clinical review. *World J Gastroenterol* 20 (17):4934–4947.

Ricca, V., E. Mannucci, B. Mezzani, M. Di Bernardo, T. Zucchi, A. Paionni, G. P. Placidi, C. M. Rotella, and C. Faravelli. 2001. Psychopathological and clinical features of outpatients with an eating disorder not otherwise specified. *Eat Weight Disord* 6 (3):157–165.

Ring, J., and D. Vieluf. 1991. Adverse reactions to food. *Curr Probl Dermatol* 20:187–202.

Roberfroid, M. 2007. Prebiotics: The concept revisited. *J Nutr* 137 (3 Suppl 2):830S–837S.

Rogers, P. J., and H. J. Smit. 2000. Food craving and food "addiction": A critical review of the evidence from a biopsychosocial perspective. *Pharmacol Biochem Behav* 66 (1):3–14.

Rubio-Tapia, A., J. F. Ludvigsson, T. L. Brantner, J. A. Murray, and J. E. Everhart. 2012. The prevalence of celiac disease in the United States. *Am J Gastroenterol* 107 (10):1538–1544; quiz 1537, 1545.

Sampson, H. A. 1996. Epidemiology of food allergy. *Pediatr Allergy Immunol* 7 (9 Suppl):42–50.

Sapone, A., J. C. Bai, C. Ciacci, J. Dolinsek, P. H. Green, M. Hadjivassiliou, K. Kaukinen et al. 2012. Spectrum of gluten-related disorders: Consensus on new nomenclature and classification. *BMC Med* 10:13.

Scaldaferri, F., V. Gerardi, L. R. Lopetuso, F. Del Zompo, F. Mangiola, I. Boskoski, G. Bruno et al. 2013. Gut microbial flora, prebiotics, and probiotics in IBD: Their current usage and utility. *Biomed Res Int* 2013:435268.

Sheehan, A. L., B. F. Warren, M. W. Gear, and N. A. Shepherd. 1992. Fat-wrapping in Crohn's disease: Pathological basis and relevance to surgical practice. *Br J Surg* 79 (9):955–958.

Shepherd, S. J., M. C. Lomer, and P. R. Gibson. 2013. Short-chain carbohydrates and functional gastrointestinal disorders. *Am J Gastroenterol* 108 (5):707–717.

Shepherd, S. J., F. C. Parker, J. G. Muir, and P. R. Gibson. 2008. Dietary triggers of abdominal symptoms in patients with irritable bowel syndrome: Randomized placebo-controlled evidence. *Clin Gastroenterol Hepatol* 6 (7):765–771.

Sicherer, S. H., A. Munoz-Furlong, A. W. Burks, and H. A. Sampson. 1999. Prevalence of peanut and tree nut allergy in the US determined by a random digit dial telephone survey. *J Allergy Clin Immunol* 103 (4):559–562.

Soares, R. L. 2014. Irritable bowel syndrome: A clinical review. *World J Gastroenterol* 20 (34):12144–12160.

Spehlmann, M. E., A. Z. Begun, E. Saroglou, F. Hinrichs, U. Tiemann, A. Raedler, and S. Schreiber. 2012. Risk factors in German twins with inflammatory bowel disease: Results of a questionnaire-based survey. *J Crohns Colitis* 6 (1):29–42.

Spiegel, B. M., I. M. Gralnek, R. Bolus, L. Chang, G. S. Dulai, E. A. Mayer, and B. Naliboff. 2004. Clinical determinants of health-related quality of life in patients with irritable bowel syndrome. *Arch Intern Med* 164 (16):1773–1780.

Spielmans, G. I., S. G. Benish, C. Marin, W. M. Bowman, M. Menster, and A. J. Wheeler. 2013. Specificity of psychological treatments for bulimia nervosa and binge eating disorder? A meta-analysis of direct comparisons. *Clin Psychol Rev* 33 (3):460–469.

Strobel, S. 1993. Epidemiology of food sensitivity in childhood—With special reference to cow's milk allergy in infancy. *Monogr Allergy* 31:119–130.

Trynka, G., K. A. Hunt, N. A. Bockett, J. Romanos, V. Mistry, A. Szperl, S. F. Bakker et al. 2011. Dense genotyping identifies and localizes multiple common and rare variant association signals in celiac disease. *Nat Genet* 43 (12):1193–1201.

Ueda, Y., Y. Kawakami, D. Kunii, H. Okada, M. Azuma, D. S. Le, and S. Yamamoto. 2008. Elevated concentrations of linoleic acid in erythrocyte membrane phospholipids in patients with inflammatory bowel disease. *Nutr Res* 28 (4):239–244.

Verdu, E. F., D. Armstrong, and J. A. Murray. 2009. Between celiac disease and irritable bowel syndrome: The "no man's land" of gluten sensitivity. *Am J Gastroenterol* 104 (6):1587–1594.

Virta, L. J., M. Ashorn, and K. L. Kolho. 2013. Cow's milk allergy, asthma, and pediatric IBD. *J Pediatr Gastroenterol Nutr* 56 (6):649–651.

Vitek, L. 2015. Bile acid malabsorption in inflammatory bowel disease. *Inflamm Bowel Dis* 21 (2):476–483.

Voitk, A. J., V. Echave, J. H. Feller, R. A. Brown, and F. N. Gurd. 1973. Experience with elemental diet in the treatment of inflammatory bowel disease. Is this primary therapy? *Arch Surg* 107 (2):329–333.

Weakley, F. L., and R. B. Turnbull. 1971. Recognition of regional ileitis in the operating room. *Dis Colon Rectum* 14 (1):17–23.

Wessely, S., and P. D. White. 2004. There is only one functional somatic syndrome. *Br J Psychiatry* 185:95–96.

Whitehead, W. E., O. Palsson, and K. R. Jones. 2002. Systematic review of the comorbidity of irritable bowel syndrome with other disorders: What are the causes and implications? *Gastroenterology* 122 (4):1140–1156.

Wuthrich, B., C. Schindler, P. Leuenberger, and U. Ackermann-Liebrich. 1995. Prevalence of atopy and pollinosis in the adult population of Switzerland (SAPALDIA study). Swiss Study on Air Pollution and Lung Diseases in Adults. *Int Arch Allergy Immunol* 106 (2):149–156.

Young, E., M. D. Stoneham, A. Petruckevitch, J. Barton, and R. Rona. 1994. A population study of food intolerance. *Lancet* 343 (8906):1127–1130.

Zeiger, R. S., and S. Heller. 1995. The development and prediction of atopy in high-risk children—Follow-up at age 7 years in a prospective randomized study of combined maternal and infant food allergen avoidance. *J Allergy Clin Immunol* 95 (6):1179–1190.

5 Approach to the Overweight and Obese Patient

The Elephant in the Room

5.1 INTRODUCTION

In Chapters 2 and 5, a diet and lifestyle program for the general population designed to maintain healthy body composition on an individual basis is described. A key principle centered on dietary protein at levels greater than those generally recognized as required by government agencies. The physiology behind this idea centered on matching protein intake to the energetics and composition of the body. Many of those so-called healthy individuals in industrialized countries, even at normal body mass index (BMI) and waist circumference, are already overfat to some degree due to a sedentary lifestyle and unbalanced nutrition (Thomas et al. 2012). In this chapter, the overtly or obviously obese patient based on BMI criteria presenting to primary care practices is the focus of discussion. While overfatness is a hidden epidemic requiring increased vigilance toward prevention, the obviously obese require a coordinated program of care.

Often, obese patients have been left untreated in primary care, since they represented too great a challenge for the typical practitioner with limited time. Instead of dealing with the underlying obesity, palliative medications would be prescribed to deal with the cardiometabolic and endocrine issues associated with obesity (Goodfellow et al. 2016). These metabolic consequences are due to excess body fat and not excess body weight.

In fact, among the obviously obese there is a significant subpopulation of metabolically healthy individuals (Lopez-Garcia et al. 2016) who will respond to diet and exercise with greater short-term weight loss than the mildly overweight, because they tend to have greater resting metabolic rates due to their increased lean body mass. These patients have less excess body fat than expected based simply on their body weight. In childhood and adolescence, visibly obese children are often ridiculed by their peers and suffer social and psychological trauma (Udo and Grilo 2016). However, from a metabolic point of view, they may be as healthy as many lean patients except for the orthopedic stress to their joints due to their excess weight. As they age, muscle atrophy and worsening hips, knees, and back often lead to reduced physical activity and increased food intake, resulting in rapid weight and fat gain, with resulting metabolic problems. Cardiopulmonary issues, including those linked to sleep apnea and hypertension, are frequent comorbid conditions. The central role that obesity plays in many organ system diseases in these patients is discussed in several of the later chapters, but this chapter concentrates on the early recognition of these at-risk metabolically normal obese individuals and the treatment of the already obese patient at risk for the metabolic syndrome (MetS), diabetes, heart disease, and hypertension.

5.2 PATHOPHYSIOLOGY OF OBESITY

While the incidence of obesity in the United States has been increasing since the early decades of the last century, dramatic accelerations worldwide have been described over the past four decades (Zimmet et al. 2001; Caballero 2007), as significant changes in diet and lifestyle have led to what is called an obesogenic environment. According to figures announced in 2015 by the World Obesity

Federation, it is suggested that 2.7 billion adults worldwide will be overweight by 2025 if current trends continue (World Obesity Federation 2016). This is a 35% increase from 2.0 billion in 2014.

The current epidemic of obesity is caused primarily by an environment that promotes excess food intake and discourages physical activity. This is a global epidemic, as Western ideals and lifestyles are being adopted in urban and rural settings worldwide. Although humans have evolved excellent physiological mechanisms to defend against starvation and infection associated with calorie restriction, they have only weak physiological mechanisms to defend against body weight gain when food is abundant and exercise is limited. The excessive consumption of energy-dense foods rich in salt, fat, and sugar, in combination with sedentary lifestyles, urbanization, and socioeconomic-dependent limited access to a healthy diet (Misra and Khurana 2008), underpins the global obesity epidemic.

Why is this so prevalent? To understand the commonality of obesity, it is important to understand the genetic and epigenetic basis underlying the evolution of humankind. The adaptation to starvation involves a switch to a fat-fuel economy after the glycogen stores in the liver and muscle are exhausted, which usually occurs after just 3 days (Cahill 2006). Once carbohydrate stores are exhausted, the primary way that the brain and red blood cells can get the glucose they need is to break down body protein from cells and muscles. At first, about 75 g of body protein is broken down per day, but over several weeks, this amount is reduced to about 20 g/day, as the brain begins to use ketone bodies made from fatty acids for energy, reducing the amount of glucose needed by breaking down muscle and other body proteins. So, the primary goal of the adaptation to starvation is to reduce the rate at which protein is broken down. With adequate hydration and vitamins, starving individuals can survive about 6 months with no food intake. If the adaptation to starvation is inhibited, then survival is only possible for about 60 days. If, in addition, there is active inflammation due to tumor, trauma, or infection, survival may be only about 30 days.

These different durations of survival all have one thing in common. They occur when the pre-illness body protein is reduced by 50% (Muller et al. 2015). At that point, there is impairment of delayed cell hypersensitivity and immune function, so that death usually results from infection and sepsis.

Since starvation and infection have been the greatest nutrition-related threats to human survival over the last 100,000 years, it is reasonable that genetic evolution and epigenetic changes would seek to maximize lean body mass as long as adequate protein was available in the environment.

There is great variability in BMI values, which have their origin in genetics and epigenetic differences among individuals (Bouchard 2008; Fleisch et al. 2012; van Vliet-Ostaptchouk et al. 2012). While BMI is taken as a practical index of obesity, it clearly fails to account for variations in lean body mass and fat mass among individuals from different ethnic groups and nutritional environments.

A BMI cutoff of 30 kg/m^2 is generally used to define medical obesity (WHO 2013). The BMI threshold has been assessed by the risk for morbidity and mortality in populations of European ancestry (de Gonzalez et al. 2010). Using a single standard cutoff value to define obesity has been questioned, and ethnic-specific BMI cutoffs have been proposed (Evans et al. 2006; Romero-Corral et al. 2008; Rahman and Berenson 2010). In Asian populations, increased disease risks occur at normal BMI values of 20–25 kg/m^2 (Yang et al. 2010).

A BMI paradox in the survival of patients with congestive heart failure where greater BMI predicts better survival has been attributed to the increased lean body mass in some patients (Curtis et al. 2005).

It has long been known that increased BMI confers a survival benefit for obese individuals compared with lean individuals based on their increased lean body mass and fat mass. The familial aggregation of body size was first reported by Sir Francis Galton in 1894 (Galton 1894). Since then, family history of obesity has become a well-established risk factor for childhood obesity. Studies indicate that parental BMI or overweight or obesity status is associated with BMI or the risk of overweight or obesity in children, and is an important predictor of obesity in adulthood (Danielzik et al. 2002, 2004; Oliveira et al. 2007; Birbilis et al. 2013). The ethnic-dependent pattern of obesity prevalence further supports the heritability of obesity, which could be explained in part by specific lifestyles or environmental exposures. In fact, most studies have demonstrated an important contribution of both genes and environment (Muller et al. 2010).

Another important feature of lean body mass is that it is the strongest predictor of resting energy expenditure, which in turn accounts for more than 75% of total calories burned per day, with the remainder being related to exercise, dietary thermogenesis, brown fat cell metabolism, and a small amount of measurable adaptive thermogenesis (Deriaz et al. 1992). Overnutrition increases energy expenditure via putative effects on brown fat, and this effect, which has been controversial, is called "luxuskonsumption" (Ravussin et al. 1985). Undernutrition decreases energy expenditure. With very low-calorie diets, about a 10–15% decrease in energy expenditure has been ascribed to adaptive thermogenesis (Major et al. 2007).

5.2.1 Genetic and Environmental Interactions in Obesity

The completion of the human genome sequence, combined with high-throughput methodological advances in the laboratory, has led to the identification of a large number of genes modulating both BMI and the tendency to gain weight in an obesogenic environment.

Monogenic obesity syndromes are very rare and characterized by mental retardation, dysmorphic features, and specific abnormalities in various organs, in addition to obesity (Waalen 2014). More than 30 monogenic syndromes have been reported in the literature, of which many have not been genetically elucidated (Garver et al. 2013). The most famous of these is the Prader–Willi syndrome, first reported in 1956 by Andrea Prader. This syndrome has an incidence of 1 in 15,000–30,000 individuals (Cassidy and Driscoll 2009). Common characteristics include hypotonia, feeding difficulties, poor growth, and delayed development in the first year of life, followed by hyperphagia, childhood obesity, short stature, and cognitive disability (Cassidy and Driscoll 2009).

Nonsyndromic monogenic obesity refers to a single gene disorder that leads to a highly penetrant form of the disease. A frameshift homozygous mutation in the leptin (*LEP*) gene resulting in truncated transcription of leptin was first discovered in 1997 in two severely obese cousins within a highly consanguineous family of Pakistani origin (Montague et al. 1997). Other reports have confirmed this initial discovery in additional patients with no detectable leptin, in Pakistan, Turkey, and Egypt (Gibson et al. 2004; Mazen et al. 2009). Two patients with severe early-onset obesity with a homozygous *LEP* mutation exhibited detectable circulating leptin levels, indicating that the mutation affects protein function rather than expression, leading to an inactive leptin protein (Wabitsch et al. 2015). Clinical manifestations of patients with mutations in *LEP* or leptin receptor (*LEPR*) include rapid weight gain within the first year of life, severe hyperphagia, and intolerant behavior when presented with food restrictions (Farooqi et al. 2002). Onset of puberty is often delayed due to hypogonadotrophic hypogonadism (Farooqi et al. 2007).

There was a great deal of excitement when the *ob/ob* mouse was found to have leptin deficiency due to a mutation in the leptin gene. This led to the identification and synthesis of leptin, and its administration led to resolution of obesity in mice with the genetic lesion, as well as in mice fed a high-fat or high-sugar cafeteria diet. Clinical studies of leptin administration in humans only resulted in reversal of obesity in individuals with the rare genetic defects described above, but not in most individuals with typical obesity (Heymsfield et al. 1999). The reason for this is that obese humans are resistant to leptin. Leptin has more to do with the adaptation to starvation than it does with obesity.

During fasting, or when food intake is decreased, leptin levels decrease, leading to increased food intake and decreased physical activity. Low leptin levels account in part for the ability of prisoners of war to regain weight rapidly as they undergo refeeding. Similarly, leptin levels are low in obese individuals after weight reduction (Mantzoros et al. 2011). Obese individuals have a requirement for more calories due to their increased lean body mass compared with lean individuals. When they eat to meet this energy requirement with the available foods in industrialized countries, they

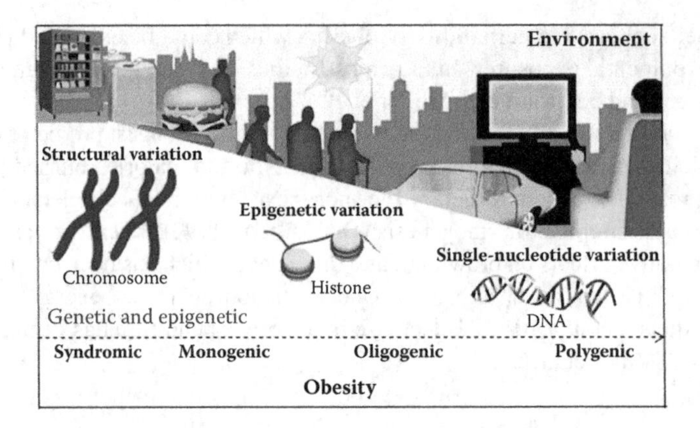

FIGURE 5.1 **(See color insert.)** Contribution of genetic, epigenetic, and environmental stimuli to obesity. In monogenic and syndromic obesity, a single gene mutation could result in severe obesity, irrespective of environmental stimuli. However, in cases of oligogenic and polygenic obesity, environmental factors can exacerbate the progression of obesity if the individuals have a genetic predisposition to weight gain. (Reprinted from Pigeyre, M. et al., *Clin. Sci.*, 130, 943–986, 2016.)

get additional calories from hidden fats and sugars, leading to weight gain. As discussed below, by supplementing the diet with additional protein and cutting added sugars and hidden fats, this problem can be addressed in programs directed at the prevention and treatment of obesity.

As shown in Figure 5.1, polygenic obesity is the most common form and has a very significant interaction with the environment, and the genetic underpinnings of this relationship are complex, with multiple genetic and epigenetic influences, as well as single-nucleotide polymorphisms associated with this heterogeneous and common phenotype. The much rarer monogenic and oligogenic forms have a greater genetic component. Research in this area continues in the hope of finding personalized approaches to obesity. However, as discussed below, the amount of genetic information in the human genome is dwarfed by what is found in the gut microbiome, and there is increasing evidence of the importance of microflora in the etiology of obesity, even in genetically identical twins.

5.2.2 Biological Signals Regulating Food Intake

Despite variations in the amounts and types of foods eaten each day, the body maintains a relatively constant body weight. As already discussed, most of the physiology of obesity is directed at the adaptation to starvation. However, the gastrointestinal (GI) tract has mechanisms to protect itself from the overconsumption of foods in a meal. While a vast number of people eat even when they are not hungry, there are well-defined signals from the gut to the brain that cause satiety. Satiety refers to processes that end meals in order to limit meal size (Blundell and Halford 1994; Smith 1998). After a meal, these signals can affect the time to the next meal, regulating the number of meals per day, which is also entrained by learned habits (Strubbe and Woods 2004). A combination of neural and endocrine signals originates in the gut in response to mechanical and chemical properties of ingested food. While these signals end an ongoing meal, they do not delay the onset of the next meal or food intake between meals, including snacks (Strubbe and Woods 2004).

By affecting intestinal motility and secretion of digestive enzymes, the satiety signals assist the GI tract in carrying out its primary function of nutrient digestion and absorption. Some signals directly affect GI motility and secretion and restrict the rate at which nutrients reach the gut (Gibbs et al. 1973). Meals are stopped before gastric capacity is filled. The stomach has a large maximal capacity, which is a major reason that the gastric bubble intervention of the 1990s failed.

The signals from the distention of the stomach and peptides released from gutendocrine cells travel to the hindbrain via the vagus nerve and the bloodstream, respectively. Pathways relaying short-acting satiation signals from the gut to the hindbrain also interact at several levels with long-acting adiposity hormones involved in body weight regulation, such as leptin and insulin. Through multifaceted mechanisms, adiposity hormones function as gain-setters to modulate the sensitivity of vagal and hindbrain responses to GI satiation signals. Adiposity hormones thereby regulate short-term food intake in order to achieve long-term energy balance (Figure 5.2) (Schwartz et al. 2000; Morton et al. 2006).

Ghrelin is a peptide produced in the stomach and proximal small intestine. It gets its strange name from its ability to release growth hormone, but its main function is to work exactly the opposite of the satiety hormones (Cummings et al. 2005). It increases rather than decreases food intake (Tschop et al. 2000). Ghrelin increases GI motility and decreases insulin secretion, resulting in increased hunger between meals, and then it decreases after meals.

The ileal brake is a feedback phenomenon whereby ingested food activates distal-intestinal signals that inhibit proximal GI motility and gastric emptying (Pironi et al. 1993). It is mediated by neural mechanisms and several peptides that are also implicated in satiation. These signals act to put a behavior brake on eating to supplement the ileal brake's actions and reduce the rate of nutrient entry into the bloodstream (Strader and Woods 2005). Glucagon-like peptide 1 (GLP-1) is cleaved from proglucagon, expressed in the gut, pancreas, and brain (Drucker 2006). Other proglucagon products include glucagon (a counterregulatory hormone), GLP-2 (an intestinal growth factor), glicentin (a gastric acid inhibitor), and oxyntomodulin. The strongest evidence for satiety effects have been found for GLP-1 and oxyntomodulin. Like GLP-1, oxyntomodulin is a proglucagon-derived peptide secreted from distal-intestinal L-cells in proportion to ingested calories. PYY is produced mainly by distal-intestinal L-cells, most of which coexpress GLP-1. It is secreted after meals in proportion to caloric load, with a macronutrient potency of lipids being greater than that of carbohydrates, which is greater than that of proteins (Degen et al. 2005).

This brief discussion was not meant to be comprehensive, but to indicate the complexity of the regulation of food intake by endocrine glands, fat cells, and the GI tract, which has been called the second brain due to its ongoing communication with the brain through the vagus nerve. There are

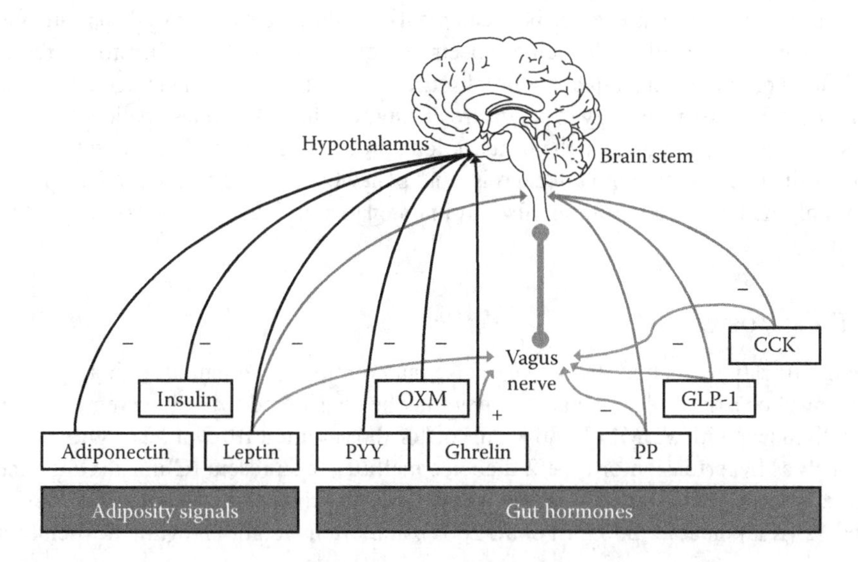

FIGURE 5.2 Energy homeostasis is controlled by peripheral signals from adipose tissue, the pancreas, and the GI tract. Peripheral signals from the gut include peptide YY (PYY), oxyntomodulin (OXM), ghrelin, pancreatic polypeptide (PP), GLP-1, and cholecystokinin (CCK). These gut-derived peptides and adiposity signals influence central circuits in the hypothalamus and brain stem to produce a negative (–) or positive (+) effect on energy balance. Thus, the drive to eat and energy expenditure are adjusted so that over time, body weight remains stable. (Reprinted from Stanley, S. et al., *Physiol. Rev.*, 85, 1131–1158, 2005.)

numerous ongoing discoveries of factors affecting food intake and energy expenditure not only in the brain, but also in the gut, liver, and muscles. As is the nature of academics, each of these factors, like leptin, is hailed as the cure for obesity. The main thing to understand from all this is that the regulation of food intake is complex since it is vital to survival, especially survival from starvation (Figure 5.2).

Attempts to alter this system through drugs that target individual factors and surgery that bypasses the digestive tract have been largely unsuccessful for two reasons. First, there are multiple feedback systems that can block any effect of a drug on one system. A drug that is truly effective on this system would also be toxic by inhibiting the adaptation to starvation. Second, the hedonic inputs to food intake and food addiction overcome the effects of these attempted medical and surgical cures since people eat when they are not hungry. The available drugs and surgical approaches will be discussed briefly, but they are often ineffective or toxic choices of last resort, rather than the initial or preventive treatment of obesity, which should always be based on diet and lifestyle. Psychology trumps physiology every time, and there are major behavioral inputs to food intake that require a combined physical and behavioral treatment approach.

5.2.3 Protein Is the Most Satiating Macronutrient

A great deal of research has established that protein-enriched meal replacements are effective in weight loss and weight maintenance largely through the effects of protein on satiety. In comparison with carbohydrate and fat, protein is the most satiating macronutrient, and when combined with resistance exercise, it preserves lean body mass during weight loss (Leidy et al. 2007). In the DIOGENES trial that spanned eight countries in Europe, a high-protein, low-glycemic-index diet was the only one of five possible combinations of control and high- and low-protein or high- and low-glycemic-index diets to maintain weight over 6 months following successful loss of weight over 8 weeks (McConnon et al. 2013). High-protein diets have also been shown to have positive effects on mood and cognitive function (Spring et al. 1983; Jakobsen et al. 2011; Zeng et al. 2011). Both in the short term and over the long term, protein is the most satiating macronutrient, even as snacks between meals (Lieberman et al. 1986). While most snack foods are high in fat, salt, and sugar, a study of high-protein soy snacks eaten between meals by adolescents improved appetite, satiety, and diet quality while beneficially influencing aspects of mood and cognition. Therefore, prescribing the right amount of protein from plant and animal sources is key to controlling hunger, and maintaining lean body mass and resting energy expenditure during weight loss in obese patients.

Just as no drug is a cure-all (see the next section), protein has an important role to play, but must be eaten within a daily diet plan with exercise and behavior change designed to have its maximum effect not only on hunger control, but also on maintenance of lean body mass and resting energy expenditure.

5.2.4 Drugs for Obesity

Lifestyle modifications such as diet and exercise intervention are essential for both prevention and management of obesity, and pharmacotherapy may be considered if the interventions are ineffective for individuals with a BMI of ≥30 kg/m^2 or for those with a BMI of ≥27 kg/m^2 when comorbidities, such as hypertension or type 2 diabetes mellitus, are present (Clinical Guidelines 1998). However, antiobesity drugs are a frequent adjunct, because these interventions have limited long-term success (Kaukua et al. 2003; Li et al. 2005), and often weight is regained when treatment is discontinued.

Phentermine is one of the centrally acting appetite-suppressant drugs of the β-phenethylamine family, which was approved for short-term (up to 3 months) use in the treatment of obesity by the U.S. Food and Drug Administration (FDA) in 1959 and remains available today. There are little data from large randomized controlled trials (RCTs) relating to the long-term efficacy or safety of phentermine, especially when used as monotherapy (Li et al. 2005).

As a substitute for phentermine, caffeine and green tea can help to increase mental energy and mobilize fat, and represent an alternative since phentermine is only approved for short-term use in the United States (Hursel and Westerterp-Plantenga 2013). In 2000, the European Medicines Agency (EMA) recommended the market withdrawal of phentermine due to an unfavorable risk-to-benefit ratio.

In the 1990s, fenfluramine and dexfenfluramine were withdrawn from the market because of heart valve damage (Connolly et al. 1997). The initial description including thickened valves was previously associated with endomyocarditis of starvation and pulmonary hypertension. Subsequent studies showed that the effects were largely reversed on discontinuation of the combination, which is no longer available (Mast et al. 2001).

The first selective endocannabinoid CB1 receptor blocker, rimonabant, was developed due to the idea that the reward circuits in the brain motivated eating in the absence of true hunger. By reducing the pleasure of eating, this drug was supposed to lead to weight loss. However, the drug was never approved by the U.S. FDA due to an increased risk of psychiatric adverse events, including depression, anxiety, and suicidal ideation (Christensen et al. 2007). Subsequently, rimonabant was withdrawn from the European market in 2009.

Sibutramine, a selective noradrenaline and serotonin reuptake inhibitor, was widely used after approval by the U.S. FDA in 1997. Sibutramine inhibited the decreases in blood pressure observed with weight loss but did not increase blood pressure. Nonetheless, there was concern expressed for cardiovascular risk associated with the use of this drug. Ultimately, sibutramine was withdrawn from the market voluntarily by the manufacturer (James et al. 2010).

For completeness, here are the other commonly prescribed and approved drugs that are rarely used by primary care physicians, and are largely restricted to bariatric or obesity medicine specialists.

Diethypropion is a sympathomimetic appetite suppressant available as a 25 mg immediate-release form or a 75 mg sustained-release form. The 25 mg form is taken 30 minutes before meals (Cercato et al. 2009). There is some concern about habituation to the use of this drug, which is contraindicated in individuals with cardiovascular disease (Cercato et al. 2009).

Combinations of drugs already approved for other indications have also been a source of new pharmacological approaches to obesity. A combination of naltrexone and burproprion has been approved and is based on the idea that addiction medicine is relevant to obesity. Both drugs have been used individually for addictions, including smoking and drug addiction (Apovian et al. 2013). Topiramate has been used alone and in combination with phentermine for the treatment of obesity (Shin and Gadde 2013; Paravattil et al. 2016). This drug was first discovered to be an antiseizure medication without the weight gain side effects of other commonly used antiseizure medications. Subsequently, weight loss was demonstrated in clinical trials.

Lorcaserin was developed due to its similarity to fenfluramine in an attempt to develop a serotonin-active agent without the side effects of fenfluramine (Apovian et al. 2016). The FDA approved two combination drugs for weight loss consisting of combinations of drugs already approved for other indications, including naltrexone combined with bupropion and topiramate with phentermine. In addition, they approved lorcaserin, which was similar to fenfluramine but had extensive research done demonstrating cardiovascular safety. In the end, the FDA approved these drugs given the health impacts of obesity on diabetes, heart disease, and many other diseases realizing that there were no approved drugs for this common condition increasingly becoming recognized by the public other than orlistat, which blocks fat absorption (Azebu 2014).

5.2.5 Surgical Approaches to Obesity

Surgery is attractive to obese and overweight patients since they can turn over this difficult problem to a surgeon. The appeal cannot be overestimated, as indicated by the popularity of many surgical approaches, including the lap-band, gastric sleeve, and Roux-en-Y bypass. A full description of the surgeries is outside the scope of this review. However, the unrealistic expectations of patients undergoing surgery for obesity have been well documented (Li and Heber 2014).

The amount of bariatric surgery being performed in the United States has changed dramatically over the past two decades. Between 2009 and 2012, the number of inpatient bariatric operations ranged from 81,005 to 114,780 cases annually (Nguyen et al. 2016). During this time period, the annual rate of bariatric procedures was highest for 2012, at 47.3 procedures per 100,000 adults. The bariatric surgery approach most commonly performed continues to be laparoscopic, ranging from 93.1% to 97.1%. In 2012, there was a precipitous reduction in the number of gastric bypass and gastric banding operations, which were replaced by an increase in the number of sleeve gastrectomy operations. The in-hospital mortality rate remains low, ranging from 0.07% to 0.10% overall, but is clearly higher in compromised patients. Therefore, surgery should be a last resort after other options have been exhausted, including a medically supervised very low-calorie diet as part of a multidisciplinary approach, which can also result in rapid weight loss to resolve medical issues.

5.3 IMPACT OF EXCESS BODY FAT ON HEALTH

The reason that the chapter title includes the phrase "The Elephant in the Room" is that excess fat in the abdomen, via its effects on metabolism and inflammation, is an important factor in the etiology and progression of many of the most common diseases in the primary care office, and yet it is rarely addressed in the process of prevention and treatment of the common chronic diseases described next. The interaction of nutrition with some of these conditions is detailed further in separate chapters, but the following subsections indicate the strength of the associations of these common age-related chronic diseases to unbalanced nutrition and a sedentary lifestyle, which leads to the accumulation of excess body fat.

5.3.1 Type 2 Diabetes Mellitus

Type 2 diabetes mellitus is the disease most closely associated with excess body fat. It is linked to visceral obesity and inflammation and follows the epidemic of obesity so closely that the term *diabesity* has been applied to this condition. Epidemiological studies using BMI have developed convincing evidence of this association. The Nurses' Health Study of 114,000 women followed for 14 years demonstrated that the risk of developing type 2 diabetes was 93 times higher among women who had a BMI of 35 or higher at the start of the study than among women with BMIs lower than 22 (Colditz et al. 1995). This risk factor is well out of the range of all other obesity-associated diseases, which typically are four to six times more common in obese than lean individuals. Weight gain during adulthood also increases diabetes risk, even among women with BMIs in the healthy range, pointing to the known association of type 2 diabetes with abdominal visceral fat. The Health Professionals Follow-Up Study found a similar association in men (Koh-Banerjee et al. 2004). Moderate weight loss can prevent or delay the start of diabetes in people who are at high risk (Tuomilehto et al. 2001; Knowler et al. 2002; Li et al. 2008).

5.3.2 Hypertension and Renal Disease

Abdominal visceral obesity is a major cause of hypertension, accounting for 65–75% of the risk for human primary or essential hypertension (Hall et al. 2015). Increased renal tubular sodium reabsorption plays a significant role in initiating obesity-induced hypertension, but this condition is mediated by several interrelated factors, including (1) physical compression of the kidneys due to excessive fat in and around the kidneys, (2) activation of the renin–angiotensin–aldosterone system by angiotensinogen secreted from adipocytes, and (3) increased sympathetic nervous system activity. Chronic obesity hypertension leads to renal injury. At this point, obesity-associated hypertension becomes more difficult to control, often requiring multiple antihypertensive drugs and treatment of other risk factors, including dyslipidemia, diabetes mellitus, and inflammation. The interaction of nutrition and renal disease is complex and will be dealt with in detail in Chapter 12.

5.3.3 Cardiovascular Diseases: Coronary Artery Disease and Stroke

Cardiovascular disease is the leading cause of death in patients with type 2 diabetes mellitus and obesity (Cho et al. 2002) and in those with chronic kidney disease (CKD) (Briasoulis and Bakris 2013), which is also associated with obesity. Diabetes and CKD are known independent risk factors for cardiovascular death, and patients with CKD are more likely to die from cardiovascular causes than to progress to end-stage renal disease. Diabetes increases the risk of cardiovascular disease, including coronary artery disease (CAD), stroke, peripheral artery disease, and heart failure (Boccara and Cohen 2004). The progression from diabetes to renal failure to heart disease–related death is an all too common scenario among patients seen in primary care. While common diseases occur frequently, in this case, these common diseases have a common etiology in excess abdominal visceral fat.

Numerous studies have demonstrated a direct association between excess body weight and CAD. While not perfect, since BMI is based on both lean body mass and fat mass, the correlations and associations in these large studies send a clear message. The BMI-CAD Collaboration Investigators conducted a meta-analysis of 21 long-term studies that followed more than 300,000 participants for an average of 16 years. Study participants who were overweight had a 32% higher risk of developing CAD than participants who were at a normal weight; those who were obese had an 81% higher risk (Bogers et al. 2007). Although adjustment for blood pressure and cholesterol levels slightly lowered the risk estimates, they remained highly significant for obesity. The investigators estimated that the effect of excess weight on blood pressure and blood cholesterol accounts for only about half of the obesity-related increased risk of coronary heart disease.

Since the vast majority of patients with type 2 diabetes are obese, these various disease conditions are closely interrelated to diet and lifestyle. Ischemic (clot-caused) stroke and CAD share many of the same disease processes and risk factors. A meta-analysis of 25 prospective cohort studies with 2.3 million participants demonstrated a direct, graded association between excess weight and stroke risk. Overweight increased the risk of ischemic stroke by 22%, and obesity increased it by 64%. There was no significant relationship between overweight or obesity and hemorrhagic (bleeding-caused) stroke, however (Strazzullo et al. 2010). A repeat analysis that statistically accounted for blood pressure, cholesterol, and diabetes weakened the associations, suggesting that these factors mediate the effect of obesity on stroke.

In a meta-analysis of 26 observational studies that included 390,000 men and women, several racial and ethnic groups, and samples from the United States and other countries, obesity was significantly associated with death from cardiovascular disease. Women with BMIs of 30 or higher had a 62% greater risk of dying early from heart disease, and also had a 53% higher risk of dying early from any type of cardiovascular disease, than women who had BMIs in the normal range (18.5–24.9). Men with BMIs of 30 or higher had similarly elevated risks (McGee and Diverse Populations Collaboration 2005).

Modest diet and lifestyle changes leading to a weight loss of 5–10% of body weight have been shown to lower blood pressure, LDL cholesterol, and triglycerides, and improve other cardiovascular risk factors (de las Fuentes et al. 2009; Dengo et al. 2010; Look AHEAD Research Group and Wing 2010).

5.3.4 Obesity and Cancer

The association between obesity and cancer is not quite as clear as that for diabetes and cardiovascular disease. This is due in part to the fact that cancer is not a single disease but a collection of individual diseases.

Cancer incidence varies among populations, organs, and tissues, and sometimes it is not possible to explain tumor occurrence by known potential determinants, such as environmental exposure, pathogens, or inherited genes. It is impossible to predict exactly who will develop a cancer and who will not. We know that several "risk factors" may increase the chance of getting cancer, and that risk increases with age. However, even with that in mind, only a subset of cancers can be explained based on diet and lifestyle.

In a paper published in the journal *Science*, Tomasetti and Vogelstein (2015) stated that most cancers are "due to bad luck," which refers to "random mutations arising in stem cells." As the number of mutations in all cells increase over time, age is a clear risk factor for cancer, so that studies looking at risk always look at age-adjusted cancer rates. Among patients, the idea that nothing can be done to prevent cancer is prevalent, and many patients take this to mean that they can live an unhealthy lifestyle with no impact on their risk of cancer.

In response to this hypothesis, researchers at the National Cancer Institute pointed out that there are many known factors that can influence cancer incidence, which can be summarized as age; sex; ethnic origin; geographic location; inheritance of susceptibility genes; overweight and obesity; lifestyle; exposure to carcinogens, including chemical; and physical and infectious agents, such as viruses or bacteria (Albini et al. 2015). Breast cancer risk is influenced by age at menarche, parity, hormonal status, and lactation. Prostate cancers, which account for about one-third of all male cancers, have few stem cells involved and have a clear relationship to diet and lifestyle. Many influential factors are still unknown, as are potential interactions among multiple factors.

A 2012 report from the Centers for Disease Control and Prevention highlighted the increased cancer risk associated with excess weight (overweight or obesity) and lack of sufficient physical activity (<150 minutes of physical activity per week). Death rates from all cancers combined decreased from 1999 to 2008, continuing a decline that began in the early 1990s, among both men and women in most racial and ethnic groups. Death rates decreased from 1999 to 2008 for most cancer sites, including the four most common cancers (lung, colorectal, breast, and prostate). The incidence of prostate and colorectal cancers also decreased from 1999 to 2008. Lung cancer incidence declined from 1999 to 2008 among men and from 2004 to 2008 among women. Breast cancer incidence decreased from 1999 to 2004, but was stable from 2004 to 2008.

Incidence increased for several cancers, including pancreas, kidney, and adenocarcinoma of the esophagus, which are all associated with excess weight. Although improvements are reported in the U.S. cancer burden, excess weight and lack of sufficient physical activity contribute to the increased incidence of many cancers, adversely affect quality of life for cancer survivors, and may worsen prognosis for several cancers. The report highlighted the importance of efforts to promote healthy weight and sufficient physical activity in reducing the cancer burden in the United States.

5.3.5 Obesity and Depression

Obesity and depression so frequently coexist, especially atypical depression, that the important clinical decision is to determine whether depression is secondary to obesity or, alternatively, driving overeating and a sedentary lifestyle. An analysis of 17 cross-sectional studies found that people who were obese were more likely to have depression than people with healthy weights (de Wit et al. 2010). The studies did not determine whether obesity increases the risk of depression or depression increases the risk of obesity. A meta-analysis of 15 long-term studies that followed 58,000 participants for up to 28 years found that people who were obese at the start of the study had a 55% higher risk of developing depression by the end of the follow-up period, and people who had depression at the start of the study had a 58% higher risk of becoming obese (Luppino et al. 2010). Possible mechanisms linking obesity and depression include inflammation, changes in the hypothalamic–pituitary–adrenal axis, insulin resistance, and social or cultural factors.

5.3.6 Obesity and Infertility

Polycystic ovarian syndrome (PCOS) was classically characterized by obesity, hirsutism, and infertility. It has been attributed to compensatory hyperinsulinemia due to insulin resistance. Elevated insulin levels have been thought to promote hyperandrogenism. However, physiological insulin infusion has no effect on androgen levels in PCOS (Gonzalez 2015). The cause of hyperandrogenism and ovarian dysfunction in the 30–50% of women with PCOS who are of normal weight and lack insulin resistance remains unexplained. Inflammation may also play a role in insulin resistance when present in PCOS, and visceral fat may not have been detected in those studies of PCOS where BMI is the sole measure of obesity utilized. Inflammation in PCOS is likely the result of excess abdominal adiposity.

The association between obesity and female infertility is represented by a classic U-shaped curve. In the Nurses' Health Study, infertility was lowest in women with BMIs between 20 and 24, and increased with lower and higher BMIs (Rich-Edwards et al. 2002). Eating disorders, malnutrition, and excessive exercise can all lead to infertility. About 25% of ovulatory infertility in the United States may be attributable to obesity. During pregnancy, obesity increases the risk of early and late miscarriage, gestational diabetes, preeclampsia, and complications during labor and delivery (Huda et al. 2010). It also slightly increases the chances of bearing a child with congenital anomalies (Stothard et al. 2009). One small randomized trial suggests that modest weight loss improves fertility in obese women (Clark et al. 1995).

In normal-weight males, the incidence of low sperm count and poor sperm motility were each increased with increasing BMI, by 5.3% and 4.5%, respectively. In obese men, these fertility parameters were increased by 15.6% and 13.3%, respectively (Hammoud et al. 2008). In contrast, a study by Chavarro and colleagues (2010) found little effect of body weight on semen quality, except at the highest BMIs (above 35), despite major differences in reproductive hormone levels with increasing weight.

Erectile dysfunction may also be affected by obesity. Data from the Health Professionals Follow-Up Study (Bacon et al. 2006), the National Health and Nutrition Examination Survey (NHANES) (Saigal et al. 2006), and the Massachusetts Male Aging Study (Johannes et al. 2000) indicate that the odds of developing erectile dysfunction increase with increasing BMI. Of note, weight loss appears to be mildly helpful in maintaining erectile function (Wing et al. 2010).

Obese women are less likely than normal-weight women to report having had a sexual partner in the preceding 12 months, but the prevalence of sexual dysfunction is similar in lean and obese women (Bajos et al. 2010). Obese women have been found to have lower scores on the Female Sexual Function Index and problems with arousal, orgasm, and satisfaction (Esposito et al. 2007).

5.3.7 Obesity and Pulmonary Diseases: Sleep Apnea and Asthma

Obesity very commonly leads to sleep apnea and impaired sleep quality, which can in turn perpetuate overweight and obesity. Concomitant treatment of sleep apnea with continuous positive airway pressure can both improve sleep quality and aid in weight reduction. Sleep questionnaire responses and the presence of snoring can be used to screen for sleep apnea in the obese patient (Raman et al. 2016).

Obesity impairs respiratory function via mechanical and metabolic pathways. Accumulation of abdominal fat can limit the descent of the diaphragm and lung expansion. Visceral fat can also reduce the flexibility of the chest wall, reduce respiratory muscle strength, and narrow airways in the lungs (McClean et al. 2008). Cytokines generated by the low-grade inflammatory state that accompanies obesity may also impede lung function.

In a meta-analysis of seven prospective studies that included 333,000 subjects, obesity was a major contributor to obstructive sleep apnea, which is estimated to affect approximately one in five adults. One in 15 adults has moderate or severe obstructive sleep apnea. This condition is associated with daytime sleepiness, accidents, hypertension, cardiovascular disease, and premature mortality. Between 50% and 75% of individuals with obstructive sleep apnea are obese (McClean et al. 2008). Clinical trials suggest that modest weight loss can be helpful when treating sleep apnea (Tuomilehto et al. 2009; Nerfeldt et al. 2010).

Asthma is now understood to be an inflammatory disease, with the bronchoconstriction that occurs no longer being the only therapeutic target. Obesity most likely, through inflammation, is linked to asthma pathophysiology (Beuther and Sutherland 2007).

5.3.8 Obesity in Aging and Brain Health

A recent systematic review and meta-analysis suggests a positive association between obesity in midlife and later dementia, but the opposite in late life (Pedditizi et al. 2016). The influence of obesity on dementia has been a subject of controversy for many years. A meta-analysis of studies suggest that obesity and central obesity seem to play an independent role in the etiology of Alzheimer's disease and in some cases of vascular dementia, even when sociodemographic, lifestyle, and health-related comorbid factors are controlled (Beydoun et al. 2008). Overall, there seems to be a U-shaped relation between BMI status and dementia, with both obesity and underweight increasing the risk of dementia. Whether weight reduction in midlife reduces risk is worthy of further study. A short-term healthy lifestyle program combining mental and physical exercise, stress reduction, and healthy diet was associated with significant effects on cognitive function and brain metabolism (Small et al. 2006).

5.3.9 Obesity and Musculoskeletal Disorders

Among the most common complaints of markedly obese patients are knee pain, back pain, and ankle pain. Excess weight places significant mechanical and metabolic strains on bones, muscles, and joints. Osteoarthritis of the knee and hip is positively associated with obesity, and obese patients account for one-third of all joint replacement operations (Anandacoomarasamy et al. 2008). Obesity also increases the risk of back pain, lower limb pain, and disability due to musculoskeletal conditions.

5.3.10 Obesity and Fatty Liver Disease

Nonalcoholic fatty liver disease is the most common liver disease worldwide, progressing from simple steatosis to fibrosis and nonalcoholic steatohepatitis (NASH). As NASH advances, it leads in some cases to cirrhosis and hepatocellular carcinoma (Katsiki et al. 2016). Inflammation, oxidative stress, and insulin resistance are involved in the development and progression of these conditions. Fatty liver has been associated with obesity, dyslipidemia, hyperglycemia, and hypertension.

5.3.11 Gallstones and Gout

A number of additional health outcomes have been linked to excess weight. These include the development of gallstones in men (Tsai et al. 2004) and women (Stampfer et al. 1992), as well as gout (Choi et al. 2005; Bhole et al. 2010).

5.3.12 Bottom Line on Obesity and Health

Obesity harms virtually every aspect of health, from contributing to chronic conditions, such as diabetes and cardiovascular disease, to interfering with sexual function, breathing, mood, and social interactions. Prevention of obesity—beginning at an early age and extending across the life span—could vastly improve individual and public health, reduce suffering, and save billions of dollars each year in health care costs.

5.4 DETERMINING THE OBESITY PHENOTYPE

This chapter deals with both overweight and obese patients who are obviously overweight or obese. That weight is most likely a combination of excess fat and increased lean body mass in most obese and obviously overweight patients. As we saw in Chapter 2, many individuals who appear to be of normal weight have excess body fat. Attempts to divide up the obese, overweight, normal weight with excess body fat, and overweight with excess lean body mass fall under the general area of obesity phenotypes or body shape. The latter classifications have been expanded by the clothing industry into a large number of fashion shapes, such as rectangles, triangles, pear shape, and apple shape, for the purposes of design. That type of classification is not what will be reviewed here. Rather, the impact of obesity phenotypes on obesity-associated diseases and the need to customize and personalize approaches to treatment and prevention are the focus of the balance of this chapter.

While BMI has generally been the most widely used tool to screen for obesity, about 10–25% of those patients classified as obese (Bluher 2010) and a subgroup of clearly obese patients (Soverini et al. 2010) are not affected by metabolic changes, such as those defining MetS, type 2 diabetes, or hyperlipidemia (Brochu et al. 2001; Karelis et al. 2005; Stefan et al. 2008; Wildman et al. 2008). These metabolically healthy obese patients are insulin sensitive and have increased lean body mass. They typically have normal blood pressure, a favorable lipid profile, a lower proportion of visceral fat, less liver fat, and a normal glucose metabolism despite having excess body fat (Reaven et al. 1996; Ruderman et al. 1998; Sims 2001; Karelis et al. 2004a,b; Aguilar-Salinas et al. 2008; Lynch et al. 2009; Messier et al. 2010). At the other end of the spectrum, there are many normal-weight individuals with metabolic changes characteristic of obesity (Conus et al. 2007). These patients are called "metabolically obese, normal-weight individuals." Thus, obesity consists of different subtypes with different metabolic profiles (Figure 5.3).

The survey from Figure 5.3 included 205 individuals (80 men and 125 women) of normal weight who had MetS and 94 obese individuals (27 men and 67 women) without MetS (Pajunen et al. 2011). MetS was defined by three or more of the following five components: increased waist circumference (≥94 cm in men and ≥80 cm in women), hypertriglyceridemia (≥1.7 mmol/L), HDL cholesterol level of <1.0 mmol/L in men or <1.3 mmol/L in women, elevated blood pressure (systolic ≥130 mmHg and/or diastolic ≥85 mmHg) or antihypertensive drug treatment or history of hypertension, and elevated fasting plasma glucose of ≥5.6 mmol/L or drug treatment.

A metabolically healthy but obese phenotype was observed in 9.2% of obese men and in 16.4% of obese women (Figure 5.3). Among all participants, the prevalence of healthy obesity was 2.0% among men and 4.5% among women. Of the normal-weight individuals, 20.4% of men and 23.8% of women had MetS. These data clearly demonstrate that it is important to determine the metabolic phenotype in patients regardless of whether BMI categorization indicates normal weight, overweight, or obesity.

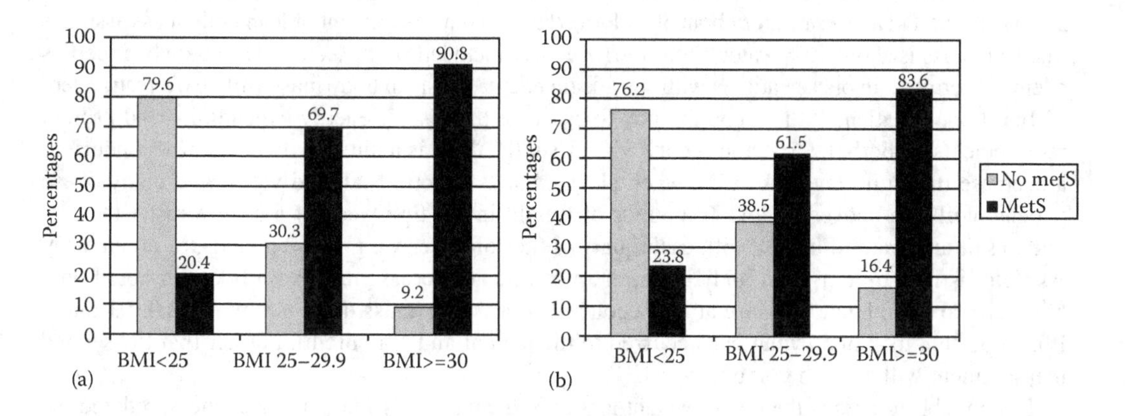

FIGURE 5.3 Prevalence of persons with and without MetS within each BMI category among men (a) and among women (b) (total 100% within the BMI class). (Reprinted from Pajunen, P. et al., *BMC Public Health*, 11, 754, 2011.)

Having tackled the metabolic aspects of obesity phenotypes based on weight or BMI, it is also important to consider what the patient perceives. The body image is the perception of patients about their weight, which refers to their ability to estimate the size and shape of the body. The difference between a person's perception of his or her body size and ideal body size is related to body satisfaction (Dounchis et al. 2001). Body image dissatisfaction and distortion are common among obese patients, so a reality check based on body composition measurements is warranted, along with a discussion of an appropriate target weight.

Body weight and body image are often considered as one by patients, but they can be very different. Assessments of weight loss expectations by asking subjects to indicate their "dream" weight, weight values that they would be "happy" with, body weights they would consider "acceptable," and those they would be "disappointed" with at the end of a weight loss intervention have been used to study the impact of body image on the success of weight loss and weight maintenance (Foster et al. 1997). Having a realistic body image is a pretreatment variable significantly associated with successful weight loss and weight maintenance (Traverso et al. 2000; Schwartz and Brownell 2004). Unrealistic weight loss expectations can result in weight management failure and dropping out of treatment regimens (Fowler et al. 1985; Bennett and Jones 1986; McLean et al. 2016).

Negative body image and quality of life are closely linked with obesity (Brown et al. 1990), and compared with normal-weight individuals, obese patients are more dissatisfied and preoccupied with physical appearance, and avoid more social situations because of their appearance concerns (Ramirez and Rosen 2001). Overall, body image dissatisfaction has been described as the most consistent psychosocial consequence of obesity (Sarwer et al. 2005).

5.5 ESTIMATING ENERGY EXPENDITURE AND PROTEIN REQUIREMENTS

One of the great advantages of bioelectrical impedance analysis is that the amount of lean mass is measured directly with an accuracy of about 95%. It is sometimes called fat-free mass, and it is the only directly measured body composition parameter, since lean mass is about 70% water, which conducts electricity, while fat is an insulator that acts as an electrical capacitor. All the other estimates, such as percent body fat, are derived from the total body weight and the lean body mass through calculations. The algorithms for even lean body mass differ among different manufacturers, and all these equations incorporate weight, height, age, and gender.

Nonetheless, the lean body mass serves as a means to provide personalized information to patients, including estimates of resting energy expenditure, rate of weight loss on set number of calories eaten each day, and a range of target weights based on body fat, which is approximate.

The resting energy expenditure is directly related to lean body mass, so that 1 pound of lean mass on average burns 14 calories/day, or about 30 calories/kg. Since measurement of lean body mass assumes that lean mass is about 70% water, fluid is erroneously included in the lean body mass when there is edema. Therefore, in obese patients with significant edema, the lean body mass will be overestimated.

In all obese patients, it is a good policy to estimate the resting energy expenditure and protein requirements on both the first and second visit. Usually, there is a diuresis that occurs secondary to a decrease in insulin levels. Insulin, when elevated, acts to retain salt and water, and many obese patients will lose between 5 and 10 pounds of weight in the first week of a calorie-restricted diet due to salt and water diuresis, with each quart or liter of water weighing 2 pounds, or about 1 kg. As water is measured as lean body mass, there can be an increase in percent body fat noted on a bioelectrical impedance measure at the second visit, as water mass decreases more than fat mass. It is important to explain what has occurred to the patient and reassure him or her that the second measurement will be used going forward.

It is possible to predict the rate of weight loss once the lean body mass has been measured and the resting energy expenditure calculated after the first week (Korth et al. 2007). For every 500 calories below the resting energy expenditure recommended in the nutrition intervention, there will be a weight loss of about 1 pound/week.

The resting energy expenditure can also be helpful in communicating to patients that you understand their weight history. A female patient with a resting energy expenditure of 1200 calories/day is someone who has dieted religiously with poor weight loss results, but may not have added in daily exercise to boost her metabolism. On the other hand, a large man who burns 2500 calories/day at rest and loves to eat red meat may be someone who has no trouble losing weight but has never worked very hard at maintaining a healthy body weight over time. By simply cutting his steak in half, he can lose 15 or 20 pounds, but inevitably, the weight is regained as his eating habits return over time, to include high-fat, high-sugar foods. The concept that he can get away with eating more calories due to a high resting metabolic rate contributes to the notion that he is not vulnerable to gaining weight.

This collection of potential educational information for patients derived from a simple measurement will also help establish your expertise in the eyes of your patients. The greater their confidence in your guidance, the greater is the likelihood that they will be successful in a specific weight management intervention.

5.6 PROVIDING STRUCTURED DIET PROGRAMS THAT INCLUDE CHOICE

For many obese patients, a highly structured diet using meal replacements and portion-controlled food is desirable. While for many individuals, including food is essential, as a single meal, the idea that you are simply going to get someone to lose large amounts of excess body fat with minimal changes to his or her diet and lifestyle is not realistic.

A highly structured program will lead to the most predictable rates of weight loss and provide an opportunity for education on weight maintenance after weight loss. While some patients will tolerate a diet of complete meal replacements classically used in very low-calorie diets, others want at least one meal per day. The experience of more than 2000 patients with obesity, prediabetes, or diabetes demonstrated comparable rates of weight loss using the diet program described below (Li et al. 2014).

At the University of California, Los Angeles (UCLA) Risk Factor Obesity Clinic, we utilize two different meal replacements. One of the formulas provides 100 calories with 15 g of protein, 10 g of carbohydrate, and no fat, and the other provides 142 calories with 25 g of protein, about 10 g of carbohydrate, and no fat. Using these formulas, the following typical examples apply:

- A woman, 62 inches tall, weighing 150 pounds, with 100 pounds of lean body mass. At a resting energy expenditure of 1400 calories/day, she would be prescribed seven servings of the 100-calorie supplement, delivering 700 calories and 105 g of protein. She would be expected to lose about 1.5 pounds/week to a target weight she would help to choose of between 120 and 130 pounds.
- The same woman returns 3 weeks later and complains that she can no longer live on shakes alone. She wants to have one meal. Her plan would now shift to four meal replacements of 100 calories each and one meal of about 500 calories. This would reduce her rate of weight loss to 1 pound/week. The meal should be structured to include a 25 g portion of protein, such as 4 ounces of chicken, tofu, or fish; 2 cups of steamed vegetables; and a salad seasoned with lemon or rice vinegar. An alternative for some patients will be a frozen dinner and salad.
- A man, 71 inches tall, weighing 240 pounds, with a lean body mass of 175 pounds, would be prescribed 175 g of protein from seven 25 g protein shakes, each at about 140 calories, for a total calorie intake of about 1000 calories/day. At a resting energy expenditure of 2450 calories/day, he will lose about 3 pounds/week to a target weight of 210–220 pounds.
- This man simply cannot stand having just liquids after 1 week. However, given his high resting energy expenditure, you have the ability to provide him with a food meal that is carefully constructed with a 50 g portion of protein (8 ounces of chicken breast, turkey,

or ocean-caught fish), providing 280 calories, in combination with steamed vegetables and a salad with rice or wine vinegar, providing about 500 calories in total. This would eliminate two of the protein shakes, or 280 calories, making the net increase in total calorie intake about 220 calories, which will only reduce the rate of weight loss by ½ pound/week. Of course, exercise daily will increase lean body mass in men and reduce fat mass in comparison with simply restricting calories.

Once the target weight range is reached, the diet can be liberalized so that there is only one shake per day taken at breakfast. Patients who regain their weight can reenter the very low-calorie or low-calorie diet intervention multiple times and still expect to lose weight at the same rate as they did initially (Li et al. 2007). This information can be very helpful to patients fearing failure after multiple weight loss attempts. I usually tell them to plan to reenter if they regain their weight, noting that Mark Twain reportedly tried to stop smoking 10 times. Attendance at weekly group meetings and regular physical activity, as discussed in the next section, will help with weight maintenance and internalization of new diet and lifestyle habits. In terms of diets for weight maintenance in the long term, the DIOGENES trial has shown a high-protein, low-glycemic-index diet to lead to weight maintenance over 6 months after an 8-week weight loss on a very low-calorie diet, while high-protein, high-glycemic-index and low-protein with either high- or low-glycemic-index foods led to weight regain (Aller et al. 2014).

5.7 LEISURE TIME PHYSICAL ACTIVITY AND EXERCISE

Reductions in energy expenditure, secondary to sedentary lifestyles, have been identified as a key factor in the obesity epidemic (Peters et al. 2002; Wareham et al. 2005). Both leisure time physical activity and exercise that are associated with bodily movement result in increased energy expenditure and account for the variation in daily energy expenditure among individuals with similar lean body mass.

Given the reduction in the requirement for physical activity at work and for activities of daily living over the past several decades (Church et al. 2011; Archer et al. 2013), exercise during leisure time has become an important component of total physical activity and total daily energy expenditure (Westerterp 2003). While physical activity includes leisure time and work-related or transport-related movement, exercise consists of planned and structured physical activities (Caspersen et al. 1985). A recent meta-analysis showed that exercise and sport have a stronger association with mortality than do occupational or transport-related physical activity (Samitz et al. 2011).

Aerobic exercise has been associated with an increase in energy expenditure in young adults (Westerterp 2008). However, differences in exercise type should be considered in terms of both energy expenditure during exercise and the differential effect on energy expenditure after exercise. Aerobic exercise has been shown to increase resting energy expenditure for up to 19 hours after exercise (Hunter et al. 2006), while resistance exercise has been associated with an increase in functional capacity, which could secondarily lead to an increase in total energy expenditure by enabling an increase in total physical activity (Hunter et al. 2000; Levinger et al. 2007).

An example of how lifestyle can affect physical activity is an Australian study of time spent sitting in a car commuting (Sugiyama et al. 2016). Among 2800 participants in this study, prolonged time spent sitting in cars, in particular more than 1 hour/day, was associated with higher total and central adiposity and a more adverse cardiometabolic risk profile.

Twin studies of 10 pairs of twins showed a 31% higher amount of intra-abdominal fat measure by MRI in inactive twins over the prior 3 years compared with active twins (Rottensteiner et al. 2016).

The only major component of daily energy expenditure that can be voluntarily influenced is physical activity through the replacement of sedentary activities by various kinds of muscle motor activity, from standing rather than sitting to walking, running, swimming, or bicycling. Walking or bicycling instead of driving a car for short trips would expend additional calories while traveling the same distance.

Despite the physiological increase in energy expenditure that occurs and the role that physical activity plays in addressing obesity from a behavioral viewpoint, it appears to produce only modestly increased weight losses beyond those caused by dietary measures alone, and these effects are variable among different individuals (Stefanick 1993). In numerous studies where increased physical activity is the only intervention, or in which it was added to dietary restriction, the component of weight loss ascribable to exercise has been modest (Hunter et al. 2010).

Despite the observations of small effects on weight loss, observational studies have developed evidence that physical activity can help prevent weight regain after an initial sizable weight loss (Schoeller et al. 1997; Klem et al. 2000; Wing and Hill 2001; Weinsier et al. 2002; Nelson et al. 2007). These studies examined the effects of exercise in people who had lost between 30 and 50 pounds with maintained weight over several years. These studies used the technique of doubly labeled water, which depends on the ratio of carbon-14 and oxygen-18 measured in urine samples, together with a measure of the respiratory quotient (RQ), which is the ratio of the carbon dioxide production to oxygen utilization (Schoeller et al. 1997). This method measures total energy expenditure encompassing both changes in dietary intake and exercise. Extrapolation from these carefully conducted studies has led to the concept that 60–90 minutes of moderate-intensity physical activity per day may be necessary for weight maintenance after weight loss.

When writing an exercise prescription for moderate-intensity physical activity, it is important to be able to be somewhat specific, rather than simply saying "exercise more." One method for estimating energy expenditure during physical activity is the metabolic equivalent (MET) (Ainsworth et al. 2000a). One MET represents the energy expended while sitting quietly. Walking at 3 mph on a flat, hard surface will lead to the expenditure of about 3.3 METs. Jogging or running on a flat surface at a pace in which a mile is completed in about 12 minutes (about 5 mph) will expend approximately 8 METs (Table 5.1).

For example, a person who walked at 3 mph for 30 minutes would accumulate 99 MET-minutes of credited activity, which over 5 days/week would total 495 MET-minutes. If the patient jogged at 5 mph for 20 minutes, he or she would accumulate 160 MET-minutes (8 METs × 20 minutes = 160 MET-minutes). He or she could do this higher level of activity for only 20 minutes on 3 days and derive the same benefit. The advantage of dosing exercise recommendations in this way is that it provides flexibility to patients in both meeting their needs and assessing the effectiveness of their overall activities. While the subject has been previously discussed in terms of general recommendations for a healthy population, the intensity of the recommendation for the maintenance of weight in the obese population requires greater attention. When combining moderate- and vigorous-intensity activity to meet the exercise recommendations for prevention of weight regain, the minimum goal should be in the range of 450–750 MET-minutes/week. These values are based on the MET range of 3–6 for moderate-intensity activity and 150 minutes/week (3 METs × 150 minutes = 450 MET-minutes and 6 METs × 150 minutes = 750 MET-minutes).

Obese patients should start at the lower end of this range at the beginning of any prescribed activity program and slowly advance to the higher activity levels as they become more fit.

Personalized lifestyle change is vital in facilitating a physical activity prescription over the long term (Kahn et al. 2002). To achieve long-term changes in behavior, medical, behavioral, social, and environmental factors need to be comprehensively addressed (Sallis et al. 2002). Obese individuals often have increased lean mass, but maintaining or increasing lean mass can help to maintain energy expenditure after weight loss and will also have functional benefits on the activities of daily living. Resistance training at least twice per week provides a safe and effective method to improve muscular strength and endurance (Pollock et al. 2000). It is recommended that 8–10 exercises be performed on two or more nonconsecutive days each week using the major muscles. A resistance (weight) should be used that results in substantial fatigue after 8–12 repetitions of each exercise. Primary care professionals can broaden their advice to patients beyond the traditional prescriptive program based on medical clearance and supervision by encouraging them to accumulate moderate-intensity physical activity. Different activities should be identified that meet each person's interests, needs, schedule, and environment, and take into consideration family, work, and social

TABLE 5.1
MET Values for a Variety of Physical Activities That Are of Light, Moderate, or Vigorous Intensity

Light, <3.0 METs	Moderate, 3.0–6.0 METs	Vigorous, >6.0 METs
Walking Walking slowly around home, store, or office = 2.0[a]	Walking Walking 3.0 mph = 3.3[a] Walking at a very brisk pace (4 mph) = 5.0[a]	Walking, jogging, and running Walking at a very brisk pace (4.5 mph) = 6.3[a] Walking/hiking at moderate pace and grade with no or light pack (<10 pounds) = 7.0 Hiking at steep grades and pack 10–42 pounds = 7.5–9.0 Jogging at 5 mph = 8.0[a] Jogging at 6 mph = 10.0[a] Running at 7 mph = 11.5[a]
Household and occupation Sitting—using computer work at desk, using light hand tools = 1.5 Standing—performing light work such as making bed, washing dishes, ironing, preparing food, or working as a store clerk = 2.0–2.5	Cleaning—heavy: Washing windows or car, cleaning garage = 3.0 Sweeping floors or carpet, vacuuming, mopping = 3.0–3.5 Carpentry—general = 3.6 Carrying and stacking wood = 5.5 Mowing lawn—pushing power mower = 5.5	Shoveling sand, coal, etc. = 7.0 Carrying heavy loads, such as bricks = 7.5 Heavy farming, such as baling hay = 8.0 Shoveling, digging ditches = 8.5
Leisure time and sports Arts and crafts, playing cards = 1.5 Billards = 2.5 Boating—power = 2.5 Croquet = 2.5 Darts = 2.5 Fishing—sitting = 2.5 Playing most musical instruments = 2.0–2.5	Badminton—recreational = 4.5 Basketball—shooting around = 4.5 Bicycling—on flat: Light effort (10–12 mph) = 6.0 Dancing—ballroom slow = 3.0; ballroom fast = 4.5 Fishing from riverbank and walking = 4.0 Golf—walking and pulling clubs = 4.3 Sailing boat, wind surfing = 3.0 Swimming leisurely = 6.0[b] Table tennis = 4.0 Tennis doubles = 5.0 Volleyball—noncompetitive = 3.0–4.0	Basketball game = 8.0 Bicycling—on flat: Moderate effort (12–14 mph) = 8.0; fast (14–16 mph) = 10 Skiing cross-country—slow (2.5 mph) = 7.0; fast (5.0–7.9 mph) = 9.0 Soccer—casual = 7.0; competitive = 10.0 Swimming—moderate/hard = 8–11[b] Tennis singles = 8.0 Volleyball—competitive at gym or beach = 8.0

Source: Adapted from Ainsworth, B. E. et al., *Med. Sci. Sports Exerc.*, 32(9), S498–S504, 2000b; Haskell, W. L. et al., *Med. Sci. Exec.*, 39(8), 1423–1434, 2007.

[a] On flat, hard surface.

[b] MET values can vary substantially from person to person during swimming as a result of different strokes and skin levels.

commitments. It is also helpful to have options for travel, such as portable exercise bands, and strategies for exercising indoors when there is bad weather. Materials for patient education and counseling are available from the National Institutes of Health (U.S. Department of Health and Human Services 2006), the American College of Sports Medicine (2003), and the American Heart Association (2016).

For primary care professionals, the challenge is to increase their professional credibility with patients in the areas of nutrition and exercise by advising patients to undertake physical activity programs that are designed to overcome barriers to long-term adherence, using effective behavioral management and environmental change strategies, so that more patients can benefit from a healthy active lifestyle.

5.8 BEHAVIORAL STRATEGIES THAT WORK

Government advisory groups in the United States have recommended that clinicians screen all adults for obesity and offer intensive multicomponent behavioral interventions to affected individuals, either by providing such treatment themselves or by referring patients to appropriate interventions (Moyer 2012). Reimbursement for these services has been authorized by the U.S. Centers for Medicare and Medicaid Services. Specifically, reimbursement is contingent on the provision of intensive behavioral counseling to obese seniors in primary care practice delivered by physicians, nurse practitioners, or physician assistants from the practice (Jacques et al. 2011). It was recommended that practitioners provide brief (15 minutes) weekly counseling sessions for the first month, followed by every-other-week visits for an additional 5 months. Patients who lose more than 3 kg in the first 6 months (in these 14 sessions) are eligible for six additional monthly visits.

The provision of behavioral weight loss counseling in primary care practices has been met with limited success, in most cases producing mean weight losses of only 1–3 kg in 6–24 months. These modest weight losses were most likely secondary to the infrequent treatment contacts, typically at monthly to quarterly intervals, as well as to the brief duration of visits, usually lasting only 10–15 minutes. This low-intensity behavioral treatment may be all that can be practically delivered in busy outpatient practices.

On the other hand, studies with greater intensity in academic medical centers have produced weight losses of 7–10%. It is not fair to compare the results of underfunded pilot studies conducted in primary care with findings in well-funded research settings that may not be generalizable (Leblanc et al. 2011).

A more practical approach for primary care practices may be remotely delivered, high-intensity behavioral weight loss counseling. It has been demonstrated that 12 weekly telephone sessions of 20 minutes each, followed by monthly calls, induced a mean loss of 6.1 kg at 6 months and 4.6 kg at 24 months. These losses were similar to those found with face-to-face interventions that combined both group and individual visits.

A number of other trials, outside of primary care practices, using telephone-based counseling alone, have found results comparable to those of on-site interventions (Logue et al. 2005; Donnelly et al. 2007; Perri et al. 2008). Remotely delivered lifestyle counseling, whether provided by a primary care practice or by a call center with which it has contracted, would appear to be a very convenient option for patients. More importantly, it would support primary care practices so that they could offer intensive behavioral counseling without overwhelming practice schedules.

5.8.1 Widely Accepted Behavioral Strategies

Clearly, behavioral interventions are very personal, and what is appropriate for one person may not be for another. Nonetheless, there are some general principles that apply to behavior change that may already be familiar to you. However, the key to successful behavioral intervention is following a stages of change or transtheoretical model for behavior change, popularized by Prochaska and DiClemente (Velicer et al. 1990) and widely accepted in the psychology and social services community not only for obesity but also for smoking cessation, drug addiction, and alcoholism.

The stages of change are as follows: (1) precontemplation (unaware of the problem), (2) contemplation (aware of the problem and wants to change), (3) preparation (intends to take action), (4) action (practices the desired behavior), and (5) maintenance (works to sustain behavior change). For stage 1, it is important to point out issues around obesity and overweight in a health context. The psychosocial morbidity of obesity makes patients extremely sensitive, and leading a careful conversation to draw out the awareness of the patient is helpful and is called motivational interviewing in the obesity literature. For stage 2, there is a common 10-point scale used to determine readiness to change. For stage 3, it is important to establish a date to begin the new changed behaviors. For stage 4, the actions have to be very simple. Sometimes, there is too much nutrition information given, so that patients are confused as to what to do. I typically provide them with a "trigger foods list" that contains the foods they should not eat and, together with a dietitian, develop a daily diet at a personalized calorie level in the form of a daily menu of foods to eat.

As noted in Figure 5.4, relapse can occur at any one of the stages of change. Addiction theory, which includes relapse prevention, plays a role in the maintenance of new behaviors that promote weight maintenance. Relapse prevention incorporates a number of approaches, but is based on the idea that behavior lapses are extremely common and have an antecedent cause and a consequence. Charting lapses is the first step in prevention. The ABC theory of antecedents, behaviors, and consequences can help patients identify the motivators of the lapse. A series of lapses is called a relapse, and continued relapses lead to collapse.

Even when collapse occurs, patients should be encouraged to initiate the process again by getting ready to change. As already reviewed, there is no reason that patients will not be able to change again. It is helpful to indicate that one of the hardest things for patients to accomplish is behavior changes, and that multiple attempts are not uncommon. Allaying fear of failure is an important part of encouraging patients to undertake a new diet and lifestyle for weight management.

Cognitive behavioral therapy engages the thinking brain to control emotional urges around eating. This often requires blending nutritional and behavioral approaches. While there is some dietary composition research reviewed in Chapter 2 with regard to the benefits of a high-protein and low-glycemic-index diet in promoting weight maintenance after weight loss, there is clearly much more at work in maintenance. Psychology trumps physiology as patients snack on high-fat, high-sugar foods out of habit, in response to stress, or simply because of boredom. Teaching patients to get into a daily rhythm of eating and exercise in which they recognize hunger and thirst normally is important. Hunger is driven by gut hormones and nutrient signals and is heralded by stomach rumbles and a sensation of emptiness. Stimulus control, stress reduction, and social support are important components of an integrated behavioral approach. Stimulus control is simply planning appropriately for future events. The simple example is that if you know that you are going to step on a cold floor in the morning, put out slippers at the side of your bed the night before. In planning the diet, packing foods for trips or deciding on healthy dinners in advance to avoid excessive restaurant eating or fast-food eating at the last moment is an important strategy for weight maintenance.

Much snacking behavior is simply an attempt to avoid the natural feelings of hunger. Sometimes, if the snack is healthy, such as nuts or a small protein snack in the afternoon, this can be helpful in

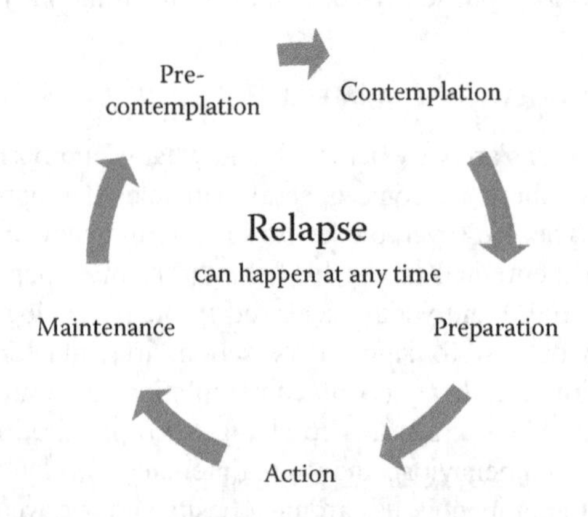

FIGURE 5.4 Stages of change. (Adapted from Prochaska, J. O., and C. C. DiClemente, *J. Consult. Clin. Psychol.*, 51(3), 390–395, 1983 and described in detail in the text.)

maintaining a daily pattern of eating. On the other hand, night snacking, which occurs in about a quarter of obese patients, is associated with excessive snack food consumption. The food industry over the last 40 years has promoted snacking through the development of many snack foods listed in the trigger food list:

1. Colas: A can of cola or soda has 150 calories; a big drink has more than 600! Have plain water or mineral water with a slice of lemon or lime. Have fruit instead of fruit juices or flavor water with juice to reduce calories, but recognize that some fruit juices can provide phytonutrients (tomato, pomegranate, and orange juices), in addition to vitamins, minerals, and water. Fruit juices are often only partially made with fruit juice. Some guava juices are only 15% juice, but have high-fructose corn syrup added for sweetness so that they provide 150 calories in 8 ounces. Using 100% fruit juices is a way to avoid this issue.
2. Snack chips and movie popcorn: A small bag of potato chips or corn chips can have as many as 400 calories. At a restaurant, a basket of corn chips can have as many as 550 calories. Movie popcorn with added oil can have 1200 calories in a large serving. Air-popped popcorn will have much fewer calories.
3. Bread and pastries: There are more than 1200 calories in the typical loaf of bread. Choose a high-fiber bread with about 80 calories/slice. Bread should be limited to one or two slices per day. Ordering bread before a restaurant meal and then ordering a second serving is a very common stress-related behavior.
4. Frozen yogurt, ice cream, cakes, and pastries: These desserts add lots of extra calories as fat and sugar. Even the fat-free versions pack in many extra calories as sugar with too little protein. Mixed fruits are an excellent dessert choice even when dressed with a small amount of chocolate or cream.
5. Cheese and pizza: Hard cheese has up to 80% fat, and even nonfat cheese is 80 calories/slice. American pizza is a popular trigger food composed largely of fat and refined carbohydrates that is sold based on the taste provided by added oil, salt, and sugar with little protein. In Italy, thin-crust pizza made without the added oil of deep-dish pizza is a healthier alternative. This type of pizza is also available in restaurants in the United States, but not typically in large fast-food pizza franchises.
6. Red meat and fatty fish: One of the easiest ways to reduce excess calories is by limiting consumption of red meat and fatty fish. Red meat includes veal, beef, pork, and lamb. One 14-ounce cut of prime rib has about 1500 calories and 50 g of fat. That is the total of fat and calories many women require daily. A fast-food burger, milkshake, and fries have about 1300 calories and about 50% fat calories. Substituting skinless white meat of chicken or white meat of turkey for red meat will reduce calories while maintaining protein intake. If it will help those who enjoy savory tastes, suggest putting steak sauce on chicken to imitate the taste of seasoned red meat. Dark poultry meat is higher in fat than white meat and can have as much fat as some types of red meat. Dark poultry meat is included in many restaurant dishes to reduce tastes, and is preferred in many Asian recipes. However, white meat of chicken or turkey or firm tofu is easily incorporated into many recipes without reducing taste. Salmon, trout, and catfish that are farm fed are high in total fat. While the content of omega-3 fatty acids is similar in farmed and ocean-caught salmon, the farmed variety have twice as much omega-6, in addition to omega-3. Substituting halibut, cod, sole, canned white tuna packed in water, orange roughy, red snapper, or Hawaiian fish will reduce calorie and fat intake. Shrimp, scallops, lobster, and crab are also low in fat and have healthy omega-3.
7. Mayonnaise, margarine, and butter: There is no daily margarine requirement. Even the fat-free varieties (like ultra-fat-free margarine) are 100% fat. According to the law, these can be labeled as fat-free because they have less than 0.5 g of fat/serving. Reducing bread intake, which can be a trigger food, is important, but as a regular behavior, adding

margarine, mayonnaise, or butter to bread adds little additional taste and needless extra calories.

8. Salad dressing: Chinese chicken salad, prepared in many restaurants with dressing, can provide up to 1000 calories. Both creamy and oil-based salad dressings provide, on average, 150 calories and 10–20 g of fat/ounce. Dressings, including so-called low-fat varieties add significant calories to salads, and their portion control is often problematic. Balsamic vinegar, rice vinegar, lemon, and wine vinegar are good alternatives. Salads with dark green lettuce, tomatoes, alfalfa sprouts, green pepper, and other vegetables will add taste variety, so the taste of the salad is not dependent on salad dressing.
9. Rice, beans, and nuts: Rice and beans both provide about 250 calories/cup. Substituting seasoned vegetables without butter for rice will reduce calories. Peanuts and some other nuts can be a trigger food, depending on the context in which they are eaten. Having 2 ounces of pistachios, almonds, peanuts, or walnuts as a snack is a healthy choice as long as there is a small portion package with listed calories. However, having large portions of rice, beans, or nuts can add calories in significant amounts to the diet.

5.9 FOLLOW-UP AND SOCIAL SUPPORT

Follow-up of patients with frequent contact is one of the greatest challenges for primary care weight management. Self-help and group support programs directed by educated lay health coaches are a resource that can be employed to address this vexing issue. The increasing prevalence of obesity and overweight has been mirrored by a parallel increase in the number of programs utilizing group support. Research evaluating these programs is limited compared with the large numbers of individuals participating and the research available on weight management in clinical settings.

Weight Watchers was incorporated in 1963 to become a commercial weight loss program based on groups of individuals coming together for self-help. As it developed, Weight Watchers incorporated a structured diet and exercise plan within a strong behavioral program designed by experts in the field. Weight Watchers maintained a fee schedule affordable to lower- and middle-income persons. Early in its history, Weight Watchers became a convenient database for researchers who were no doubt attracted by its large membership (Misovich 1973; Stuart and Guire 1978; Hall et al. 1986; Andreen and Kohler 1992). Evaluative research of the program progressed from descriptive reports of participant weight loss (Williams and Duncan 1976; Lowe et al. 2001) to a short-term (4 weeks) study of weight loss by program participants compared with a self-help group (Lowe et al. 1999), and finally to a randomized controlled study reporting results at 26 weeks and 2 years (Heshka et al. 2000, 2003).

Take Off Pounds Sensibly (TOPS) was founded in 1948, providing peer group support to overweight people. It does not advocate any particular diet, leaving that decision to the participant and his or her physician. TOPS has grown to include 10,300 chapters with more than 200,000 members. Strictly speaking, TOPS is not a commercial program because it is a nonprofit organization whose member fees ($20.00 per year in the United States) are used to pay organizational expenses and obesity research (to date, $5.4 million has been spent to fund obesity research by well-known basic and clinical scientists). The program consists of weekly meetings, which include a weigh-in, followed by a group discussion during which members talk about their weight loss efforts and give each other encouragement to continue.

In 1970, Stunkard published a descriptive study of the weight loss achieved by 485 members enrolled in 22 chapters in West Philadelphia (Stunkard et al. 1970). This study had two interesting findings: (1) 28% of TOPS participants lost more than 20 pounds, roughly equal to the weight loss reported in the literature up to that time by medical programs, and (2) there was wide variation in the average weight loss of individual chapters, suggesting that an unidentified program component might be playing a part in the success or lack of success by individual chapters. However, this was a cross-sectional study of active participants, saying little about the longer-term success of active participants or of those who chose to drop out. Nevertheless, the data seemed to indicate that TOPS was as successful as medically based programs. The variability in the success rate of individual chapters was thought to possibly reflect important interchapter differences in program content and presentation that, if identified, could provide insight on ways to improve the efficacy of weight loss programs.

A follow-up study of the same chapters published 4 years later (Garb and Stunkard 1974) cast a different light on the success of the TOPS program, and dampened hope that an analysis of interchapter variability (noted in the first study) would lead to new insights on ways to structure more effective weight loss programs. In this study, the authors found that the average weight loss of active members was similar between the earlier and later studies (15 and 14.2 pounds), but that dropouts were very high, 47% at 1 year and 70% at 2 years. Dropouts were also found to lose a lesser amount of weight than those who remained with the program. Thus, the success of active participants did not reflect the overall success of the program. The second survey showed less variability in weight loss between chapters. Also, the rank order of chapters had changed from the first survey. Thus, it appeared that the differences in weight loss between chapters were not due to programmatic differences, but rather to differences in the characteristics of their participants. Although these two studies do not substantiate the weight loss efficacy of the TOPS program for most of its enrollees, it should be said that TOPS is one of the least expensive programs available to people seeking support in losing weight.

Herbalife International was founded in 1980 and distributed weight management products, including meal replacements, through direct sales methods. Beginning in 2001, Dr. Enrique Varella, a college professor and independent businessman with Herbalife International, originated the idea of a nutrition club to enable groups of up to about 20 individuals to afford to consume a daily meal replacement shake in a group setting, even if they could not afford to buy the usual product containing about 30 servings of the product. As this model evolved, it became clear that many subjects who experienced positive results wanted to start their own clubs. The club directors would train them in the preparation of shakes and proper social interactions in the clubs, and the number of clubs grew progressively. A unique feature of the club is that individuals do not pay for product directly. Rather, they join the club for a daily affordable fee comparable to what would have been spent on a high-fat breakfast. A nutrition education program is currently being pilot tested in Mexico that involves simplified education on general public health and nutrition. The number of clubs is currently approximately 100,000 worldwide. Herbalife members from other countries have come to Mexico to learn how to establish this type of club. The clubs grow organically, with high rates of retention in the long term addressing one of the key deficits of earlier versions of group weight loss programs.

These group programs are community resources for referral of weight management patients in primary care. Alternatively, these groups could be started under the auspices of the primary care practice in unused space in the office on nights and weekends. This approach combines the social support provided by these group programs with medical supervision.

Individual-focused education strategies have been limited in effecting behavior change and improving health outcomes (Bouchard 2008). Despite numerous preventive efforts regarding dietary behavior and chronic diseases, obesity and associated chronic conditions continue to increase in prevalence. Identifying unhealthy behaviors and developing educational strategies to change fail to include contextual and environmental influences (Bouchard 2008; Misra and Khurana 2008; Fleisch et al. 2012; van Vliet-Ostaptchouk et al. 2012; Muller et al. 2015; World Obesity Federation 2016). Yet, few studies have investigated individuals' perceptions of the relationship between their environment and diet and physical activity behaviors (Bouchard 2008). A number of groups have recognized the impact of cultural context and socioeconomic factors in obesity. Figure 5.5 summarizes one such effort attempting to clarify the relationship between the environment and lifestyle behaviors.

The framework shown in Figure 5.5 organizes the various factors working on the individual obese or overweight patient, including multiple levels where social support has influences on eating behavior and physical activity.

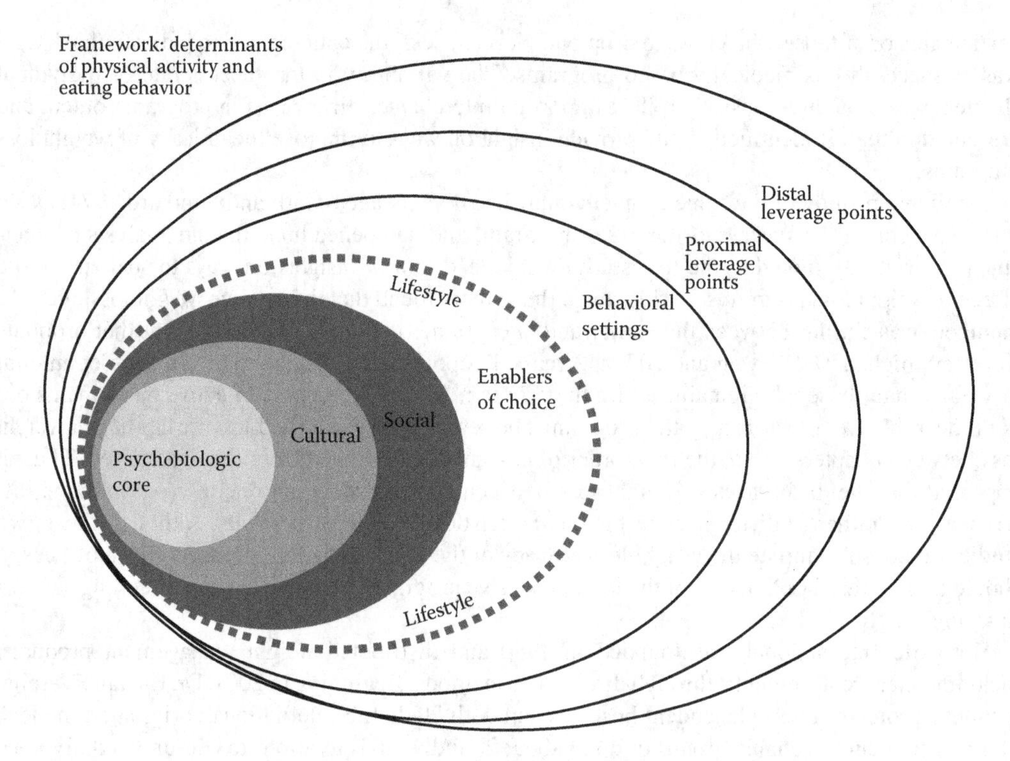

FIGURE 5.5 Determinants of physical activity and eating behavior. (Reprinted from Booth, S. L. et al., *Nutr. Rev.*, 59 (3 Pt. 2), S21–S39, 2001.)

We have extensively discussed the psychobiological core of the individual. The factors in this core include the genetically programmed metabolism and behaviors related to eating and physical activity. Early conditioned behaviors and experiences can lead to identifiable behavioral and metabolic phenotypes expressed within a given environment. The psychobiologic core also includes current health conditions.

The cultural core includes personal values and beliefs that are influenced by cultural factors and immediate social and cultural settings.

The societal core includes how society views the individual and how the individual views society. In other words, how society views the individual also influences how the individual views himself or herself.

Enablers of choice are the most proximal factors affecting food choices and physical activity and are seen as barriers to change.

Current lifestyle is a mixture of the present physical activity and eating behaviors, as well as the aspirational behaviors. Therefore, these are also the factors that are the focus of lifestyle change.

Behavior settings comprise the physical and social settings in which physical activity and eating behaviors take place and where choices are made within a situational context.

Proximal leverage points include controllers of the structure and features of the microenvironment that affect the physical activity and eating behavior choices.

Distal leverage points include the behavior settings and environments influenced by additional direct or indirect factors, for example, snack foods that consumers purchase or are exposed to, along with the laws, policies, economics, and politics affecting their sale. The distal leverage points also include media effects on attitudes, beliefs, and knowledge about eating behaviors and physical activity.

This is one of many such models, but it displays the complexity of individual behavior and many of the reasons our medical prevention and treatment models are not as successful as we would like in many patients. The primary care practice is only one of many influences, but the hope is that providing social support and follow-up will help many patients change their lifestyle behaviors.

REFERENCES

Aguilar-Salinas, C. A., E. G. Garcia, L. Robles, D. Riano, D. G. Ruiz-Gomez, A. C. Garcia-Ulloa, M. A. Melgarejo et al. 2008. High adiponectin concentrations are associated with the metabolically healthy obese phenotype. *J Clin Endocrinol Metab* 93 (10):4075–4079.

Ainsworth, B. E., W. L. Haskell, M. C. Whitt, M. L. Irwin, A. M. Swartz, S. J. Strath, W. L. O'Brien et al. 2000a. Compendium of physical activities: An update of activity codes and MET intensities. *Med Sci Sports Exerc* 32 (9 Suppl):S498–S504.

Albini, A., S. Cavuto, G. Apolone, and D. M. Noonan. 2015. Strategies to prevent "bad luck" in cancer. *J Natl Cancer Inst* 107 (10):djv213.

Aller, E. E., T. M. Larsen, H. Claus, A. K. Lindroos, A. Kafatos, A. Pfeiffer, J. A. Martinez et al. 2014. Weight loss maintenance in overweight subjects on ad libitum diets with high or low protein content and glycemic index: The DIOGENES trial 12-month results. *Int J Obes (Lond)* 38 (12):1511–1517.

American College of Sports Medicine. 2003. *ACSM Fitness Book*. Indianapolis: American College of Sports Medicine.

American Heart Association. 2016. Fitness basics. Dallas, TX: American Heart Association. https://www.heart.org/HEARTORG/HealthyLiving/PhysicalActivity/FitnessBasics/Fitness-Basics_UCM_462340_SubHomePage.jsp#.

Anandacoomarasamy, A., I. Caterson, P. Sambrook, M. Fransen, and L. March. 2008. The impact of obesity on the musculoskeletal system. *Int J Obes (Lond)* 32 (2):211–222.

Andreen, I., and B. Kohler. 1992. Effects of Weight Watchers' diet on salivary secretion rate, buffer effect and numbers of mutans streptococci and lactobacilli. *Scand J Dent Res* 100 (2):93–97.

Apovian, C. M., L. Aronne, D. Rubino, C. Still, H. Wyatt, C. Burns, D. Kim, E. Dunayevich, and COR-II Study Group. 2013. A randomized, phase 3 trial of naltrexone SR/bupropion SR on weight and obesity-related risk factors (COR-II). *Obesity (Silver Spring)* 21 (5):935–943.

Apovian, C., K. Palmer, R. Fain, C. Perdomo, and D. Rubino. 2016. Effects of lorcaserin on fat and lean mass loss in obese and overweight patients without and with type 2 diabetes mellitus: The BLOSSOM and BLOOM-DM studies. *Diabetes Obes Metab* 18 (9):945–948.

Archer, E., R. P. Shook, D. M. Thomas, T. S. Church, P. T. Katzmarzyk, J. R. Hebert, K. L. McIver, G. A. Hand, C. J. Lavie, and S. N. Blair. 2013. 45-Year trends in women's use of time and household management energy expenditure. *PLoS One* 8 (2):e56620.

Azebu, L. M. 2014. The FDA's risk/benefit calculus in the approvals of Qsymia and Belviq: Treating an obesity epidemic while avoiding another fen-phen. *Food Drug Law J* 69 (1):87–111, ii–iii.

Bacon, C. G., M. A. Mittleman, I. Kawachi, E. Giovannucci, D. B. Glasser, and E. B. Rimm. 2006. A prospective study of risk factors for erectile dysfunction. *J Urol* 176 (1):217–221.

Bajos, N., K. Wellings, C. Laborde, C. Moreau, and CSF Group. 2010. Sexuality and obesity, a gender perspective: Results from French national random probability survey of sexual behaviours. *BMJ* 340:c2573.

Bennett, G. A., and S. E. Jones. 1986. Dropping out of treatment for obesity. *J Psychosom Res* 30 (5):567–573.

Beuther, D. A., and E. R. Sutherland. 2007. Overweight, obesity, and incident asthma: A meta-analysis of prospective epidemiologic studies. *Am J Respir Crit Care Med* 175 (7):661–666.

Beydoun, M. A., H. A. Beydoun, and Y. Wang. 2008. Obesity and central obesity as risk factors for incident dementia and its subtypes: A systematic review and meta-analysis. *Obes Rev* 9 (3):204–218.

Bhole, V., M. de Vera, M. M. Rahman, E. Krishnan, and H. Choi. 2010. Epidemiology of gout in women: Fifty-two-year followup of a prospective cohort. *Arthritis Rheum* 62 (4):1069–1076.

Birbilis, M., G. Moschonis, V. Mougios, and Y. Manios. 2013. Obesity in adolescence is associated with perinatal risk factors, parental BMI and sociodemographic characteristics. *Eur J Clin Nutr* 67 (1):115–121.

Bluher, M. 2010. The distinction of metabolically "healthy" from "unhealthy" obese individuals. *Curr Opin Lipidol* 21 (1):38–43.

Blundell, J. E., and J. C. G. Halford. 1994. Regulation of nutrient supply—The brain and appetite control. *Proc Nutr Soc* 53 (2):407–418.

Boccara, F., and A. Cohen. 2004. Interplay of diabetes and coronary heart disease on cardiovascular mortality. *Heart* 90 (12):1371–1373.

Bogers, R. P., W. J. Bemelmans, R. T. Hoogenveen, H. C. Boshuizen, M. Woodward, P. Knekt, R. M. van Dam et al. 2007. Association of overweight with increased risk of coronary heart disease partly independent of blood pressure and cholesterol levels: A meta-analysis of 21 cohort studies including more than 300 000 persons. *Arch Intern Med* 167 (16):1720–1728.

Booth, S. L., J. F. Sallis, C. Ritenbaugh, J. O. Hill, L. L. Birch, L. D. Frank, K. Glanz et al. 2001. Environmental and societal factors affect food choice and physical activity: Rationale, influences, and leverage points. *Nutr Rev* 59 (3 Pt 2):S21–S39; discussion S57–S65.

Bouchard, C. 2008. Gene–environment interactions in the etiology of obesity: Defining the fundamentals. *Obesity* 16:S5–S10.

Briasoulis, A., and G. L. Bakris. 2013. Chronic kidney disease as a coronary artery disease risk equivalent. *Curr Cardiol Rep* 15 (3):340.

Brochu, M., A. Tchernof, I. J. Dionne, C. K. Sites, G. H. Eltabbakh, E. A. Sims, and E. T. Poehlman. 2001. What are the physical characteristics associated with a normal metabolic profile despite a high level of obesity in postmenopausal women? *J Clin Endocrinol Metab* 86 (3):1020–1025.

Brown, T. A., T. F. Cash, and P. J. Mikulka. 1990. Attitudinal body-image assessment: Factor analysis of the Body-Self Relations Questionnaire. *J Pers Assess* 55 (1–2):135–144.

Caballero, B. 2007. The global epidemic of obesity: An overview. *Epidemiol Rev* 29:1–5.

Cahill, G. F., Jr. 2006. Fuel metabolism in starvation. *Annu Rev Nutr* 26:1–22.

Caspersen, C. J., K. E. Powell, and G. M. Christenson. 1985. Physical activity, exercise, and physical fitness: Definitions and distinctions for health-related research. *Public Health Rep* 100 (2):126–131.

Cassidy, S. B., and D. J. Driscoll. 2009. Prader-Willi syndrome. *Eur J Hum Genet* 17 (1):3–13.

Cercato, C., V. A. Roizenblatt, C. C. Leanca, A. Segal, A. P. Lopes Filho, M. C. Mancini, and A. Halpern. 2009. A randomized double-blind placebo-controlled study of the long-term efficacy and safety of diethylpropion in the treatment of obese subjects. *Int J Obes (Lond)* 33 (8):857–865.

Chavarro, J. E., T. L. Toth, D. L. Wright, J. D. Meeker, and R. Hauser. 2010. Body mass index in relation to semen quality, sperm DNA integrity, and serum reproductive hormone levels among men attending an infertility clinic. *Fertil Steril* 93 (7):2222–2231.

Cho, E., E. B. Rimm, M. J. Stampfer, W. C. Willett, and F. B. Hu. 2002. The impact of diabetes mellitus and prior myocardial infarction on mortality from all causes and from coronary heart disease in men. *J Am Coll Cardiol* 40 (5):954–960.

Choi, H. K., K. Atkinson, E. W. Karlson, and G. Curhan. 2005. Obesity, weight change, hypertension, diuretic use, and risk of gout in men: The Health Professionals Follow-Up Study. *Arch Intern Med* 165 (7):742–748.

Christensen, R., P. K. Kristensen, E. M. Bartels, H. Bliddal, and A. Astrup. 2007. Efficacy and safety of the weight-loss drug rimonabant: A meta-analysis of randomised trials. *Lancet* 370 (9600):1706–1713.

Church, T. S., D. M. Thomas, C. Tudor-Locke, P. T. Katzmarzyk, C. P. Earnest, R. Q. Rodarte, C. K. Martin, S. N. Blair, and C. Bouchard. 2011. Trends over 5 decades in U.S. occupation-related physical activity and their associations with obesity. *PLoS One* 6 (5):e19657.

Clark, A. M., W. Ledger, C. Galletly, L. Tomlinson, F. Blaney, X. Wang, and R. J. Norman. 1995. Weight loss results in significant improvement in pregnancy and ovulation rates in anovulatory obese women. *Hum Reprod* 10 (10):2705–2712.

Clinical guidelines on the identification, evaluation, and treatment of overweight and obesity in adults—The evidence report. National Institutes of Health. 1998. *Obes Res* 6 (Suppl 2):51S–209S.

Colditz, G. A., W. C. Willett, A. Rotnitzky, and J. E. Manson. 1995. Weight gain as a risk factor for clinical diabetes mellitus in women. *Ann Intern Med* 122 (7):481–486.

Connolly, H. M., J. L. Crary, M. D. McGoon, D. D. Hensrud, B. S. Edwards, W. D. Edwards, and H. V. Schaff. 1997. Valvular heart disease associated with fenfluramine-phentermine. *N Engl J Med* 337 (9):581–588.

Conus, F., R. Rabasa-Lhoret, and F. Peronnet. 2007. Characteristics of metabolically obese normal-weight (MONW) subjects. *Appl Physiol Nutr Metab* 32 (1):4–12.

Cummings, D. E., K. E. Foster-Schubert, and J. Overduin. 2005. Ghrelin and energy balance: Focus on current controversies. *Curr Drug Targets* 6 (2):153–169.

Curtis, J. P., J. G. Selter, Y. Wang, S. S. Rathore, I. S. Jovin, F. Jadbabaie, M. Kosiborod, E. L. Portnay, S. I. Sokol, F. Bader, and H. M. Krumholz. 2005. The obesity paradox: Body mass index and outcomes in patients with heart failure. *Arch Intern Med* 165 (1):55–61.

Danielzik, S., M. Czerwinski-Mast, K. Langnase, B. Dilba, and M. J. Muller. 2004. Parental overweight, socioeconomic status and high birth weight are the major determinants of overweight and obesity in 5–7 y-old children: Baseline data of the Kiel Obesity Prevention Study (KOPS). *Int J Obes Relat Metab Disord* 28 (11):1494–1502.

Danielzik, S., K. Langnase, M. Mast, C. Spethmann, and M. J. Muller. 2002. Impact of parental BMI on the manifestation of overweight 5–7 year old children. *Eur J Nutr* 41 (3):132–138.
Degen, L., S. Oesch, M. Casanova, S. Graf, S. Ketterer, J. Drewe, and C. Beglinger. 2005. Effect of peptide YY3-36 on food intake in humans. *Gastroenterology* 129 (5):1430–1436.
de Gonzalez, A. B., P. Hartge, J. R. Cerhan, A. J. Flint, L. Hannan, R. J. MacInnis, S. C. Moore et al. 2010. Body-mass index and mortality among 1.46 million white adults. *N Engl J Med* 363 (23):2211–2219.
de las Fuentes, L., A. D. Waggoner, B. S. Mohammed, R. I. Stein, B. V. Miller 3rd, G. D. Foster, H. R. Wyatt, S. Klein, and V. G. Davila-Roman. 2009. Effect of moderate diet-induced weight loss and weight regain on cardiovascular structure and function. *J Am Coll Cardiol* 54 (25):2376–2381.
Dengo, A. L., E. A. Dennis, J. S. Orr, E. L. Marinik, E. Ehrlich, B. M. Davy, and K. P. Davy. 2010. Arterial destiffening with weight loss in overweight and obese middle-aged and older adults. *Hypertension* 55 (4):855–861.
Deriaz, O., G. Fournier, A. Tremblay, J. P. Despres, and C. Bouchard. 1992. Lean-body-mass composition and resting energy expenditure before and after long-term overfeeding. *Am J Clin Nutr* 56 (5):840–847.
de Wit, L., F. Luppino, A. van Straten, B. Penninx, F. Zitman, and P. Cuijpers. 2010. Depression and obesity: A meta-analysis of community-based studies. *Psychiatry Res* 178 (2):230–235.
Donnelly, J. E., B. K. Smith, L. Dunn, M. M. Mayo, D. J. Jacobsen, E. E. Stewart, C. Gibson, and D. K. Sullivan. 2007. Comparison of a phone vs clinic approach to achieve 10% weight loss. *Int J Obes (Lond)* 31 (8):1270–1276.
Dounchis, J. Z., H. A. Hayden, and D. E. Wilfley. 2001. Obesity, body image, and eating disorders in ethnically diverse children and adolescents. In *Body Image, Eating Disorders, and Obesity in Youth: Assessment, Prevention, and Treatment*, ed. J. K. Thompson and L. Smolak, 67–98. Washington, DC: American Psychological Assocation.
Drucker, D. J. 2006. The biology of incretin hormones. *Cell Metab* 3 (3):153–165.
Esposito, K., M. Ciotola, F. Giugliano, C. Bisogni, B. Schisano, R. Autorino, L. Cobellis, M. De Sio, N. Colacurci, and D. Giugliano. 2007. Association of body weight with sexual function in women. *Int J Impot Res* 19 (4):353–357.
Evans, E. M., D. A. Rowe, S. B. Racette, K. M. Ross, and E. McAuley. 2006. Is the current BMI obesity classification appropriate for black and white postmenopausal women? *Int J Obes (Lond)* 30 (5):837–843.
Farooqi, I. S., G. Matarese, G. M. Lord, J. M. Keogh, E. Lawrence, C. Agwu, V. Sanna et al. 2002. Beneficial effects of leptin on obesity, T cell hyporesponsiveness, and neuroendocrine/metabolic dysfunction of human congenital leptin deficiency. *J Clin Invest* 110 (8):1093–1103.
Farooqi, I. S., T. Wangensteen, S. Collins, W. Kimber, G. Matarese, J. M. Keogh, E. Lank et al. 2007. Clinical and molecular genetic spectrum of congenital deficiency of the leptin receptor. *N Engl J Med* 356 (3):237–247.
Fleisch, A. F., R. O. Wright, and A. A. Baccarelli. 2012. Environmental epigenetics: A role in endocrine disease? *J Mol Endocrinol* 49 (2):R61–R67.
Foster, G. D., T. A. Wadden, R. A. Vogt, and G. Brewer. 1997. What is a reasonable weight loss? Patients' expectations and evaluations of obesity treatment outcomes. *J Consult Clin Psychol* 65 (1):79–85.
Fowler, J. L., M. J. Follick, D. B. Abrams, and K. Rickard-Figueroa. 1985. Participant characteristics as predictors of attrition in worksite weight loss. *Addict Behav* 10 (4):445–448.
Galton, F. 1894. *Natural Inheritance*. London: Macmillan.
Garb, J. R., and A. J. Stunkard. 1974. Effectiveness of a self-help group in obesity control—Further assessment. *Arch Intern Med* 134 (4):716–720.
Garver, W. S., S. B. Newman, D. M. Gonzales-Pacheco, J. J. Castillo, D. Jelinek, R. A. Heidenreich, and R. A. Orlando. 2013. The genetics of childhood obesity and interaction with dietary macronutrients. *Genes Nutr* 8 (3):271–287.
Gibbs, J., R. C. Young, and G. P. Smith. 1973. Cholecystokinin elicits satiety in rats with open gastric fistulas. *Nature* 245 (5424):323–325.
Gibson, W. T., I. S. Farooqi, M. Moreau, A. M. DePaoli, E. Lawrence, S. O'Rahilly, and R. A. Trussell. 2004. Congenital leptin deficiency due to homozygosity for the Delta 133G mutation: Report of another case and evaluation of response to four years of leptin therapy. *J Clin Endocrinol Metab* 89 (10):4821–4826.
Gonzalez, F. 2015. Nutrient-induced inflammation in polycystic ovary syndrome: Role in the development of metabolic aberration and ovarian dysfunction. *Semin Reprod Med* 33 (4):276–286.
Goodfellow, J., S. Agarwal, F. Harrad, D. Shepherd, T. Morris, A. Ring, N. Walker, S. Rogers, and R. Baker. 2016. Cluster randomised trial of a tailored intervention to improve the management of overweight and obesity in primary care in England. *Implement Sci* 11:77.

Hall, A., J. Leibrich, F. H. Walkey, and G. Welch. 1986. Investigation of "weight pathology" of 58 mothers of anorexia nervosa patients and 204 mothers of schoolgirls. *Psychol Med* 16 (1):71–76.

Hall, J. E., J. M. do Carmo, A. A. da Silva, Z. Wang, and M. E. Hall. 2015. Obesity-induced hypertension: Interaction of neurohumoral and renal mechanisms. *Circ Res* 116 (6):991–1006.

Hammoud, A. O., N. Wilde, M. Gibson, A. Parks, D. T. Carrell, and A. W. Meikle. 2008. Male obesity and alteration in sperm parameters. *Fertil Steril* 90 (6):2222–2225.

Haskell, W. L., I. M. Lee, R. R. Pate, K. E. Powell, S. N. Blair, B. A. Franklin, C. A. Macera, G. W. Heath, P. D. Thompson, and A. Bauman. 2007. Physical activity and public health: Updated recommendation for adults from the American College of Sports Medicine and the American Heart Association. *Med Sci Sports Exerc* 39 (8):1423–1434.

Heshka, S., J. W. Anderson, R. L. Atkinson, F. L. Greenway, J. O. Hill, S. D. Phinney, R. L. Kolotkin, K. Miller-Kovach, and F. X. Pi-Sunyer. 2003. Weight loss with self-help compared with a structured commercial program: A randomized trial. *JAMA* 289 (14):1792–1798.

Heshka, S., F. Greenway, J. W. Anderson, R. L. Atkinson, J. O. Hill, S. D. Phinney, K. Miller-Kovach, and F. Xavier Pi-Sunyer. 2000. Self-help weight loss versus a structured commercial program after 26 weeks: A randomized controlled study. *Am J Med* 109 (4):282–287.

Heymsfield, S. B., A. S. Greenberg, K. Fujioka, R. M. Dixon, R. Kushner, T. Hunt, J. A. Lubina, J. Patane, B. Self, P. Hunt, and M. McCamish. 1999. Recombinant leptin for weight loss in obese and lean adults—A randomized, controlled, dose-escalation trial. *JAMA* 282 (16):1568–1575.

Huda, S. S., L. E. Brodie, and N. Sattar. 2010. Obesity in pregnancy: Prevalence and metabolic consequences. *Semin Fetal Neonatal Med* 15 (2):70–76.

Hunter, G. R., D. W. Brock, N. M. Byrne, P. C. Chandler-Laney, P. Del Corral, and B. A. Gower. 2010. Exercise training prevents regain of visceral fat for 1 year following weight loss. *Obesity (Silver Spring)* 18 (4):690–695.

Hunter, G. R., N. M. Byrne, B. A. Gower, B. Sirikul, and A. P. Hills. 2006. Increased resting energy expenditure after 40 minutes of aerobic but not resistance exercise. *Obesity (Silver Spring)* 14 (11):2018–2025.

Hunter, G. R., C. J. Wetzstein, D. A. Fields, A. Brown, and M. M. Bamman. 2000. Resistance training increases total energy expenditure and free-living physical activity in older adults. *J Appl Physiol (1985)* 89 (3):977–984.

Hursel, R., and M. S. Westerterp-Plantenga. 2013. Catechin- and caffeine-rich teas for control of body weight in humans. *Am J Clin Nutr* 98 (6 Suppl):1682S–1693S.

Jacques, L., T. S. Jensen, J. Schafer, S. McClain, and J. Chin. 2011. Decision memo for intensive behavioral therapy for obesity (CAG-00423N). Baltimore, MD: Centers for Medicare and Medicaid Services. https://www.cms.gov/medicare-coverage-database/details/nca-decision-memo.aspx?NCAId=253.

Jakobsen, L. H., J. Kondrup, M. Zellner, I. Tetens, and E. Roth. 2011. Effect of a high protein meat diet on muscle and cognitive functions: A randomised controlled dietary intervention trial in healthy men. *Clin Nutr* 30 (3):303–311.

James, W. P., I. D. Caterson, W. Coutinho, N. Finer, L. F. Van Gaal, A. P. Maggioni, C. Torp-Pedersen et al. 2010. Effect of sibutramine on cardiovascular outcomes in overweight and obese subjects. *N Engl J Med* 363 (10):905–917.

Johannes, C. B., A. B. Araujo, H. A. Feldman, C. A. Derby, K. P. Kleinman, and J. B. McKinlay. 2000. Incidence of erectile dysfunction in men 40 to 69 years old: Longitudinal results from the Massachusetts male aging study. *J Urol* 163 (2):460–463.

Kahn, E. B., L. T. Ramsey, R. C. Brownson, G. W. Heath, E. H. Howze, K. E. Powell, E. J. Stone, M. W. Rajab, and P. Corso. 2002. The effectiveness of interventions to increase physical activity. A systematic review. *Am J Prev Med* 22 (4 Suppl):73–107.

Karelis, A. D., M. Brochu, R. Rabasa-Lhoret, D. Garrel, and E. T. Poehlman. 2004a. Clinical markers for the identification of metabolically healthy but obese individuals. *Diabetes Obes Metab* 6 (6):456–457.

Karelis, A. D., M. Faraj, J. P. Bastard, D. H. St.-Pierre, M. Brochu, D. Prud'homme, and R. Rabasa-Lhoret. 2005. The metabolically healthy but obese individual presents a favorable inflammation profile. *J Clin Endocrinol Metab* 90 (7):4145–4150.

Karelis, A. D., D. H. St.-Pierre, F. Conus, R. Rabasa-Lhoret, and E. T. Poehlman. 2004b. Metabolic and body composition factors in subgroups of obesity: What do we know? *J Clin Endocrinol Metab* 89 (6):2569–2575.

Katsiki, N., D. P. Mikhailidis, and C. S. Mantzoros. 2016. Non-alcoholic fatty liver disease and dyslipidemia: An update. *Metabolism* 65 (8):1109–1123.

Kaukua, J., T. Pekkarinen, T. Sane, and P. Mustajoki. 2003. Health-related quality of life in obese outpatients losing weight with very-low-energy diet and behaviour modification—A 2-y follow-up study. *Int J Obes Relat Metab Disord* 27 (10):1233–1241.

Klem, M. L., R. R. Wing, W. Lang, M. T. McGuire, and J. O. Hill. 2000. Does weight loss maintenance become easier over time? *Obes Res* 8 (6):438–444.

Knowler, W. C., E. Barrett-Connor, S. E. Fowler, R. F. Hamman, J. M. Lachin, E. A. Walker, D. M. Nathan, and Diabetes Prevention Program Research Group. 2002. Reduction in the incidence of type 2 diabetes with lifestyle intervention or metformin. *N Engl J Med* 346 (6):393–403.

Koh-Banerjee, P., Y. Wang, F. B. Hu, D. Spiegelman, W. C. Willett, and E. B. Rimm. 2004. Changes in body weight and body fat distribution as risk factors for clinical diabetes in US men. *Am J Epidemiol* 159 (12):1150–1159.

Korth, O., A. Bosy-Westphal, P. Zschoche, C. C. Gluer, M. Heller, and M. J. Muller. 2007. Influence of methods used in body composition analysis on the prediction of resting energy expenditure. *Eur J Clin Nutr* 61 (5):582–589.

Leblanc, E. S., E. O'Connor, E. P. Whitlock, C. D. Patnode, and T. Kapka. 2011. Effectiveness of primary care-relevant treatments for obesity in adults: A systematic evidence review for the U.S. Preventive Services Task Force. *Ann Intern Med* 155 (7):434–447.

Leidy, H. J., N. S. Carnell, R. D. Mattes, and W. W. Campbell. 2007. Higher protein intake preserves lean mass and satiety with weight loss in pre-obese and obese women. *Obesity* 15 (2):421–429.

Levinger, I., C. Goodman, D. L. Hare, G. Jerums, and S. Selig. 2007. The effect of resistance training on functional capacity and quality of life in individuals with high and low numbers of metabolic risk factors. *Diabetes Care* 30 (9):2205–2210.

Li, G., P. Zhang, J. Wang, E. W. Gregg, W. Yang, Q. Gong, H. Li et al. 2008. The long-term effect of lifestyle interventions to prevent diabetes in the China Da Qing Diabetes Prevention Study: A 20-year follow-up study. *Lancet* 371 (9626):1783–1789.

Li, Z., and D. Heber. 2014. Managing weight loss expectations: The challenge and the opportunity. *JAMA* 311 (13):1348–1349.

Li, Z., K. Hong, E. Wong, M. Maxwell, and D. Heber. 2007. Weight cycling in a very low-calorie diet programme has no effect on weight loss velocity, blood pressure and serum lipid profile. *Diabetes Obes Metab* 9 (3):379–385.

Li, Z., M. Maglione, W. Tu, W. Mojica, D. Arterburn, L. R. Shugarman, L. Hilton, M. Suttorp, V. Solomon, P. G. Shekelle, and S. C. Morton. 2005. Meta-analysis: Pharmacologic treatment of obesity. *Ann Intern Med* 142 (7):532–546.

Li, Z., C. H. Tseng, Q. Li, M. L. Deng, M. Wang, and D. Heber. 2014. Clinical efficacy of a medically supervised outpatient high-protein, low-calorie diet program is equivalent in prediabetic, diabetic and normoglycemic obese patients. *Nutr Diabetes* 4:e105.

Lieberman, H. R., B. J. Spring, and G. S. Garfield. 1986. The behavioral effects of food constituents: Strategies used in studies of amino acids, protein, carbohydrate and caffeine. *Nutr Rev* 44 (Suppl):61–70.

Logue, E., K. Sutton, D. Jarjoura, W. Smucker, K. Baughman, and C. Capers. 2005. Transtheoretical model-chronic disease care for obesity in primary care: A randomized trial. *Obes Res* 13 (5):917–927.

Look AHEAD Research Group and R. R. Wing. 2010. Long-term effects of a lifestyle intervention on weight and cardiovascular risk factors in individuals with type 2 diabetes mellitus: Four-year results of the Look AHEAD trial. *Arch Intern Med* 170 (17):1566–1575.

Lopez-Garcia, E., P. Guallar-Castillon, E. Garcia-Esquinas, and F. Rodriguez-Artalejo. 2016. Metabolically healthy obesity and health-related quality of life: A prospective cohort study. *Clin Nutr.* DOI: 10.1016/j.clnu.2016.04.028.

Lowe, M. R., K. Miller-Kovach, N. Frye, and S. Phelan. 1999. An initial evaluation of a commercial weight loss program: Short-term effects on weight, eating behavior, and mood. *Obes Res* 7 (1):51–59.

Lowe, M. R., K. Miller-Kovach, and S. Phelan. 2001. Weight-loss maintenance in overweight individuals one to five years following successful completion of a commercial weight loss program. *Int J Obes Relat Metab Disord* 25 (3):325–331.

Luppino, F. S., L. M. de Wit, P. F. Bouvy, T. Stijnen, P. Cuijpers, B. W. Penninx, and F. G. Zitman. 2010. Overweight, obesity, and depression: A systematic review and meta-analysis of longitudinal studies. *Arch Gen Psychiatry* 67 (3):220–229.

Lynch, L. A., J. M. O'Connell, A. K. Kwasnik, T. J. Cawood, C. O'Farrelly, and D. B. O'Shea. 2009. Are natural killer cells protecting the metabolically healthy obese patient? *Obesity (Silver Spring)* 17 (3):601–605.

Major, G. C., E. Doucet, P. Trayhurn, A. Astrup, and A. Tremblay. 2007. Clinical significance of adaptive thermogenesis. *Int J Obes* 31 (2):204–212.

Mantzoros, C. S., F. Magkos, M. Brinkoetter, E. Sienkiewicz, T. A. Dardeno, S. Y. Kim, O. P. R. Hamnvik, and A. Koniaris. 2011. Leptin in human physiology and pathophysiology. *Am J Physiol Endocrinol Metab* 301 (4):E567–E584.

Mast, S. T., J. G. Jollis, T. Ryan, K. J. Anstrom, and J. L. Crary. 2001. The progression of fenfluramine-associated valvular heart disease assessed by echocardiography. *Ann Intern Med* 134 (4):261–266.

Mazen, I., M. El-Gammal, M. Abdel-Hamid, and K. Amr. 2009. A novel homozygous missense mutation of the leptin gene (N103K) in an obese Egyptian patient. *Mol Genet Metab* 97 (4):305–308.

McClean, K. M., F. Kee, I. S. Young, and J. S. Elborn. 2008. Obesity and the lung. 1. Epidemiology. *Thorax* 63 (7):649–654.

McConnon, A., G. W. Horgan, C. Lawton, J. Stubbs, R. Shepherd, A. Astrup, T. Handjieva-Darlenska et al. 2013. Experience and acceptability of diets of varying protein content and glycemic index in an obese cohort: Results from the Diogenes trial. *Eur J Clin Nutr* 67 (9):990–995.

McGee, D. L., and Diverse Populations Collaboration. 2005. Body mass index and mortality: A meta-analysis based on person-level data from twenty-six observational studies. *Ann Epidemiol* 15 (2):87–97.

McLean, R. C., D. S. Morrison, R. Shearer, S. Boyle, and J. Logue. 2016. Attrition and weight loss outcomes for patients with complex obesity, anxiety and depression attending a weight management programme with targeted psychological treatment. *Clin Obes* 6 (2):133–142.

Messier, V., A. D. Karelis, M. E. Robillard, P. Bellefeuille, M. Brochu, J. M. Lavoie, and R. Rabasa-Lhoret. 2010. Metabolically healthy but obese individuals: Relationship with hepatic enzymes. *Metabolism* 59 (1):20–24.

Misovich, S. 1973. Birth order, affiliation, and membership in Weight Watchers. *Psychol Rep* 32 (1):94.

Misra, A., and L. Khurana. 2008. Obesity and the metabolic syndrome in developing countries. *J Clin Endocrinol Metab* 93 (11 Suppl 1):S9–S30.

Montague, C. T., I. S. Farooqi, J. P. Whitehead, M. A. Soos, H. Rau, N. J. Wareham, C. P. Sewter et al. 1997. Congenital leptin deficiency is associated with severe early-onset obesity in humans. *Nature* 387 (6636):903–908.

Morton, G. J., D. E. Cummings, D. G. Baskin, G. S. Barsh, and M. W. Schwartz. 2006. Central nervous system control of food intake and body weight. *Nature* 443 (7109):289–295.

Moyer, V. A. 2012. Screening for and management of obesity in adults: U.S. Preventive Services Task Force recommendation statement. *Ann Intern Med* 157 (5):373–378.

Muller, M. J., A. Bosy-Westphal, and M. Krawczak. 2010. Genetic studies of common types of obesity: A critique of the current use of phenotypes. *Obes Rev* 11 (8):612–618.

Muller, M. J., J. Enderle, M. Pourhassan, W. Braun, B. Eggeling, M. Lagerpusch, C. C. Gluer, J. J. Kehayias, D. Kiosz, and A. Bosy-Westphal. 2015. Metabolic adaptation to caloric restriction and subsequent refeeding: The Minnesota Starvation Experiment revisited. *Am J Clin Nutr* 102 (4):807–819.

Nelson, M. E., W. J. Rejeski, S. N. Blair, P. W. Duncan, J. O. Judge, A. C. King, C. A. Macera, and C. Castaneda-Sceppa. 2007. Physical activity and public health in older adults: Recommendation from the American College of Sports Medicine and the American Heart Association. *Med Sci Sports Exerc* 39 (8):1435–1445.

Nerfeldt, P., B. Y. Nilsson, L. Mayor, J. Udden, and D. Friberg. 2010. A two-year weight reduction program in obese sleep apnea patients. *J Clin Sleep Med* 6 (5):479–486.

Nguyen, N. T., S. Vu, E. Kim, N. Bodunova, and M. J. Phelan. 2016. Trends in utilization of bariatric surgery, 2009–2012. *Surg Endosc* 30 (7):2723–2727.

Oliveira, A. M., A. C. Oliveira, M. S. Almeida, N. Oliveira, and L. Adan. 2007. Influence of the family nucleus on obesity in children from northeastern Brazil: A cross-sectional study. *BMC Public Health* 7:235.

Pajunen, P., A. Kotronen, E. Korpi-Hyovalti, S. Keinanen-Kiukaanniemi, H. Oksa, L. Niskanen, T. Saaristo et al. 2011. Metabolically healthy and unhealthy obesity phenotypes in the general population: The FIN-D2D Survey. *BMC Public Health* 11:754.

Paravattil, B., K. J. Wilby, and R. Turgeon. 2016. Topiramate monotherapy for weight reduction in patients with type 2 diabetes mellitus: A systematic review and meta-analysis. *Diabetes Res Clin Pract* 114:9–14.

Pedditizi, E., R. Peters, and N. Beckett. 2016. The risk of overweight/obesity in mid-life and late life for the development of dementia: A systematic review and meta-analysis of longitudinal studies. *Age Ageing* 45 (1):14–21.

Perri, M. G., M. C. Limacher, P. E. Durning, D. M. Janicke, L. D. Lutes, L. B. Bobroff, M. S. Dale, M. J. Daniels, T. A. Radcliff, and A. D. Martin. 2008. Extended-care programs for weight management in rural communities: The treatment of obesity in underserved rural settings (TOURS) randomized trial. *Arch Intern Med* 168 (21):2347–2354.

Peters, J. C., H. R. Wyatt, W. T. Donahoo, and J. O. Hill. 2002. From instinct to intellect: The challenge of maintaining healthy weight in the modern world. *Obes Rev* 3 (2):69–74.

Pigeyre, M., F. T. Yazdi, Y. Kaur, and D. Meyre. 2016. Recent progress in genetics, epigenetics and metagenomics unveils the pathophysiology of human obesity. *Clin Sci (Lond)* 130 (12):943–986.

Pironi, L., V. Stanghellini, M. Miglioli, R. Corinaldesi, R. Degiorgio, E. Ruggeri, C. Tosetti et al. 1993. Fat-induced ileal brake in humans—A dose-dependent phenomenon correlated to the plasma-levels of peptide-YY. *Gastroenterology* 105 (3):733–739.

Pollock, M. L., B. A. Franklin, G. J. Balady, B. L. Chaitman, J. L. Fleg, B. Fletcher, M. Limacher, I. L. Pina, R. A. Stein, M. Williams, and T. Bazzarre. 2000. Resistance exercise in individuals with and without cardiovascular disease—Benefits, rationale, safety, and prescription—An advisory from the Committee on Exercise, Rehabilitation, and Prevention, Council on Clinical Cardiology, American Heart Association. *Circulation* 101 (7):828–833.

Prochaska, J. O., and C. C. DiClemente. 1983. Stages and processes of self-change of smoking: Toward an integrative model of change. *J Consult Clin Psychol* 51 (3): 390–395.

Rahman, M., and A. B. Berenson. 2010. Accuracy of current body mass index obesity classification for white, black, and Hispanic reproductive-age women. *Obstet Gynecol* 115 (5):982–988.

Raman, V. T., M. Splaingard, D. Tumin, J. Rice, K. R. Jatana, and J. D. Tobias. 2016. Utility of screening questionnaire, obesity, neck circumference, and sleep polysomnography to predict sleep-disordered breathing in children and adolescents. *Paediatr Anaesth* 26 (6):655–664.

Ramirez, E. M., and J. C. Rosen. 2001. A comparison of weight control and weight control plus body image therapy for obese men and women. *J Consult Clin Psychol* 69 (3):440–446.

Ravussin, E., Y. Schutz, K. J. Acheson, M. Dusmet, L. Bourquin, and E. Jequier. 1985. Short-term, mixed-diet overfeeding in man—No evidence for luxuskonsumption. *Am J Physiol* 249 (5):E470–E477.

Reaven, G. M., H. Lithell, and L. Landsberg. 1996. Hypertension and associated metabolic abnormalities—The role of insulin resistance and the sympathoadrenal system. *N Engl J Med* 334 (6):374–381.

Rich-Edwards, J. W., D. Spiegelman, M. Garland, E. Hertzmark, D. J. Hunter, G. A. Colditz, W. C. Willett, H. Wand, and J. E. Manson. 2002. Physical activity, body mass index, and ovulatory disorder infertility. *Epidemiology* 13 (2):184–190.

Romero-Corral, A., V. K. Somers, J. Sierra-Johnson, R. J. Thomas, M. L. Collazo-Clavell, J. Korinek, T. G. Allison, J. A. Batsis, F. H. Sert-Kuniyoshi, and F. Lopez-Jimenez. 2008. Accuracy of body mass index in diagnosing obesity in the adult general population. *Int J Obes (Lond)* 32 (6):959–966.

Rottensteiner, M., T. Leskinen, E. Jarvela-Reijonen, K. Vaisanen, S. Aaltonen, J. Kaprio, and U. M. Kujala. 2016. Leisure-time physical activity and intra-abdominal fat in young adulthood: A monozygotic co-twin control study. *Obesity (Silver Spring)* 24 (5):1185–1191.

Ruderman, N., D. Chisholm, X. Pi-Sunyer, and S. Schneider. 1998. The metabolically obese, normal-weight individual revisited. *Diabetes* 47 (5):699–713.

Saigal, C. S., H. Wessells, J. Pace, M. Schonlau, T. J. Wilt, and Project Urologic Diseases in America. 2006. Predictors and prevalence of erectile dysfunction in a racially diverse population. *Arch Intern Med* 166 (2):207–212.

Sallis, J. F., K. Kraft, and L. S. Linton. 2002. How the environment shapes physical activity—A transdisciplinary research agenda. *Am J Prev Med* 22 (3):208.

Samitz, G., M. Egger, and M. Zwahlen. 2011. Domains of physical activity and all-cause mortality: Systematic review and dose-response meta-analysis of cohort studies. *Int J Epidemiol* 40 (5):1382–1400.

Sarwer, D. B., J. K. Thompson, and T. F. Cash. 2005. Body image and obesity in adulthood. *Psychiatr Clin* 28 (1):69–87.

Schoeller, D. A., K. Shay, and R. F. Kushner. 1997. How much physical activity is needed to minimize weight gain in previously obese women? *Am J Clin Nutr* 66 (3):551–556.

Schwartz, M. B., and K. D. Brownell. 2004. Obesity and body image. *Body Image* 1 (1):43–56.

Schwartz, M. W., S. C. Woods, D. Porte, R. J. Seeley, and D. G. Baskin. 2000. Central nervous system control of food intake. *Nature* 404 (6778):661–671.

Shin, J. H., and K. M. Gadde. 2013. Clinical utility of phentermine/topiramate (Qsymia) combination for the treatment of obesity. *Diabetes Metab Syndr Obes* 6:131–139.

Sims, E. A. 2001. Are there persons who are obese, but metabolically healthy? *Metabolism* 50 (12): 1499–1504.

Small, G. W., D. H. Silverman, P. Siddarth, L. M. Ercoli, K. J. Miller, H. Lavretsky, B. C. Wright, S. Y. Bookheimer, J. R. Barrio, and M. E. Phelps. 2006. Effects of a 14-day healthy longevity lifestyle program on cognition and brain function. *Am J Geriatr Psychiatry* 14 (6):538–545.

Smith, G. P. 1998. *Satiation: From Gut to Brain*. New York: Oxford University Press.

Soverini, V., S. Moscatiello, N. Villanova, E. Ragni, S. Di Domizio, and G. Marchesini. 2010. Metabolic syndrome and insulin resistance in subjects with morbid obesity. *Obes Surg* 20 (3):295–301.

Spring, B., O. Maller, J. Wurtman, L. Digman, and L. Cozolino. 1983. Effects of protein and carbohydrate meals on mood and performance—Interactions with sex and age. *J Psychiatr Res* 17 (2):155–167.

Stampfer, M. J., K. M. Maclure, G. A. Colditz, J. E. Manson, and W. C. Willett. 1992. Risk of symptomatic gallstones in women with severe obesity. *Am J Clin Nutr* 55 (3):652–658.

Stanley, S., K. Wynne, B. McGowan, and S. Bloom. 2005. Hormonal regulation of food intake. *Physiol Rev* 85 (4):1131–1158.

Stefan, N., K. Kantartzis, J. Machann, F. Schick, C. Thamer, K. Rittig, B. Balletshofer, F. Machicao, A. Fritsche, and H. U. Haring. 2008. Identification and characterization of metabolically benign obesity in humans. *Arch Intern Med* 168 (15):1609–1616.

Stefanick, M. L. 1993. Exercise and weight control. *Exerc Sport Sci Rev* 21:363–396.

Stothard, K. J., P. W. Tennant, R. Bell, and J. Rankin. 2009. Maternal overweight and obesity and the risk of congenital anomalies: A systematic review and meta-analysis. *JAMA* 301 (6):636–650.

Strader, A. D., and S. C. Woods. 2005. Gastrointestinal hormones and food intake. *Gastroenterology* 128 (1):175–191.

Strazzullo, P., L. D'Elia, G. Cairella, F. Garbagnati, F. P. Cappuccio, and L. Scalfi. 2010. Excess body weight and incidence of stroke: Meta-analysis of prospective studies with 2 million participants. *Stroke* 41 (5):e418–e426.

Strubbe, J. H., and S. C. Woods. 2004. The timing of meals. *Psychol Rev* 111 (1):128–141.

Stuart, R. B., and K. Guire. 1978. Some correlates of the maintenance of weight lost through behavior modification. *Int J Obes* 2 (3):225–235.

Stunkard, A., H. Levine, and S. Fox. 1970. The management of obesity. Patient self-help and medical treatment. *Arch Intern Med* 125 (6):1067–1072.

Sugiyama, T., K. Wijndaele, M. J. Koohsari, S. K. Tanamas, D. W. Dunstan, and N. Owen. 2016. Adverse associations of car time with markers of cardio-metabolic risk. *Prev Med* 83:26–30.

Thomas, E. L., J. R. Parkinson, G. S. Frost, A. P. Goldstone, C. J. Dore, J. P. McCarthy, A. L. Collins, J. A. Fitzpatrick, G. Durighel, S. D. Taylor-Robinson, and J. D. Bell. 2012. The missing risk: MRI and MRS phenotyping of abdominal adiposity and ectopic fat. *Obesity (Silver Spring)* 20 (1):76–87.

Tomasetti, C., and B. Vogelstein. 2015. Variation in cancer risk among tissues can be explained by the number of stem cell divisions. *Science* 347 (6217):78–81.

Traverso, A., G. Ravera, V. Lagattolla, S. Testa, and G. F. Adami. 2000. Weight loss after dieting with behavioral modification for obesity: The predicting efficiency of some psychometric data. *Eat Weight Disord* 5 (2):102–107.

Tsai, C. J., M. F. Leitzmann, W. C. Willett, and E. L. Giovannucci. 2004. Prospective study of abdominal adiposity and gallstone disease in US men. *Am J Clin Nutr* 80 (1):38–44.

Tschop, M., D. L. Smiley, and M. L. Heiman. 2000. Ghrelin induces adiposity in rodents. *Nature* 407 (6806):908–913.

Tuomilehto, H. P., J. M. Seppa, M. M. Partinen, M. Peltonen, H. Gylling, J. O. Tuomilehto, E. J. Vanninen et al. 2009. Lifestyle intervention with weight reduction: First-line treatment in mild obstructive sleep apnea. *Am J Respir Crit Care Med* 179 (4):320–327.

Tuomilehto, J., J. Lindstrom, J. G. Eriksson, T. T. Valle, H. Hamalainen, P. Ilanne-Parikka, S. Keinanen-Kiukaanniemi et al. 2001. Prevention of type 2 diabetes mellitus by changes in lifestyle among subjects with impaired glucose tolerance. *N Engl J Med* 344 (18):1343–1350.

Udo, T., and C. M. Grilo. 2016. Perceived weight discrimination, childhood maltreatment, and weight gain in U.S. adults with overweight/obesity. *Obesity (Silver Spring)* 24 (6):1366–1372.

U.S. Department of Health and Human Services, National Institutes of Health, National Heart, Lung, and Blood Institute. 2006. Your guide to physical activity and your heart. NIH Publication 06-5714. Washington, DC: U.S. Department of Health and Human Services.

van Vliet-Ostaptchouk, J. V., H. Snieder, and V. Lagou. 2012. Gene–lifestyle interactions in obesity. *Curr Nutr Rep* 1:184–196.

Velicer, W. F., C. C. Diclemente, J. S. Rossi, and J. O. Prochaska. 1990. Relapse situations and self-efficacy: An integrative model. *Addict Behav* 15 (3):271–283.

Waalen, J. 2014. The genetics of human obesity. *Transl Res* 164 (4):293–301.

Wabitsch, M., J. B. Funcke, B. Lennerz, U. Kuhnle-Krahl, G. Lahr, K. M. Debatin, P. Vatter, P. Gierschik, B. Moepps, and P. Fischer-Posovszky. 2015. Biologically inactive leptin and early-onset extreme obesity. *N Engl J Med* 372 (1):48–54.

Wareham, N. J., E. M. van Sluijs, and U. Ekelund. 2005. Physical activity and obesity prevention: A review of the current evidence. *Proc Nutr Soc* 64 (2):229–247.

Weinsier, R. L., G. R. Hunter, R. A. Desmond, N. M. Byrne, P. A. Zuckerman, and B. E. Darnell. 2002. Free-living activity energy expenditure in women successful and unsuccessful at maintaining a normal body weight. *Am J Clin Nutr* 75 (3):499–504.

Westerterp, K. R. 2003. Impacts of vigorous and non-vigorous activity on daily energy expenditure. *Proc Nutr Soc* 62 (3):645–650.

Westerterp, K. R. 2008. Physical activity as determinant of daily energy expenditure. *Physiol Behav* 93 (4–5):1039–1043.

WHO (World Health Organization). 2013. Obesity and overweight. Fact sheet 311. Geneva: WHO.

Wildman, R. P., P. Muntner, K. Reynolds, A. P. McGinn, S. Rajpathak, J. Wylie-Rosett, and M. R. Sowers. 2008. The obese without cardiometabolic risk factor clustering and the normal weight with cardiometabolic risk factor clustering: Prevalence and correlates of 2 phenotypes among the US population (NHANES 1999–2004). *Arch Intern Med* 168 (15):1617–1624.

Williams, A. E., and B. Duncan. 1976. A commercial weight-reducing organization: A critical analysis. *Med J Aust* 1 (21):781–785.

Wing, R. R., and J. O. Hill. 2001. Successful weight loss maintenance. *Annu Rev Nutr* 21:323–341.

Wing, R. R., R. C. Rosen, J. L. Fava, J. Bahnson, F. Brancati, I. N. Gendrano III, A. Kitabchi, S. H. Schneider, and T. A. Wadden. 2010. Effects of weight loss intervention on erectile function in older men with type 2 diabetes in the Look AHEAD trial. *J Sex Med* 7 (1 Pt 1):156–165.

World Obesity Federation. 2016. World obesity day 2015 statistics. London: World Obesity Federation. http://www.worldobesity.org/site_media/uploads/World_Obsesity_Day_Press_Release.pdf.

Yang, W. Y., J. M. Lu, J. P. Weng, W. P. Jia, L. N. Ji, J. Z. Xiao, Z. Y. Shan et al. 2010. Prevalence of diabetes among men and women in China. *N Engl J Med* 362 (12):1090–1101.

Zeng, Y.-C., S.-M. Li, G.-L. Xiong, H.-M. Su, and J.-C. Wan. 2011. Influences of protein to energy ratios in breakfast on mood, alertness and attention in the healthy undergraduate students. *Health* 3 (6):383.

Zimmet, P., K. G. Alberti, and J. Shaw. 2001. Global and societal implications of the diabetes epidemic. *Nature* 414 (6865):782–787.

6 Evolution of Type 2 Diabetes Mellitus

6.1 INTRODUCTION

While the majority of obese and insulin-resistant individuals do not develop type 2 diabetes mellitus (T2DM), it is estimated that 20% or more of obese individuals will develop type 2 diabetes (T2DM) in their lifetime. This chapter provides the background science on how those who develop T2DM or "diabesity" differ from the majority of obese individuals. Diabetes and prediabetes affect half of the population of the state of California (Babey et al. 2016) and about half the population in China (Xu et al. 2013). These statistics are likely to be repeated elsewhere in the world and represent both an economic and a global health disaster in the making. The ability of diet and lifestyle, in combination with the long-established, off-patent, and safe drug metformin, to reduce the rate of progression of T2DM with benefits on cardiovascular mortality will be the emphasis of the intervention approach recommended here. The issues previously reviewed in Chapter 2 on dietary recommendations and in Chapter 5 on obesity treatment will not be repeated here, but those considerations fully apply to the individuals with obesity who are at risk of T2DM.

Insulin resistance is very common and may have benefits for the adaptation to starvation. However, individuals predisposed to T2DM have additional factors that mediate the risk to develop T2DM, including reduced pancreatic β-cell mass at birth or in childhood, which when faced with the ongoing demand for insulin related to hyperglycemia results in the death of β-cells and ultimately leads to T2DM. Predispositions to oxidant stress and inflammation also likely play a role at a cellular and systemic level (Marseglia et al. 2015).

Analytical methodologies such as genetic profiling and genome-wide scans have largely failed to establish a genetic cause for most T2DM, while risk factors are clearly recognized. Age, family history of diabetes, gestational diabetes, obesity, physical inactivity, hypertension, and hyperlipidemia are all risk factors for the development of T2DM. While the genetic findings are still inconclusive, there is an appreciation for the role of insulin-associated polypeptide (IAPP), inflammation, obesity, oxidant stress, and toxicity from glucose and lipids in promoting the demise of β-cells and the development of diabetes. In this chapter, the genetic, social, economic, and nutritional factors increasing risk are reviewed, with the hope that this knowledge will lead to earlier screening and intervention with nutrition and increased physical activity to help prevent progression to diabetes.

6.2 SOCIAL AND ECONOMIC DETERMINANTS OF RISK

Social and economic factors driving the diabetes epidemic globally are also contributing to an increase in the prevalence of T2DM. Existing data support the concept that the global increase in diabetes prevalence is due to macroeconomic and lifestyle factors associated with the observation that for the first time in human history, there are more overweight than underweight people in the world.

The global nutrition transition has resulted in a greater number of overweight than underweight individuals in most lower- and middle-income countries around the world, especially in urban areas (Mendez et al. 2005; Alexandratos 2006; Popkin 2006; Monteiro et al. 2007; Kearney 2010; Subramanyam et al. 2010). Changes in global per capita food intake in many countries and an increased proportion of food intake derived from energy-dense and fatty foods have contributed to the epidemic of obesity (Bell et al. 2002; Alexandratos 2006; Popkin 2006; Kearney 2010; Ng and Popkin 2012; Wang et al. 2012; Marseglia et al. 2015). Means of transportation (Misra and Khurana 2008), types of employment, and selected leisure activities have all become more sedentary, contributing to an imbalance of energy intake and expenditure (Bell et al. 2002; Zhai et al. 2007; Ng and Popkin 2012). Macroeconomic factors, including economic development, urbanization, foreign investment, and trade liberalization, have contributed to shifting patterns of diet, physical activity, and stress and poor sleep patterns (Popkin 2006; Misra and Khurana 2008). Economic development and increases in per capita income are associated with increased consumption of energy-dense foods (Zhai et al. 2007). Moreover, economic development is associated with a faster rate of growth in the prevalence of overweight among lower-income groups in many countries where obesity was rare just 20 years ago (Jones-Smith et al. 2011, 2012). Urbanization increases access to processed diets, limits opportunities for physical activity, and exposes people to pervasive food advertising and subliminal marketing messages. These social and economic factors in combination promote a sedentary lifestyle associated with reduced energy expenditure and increased calorie intake, which work in opposition to the universal human adaptation to food scarcity and mandatory physical activity, rather than excess food supplies and labor-saving devices, including automobiles, kitchen appliances, and air conditioning (Misra and Khurana 2008). The globalization of the world's economies through foreign investment in developing countries, in combination with free trade agreements (Hawkes 2005), has reshaped the global market for food, particularly in developing lower- and middle-income countries, by competing with and often displacing traditional agricultural practices while facilitating the processing, distribution, and marketing of lower-cost, energy-dense food (Popkin et al. 2012; Stuckler et al. 2012).

6.3 MINORITY HEALTH DISPARITIES AND RISK FACTORS IN THE UNITED STATES

African Americans have been demonstrated to have a 1.9-fold higher incidence of T2DM than Caucasians (Cowie et al. 2009), and this difference is found in all age groups (Cowie et al. 2006). The higher prevalence of T2DM in U.S. African Americans compared with Caucasians may be due to a higher frequency of risk factors or a higher inherent susceptibility to T2DM, or it may be that the risk factors have a greater pathophysiological effect. Although most risk factors are more common in African Americans, this higher frequency does not completely explain the racial disparity in the prevalence of T2DM. After adjustment for all risk factors by logistic regression, an elevated risk of diabetes in African Americans is particularly evident at higher obesity levels. The risk for developing diabetes was 70% higher in African Americans at 150 percent of desirable weight in comparison to Caucasians with the same degree of overweight (95% confidence interval 1.1–2.8). The risk of diabetes associated with obesity is greater in African-American women than men. The odds of developing diabetes in this group were sevenfold higher at a percentage of desirable weight of 150 versus Caucasians with the same degree of overweight.

The possibility of racial differences in metabolic adaptation to obesity highlights the importance of preventing this condition among African Americans, particularly women.

Hispanic Americans, who represent the largest minority population in the United States, are also at increased risk for obesity and diabetes (Yracheta et al. 2015). Both genetic and environmental factors might account for their increased risk for these conditions. Excessive intake of sugary beverages has been highlighted as an important contributory cause in this population. Studies focusing on decreasing the intake of sugary beverages among Hispanic Americans could potentially reduce renal and cardiovascular complications in this population.

T2DM is an increasing concern among Asian Americans, the fastest-growing ethnic group in the United States. The U.S. Centers for Disease Control has determined that the age-adjusted prevalence of T2DM for Asian Americans is 9%, placing them at moderate risk. However, different levels of risk emerge when Asian American ethnic groups are examined separately. Filipino, Pacific Islander, Japanese, and South Asian groups are consistently described as having the highest prevalence of diabetes (Nguyen et al. 2015b). For many years, health services for Asian American populations have been affected by the myth that Asian Americans are self-sufficient and well educated, and have lower burdens of disease (Chen and Hawks 1995; Tendulkar et al. 2012). This myth of a so-called model minority was perpetuated by the lack of reliable data that often lumped Asian Americans into one large category, when in fact they represent a varied and heterogeneous group.

6.4 ADAPTATION TO STARVATION SETS THE STAGE FOR T2DM

When deprived of food, a metabolic adaptation is triggered by a series of hormonal adaptations, including a decrease in insulin that results in the utilization of fat, rather than glucose, for energy. Since protein breakdown is required for the synthesis of glucose after the first 3 days of starvation, after which glycogen stores of only 1200 calories are depleted and the red cells and brain continue to require glucose, the adaptation to starvation has been key to human survival in times of famine and food shortages throughout history. Multiple observations have shown that when body cell mass is reduced to 50% of preillness levels, life ends regardless of whether the cause was starvation, trauma, tumor, or surgical complications. A second threat to the survival of ancient man was death from infection. This latter threat is key to understanding the benefits of activating the immune system during starvation, as well as understanding that a negative skin tuberculin test in malnourished patients is a sign of a nutritionally compromised immune system and the breakdown of this part of the adaptation to starvation. Women have both gynoid and visceral fat, while men have only visceral fat. The visceral fat is the store of fat most rapidly mobilized during starvation, but it is also a limited store of fat, with excess fat being deposited ectopically primarily in the liver.

The common occurrence of insulin resistance when energy stores are overloaded in the overweight and obese patient has stimulated the notion that relative insulin resistance as insulin levels drop during starvation may have some survival benefit, accounting for its commonality. Energy storage, mainly as glycogen in liver and triglycerides in adipose tissue, is regulated by the anabolic actions of insulin. On the other hand, mobilization of stored energy during infection, trauma, or stress is served by the temporary inhibition of insulin action in target tissues by pro-inflammatory cytokines and stress hormones. Theoretically, individuals with greater insulin resistance would have even more efficient mobilization of fat stores during starvation, extending survival (Tsatsoulis et al. 2013; Babey et al. 2016).

In the current obesogenic environments of much of the industrialized and developing world, high energy intake, low physical activity, and chronic stress favor the storage of surplus fat in adipose tissue depots that far exceeds their storage capacity and results in the export of triglycerides into the circulation from the liver. Lipid overload in visceral fat initiates an inflammatory response and adipocyte dysfunction with resultant low-grade systemic inflammation and lipid overflow to peripheral tissues. In turn, inflammatory cytokines and lipid metabolites, accumulated in liver and muscle cells, activate the mechanism of insulin resistance, as would occur in the case of infection or stress. The same factors, together with the ensuing insulin resistance, put a burden on pancreatic β-cell insulin synthesis and secretion, leading to cellular death (Costes et al. 2013; Xu et al. 2013). In individuals beginning life with reduced pancreatic β-cell mass, the ongoing demand for insulin ultimately leads to T2DM, while oxidation of lipids and inflammation lead to cardiovascular disease (Lee et al. 2012; Marseglia et al. 2015).

The physiology of starvation and its undoing by excess calorie intake and sedentary lifestyles provide a framework for the notion that insulin resistance evolved as a physiological adaptive mechanism in human survival, and that the same mechanism is inappropriately activated on a chronic basis in the current environment, leading to the manifestations of the metabolic syndrome. While this syndrome is extremely common, it is not universal, and there are healthy obese individuals and unhealthy thin-appearing individuals with excess visceral fat who do not develop T2DM. The current science on the factors promoting pancreatic burnout is rapidly providing a coherent picture on why some people develop T2DM while others do not.

6.5 PANCREATIC β-CELL EXHAUSTION AND THE DEVELOPMENT OF T2DM

T2DM is characterized by a reduction of β-cell mass with aging and accumulation of islet amyloid derived from IAPP in the pancreatic islets (Kloppel et al. 1985). Islet amyloid deposition can occur in up to 80% of patients with diabetes mellitus and is thought to be a key factor in triggering β-cell destruction when misfolding of the protein occurs (Clark and Nilsson 2004). IAPP is a 37-amino-acid peptide synthesized and secreted with insulin from pancreatic β-cells. It functions as a short-loop feedback to insulin secretion and regulating glucose levels. It inhibits the effects of insulin, as well as arginine-stimulated glucagon release by α-cells (Young et al. 1995; Nguyen et al. 2015a). In addition, IAPP has been demonstrated to have other physiological functions, such as sleep and appetite regulation via the gut–brain axis, and it functions as a growth factor to maintain β-cell mass (Wookey et al. 2006). The incidence of T2DM is considered to increase with age because of the reduced proliferative capacity and increased apoptosis rate of β-cells, which can also lead to higher rates of IAPP aggregation (Gunasekaran and Gannon 2011).

Human IAPP (h-IAPP) is only identified histologically at autopsy or in surgical specimens, but pancreatic β-cell apoptosis and the induction of diabetes have been confirmed in h-IAPP transgenic rat and mouse models, supporting the idea that amyloids are associated with the induction and progression of diabetes (Butler et al. 2004). Indeed, an h-IAPP transgenic model formed toxic IAPP oligomers that eventually generated endoplasmic reticulum stress-induced apoptosis and characteristics of T2DM, including hyperglycemia, impaired insulin secretion, insulin resistance, and hyperglucagonemia (Matveyenko and Butler 2006a; Huang et al. 2007).

IAPP aggregates have been shown to induce inflammation in islets of Langerhans. IAPP aggregates were observed in macrophages present in pancreatic tissues of biopsy samples from T2DM patients, as well as in diabetic monkeys, cats, and transgenic h-IAPP mice (de Koning et al. 1998). These macrophages could not efficiently remove the IAPP aggregates, but internalization of IAPP aggregates led to secretion of multiple inflammatory cytokines, including interleukin 1β (IL-1β) in cell culture studies (Gitter et al. 2000; Yates et al. 2000; Westwell-Roper et al. 2011, 2014). A threefold increased risk of developing diabetes has been demonstrated in individuals with elevated levels of both IL-1β and IL-6, but not IL-6 alone (Spranger et al. 2003), suggesting that an inherited brisk inflammatory response contributes to the pathogenesis of diabetes. Within immune cells from the bone marrow, phagocytized h-IAPP oligomers activate the NLRP3 inflammasome, leading to IL-1β secretion (Masters et al. 2010). Moreover, a recent study indicated that h-IAPP oligomers induce a pro-inflammatory response in islet resident macrophages, including IL-1β secretions, leading to islet dysfunction in the transgenic h-IAPP mouse model (Westwell-Roper et al. 2015).

The presence of misfolded IAPP aggregates deposited in the pancreatic islets of patients with T2DM and the loss of β-cells is well established. The key question is whether these aggregates are simply bystanders that accumulate as a result of the tissue damage during the disease, or they actually play a key role in the pathogenesis of T2DM. Amyloid deposits occur as a consequence of folding and failure to clear intracellular proteins with the propensity to form amyloid deposits. These proteins may form a variety of oligomers, the most toxic of which are those that form relatively early and interact with cellular membranes (McLaurin and Chakrabartty 1996; Janson et al. 1999). In contrast, if misfolded IAPP oligomers organize into amyloid fibrils, these are generally less toxic but also relatively inert, and as such, they tend to accumulate in the extracellular space, where they may play a role as a physical barrier and contribute to cellular dysfunction (Clark et al. 1987; Hayden et al. 2007). The diabetes field has mostly ignored the potential importance of IAPP aggregates in diabetes. Evidence in favor of a direct toxic effect of islet amyloid (Lorenzo et al. 1994) was outnumbered by studies that did not identify such toxicity (Janson et al. 1999; Butler et al. 2003b). However, toxic amyloid forms were not considered in these studies. This contrasts with the situation in neurodegenerative conditions such as Alzheimer's disease and Parkinson's disease, where elevated protein aggregates are an accepted component of disease progression, if not the causative factor. In the brain, as in the pancreas, inflammation triggered by misfolded proteins and tau tangles also appears to be part of the pathogenesis of neurodegenerative diseases.

The formation of intracellular IAPP oligomers and extracellular amyloid fibrils in humans implies that the mechanisms to prevent accumulation of misfolded proteins are overloaded. There is a threshold of IAPP expression that, if exceeded, leads to formation of IAPP oligomers, leading to the adverse consequences described (Couce et al. 1996; Janson et al. 1996; Soeller et al. 1998; Matveyenko and Butler 2006b; Huang et al. 2010). This threshold may be exceeded due to an excessive influx of IAPP at a level that exceeds the capacity of a healthy pancreatic β-cell to fold, process, and dispose of the proteins or because the threshold is decreased by other pathological factors. h-IAPP transgenic rodent models and transgenic β-cells imply that both of these mechanisms may be involved (Couce et al. 1996; Janson et al. 1996; Soeller et al. 1998; Matveyenko and Butler 2006b; Huang et al. 2010). h-IAPP transgenic mice and rats develop diabetes in a transgene dose–response manner (Janson et al. 1996), or if h-IAPP expression is increased by drug- or obesity-induced insulin resistance (Soeller et al. 1998).

The most common risk factor for T2DM is obesity. With increasing obesity, insulin resistance increases, requiring increased expression of insulin and IAPP (Mulder et al. 1995). The stress placed on the pancreatic β-cells in an individual is dependent on overall insulin demand, but also the number of β-cells that can meet this demand. The number of β-cells in humans increases during early childhood through the mechanism of β-cell replication, and then remains relatively constant through adult life once the capacity for β-cell replication declines after early childhood (Butler et al. 2003a; Meier et al. 2008; Rahier et al. 2008). An underappreciated but potentially important characteristic of β-cell mass expansion during the postnatal period is the wide range of β-cell mass that then accrues (Figure 6.1). A wide variation in the mass of pancreatic β-cell has been observed in adult humans, monkeys, pigs, and rodents (Kjems et al. 2001; Butler et al. 2003a; Matveyenko and Butler 2006a; Ritzel et al. 2006; Meier et al. 2008; Saisho et al. 2010). This variation is probably due to nutritional programing in utero (Matveyenko et al. 2010) and to genetic variations related to the adaptation to starvation (Morris et al. 2012). These adaptations through genetics and epigenetics are meant for an environment of food scarcity and end up leading to obesity and diabetes when confronted with excessive food intake or hormonal changes that promote insulin resistance.

A proposed model for the interaction of obesity-induced insulin resistance with a wide range of β-cell mass after postnatal expansion is shown in Figure 6.1. The demand for protein synthesis per

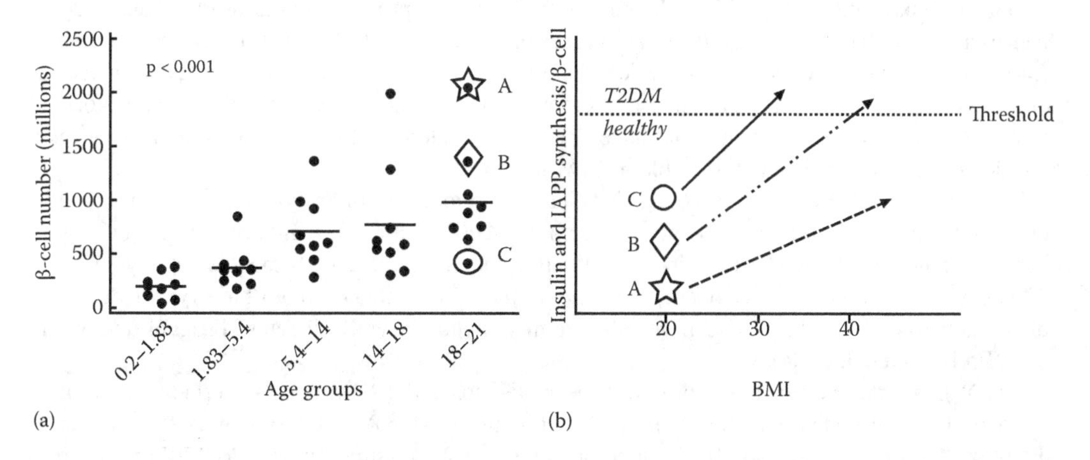

FIGURE 6.1 (a) β-Cell mass growth varies widely in childhood. The postnatal expansion of β-cell number plays a major role in establishing β-cell mass in adult humans and is highly variable between individuals. Total number of β-cells in 46 children aged 2 weeks to 21 years. Data are represented as individual data points. Individuals with high (A, star), intermediate (B, diamond), and low (C, circle) β-cell numbers are shown for consideration of β-cell workload in response to obesity in panel B. (b) The interaction of postnatal β-cell mass and body mass index (BMI) on insulin and IAPP synthetic demand is shown schematically. The risk of T2DM in individuals with high, intermediate, and low β-cell mass formed after postnatal growth incorporating the influence of obesity is shown as increasing BMI. The protein synthetic burden per β-cell increases more steeply in those with a low (individual C) than a high (individual A) number of β-cells. The burden placed on β-cells by obesity is thus higher in individual C, as is the risk to overcome the threshold for protein folding and disposal, ultimately leading to β-cell failure in T2DM. (Adapted from Costes, S. et al., *Diabetes* 62 (2), 327–335, 2013.)

β-cell of insulin and IAPP increases much more steeply in those with a low number of β-cells than in those with a high number.

6.6 GENETICS OF T2DM LINKED TO MULTIPLE RISK FACTORS

The genetics of the most common form of T2DM is complex. To date, variants in at least 65 genetic loci have been implicated in the susceptibility to T2DM, which together explain approximately 10–11% of cases (Morris et al. 2012). Many genetic studies, including single gene studies and genome-wide association studies (GWASs), aim to identify risk alleles for T2DM. Each of the variants identified by GWASs is associated with only a small increase in diabetes risk; in one analysis, even if an individual carried risk alleles at all 10 identified loci, the incremental disease risk (over noncarriers) was rather small, with risk rising only from 5% to 20% (Scott et al. 2007).

Studies of the genetics of diabetes have also supported the notion of mitochondrial oxidative dysfunction in the observed metabolic inflexibility, reduced lipid oxidation, and increased accumulation of intramyocellular lipid characteristic of insulin resistance (Kelley et al. 2002; Sreekumar et al. 2002; Mootha et al. 2003; Patti et al. 2003). It has not been determined whether these defects are critical in disease pathogenesis, or simply secondary to obesity, lipid accumulation (Crunkhorn et al. 2007), and the metabolic environment of the at-risk individual (Sreekumar et al. 2002). Additional studies in both muscle and adipose tissue from human subjects will be required to determine whether defects in mitochondrial gene expression are also a feature of isolated insulin resistance early in the course of progression to diabetes.

There is a significant amount of hereditary risk that cannot be simply explained by individual risk genes. In general, GWASs support the evidence that environmentally triggered insulin resistance interacts with genetically programmed β-cell dysfunction to precipitate diabetes. There is still a need for developing systems biology approaches to integrate comprehensive genetic information and provide new insight on gene–nutrient and gene–gene interaction in the risk for the development of T2DM.

Genetic risk profiling for T2DM does not currently have proven clinical utility (Kuehn 2010; Mihaescu et al. 2011). Genetic counseling in cases of confirmed T2DM is simply focused on family history-based recurrence risk. The American Diabetes Association recommends that before age 45, a fasting or random glucose, oral glucose tolerance test, or glycosylated hemoglobin be performed in individuals who are overweight and have one or more additional risk factors, one of which is a first-degree relative with diabetes (Table 6.1) (Mihaescu et al. 2011).

Maturity-onset diabetes of the young (MODY) is the most common type of inherited diabetes, resulting from one of several single gene defects in β-cell function. It is inherited in an autosomal dominant manner. In the classic criteria, patients typically present with diabetes at a young age (<25 years), are not necessarily obese, continue to make insulin, and do not have type 1 diabetes-related autoantibodies. They also have other family members with diabetes (Froguel and Velho 1999; Ehtisham et al. 2004).

MODY can often be mistaken for both type 1 diabetes and T2DM due to overlapping features. Thirteen different genes have been implicated in causing MODY (Ledermann 1995; Schober et al. 2009; Molven and Njolstad 2011; Bonnefond et al. 2012). Most commonly, MODY results from

TABLE 6.1
Nonmodifiable and Modifiable Risk Factors for T2DM

Nonmodifiable Risk Factors	Modifiable Risk Factors
History of gestational diabetes	Physical inactivity
Race/ethnicity	High body fat or body weight
Age over 45 years	High blood pressure
Family history of diabetes	High cholesterol

mutations in transcription factor genes, involved in the insulin secretion/β-cell development pathways (Frayling et al. 1997; Shields et al. 2010). Mutations in the *GCK* gene, encoding the enzyme glucokinase, are implicated in 32% of MODY cases (Froguel et al. 1993; Byrne et al. 1994; Matschinsky et al. 1998; Shields et al. 2008). About 10% of MODY cases are due to mutations in *HNF4A* (MODY1), encoding the transcription factor HNF4a. Some MODY families remain genetically unexplained (MODY-X), but with advancements in DNA sequencing techniques, more genes will likely be identified (Bonnefond et al. 2012). Patients with transcription factor MODY subtypes develop progressive hyperglycemia, typically in adolescence or early adulthood (Bellanne-Chantelot et al. 2011). They are at risk for diabetes-related complications if not treated, and so require appropriate monitoring, including regular eye and foot exams and screening of the urine for microalbuminuria (Velho et al. 1996).

6.6.1 Gestational Diabetes Mellitus

Gestational diabetes mellitus (GDM) is hyperglycemia first diagnosed during pregnancy, a time of insulin resistance induced by placental hormones (Kuhl 1991; Janson et al. 1999). Women diagnosed with GDM are at a significantly increased risk for developing T2DM later in life (McLaurin and Chakrabartty 1996; Lobner et al. 2006). For some women, a diagnosis of GDM may be the first recognition of preexisting T2DM, which can be asymptomatic. Maternal hyperglycemia in the third trimester, as seen with true GDM, is associated with adverse maternal, fetal, and neonatal outcomes, including macrosomia and perinatal distress, and preexisting maternal hyperglycemia increases the risk for certain congenital malformations. Therefore, diagnosis and effective treatment are essential (Clark et al. 1987; Hapo Study Cooperative Research Group et al. 2008). Treatment of GDM can include lifestyle therapy with diet and exercise, or pharmacological therapy with antidiabetic pills or insulin, depending on the degree of hyperglycemia (Hayden et al. 2007; Blumer et al. 2013). In addition, screening for diabetes is recommended 6–12 weeks postpartum given the increased risk.

GDM is often viewed not as a specific disease, but as a manifestation of underlying glucose intolerance brought out by the insulin sensitivity-challenging conditions of pregnancy, and this is borne out by association of T2DM variants with GDM (Lorenzo et al. 1994; Watanabe 2011). Family history of both GDM and T2DM can be used as a guide to estimate risk of GDM. After 10 years, women participating in the National Institutes of Health (NIH) Diabetes Prevention Program with a history of GDM and hyperglycemia assigned to placebo had a 48% higher risk of developing diabetes than women without a history of GDM with hyperglycemia. In women with a history of GDM, intensive lifestyle intervention and metformin reduced progression to diabetes compared with placebo by 35% and 40%, respectively. Among women without a history of GDM, intensive lifestyle intervention reduced the progression to diabetes by 30%, but metformin did not reduce the progression to diabetes (Butler et al. 2003b; Aroda et al. 2015). These observations suggest that women with a history of GDM have a different status than women without in terms of insulin action and developing T2DM.

6.6.2 Gene–Environment Interaction and Risk for T2DM

Risk factors for the development of T2DM include (1) family history of diabetes, implying heritable genetic polymorphisms (Barroso et al. 1999; Horikawa et al. 2000; Fajans et al. 2001; O'Rahilly et al. 2005; Florez et al. 2006; Grant et al. 2006; Owen and McCarthy 2007), and (2) both pre- and postnatal environmental factors, including suboptimal intrauterine environment resulting in epigenetic changes (Barker et al. 1993; Dabelea et al. 2000), low birth weight (Barker et al. 1993; Rich-Edwards et al. 1999), obesity (Despres 1993; Lazar 2005), inactivity (Manson et al. 1991), gestational diabetes (Buchanan and Xiang 2005), and advancing age (Lonnroth and Smith 1986) (Figure 6.2). Each of these risk factors can lead to skeletal muscle, adipose, and hepatic insulin resistance, and β-cell dysfunction. Ultimately, insulin resistance accompanied by

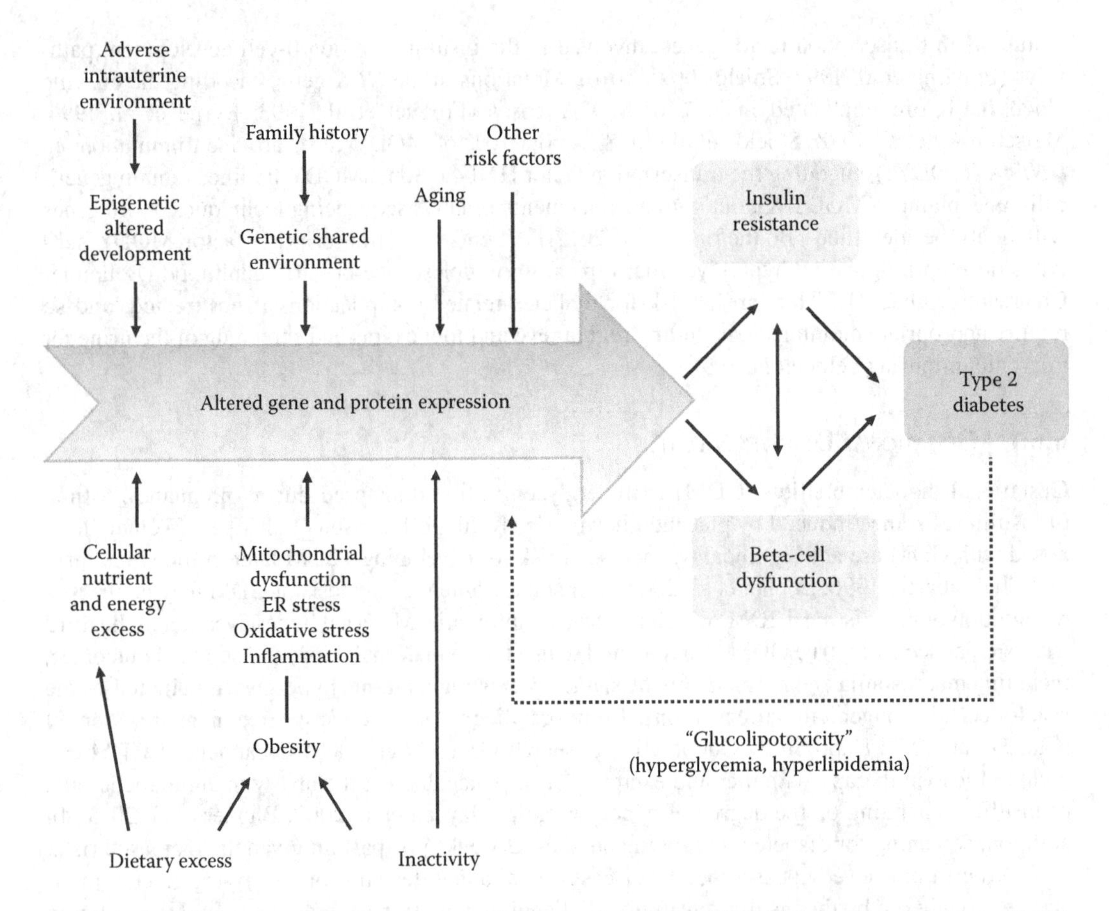

FIGURE 6.2 Multiple risk factors are involved in the pathogenesis of T2DM, including classic genetic risk (family history); prominent contribution from multiple environmental risk factors, such as a suboptimal intrauterine environment, which can impact the development of key tissues in metabolic homoeostasis; and postnatal factors, including obesity, inactivity, and aging. Together, these factors can lead to progression of insulin resistance and β-cell dysfunction, both of which are required for the ultimate development of T2DM. The pathophysiology of diabetes is further complicated by the influence of hyperglycemia and hyperlipidemia on the β-cell, creating a vicious cycle leading to β-cell decompensation in susceptible individuals. (Adapted from Jin, W., and Patti, M. E., *Clin. Sci. (Lond.)*, 116(2), 99–111, 2009.)

inadequate insulin secretory responses results in postprandial and fasting hyperglycemia. In turn, diabetes-related hyperglycemia and associated metabolic abnormalities can further alter signal transduction and gene expression (glucolipotoxicity), thus contributing to a vicious cycle (Wang et al. 1998; Patti et al. 1999).

6.6.3 Prediabetes

Prediabetes reflects failing pancreatic compensation to an underlying state of insulin resistance, most commonly caused by excess body weight or obesity. Current criteria for the diagnosis of prediabetes include impaired glucose tolerance, impaired fasting glucose, or metabolic syndrome. Any one of these factors is associated with a fivefold increase in the risk for T2DM (Garber et al. 2008).

The primary goal of prediabetes management is weight loss through a combination of increased physical activity and the creation of a caloric deficit while maintaining balanced nutrition. Loss of visceral fat reduces insulin resistance and can effectively prevent progression to diabetes, as well as improve lipids and blood pressure. However, weight loss may not directly address the pathogenesis of declining β-cell function.

Antihyperglycemic medications, such as metformin and acarbose, reduce the risk of future diabetes in prediabetic patients by 25–30%. Both medications are relatively well tolerated and safe, and they confer a cardiovascular risk benefit (Chiasson et al. 1994; U.S. Food and Drug Administration 2016). In clinical trials, thiazolidinediones prevented future development of diabetes in 60–75% of subjects with prediabetes, but this class of drugs has been associated with a number of adverse outcomes (Knowler et al. 2005; Dream Trial Investigators et al. 2006). Glucagon-like peptide 1 receptor agonists may be equally effective, but the cost and discomfort of daily injections has to date limited the application of this approach (Astrup et al. 2009).

6.7 CONCLUSION

The "thrifty gene hypothesis" suggests that human evolution has selected for genes promoting efficient food collection and nutrient storage in order to promote survival during periods of famine. In the present era of food excess, these genes would be disadvantageous because they may contribute to energy storage, impaired energy expenditure, and an increased risk for the development of T2DM (Speakman 2007).

T2DM in the United States and around the world has reached epidemic proportions. From 1980 to 2014, the number of Americans with diagnosed diabetes has increased fourfold, from 5.5 million to 22.0 million (U.S. Department of Health and Human Services 2016). The global prevalence of diabetes among adults over 18 years of age has risen from 4.7% in 1980 to 8.5% in 2014, and the incidence of diabetes is projected to continue to rise exponentially, reaching 642 million by 2040 (da Rocha Fernandes et al. 2016). Diabetes also exacts enormous personal tolls, including long-term complications of cardiovascular disease, retinopathy, neuropathy, and nephropathy.

Intimately linked with the rise in the prevalence of diabetes is the global epidemic of obesity in both highly developed industrialized countries and lower- and middle-income countries. It is estimated that in 2014, more than 1.9 billion adults, 18 years and older, were overweight. Of these, more than 600 million were obese (World Health Organization 2016). Despite the expenditure of billions of dollars on diets and health clubs, the rates of obesity continue to increase (Ogden et al. 2006). In 2004, 17.1% of children aged 2–19 years old in the United States were overweight, and 32.2% of adults over 20 years of age were obese (American Diabetes Association 2016). These findings are particularly alarming, as obesity is a major risk factor for insulin resistance and T2DM. In 2012, 86 million Americans age 20 and older had prediabetes (fasting blood glucose between 100 and 125 mg/dL). This is an increase from 79 million in 2010 (American Diabetes Association 2016). Many more individuals have insulin resistance and an unappreciated risk for T2DM. An important public health goal should be to identify individuals at high risk for the development of diabetes in order to implement prevention and early intervention strategies, including exercise, modest weight loss, and some medication, as needed (Tuomilehto et al. 2001; Knowler et al. 2002). Primary care providers can be on the front line of this effort if they familiarize themselves with the factors increasing the risks for developing T2DM and appropriate screening and intervention.

REFERENCES

Alexandratos, N. 2006. World agriculture: Towards 2030/2050. Rome: United Nations Food and Agriculture Organization.

American Diabetes Association. 2016. Diabetes statistics: Total prevalence of diabetes and pre-diabetes. Arlington, VA: American Diabetes Association. www.diabetes.org.

Aroda, V. R., C. A. Christophi, S. L. Edelstein, P. Zhang, W. H. Herman, E. Barrett-Connor, L. M. Delahanty et al. 2015. The effect of lifestyle intervention and metformin on preventing or delaying diabetes among women with and without gestational diabetes: The Diabetes Prevention Program outcomes study 10-year follow-up. *J Clin Endocrinol Metab* 100 (4):1646–1653.

Astrup, A., S. Rossner, L. Van Gaal, A. Rissanen, L. Niskanen, M. Al Hakim, J. Madsen, M. F. Rasmussen, M. E. Lean, and NN Study Group. 2009. Effects of liraglutide in the treatment of obesity: A randomised, double-blind, placebo-controlled study. *Lancet* 374 (9701):1606–1616.

Babey, S. H., J. Wolstein, A. L. Diamant, and H. Goldstein. 2016. Prediabetes in California: Nearly half of California adults on path to diabetes. *Policy Brief UCLA Cent Health Policy Res* (PB2016–1):1–8.

Barker, D. J., C. N. Hales, C. H. Fall, C. Osmond, K. Phipps, and P. M. Clark. 1993. Type 2 (non-insulin-dependent) diabetes mellitus, hypertension and hyperlipidaemia (syndrome X): Relation to reduced fetal growth. *Diabetologia* 36 (1):62–67.

Barroso, I., M. Gurnell, V. E. Crowley, M. Agostini, J. W. Schwabe, M. A. Soos, G. L. Maslen et al. 1999. Dominant negative mutations in human PPARgamma associated with severe insulin resistance, diabetes mellitus and hypertension. *Nature* 402 (6764):880–883.

Bell, A. C., K. Ge, and B. M. Popkin. 2002. The road to obesity or the path to prevention: Motorized transportation and obesity in China. *Obes Res* 10 (4):277–283.

Bellanne-Chantelot, C., D. J. Levy, C. Carette, C. Saint-Martin, J. P. Riveline, E. Larger, R. Valero et al. 2011. Clinical characteristics and diagnostic criteria of maturity-onset diabetes of the young (MODY) due to molecular anomalies of the HNF1A gene. *J Clin Endocrinol Metab* 96 (8):E1346–E1351.

Blumer, I., E. Hadar, D. R. Hadden, L. Jovanovic, J. H. Mestman, M. H. Murad, and Y. Yogev. 2013. Diabetes and pregnancy: An Endocrine Society clinical practice guideline. *J Clin Endocrinol Metab* 98 (11):4227–4249.

Bonnefond, A., J. Philippe, E. Durand, A. Dechaume, M. Huyvaert, L. Montagne, M. Marre et al. 2012. Whole-exome sequencing and high throughput genotyping identified KCNJ11 as the thirteenth MODY gene. *PLoS One* 7 (6):e37423.

Buchanan, T. A., and A. H. Xiang. 2005. Gestational diabetes mellitus. *J Clin Invest* 115 (3):485–491.

Butler, A. E., J. Jang, T. Gurlo, M. D. Carty, W. C. Soeller, and P. C. Butler. 2004. Diabetes due to a progressive defect in beta-cell mass in rats transgenic for human islet amyloid polypeptide (HIP Rat): A new model for type 2 diabetes. *Diabetes* 53 (6):1509–1516.

Butler, A. E., J. Janson, S. Bonner-Weir, R. Ritzel, R. A. Rizza, and P. C. Butler. 2003a. Beta-cell deficit and increased beta-cell apoptosis in humans with type 2 diabetes. *Diabetes* 52 (1):102–110.

Butler, A. E., J. Janson, W. C. Soeller, and P. C. Butler. 2003b. Increased beta-cell apoptosis prevents adaptive increase in beta-cell mass in mouse model of type 2 diabetes: Evidence for role of islet amyloid formation rather than direct action of amyloid. *Diabetes* 52 (9):2304–2314.

Byrne, M. M., J. Sturis, K. Clement, N. Vionnet, M. E. Pueyo, M. Stoffel, J. Takeda, P. Passa, D. Cohen, and G. I. Bell. 1994. Insulin secretory abnormalities in subjects with hyperglycemia due to glucokinase mutations. *J Clin Invest* 93 (3):1120–1130.

Chen, M. S., Jr., and B. L. Hawks. 1995. A debunking of the myth of healthy Asian Americans and Pacific Islanders. *Am J Health Promot* 9 (4):261–268.

Chiasson, J. L., R. G. Josse, J. A. Hunt, C. Palmason, N. W. Rodger, S. A. Ross, E. A. Ryan, M. H. Tan, and T. M. Wolever. 1994. The efficacy of acarbose in the treatment of patients with non-insulin-dependent diabetes mellitus. A multicenter controlled clinical trial. *Ann Intern Med* 121 (12):928–935.

Clark, A., G. J. Cooper, C. E. Lewis, J. F. Morris, A. C. Willis, K. B. Reid, and R. C. Turner. 1987. Islet amyloid formed from diabetes-associated peptide may be pathogenic in type-2 diabetes. *Lancet* 2 (8553):231–234.

Clark, A., and M. R. Nilsson. 2004. Islet amyloid: A complication of islet dysfunction or an aetiological factor in type 2 diabetes? *Diabetologia* 47 (2):157–169.

Costes, S., R. Langen, T. Gurlo, A. V. Matveyenko, and P. C. Butler. 2013. Beta-cell failure in type 2 diabetes: A case of asking too much of too few? *Diabetes* 62 (2):327–335.

Couce, M., L. A. Kane, T. D. O'Brien, J. Charlesworth, W. Soeller, J. McNeish, D. Kreutter, P. Roche, and P. C. Butler. 1996. Treatment with growth hormone and dexamethasone in mice transgenic for human islet amyloid polypeptide causes islet amyloidosis and beta-cell dysfunction. *Diabetes* 45 (8):1094–1101.

Cowie, C. C., K. F. Rust, D. D. Byrd-Holt, M. S. Eberhardt, K. M. Flegal, M. M. Engelgau, S. H. Saydah, D. E. Williams, L. S. Geiss, and E. W. Gregg. 2006. Prevalence of diabetes and impaired fasting glucose in adults in the U.S. population: National Health and Nutrition Examination Survey 1999–2002. *Diabetes Care* 29 (6):1263–1268.

Cowie, C. C., K. F. Rust, E. S. Ford, M. S. Eberhardt, D. D. Byrd-Holt, C. Li, D. E. Williams, E. W. Gregg, K. E. Bainbridge, S. H. Saydah, and L. S. Geiss. 2009. Full accounting of diabetes and pre-diabetes in the U.S. population in 1988–1994 and 2005–2006. *Diabetes Care* 32 (2):287–294.

Crunkhorn, S., F. Dearie, C. Mantzoros, H. Gami, W. S. da Silva, D. Espinoza, R. Faucette, K. Barry, A. C. Bianco, and M. E. Patti. 2007. Peroxisome proliferator activator receptor gamma coactivator-1 expression is reduced in obesity: Potential pathogenic role of saturated fatty acids and p38 mitogen-activated protein kinase activation. *J Biol Chem* 282 (21):15439–15450.

Dabelea, D., R. L. Hanson, R. S. Lindsay, D. J. Pettitt, G. Imperatore, M. M. Gabir, J. Roumain, P. H. Bennett, and W. C. Knowler. 2000. Intrauterine exposure to diabetes conveys risks for type 2 diabetes and obesity: A study of discordant sibships. *Diabetes* 49 (12):2208–2211.

da Rocha Fernandes, J., K. Ogurtsova, U. Linnenkamp, L. Guariguata, T. Seuring, P. Zhang, D. Cavan, and L. E. Makaroff. 2016. IDF Diabetes Atlas estimates of 2014 global health expenditures on diabetes. *Diabetes Res Clin Pract* 117:48–54.

de Koning, E. J., J. J. van den Brand, V. L. Mott, S. B. Charge, B. C. Hansen, N. L. Bodkin, J. F. Morris, and A. Clark. 1998. Macrophages and pancreatic islet amyloidosis. *Amyloid* 5 (4):247–254.

Despres, J. P. 1993. Abdominal obesity as important component of insulin-resistance syndrome. *Nutrition* 9 (5):452–459.

Dream Trial Investigators, H. C. Gerstein, S. Yusuf, J. Bosch, J. Pogue, P. Sheridan, N. Dinccag et al. 2006. Effect of rosiglitazone on the frequency of diabetes in patients with impaired glucose tolerance or impaired fasting glucose: A randomised controlled trial. *Lancet* 368 (9541):1096–1105.

Ehtisham, S., A. T. Hattersley, D. B. Dunger, T. G. Barrett, British Society for Paediatric Endocrinology, and Diabetes Clinical Trials Group. 2004. First UK survey of paediatric type 2 diabetes and MODY. *Arch Dis Child* 89 (6):526–529.

Fajans, S. S., G. I. Bell, and K. S. Polonsky. 2001. Molecular mechanisms and clinical pathophysiology of maturity-onset diabetes of the young. *N Engl J Med* 345 (13):971–980.

Florez, J. C., K. A. Jablonski, N. Bayley, T. I. Pollin, P. I. de Bakker, A. R. Shuldiner, W. C. Knowler, D. M. Nathan, D. Altshuler, and Diabetes Prevention Program Research Group. 2006. TCF7L2 polymorphisms and progression to diabetes in the Diabetes Prevention Program. *N Engl J Med* 355 (3):241–250.

Frayling, T. M., M. P. Bulamn, S. Ellard, M. Appleton, M. J. Dronsfield, A. D. Mackie, J. D. Baird et al. 1997. Mutations in the hepatocyte nuclear factor-1alpha gene are a common cause of maturity-onset diabetes of the young in the U.K. *Diabetes* 46 (4):720–725.

Froguel, P., and G. Velho. 1999. Molecular genetics of maturity-onset diabetes of the young. *Trends Endocrinol Metab* 10 (4):142–146.

Froguel, P., H. Zouali, N. Vionnet, G. Velho, M. Vaxillaire, F. Sun, S. Lesage et al. 1993. Familial hyperglycemia due to mutations in glucokinase. Definition of a subtype of diabetes mellitus. *N Engl J Med* 328 (10):697–702.

Garber, A. J., Y. Handelsman, D. Einhorn, D. A. Bergman, Z. T. Bloomgarden, V. Fonseca, W. T. Garvey et al. 2008. Diagnosis and management of prediabetes in the continuum of hyperglycemia: When do the risks of diabetes begin? A consensus statement from the American College of Endocrinology and the American Association of Clinical Endocrinologists. *Endocr Pract* 14 (7):933–946.

Gitter, B. D., L. M. Cox, C. D. Carlson, and P. C. May. 2000. Human amylin stimulates inflammatory cytokine secretion from human glioma cells. *Neuroimmunomodulation* 7 (3):147–152.

Grant, S. F., G. Thorleifsson, I. Reynisdottir, R. Benediktsson, A. Manolescu, J. Sainz, A. Helgason et al. 2006. Variant of transcription factor 7-like 2 (TCF7L2) gene confers risk of type 2 diabetes. *Nat Genet* 38 (3):320–323.

Gunasekaran, U., and M. Gannon. 2011. Type 2 diabetes and the aging pancreatic beta cell. *Aging (Albany NY)* 3 (6):565–575.

Hapo Study Cooperative Research Group, B. E. Metzger, L. P. Lowe, A. R. Dyer, E. R. Trimble, U. Chaovarindr, D. R. Coustan et al. 2008. Hyperglycemia and adverse pregnancy outcomes. *N Engl J Med* 358 (19):1991–2002.

Hawkes, C. 2005. The role of foreign direct investment in the nutrition transition. *Public Health Nutr* 8 (4):357–365.

Hayden, M. R., P. R. Karuparthi, C. M. Manrique, G. Lastra, J. Habibi, and J. R. Sowers. 2007. Longitudinal ultrastructure study of islet amyloid in the HIP rat model of type 2 diabetes mellitus. *Exp Biol Med (Maywood)* 232 (6):772–779.

Horikawa, Y., N. Oda, N. J. Cox, X. Li, M. Orho-Melander, M. Hara, Y. Hinokio et al. 2000. Genetic variation in the gene encoding calpain-10 is associated with type 2 diabetes mellitus. *Nat Genet* 26 (2):163–175.

Huang, C. J., T. Gurlo, L. Haataja, S. Costes, M. Daval, S. Ryazantsev, X. Wu, A. E. Butler, and P. C. Butler. 2010. Calcium-activated calpain-2 is a mediator of beta cell dysfunction and apoptosis in type 2 diabetes. *J Biol Chem* 285 (1):339–348.

Huang, C. J., C. Y. Lin, L. Haataja, T. Gurlo, A. E. Butler, R. A. Rizza, and P. C. Butler. 2007. High expression rates of human islet amyloid polypeptide induce endoplasmic reticulum stress mediated beta-cell apoptosis, a characteristic of humans with type 2 but not type 1 diabetes. *Diabetes* 56 (8): 2016–2027.

Janson, J., R. H. Ashley, D. Harrison, S. McIntyre, and P. C. Butler. 1999. The mechanism of islet amyloid polypeptide toxicity is membrane disruption by intermediate-sized toxic amyloid particles. *Diabetes* 48 (3):491–498.

Janson, J., W. C. Soeller, P. C. Roche, R. T. Nelson, A. J. Torchia, D. K. Kreutter, and P. C. Butler. 1996. Spontaneous diabetes mellitus in transgenic mice expressing human islet amyloid polypeptide. *Proc Natl Acad Sci USA* 93 (14):7283–7288.

Jin, W., and M. E. Patti. 2009. Genetic determinants and molecular pathways in the pathogenesis of type 2 diabetes. *Clin Sci (Lond)* 116 (2):99–111.

Jones-Smith, J. C., P. Gordon-Larsen, A. Siddiqi, and B. M. Popkin. 2011. Cross-national comparisons of time trends in overweight inequality by socioeconomic status among women using repeated cross-sectional surveys from 37 developing countries, 1989–2007. *Am J Epidemiol* 173 (6):667–675.

Jones-Smith, J. C., P. Gordon-Larsen, A. Siddiqi, and B. M. Popkin. 2012. Is the burden of overweight shifting to the poor across the globe? Time trends among women in 39 low- and middle-income countries (1991–2008). *Int J Obes (Lond)* 36 (8):1114–1120.

Kearney, J. 2010. Food consumption trends and drivers. *Philos Trans R Soc Lond B Biol Sci* 365 (1554):2793–2807.

Kelley, D. E., J. He, E. V. Menshikova, and V. B. Ritov. 2002. Dysfunction of mitochondria in human skeletal muscle in type 2 diabetes. *Diabetes* 51 (10):2944–2950.

Kjems, L. L., B. M. Kirby, E. M. Welsh, J. D. Veldhuis, M. Straume, S. S. McIntyre, D. Yang, P. Lefebvre, and P. C. Butler. 2001. Decrease in beta-cell mass leads to impaired pulsatile insulin secretion, reduced postprandial hepatic insulin clearance, and relative hyperglucagonemia in the minipig. *Diabetes* 50 (9):2001–2012.

Kloppel, G., M. Lohr, K. Habich, M. Oberholzer, and P. U. Heitz. 1985. Islet pathology and the pathogenesis of type 1 and type 2 diabetes mellitus revisited. *Surv Synth Pathol Res* 4 (2):110–125.

Knowler, W. C., E. Barrett-Connor, S. E. Fowler, R. F. Hamman, J. M. Lachin, E. A. Walker, D. M. Nathan, and Diabetes Prevention Program Research Group. 2002. Reduction in the incidence of type 2 diabetes with lifestyle intervention or metformin. *N Engl J Med* 346 (6):393–403.

Knowler, W. C., R. F. Hamman, S. L. Edelstein, E. Barrett-Connor, D. A. Ehrmann, E. A. Walker, S. E. Fowler, D. M. Nathan, S. E. Kahn, and Diabetes Prevention Program Research Group. 2005. Prevention of type 2 diabetes with troglitazone in the Diabetes Prevention Program. *Diabetes* 54 (4):1150–1156.

Kuehn, B. M. 2010. Inconsistent results, inaccurate claims plague direct-to-consumer gene tests. *JAMA* 304 (12):1313–1315.

Kuhl, C. 1991. Insulin secretion and insulin resistance in pregnancy and GDM. Implications for diagnosis and management. *Diabetes* 40 (Suppl 2):18–24.

Lazar, M. A. 2005. How obesity causes diabetes: Not a tall tale. *Science* 307 (5708):373–375.

Ledermann, H. M. 1995. Maturity-onset diabetes of the young (MODY) at least ten times more common in Europe than previously assumed? *Diabetologia* 38 (12):1482.

Lee, S., K. G. Birukov, C. E. Romanoski, J. R. Springstead, A. J. Lusis, and J. A. Berliner. 2012. Role of phospholipid oxidation products in atherosclerosis. *Circ Res* 111 (6):778–799.

Lobner, K., A. Knopff, A. Baumgarten, U. Mollenhauer, S. Marienfeld, M. Garrido-Franco, E. Bonifacio, and A. G. Ziegler. 2006. Predictors of postpartum diabetes in women with gestational diabetes mellitus. *Diabetes* 55 (3):792–797.

Lonnroth, P., and U. Smith. 1986. Aging enhances the insulin resistance in obesity through both receptor and postreceptor alterations. *J Clin Endocrinol Metab* 62 (2):433–437.

Lorenzo, A., B. Razzaboni, G. C. Weir, and B. A. Yankner. 1994. Pancreatic islet cell toxicity of amylin associated with type-2 diabetes mellitus. *Nature* 368 (6473):756–760.

Manson, J. E., E. B. Rimm, M. J. Stampfer, G. A. Colditz, W. C. Willett, A. S. Krolewski, B. Rosner, C. H. Hennekens, and F. E. Speizer. 1991. Physical activity and incidence of non-insulin-dependent diabetes mellitus in women. *Lancet* 338 (8770):774–778.

Marseglia, L., S. Manti, G. D'Angelo, A. Nicotera, E. Parisi, G. Di Rosa, E. Gitto, and T. Arrigo. 2015. Oxidative stress in obesity: A critical component in human diseases. *Int J Mol Sci* 16 (1):378–400.

Masters, S. L., A. Dunne, S. L. Subramanian, R. L. Hull, G. M. Tannahill, F. A. Sharp, C. Becker et al. 2010. Activation of the NLRP3 inflammasome by islet amyloid polypeptide provides a mechanism for enhanced IL-1beta in type 2 diabetes. *Nat Immunol* 11 (10):897–904.

Matschinsky, F. M., B. Glaser, and M. A. Magnuson. 1998. Pancreatic beta-cell glucokinase: Closing the gap between theoretical concepts and experimental realities. *Diabetes* 47 (3):307–315.

Matveyenko, A. V., and P. C. Butler. 2006a. Beta-cell deficit due to increased apoptosis in the human islet amyloid polypeptide transgenic (HIP) rat recapitulates the metabolic defects present in type 2 diabetes. *Diabetes* 55 (7):2106–2114.

Matveyenko, A. V., and P. C. Butler. 2006b. Islet amyloid polypeptide (IAPP) transgenic rodents as models for type 2 diabetes. *ILAR J* 47 (3):225–233.

Matveyenko, A. V., I. Singh, B. C. Shin, S. Georgia, and S. U. Devaskar. 2010. Differential effects of prenatal and postnatal nutritional environment on ss-cell mass development and turnover in male and female rats. *Endocrinology* 151 (12):5647–5656.

McLaurin, J., and A. Chakrabartty. 1996. Membrane disruption by Alzheimer beta-amyloid peptides mediated through specific binding to either phospholipids or gangliosides. Implications for neurotoxicity. *J Biol Chem* 271 (43):26482–26489.

Meier, J. J., A. E. Butler, Y. Saisho, T. Monchamp, R. Galasso, A. Bhushan, R. A. Rizza, and P. C. Butler. 2008. Beta-cell replication is the primary mechanism subserving the postnatal expansion of beta-cell mass in humans. *Diabetes* 57 (6):1584–1594.

Mendez, M. A., C. A. Monteiro, and B. M. Popkin. 2005. Overweight exceeds underweight among women in most developing countries. *Am J Clin Nutr* 81 (3):714–721.

Mihaescu, R., J. Meigs, E. Sijbrands, and A. C. Janssens. 2011. Genetic risk profiling for prediction of type 2 diabetes. *PLoS Curr* 3:RRN1208.

Misra, A., and L. Khurana. 2008. Obesity and the metabolic syndrome in developing countries. *J Clin Endocrinol Metab* 93 (11 Suppl 1):S9–S30.

Molven, A., and P. R. Njolstad. 2011. Role of molecular genetics in transforming diagnosis of diabetes mellitus. *Expert Rev Mol Diagn* 11 (3):313–320.

Monteiro, C. A., W. L. Conde, and B. M. Popkin. 2007. Income-specific trends in obesity in Brazil: 1975–2003. *Am J Public Health* 97 (10):1808–1812.

Mootha, V. K., C. M. Lindgren, K. F. Eriksson, A. Subramanian, S. Sihag, J. Lehar, P. Puigserver et al. 2003. PGC-1alpha-responsive genes involved in oxidative phosphorylation are coordinately downregulated in human diabetes. *Nat Genet* 34 (3):267–273.

Morris, A. P., B. F. Voight, T. M. Teslovich, T. Ferreira, A. V. Segre, V. Steinthorsdottir, R. J. Strawbridge et al. 2012. Large-scale association analysis provides insights into the genetic architecture and pathophysiology of type 2 diabetes. *Nat Genet* 44 (9):981–990.

Mulder, H., B. Ahren, M. Stridsberg, and F. Sundler. 1995. Non-parallelism of islet amyloid polypeptide (amylin) and insulin gene expression in rats islets following dexamethasone treatment. *Diabetologia* 38 (4):395–402.

Ng, S. W., and B. M. Popkin. 2012. Time use and physical activity: A shift away from movement across the globe. *Obes Rev* 13 (8):659–680.

Nguyen, P. T., N. Andraka, C. A. De Carufel, and S. Bourgault. 2015a. Mechanistic contributions of biological cofactors in islet amyloid polypeptide amyloidogenesis. *J Diabetes Res* 2015:515307.

Nguyen, T. H., T. N. Nguyen, T. Fischer, W. Ha, and T. V. Tran. 2015b. Type 2 diabetes among Asian Americans: Prevalence and prevention. *World J Diabetes* 6 (4):543–547.

Ogden, C. L., M. D. Carroll, L. R. Curtin, M. A. McDowell, C. J. Tabak, and K. M. Flegal. 2006. Prevalence of overweight and obesity in the United States, 1999–2004. *JAMA* 295 (13):1549–1555.

O'Rahilly, S., I. Barroso, and N. J. Wareham. 2005. Genetic factors in type 2 diabetes: The end of the beginning? *Science* 307 (5708):370–373.

Owen, K. R., and M. I. McCarthy. 2007. Genetics of type 2 diabetes. *Curr Opin Genet Dev* 17 (3):239–244.

Patti, M. E., A. J. Butte, S. Crunkhorn, K. Cusi, R. Berria, S. Kashyap, Y. Miyazaki et al. 2003. Coordinated reduction of genes of oxidative metabolism in humans with insulin resistance and diabetes: Potential role of PGC1 and NRF1. *Proc Natl Acad Sci USA* 100 (14):8466–8471.

Patti, M. E., A. Virkamaki, E. J. Landaker, C. R. Kahn, and H. Yki-Jarvinen. 1999. Activation of the hexosamine pathway by glucosamine in vivo induces insulin resistance of early postreceptor insulin signaling events in skeletal muscle. *Diabetes* 48 (8):1562–1571.

Popkin, B. M. 2006. Global nutrition dynamics: The world is shifting rapidly toward a diet linked with noncommunicable diseases. *Am J Clin Nutr* 84 (2):289–298.

Popkin, B. M., L. S. Adair, and S. W. Ng. 2012. Global nutrition transition and the pandemic of obesity in developing countries. *Nutr Rev* 70 (1):3–21.

Rahier, J., Y. Guiot, R. M. Goebbels, C. Sempoux, and J. C. Henquin. 2008. Pancreatic beta-cell mass in European subjects with type 2 diabetes. *Diabetes Obes Metab* 10 (Suppl 4):32–42.

Rich-Edwards, J. W., G. A. Colditz, M. J. Stampfer, W. C. Willett, M. W. Gillman, C. H. Hennekens, F. E. Speizer, and J. E. Manson. 1999. Birthweight and the risk for type 2 diabetes mellitus in adult women. *Ann Intern Med* 130 (4 Pt 1):278–284.

Ritzel, R. A., A. E. Butler, R. A. Rizza, J. D. Veldhuis, and P. C. Butler. 2006. Relationship between beta-cell mass and fasting blood glucose concentration in humans. *Diabetes Care* 29 (3):717–718.

Saisho, Y., A. E. Butler, E. Manesso, R. Galasso, L. Zhang, T. Gurlo, G. M. Toffolo, C. Cobelli, K. Kavanagh, J. D. Wagner, and P. C. Butler. 2010. Relationship between fractional pancreatic beta cell area and fasting plasma glucose concentration in monkeys. *Diabetologia* 53 (1):111–114.

Schober, E., B. Rami, M. Grabert, A. Thon, T. Kapellen, T. Reinehr, R. W. Holl, and DPV-Wiss Initiative of the German Working Group for Paediatric Diabetology. 2009. Phenotypical aspects of maturity-onset diabetes of the young (MODY diabetes) in comparison with type 2 diabetes mellitus (T2DM) in children and adolescents: Experience from a large multicentre database. *Diabet Med* 26 (5):466–473.

Scott, L. J., K. L. Mohlke, L. L. Bonnycastle, C. J. Willer, Y. Li, W. L. Duren, M. R. Erdos et al. 2007. A genome-wide association study of type 2 diabetes in Finns detects multiple susceptibility variants. *Science* 316 (5829):1341–1345.

Shields, B. M., S. Hicks, M. H. Shepherd, K. Colclough, A. T. Hattersley, and S. Ellard. 2010. Maturity-onset diabetes of the young (MODY): How many cases are we missing? *Diabetologia* 53 (12):2504–2508.

Shields, B. M., G. Spyer, A. S. Slingerland, B. A. Knight, S. Ellard, P. M. Clark, S. Hauguel-de Mouzon, and A. T. Hattersley. 2008. Mutations in the glucokinase gene of the fetus result in reduced placental weight. *Diabetes Care* 31 (4):753–757.

Soeller, W. C., J. Janson, S. E. Hart, J. C. Parker, M. D. Carty, R. W. Stevenson, D. K. Kreutter, and P. C. Butler. 1998. Islet amyloid-associated diabetes in obese A(vy)/a mice expressing human islet amyloid polypeptide. *Diabetes* 47 (5):743–750.

Speakman, J. R. 2007. A nonadaptive scenario explaining the genetic predisposition to obesity: The "predation release" hypothesis. *Cell Metab* 6 (1):5–12.

Spranger, J., A. Kroke, M. Mohlig, K. Hoffmann, M. M. Bergmann, M. Ristow, H. Boeing, and A. F. Pfeiffer. 2003. Inflammatory cytokines and the risk to develop type 2 diabetes: Results of the prospective population-based European Prospective Investigation into Cancer and Nutrition (EPIC)-Potsdam Study. *Diabetes* 52 (3):812–817.

Sreekumar, R., P. Halvatsiotis, J. C. Schimke, and K. S. Nair. 2002. Gene expression profile in skeletal muscle of type 2 diabetes and the effect of insulin treatment. *Diabetes* 51 (6):1913–1920.

Stuckler, D., M. McKee, S. Ebrahim, and S. Basu. 2012. Manufacturing epidemics: The role of global producers in increased consumption of unhealthy commodities including processed foods, alcohol, and tobacco. *PLoS Med* 9 (6):e1001235.

Subramanyam, M. A., I. Kawachi, L. F. Berkman, and S. V. Subramanian. 2010. Socioeconomic inequalities in childhood undernutrition in India: Analyzing trends between 1992 and 2005. *PLoS One* 5 (6):e11392.

Tendulkar, S. A., R. C. Hamilton, C. Chu, L. Arsenault, K. Duffy, V. Huynh, M. Hung, E. Lee, S. Jane, and E. Friedman. 2012. Investigating the myth of the "model minority": A participatory community health assessment of Chinese and Vietnamese adults. *J Immigr Minor Health* 14 (5):850–857.

Tsatsoulis, A., M. D. Mantzaris, S. Bellou, and M. Andrikoula. 2013. Insulin resistance: An adaptive mechanism becomes maladaptive in the current environment—An evolutionary perspective. *Metabolism* 62 (5):622–633.

Tuomilehto, J., J. Lindstrom, J. G. Eriksson, T. T. Valle, H. Hamalainen, P. Ilanne-Parikka, S. Keinanen-Kiukaanniemi et al. 2001. Prevention of type 2 diabetes mellitus by changes in lifestyle among subjects with impaired glucose tolerance. *N Engl J Med* 344 (18):1343–1350.

U.S. Department of Health and Human Services. 2016. Centers for Disease Control and Prevention diabetes data and statistics. Web publication of the U.S. Diabetes Surveillance System. Washington, DC: U.S. Department of Health and Human Services. https://www.cdc.gov/diabetes/data/.

U.S. Food and Drug Administration. 2016. FDA approves Invokana to treat type 2 diabetes—First in a new class of diabetes drugs. Washington, DC: U.S. Food and Drug Administration. http://www.fda.gov/NewsEvents/Newsroom/PressAnnouncements/ucm345848.htm.

Velho, G., M. Vaxillaire, V. Boccio, G. Charpentier, and P. Froguel. 1996. Diabetes complications in NIDDM kindreds linked to the MODY3 locus on chromosome 12q. *Diabetes Care* 19 (9):915–919.

Wang, J., R. Liu, M. Hawkins, N. Barzilai, and L. Rossetti. 1998. A nutrient-sensing pathway regulates leptin gene expression in muscle and fat. *Nature* 393 (6686):684–688.

Wang, Z., F. Zhai, B. Zhang, and B. M. Popkin. 2012. Trends in Chinese snacking behaviors and patterns and the social-demographic role between 1991 and 2009. *Asia Pac J Clin Nutr* 21 (2):253–262.

Watanabe, R. M. 2011. Inherited destiny? Genetics and gestational diabetes mellitus. *Genome Med* 3 (3):18.

Westwell-Roper, C. Y., C. A. Chehroudi, H. C. Denroche, J. A. Courtade, J. A. Ehses, and C. B. Verchere. 2015. IL-1 mediates amyloid-associated islet dysfunction and inflammation in human islet amyloid polypeptide transgenic mice. *Diabetologia* 58 (3):575–585.

Westwell-Roper, C. Y., D. L. Dai, G. Soukhatcheva, K. J. Potter, N. van Rooijen, J. A. Ehses, and C. B. Verchere. 2011. IL-1 blockade attenuates islet amyloid polypeptide-induced proinflammatory cytokine release and pancreatic islet graft dysfunction. *J Immunol* 187 (5):2755–2765.

Westwell-Roper, C. Y., J. A. Ehses, and C. B. Verchere. 2014. Resident macrophages mediate islet amyloid polypeptide-induced islet IL-1beta production and beta-cell dysfunction. *Diabetes* 63 (5):1698–1711.

Wookey, P. J., T. A. Lutz, and S. Andrikopoulos. 2006. Amylin in the periphery II: An updated mini-review. *ScientificWorldJournal* 6:1642–1655.

World Health Organization. 2016. Obesity and overweight fact sheet. Geneva: World Heath Organization. http://www.who.int/mediacentre/factsheets/fs311/en/ (updated June 20, 2016).

Xu, Y., L. Wang, J. He, Y. Bi, M. Li, T. Wang, L. Wang et al. 2013. Prevalence and control of diabetes in Chinese adults. *JAMA* 310 (9):948–959.

Yates, S. L., L. H. Burgess, J. Kocsis-Angle, J. M. Antal, M. D. Dority, P. B. Embury, A. M. Piotrkowski, and K. R. Brunden. 2000. Amyloid beta and amylin fibrils induce increases in proinflammatory cytokine and chemokine production by THP-1 cells and murine microglia. *J Neurochem* 74 (3):1017–1025.

Young, A. A., B. Gedulin, W. Vine, A. Percy, and T. J. Rink. 1995. Gastric emptying is accelerated in diabetic BB rats and is slowed by subcutaneous injections of amylin. *Diabetologia* 38 (6):642–648.

Yracheta, J. M., J. Alfonso, M. A. Lanaspa, C. Roncal-Jimenez, S. B. Johnson, L. G. Sanchez-Lozada, and R. J. Johnson. 2015. Hispanic Americans living in the United States and their risk for obesity, diabetes and kidney disease: Genetic and environmental considerations. *Postgrad Med* 127 (5):503–510.

Zhai, F., H. Wang, S. Du, Y. He, Z. Wang, K. Ge, and B. M. Popkin. 2007. Lifespan nutrition and changing socio-economic conditions in China. *Asia Pac J Clin Nutr* 16 (Suppl 1):374–382.

7 Managing Diabetes without Weight Gain

7.1 INTRODUCTION

This chapter is about managing patients with diagnosed diabetes mellitus while also encouraging a nutrition program that not only controls blood sugar but also is consistent with addressing overweight and obesity-related comorbidities, including age-related chronic diseases. Nutrition is central to the prevention and treatment of diabetes mellitus, but the confusing array of medications and the focus on glucose control have blinded the primary care practitioner to the benefits of weight management interventions for type 2 diabetes (T2DM), which are wrongly thought to be a futile exercise.

The approaches to type 1 (T1DM) and type 2 (T2DM) diabetes mellitus are different. T1DM results from an autoimmune destruction of insulin-secreting cells in the pancreas and requires insulin replacement and matching of the diet to the insulin provided (Hahr and Molitch 2008). On the other hand, T2DM is closely associated with excess adiposity and requires primary attention to weight management in prevention and treatment until the late stages of T2DM, when insulin stores are depleted (Wycherley et al. 2010).

Given the prevalence of T2DM, weight reduction and weight management in T2DM are discussed first, followed by sections on the various foods that can have a role in controlling blood sugar in patients with either T1DM or T2DM. Controlling blood sugar is an important component of treatment, but not the sole aspect of improving the quality of life of diabetes patients. Overall lifestyle change can help control risk factors for cardiovascular disease, which is heightened by the inflammation, oxidative stress, and lipid abnormalities that frequently accompany T2DM. As with other common chronic diseases, those risk factors present before diagnosis and reviewed in Chapter 5 are likely to be present at the time that these patients are diagnosed with diabetes.

7.2 DIAGNOSIS OF T2DM

The diagnosis and management of diabetes has advanced and evolved over time in response to advances in laboratory diagnosis. The management of diabetes has changed dramatically during the past several thousand years. The option preferred by the physicians consulting with the pharaoh of Egypt 3500 years ago was a mixture of "water from the bird pond," elderberry, fibers from the asit plant, milk, beer, cucumber flower, and green dates (Sanders 2002).

Diabetes mellitus in Latin translates to "sweet urine." Historically, there were two disorders that caused the production of excessive amounts of urine: diabetes mellitus and diabetes insipidus. Diabetes insipidus is due to inappropriate production of antidiuretic hormone (ADH), and the urine is not sweet. You might wonder how these physicians knew that the urine was sweet in one condition and not in the other in the absence of clinical laboratory measurements. The unpleasant fact is that they tasted the urine.

Until 1921, there was little you could do but watch a patient with T1DM and a total lack of insulin die from starvation. At that time, Banting and Best transformed T1DM from a malignant disease into a chronic disorder. Only 2 years passed between the initial experiments in dogs that led to the discovery of a pancreatic factor that could cure T1DM and its widespread human application and the awarding of the Nobel Prize in 1923. Insulin-related research was the impetus for three other Nobel Prize awards for the determination of the chemical structure of insulin by Frederick Sanger in 1958, the determination of the three-dimensional structures of insulin by Dorothy Hodgkin in 1964, and the development of the radioimmunoassay by Solomon Berson and Rosalyn Yalow in 1959–1960, which transformed the fields of endocrinology and metabolism and led to a Nobel Prize for Yalow in 1977, as Berson tragically died before receiving the award (Kahn and Roth 2004). Their key discovery using this method was that patients with T1DM had little or no insulin prior to treatment but developed anti-insulin antibodies. These anti-insulin antibodies were then mixed with radioactive insulin that had been chemically labeled with an iodine isotope. As a result of this famous experiment, it was found that that T2DM patients had not only detectable but also sometimes high levels of insulin in the face of high blood sugars.

Today, we have sophisticated diagnostic criteria for the diabetes mellitus diagnosis from the American Diabetes Association (ADA), including any of the following (ADA 2010):

1. A hemoglobin A1c (HbA1c) level of 6.5% or higher. The test should be performed in a laboratory using a method that is certified by the National Glycohemoglobin Standardization Program (NGSP) and standardized or traceable to the Diabetes Control and Complications Trial (DCCT) reference assay.
2. A fasting plasma glucose (FPG) level of 126 mg/dL (7 mmol/L) or higher. Fasting is defined as no caloric intake for at least 8 hours.
3. A 2-hour plasma glucose level of 200 mg/dL (11.1 mmol/L) or higher during a 75 g oral glucose tolerance test (OGTT).
4. A random plasma glucose of 200 mg/dL (11.1 mmol/L) or higher in a patient with classic symptoms of hyperglycemia (i.e., polyuria, polydipsia, polyphagia, and weight loss) or hyperglycemic crisis.

As you will notice, all the above methods utilize glucose for practical reasons while understanding that both T1DM and T2DM, the latter being far more common, have different etiologies, which are discussed in detail in Chapter 5. In fact, there was much confusion about the distinctions between the two diagnoses in the 1970s and 1980s. Nonetheless, the focus on glucose control has stimulated most of the drug development targeted at the treatment of diabetes.

In 1947, Jean Vague was the first to suggest that the regional distribution of body fat was a more important correlate of the complications of obesity than excess fatness (Vague 1996a,b). In the 1980s, Björntorp and Kissebah simultaneously reported convincing metabolic and epidemiological data that confirmed that the proportion of abdominal fat was a key correlate of metabolic abnormalities leading to both diabetes and atherosclerosis (Kissebah et al. 1982; Lapidus et al. 1984; Larsson et al. 1984; Ohlson et al. 1985).

As a result of this focus on glucose control, most primary care providers and endocrinologists have been focused for decades on the use of insulin to lower blood sugar. Various insulin preparations that were short acting or long acting were used in both T1DM and T2DM. A large number of drugs were also developed based on their ability to lower glucose levels. As discussed in the next section, metformin is the most widely used drug globally for the treatment of diabetes, but there are also a large array of diabetes drugs that both mystify and occupy primary care practitioners in a quest to control blood sugar while having to accept noncompliance with dietary and weight management interventions that could prove useful until the very late stages of diabetes, when insulin deficiency is the primary issue.

7.3 PHARMACOLOGICAL TREATMENT OF DIABETES: A BRIEF HISTORY

French lilac, or goat's rue (*Galega officinalis*), was used as a folk remedy for diabetes in southern and eastern Europe during medieval times (White and Campbell 2008). In the early twentieth century, the glucose-lowering compound in this plant, guanidine, was isolated and synthesized (Frank et al. 1926). It was named Synthalin in Germany and used to treat diabetes during the 1920s (Galloway 1988). These early drugs were toxic to the liver, and their use ended with the discovery of insulin. However, in the 1960s and 1970s, drugs modified to reduce toxicity included the biguanide drugs phenformin in the United States, metformin in France, and buformin in Germany (Alberti et al. 1997). Phenformin and buformin were associated with lactic acidosis, especially in elderly individuals with reduced renal function. Metformin, first introduced in 1959, was approved in the United States in the 1990s. Metformin is the most widely used glucose-lowering drug in the world (White and Campbell 2008).

Some drug companies promoted the idea that insulin was no longer the central pillar in diabetes treatment, and that there was now an oral "cure" for diabetes. Manufacturers of one of the drugs being promoted used the acronym DBI-TD for "Don't Buy Insulin Today" as a marketing slogan.

Another class of drugs lowering blood sugar are the sulfonylureas. In the 1950s, the first sulfonlyurea, tolbutamide, was marketed in Germany (Quianzon and Cheikh 2012). This was followed by the introduction of the other first-generation agents, including chlorpropamide, acetohexamide, and tolazamide. Glipizide and glyburide were more potent and were introduced in 1984. These agents had been in use in Europe for several years before this. Glimepiride, which is sometimes referred to as a third-generation agent, was released in 1995 (Quianzon and Cheikh 2012). The major side effects of the sulfonylureas are hypoglycemia and weight gain.

Thiazolidinediones, which are also known simply as "glitazones," were initially introduced to the U.S. market in 1996. These agents are peroxisome proliferator-activated receptor γ activators whose mechanisms of action are enhancement of skeletal muscle insulin sensitivity and reduction in hepatic glucose production (Inzucchi et al. 2012). These agents do not increase the risk of hypoglycemia and have a more durable effect than metformin or sulfonylureas, but the two currently available agents, pioglitazone and rosiglitazone, can cause fluid retention and must be used with caution in patients with heart failure (Inzucchi et al. 2012).

The meglitinides, also called "glinides," have a mechanism of action similar to that of the sulfonylureas but are structurally unrelated to sulfonylureas. These drugs lower blood glucose levels by stimulating insulin release from the pancreas. As with the sulfonylureas, glinide-induced insulin stimulation is dependent on functioning pancreatic β-cells (White and Campbell 2008). However, the effect of these drugs is glucose dependent and diminishes at low glucose concentrations. The glinides have a more rapid onset and a shorter duration of action than the second-generation sulfonylureas, so that multiple daily dosing is required. Repaglinide (approved in 1997) and nateglinide (approved in 2000) are the two drugs in this class (Quianzon and Cheikh 2012).

Glucagon-like peptide 1 (GLP-1) and its analogs reduce glucose levels via a glucose-linked enhancement of insulin secretion; this was first observed when it was noted that oral glucose stimulated insulin secretion to a greater extent than intravenous insulin due to gastrointestinal hormones called incretins. The short half-life of 1–2 minutes of native GLP-1 due to rapid degradation by the enzyme dipeptidyl peptidase 4 (DPP-4) led to the search for GLP-1 analogs and DPP-4 inhibitors. Exendin-4 was isolated from the salivary gland venom of the Gila monster reptile (*Heloderma suspectum*). Xenatide, a synthetically produced form of exendin-4, was the first GLP-1, in 2005. A second GLP-1 receptor agonist, liraglutide, was approved in 2010, which is modified to be long acting. In 2012, a long-acting form of exenatide that could be administered weekly was approved. Weight loss is one advantage of treatment with incretin-based agents. However, these compounds can cause significant gastrointestinal side effects, particularly early in therapy, and concerns about associations between GLP-1 receptor agonists and pancreatitis are ongoing. They are also expensive and injectable. The first DPP-4 inhibitor, called sitagliptin, could be taken orally and acted by prolonging the circulating half-life of GLP-1. It was approved in 2006 and followed by the release of saxagliptin and linagliptin. Alogliptin was approved by the Food and Drug Administration (FDA) in 2013. Vildagliptin has been approved for use in Europe but is not available in the United States. DPP-4 inhibitors are weight neutral and do not tend to cause hypoglycemia (White 2014). However, pancreatitis has been reported in patients treated with DPP-4 inhibitors (Quianzon and Cheikh 2012).

The endogenous neuroendocrine hormone amylin was discovered in 1987. Amylin is cosecreted with insulin by the β-cells in equimolar amounts. Patients with T2DM have reduced amounts of amylin, whereas patients with T1DM have essentially no amylin. The only amylin analog currently on the market is pramlintide, approved by the FDA in 2005 (Quianzon and Cheikh 2012). It delays gastric emptying, reducing postprandial glucose and glucagon and causing some weight loss. The primary side effect is nausea.

The sodium glucose cotransporter 2 (SGLT-2) inhibitors antagonize a high-capacity, low-affinity glucose transporter found primarily in the kidney (White 2010). This transporter is responsible for ~90% of glucose reabsorption in the kidney. When this transporter is antagonized, excess glucose in the renal tubules is not reabsorbed, and glucose is excreted in the urine. This results in a net loss of glucose and a reduction in hyperglycemia. In addition to reducing hyperglycemia, SGLT-2 inhibitors have also been associated with slight reductions in weight and body mass index (BMI). However, an increase in urinary or genital infections is common and is especially troublesome in female patients (Monami et al. 2014).

7.4 DIABETES AND OBESITY

It had been noted for decades that those adults with T2DM were also often overweight or obese and had poor eating habits, but that finding did not impact treatment until the obesity epidemic was recognized in the 1990s. There are now 11 different categories of medications directed at the management of hyperglycemia in patients with diabetes, which is the major focus of medical approaches to diabetes treatment. Additionally, the potential dosing and various combinations of these agents are staggering and can be bewildering to primary care providers trying to design optimum therapy regimens for a given patient.

Obesity is more than a risk factor for the development of T2DM; it is a necessary component of the pathophysiology of the disease until the very late stages, when insulin is virtually absent and type 2 has virtually become a variant of T1DM with a different origin. The most profound and alarming impact of the epidemic of obesity is the development of T2DM in large numbers of overweight and obese children and teenagers. Some pediatric endocrinologists report that up to one-third of their patients have T2DM, which was rare up until about 20 years ago.

The focus on controlling blood sugar with insulin and diet has dominated the medical and dietetic approaches to T2DM, combined with attention to the deadly complications of diabetes, including nephropathy leading to renal failure, retinopathy leading to blindness, vascular disease leading to amputations, hypertension leading to strokes and contributing to renal failure, hyperlipidemias leading to cardiovascular disease, painful neuropathies, and increased susceptibility to common infections of the skin and urine when blood sugar is >180 mg/dL. The combination of hyperlipidemia, hypertension, and elevated blood sugar affects many of these comorbid conditions. The combination is more than a statistical coincidence; it is the definition of metabolic syndrome when combined with an increased waist circumference, a marker of visceral fat. There is some attention to dietary counseling in modern diabetes practice, but it is largely related to blood sugar control. The busy diabetes specialist or primary care doctor dealing with this increasingly common disease has little or no time for counseling on weight management given all the activity described above. In this chapter, we review the consequences of the glucose-centric approach to diabetes, and provide practical suggestions for the nutritional management of T2DM patients in order to avoid weight gain, a common problem that has significant metabolic consequences and increases morbidity and mortality from this very common disease.

7.5 NUTRITION AND DIABETES MANAGEMENT

Nutrition is central to the treatment of diabetes mellitus, but the approaches to T1DM and T2DM are different. T1DM, due to the destruction of insulin-secreting cells in the pancreas, requires insulin replacement and matching of the diet to the insulin provided (Hahr and Molitch 2008). On the other hand, T2DM is closely associated with excess adiposity and requires primary attention to weight management in treatment until the late stages of T2DM, when insulin stores are depleted (Wycherley et al. 2010). Given the prevalence of T2DM, weight reduction and weight management in T2DM are discussed first, followed by sections on the various foods that can have a role in controlling blood sugar in patients with either T1DM or T2DM. Controlling blood sugar is an important component of treatment, but not the sole aspect of improving the quality of life of diabetes patients. Overall lifestyle change can help control risk factors for cardiovascular disease, which is heightened by the inflammation, oxidative stress, and lipid abnormalities that frequently accompany poor control of blood glucose.

7.5.1 Weight Management and Weight Reduction in T2DM

The vast majority of patients with T2DM have excess body fat, and about 36% are medically obese (Cowie et al. 1994). Since obesity is more common in underserved minority populations, so is T2DM (Cowie et al. 1994). T2DM results primarily from insulin resistance and increased body fat, both of which result from a gene–environment interaction (Olefsky et al. 1982; Campbell and Gerich 1990). While hyperglycemia is the hallmark of T2DM, the increased risk of cardiovascular mortality is associated with hyperlipidemia and hypertension, which occur more commonly in patients with T2DM than in the general population (Albu et al. 1995). The Action to Control Cardiovascular Risk in Diabetes (ACCORD) trial also recently showed a significant reduction in the rate of nonfatal cardiovascular events in a follow-up of its study population (Gerstein et al. 2014), but that benefit was offset by an increase in mortality in the original trial (Gerstein et al. 2008). In contrast, no reduction in the rate of cardiovascular events or in mortality was found in a follow-up of the Action in Diabetes and Vascular Disease (ADVANCE) trial (Zoungas et al. 2014). The Veterans Affairs Diabetes Trial showed that intensive glucose lowering, compared with standard therapy, did not significantly reduce the rate of major cardiovascular events among 1791 military veterans (Duckworth et al. 2009). The extended 10-year follow-up of the study participants showed that subjects who had been randomly assigned to the intensive glucose control for 5.6 years had 8.6 fewer major cardiovascular events per 1000 person-years than those assigned to standard therapy, but no improvement was seen in the rate of overall survival (Hayward et al. 2015).

Because weight reduction can decrease insulin resistance and the demands on the pancreatic β-cell to secrete insulin, weight loss is an integral and necessary component of treatment for obese individuals with T2DM. Weight loss in T2DM patients is associated with decreased insulin resistance, improved measures of glycemia, reduced serum lipids, and reduced blood pressure (Hughes et al. 1984; Henry et al. 1986; Amatruda et al. 1988).

The Diabetes Prevention Program (DPP) demonstrated long-term benefit in people with glucose intolerance from structured, intensive lifestyle programs (Wing et al. 1998; DPP 1999). In the DPP, participants randomly assigned to an intensive lifestyle intervention that included a low-fat diet, increased physical activity, educational sessions, and frequent follow-up were able to lose 7% of body weight in the first year and sustain a 5% weight loss over an average follow-up period of 3 years. DPP participants received training in diet, exercise, and behavior modification from case managers who met with them for at least 16 sessions in the first 24 weeks and monthly thereafter. With intensive lifestyle intervention, the risk of developing diabetes was reduced by 58% relative to standard care. The DPP study subjects in the intensive lifestyle group succeeded in reaching their target goal of a 7% mean weight loss by 6 months and were able to maintain that level of mean weight loss for the first 12 months (Wing et al. 1998). Subsequently, they underwent a slow weight regain, and they had a mean weight loss of 4% at the time of study termination. The placebo group maintained their weight throughout the duration of the study, with neither weight gain nor weight loss, whereas the metformin treatment group initially lost a mean of approximately 2.5% of their body weight within the first year and then regained weight during the subsequent 2 years.

The primary outcome of the DPP was the effect of the intervention strategies on the development of diabetes. Subjects with an elevated fasting plasma glucose level demonstrated an exceptionally high rate of progression to confirmed diabetes mellitus. Those study participants in the placebo group reflected the natural history of progression to diabetes and demonstrated an 11% per year incidence. This rate was reduced by 31% (to 7.8% per year) by treatment with metformin and by 58% (to 4.8% per year) by intensive lifestyle intervention. Therefore, this study demonstrated that intensive lifestyle change or metformin could delay the onset of diabetes in patients with impaired glucose tolerance and elevated fasting blood sugar. A 58% reduction in the onset of new cases of diabetes were found in a Finnish population studied in the same way (Tuomilehto et al. 2001).

The National Institutes of Health (NIH) Look Action for Health in Diabetes (AHEAD) trial, examining the impact of weight loss on cardiovascular mortality in patients with T2DM, demonstrated significant weight loss in 1 year using a combination of dietary counseling, modest exercise recommendations, and meal replacements. There were three predictors of successful weight loss: (1) use of meal replacements, (2) physical activity, and (3) recording dietary intake (Wadden et al. 2009). At diagnosis, patients are often advised to accept having a lifelong disease so that they can cope with T2DM (Delahanty et al. 2007). Sequential addition of therapies is required, and within 10 years of diagnosis, 50% of individuals are on insulin therapy (Turner et al. 1999). Therapeutic weight loss in T2DM patients has been very difficult to achieve (Milne et al. 1994; Redmon et al. 2005), and patients with T2DM have less success with maintaining their weight loss (Pi-Sunyer 2005). Many of the medications traditionally employed to control blood glucose in diabetics, including insulin, thiazolidinediones, and sulfonylureas (Fonseca 2003; Heller 2004; Del Prato and Pulizzi 2006), can result in increased body fat over time. Among the above interventions, insulin is the one associated with the greatest amount of weight gain when used as monotherapy. Two of the largest studies to demonstrate this include the DCCT (1993) and UK Prospective Diabetes Study (UKPDS) Group (1998b). Insulin sensitizers such as thiazolidinediones and insulin secretagogues such as sulfonylureas also produce weight gain as monotherapy, but not to the same extent as that found with insulin (Del Prato and Pulizzi 2006; Mori et al. 1999; Patel et al. 1999).

The effort to drive HbA1c down to prevent complications can reduce the effectiveness of weight management interventions. There is most likely no one specific reason why weight gain is an associated side effect of these hypoglycemic medications. Current proposed mechanisms include (1) reduction of glycosuria, resulting in retention of calories; (2) anabolic effects of insulin; (3) increased appetite; (4) decreased leptin production; and (5) fluid retention (Pi-Sunyer 2005). Of these, increased appetite and reduction of glycosuria appear to have the greatest effect on weight gain.

In practice, physicians focus on the control of hyperglycemia while giving inadequate or no attention to weight management through changes in diet and lifestyle because of their belief that this is an exercise in futility (Pi-Sunyer 2005). In a retrospective analysis, we examined the efficacy of diet, exercise, and lifestyle intervention programs in producing weight loss in obese patients with prediabetes or diabetes in comparison with normoglycemic obese patients enrolled in the same outpatient program and found that prediabetes and diabetes patients all lost weight as effectively with a very low-calorie diet (VLCD) or LCD over 12 months (Li et al. 2014). Therefore, there is no metabolic reason that patients with T2DM given a personalized protein-rich, calorie-controlled diet that creates a caloric deficit cannot lose weight. The reason for lack of weight loss is inevitably failure to adhere to the recommended diet and exercise.

7.5.2 Typical Modern Management of T2DM

Today, a patient with T2DM can expect to be prescribed two to three glucose-lowering agents, two drugs to control blood pressure, a statin, a low-dose aspirin, urine test strips, and lancets for testing blood glucose on a portable device. If neuropathy is present, they may also receive a prescription for gabapentin or amitriptyline to alleviate their pain. Reviewing the standard laboratory measures, including fasting blood sugars, HbA1c, fasting lipids, blood pressures, and urinary microalbumin, makes for a busy office and lots of opportunity to miss the impact of overweight and obesity, especially sarcopenic obesity, which is not evident to the naked eye. That is why a team approach beyond the physician in a cramped exam room is needed to address this disease. An integrated approach, as described in Chapter 1, is most effective and simulates the conditions of our LCD and VLCD clinic at the University of California, Los Angeles (UCLA) (Li et al. 2014).

There is confusion on what to prescribe other than metformin for most patients with T2DM and insulin for all patients with T1DM. Two recent studies attempted to address these dilemmas. However, drugs other than metformin may not contribute to a reduction in overall mortality and morbidity. A study of a very large cohort in Belgium including more than 100,000 patients with T2DM who had been prescribed metformin, a sulfonylurea, or insulin, either alone or in combination, was conducted from 2003 to 2007 (Claesen et al. 2016). In Belgium, a single-payer system supports a large database, including data on diabetes medications and outcome, including mortality. Twelve control subjects were matched to each patient, including age and diagnoses of hypertension and heart disease. Patients on metformin monotherapy had longevity similar to that of controls, while those on insulin and/or sulfonylureas did not do as well. Both patients with diabetes and controls benefited from the use of statins. There were no data reported in this study on diet or obesity. So, careful glucose management by adding more insulin and sulfonylureas was associated with greater mortality. Could the missing link here be ignorance of nutrition and physical activity effects? To what degree does the focus on drugs and glucose fail the patient?

7.5.3 Use of Metformin in T2DM

Metformin is clearly the most beneficial and widely used drug in T2DM. It is troubling that a recent study reports some disagreement among experienced prescribers on how to use this drug (Goldberg et al. 2015). Questionnaires were sent to prescribers with 5–15 years of experience asking them how they would navigate some of the most common issues that arise in the use of metformin, including lack of efficacy, reduced renal function, alcoholism, and gastrointestinal side effects. There was divided opinion on whether to increase metformin doses, add another agent, or discontinue the metformin entirely, pointing out the lack of consensus on a standard treatment regimen and the confused state of diabetes pharmacotherapy.

Metformin is the only medication for T2DM that has demonstrated reproducible benefits on cardiovascular morbidity and mortality (UK Prospective Diabetes Study [UKPDS] Group 1998a). Thus, metformin is considered first-line treatment for T2DM according to the ADA's clinical practice guidelines (ADA 2015). In the UKPDS, cardiovascular morbidity and mortality benefits were demonstrated in patients with uncontrolled diabetes who were treated daily with metformin at doses of 1700–2550 mg (UK Prospective Diabetes Study [UKPDS] Group 1998a). At these doses, metformin reduced the risk of any diabetes-related end point, myocardial infarction, and all-cause mortality by 32%, 39%, and 36%, respectively (UK Prospective Diabetes Study (UKPDS) Group 1998a). Despite these findings, manufacturer guidelines suggest that the minimum effective dose of metformin is 1500 mg/day (Bristol Myers Squibb 2009). While the optimal dose has not been established in clinical trials, the trial on which much of the evidence for cardiovascular benefit is based, the UK Prospective Diabetes Study (UKPDS 1998a,b), used a median dose of 2550 mg metformin. Establishing how the dose-effect relationship may vary at different doses and what the maximum effective dose may be is an area for future work. Despite the clear benefits on glycemic control, morbidity, and mortality, metformin prescribing remains suboptimal (Calabrese et al. 2002; Desai et al. 2012). It is estimated that metformin treatment is not initiated in nearly 50% of patients with T2DM (Berkowitz et al. 2014).

Reasons for this suboptimal prescribing are not clearly defined in the literature, but they may be attributable to fear of precipitating lactic acidosis in patients with known risk factors. Potential risk factors for lactic acidosis include chronic kidney disease, hepatic dysfunction, heart failure, chronic obstructive pulmonary disease (COPD), alcohol abuse, and a history of lactic acidosis. Although there is little information on the exact risk of lactic acidosis with metformin, data suggest that the association is negligible; one study demonstrated an incidence of 4.3 per 100,000 patient-years (Salpeter et al. 2010). Furthermore, previous studies demonstrated no increased risk of lactic acidosis with metformin use in the settings of heart failure and renal dysfunction (Eurich et al. 2013; Norwood et al. 2013; Richy et al. 2014). Despite these data, the manufacturer recommends discontinuing metformin when serum creatinine exceeds 1.5 mg/dL for men and 1.4 mg/dL for women (Bristol Myers Squibb 2009), likely because of medicolegal concerns over the risk of lactic acidosis. This fear of increased lactic acidosis risk with metformin may stem from a preexisting medication, phenformin, which was associated with fatal cases of lactic acidosis in patients and has since been removed from the market (Lipska et al. 2011). However, there is no information that clearly supports similar concerns over the use of metformin. While the majority of clinicians would stop metformin because of impaired renal function, it is unclear whether the reason is due to a perceived risk of lactic acidosis or something else, perhaps a fear of legal liability, the contraindication in the manufacturer's package insert, or unfamiliarity with the actual consequences of metformin use.

There are several major guidelines outside the United States that indicate that the glomerular filtration rate (GFR) is a better measure of kidney function than serum creatinine and should be used to assess metformin use in patients with diabetes (Chadban et al. 2010). Although creatinine clearance (using the Cockcroft–Gault equation) is typically preferred for renal drug dose adjustments, metformin dose adjustments have not been evaluated in the same fashion as most other medications; thus, GFR, which is a more accurate indicator of renal function, is preferred when dosing metformin (Lipska et al. 2011; Trinkley et al. 2014; ADA 2015).

Current prescribing practices for metformin are not optimal. In patients with uncontrolled diabetes and an HgbA1c of 8.3%, most providers (84%) chose to titrate metformin from 500 to 2000 mg daily, whereas 11% chose 1500 mg of metformin daily as an appropriate regimen. Interestingly, in a similar patient with an HgbA1c of 7.3%, 75% of providers would increase metformin from 1500 to 2000 mg daily, whereas 18% of providers would choose to add a sulfonylurea. Of providers, 50% followed the metformin manufacturer's recommendations to discontinue metformin use when the serum creatinine is >1.5 mg/dL. The other 50% of providers accepted the GFR as a better indicator of when to discontinue metformin use, but there seems to be no consensus among providers on what the GFR cutoff should be. In patients taking 1750 mg of metformin daily with either hepatic dysfunction or heart failure, there was great variation in provider prescribing attitudes and no notable trends. For patients with COPD, however, 90% of providers did not alter the patient's metformin therapy. In patients with alcoholism, 59% of providers would not alter metformin dosing, but many providers would alter the dose recommended based on varying degrees of alcohol use. For patients with current or a history of lactic acidosis, provider attitudes were inconsistent. Much more needs to be done so that more patients with diabetes can benefit from metformin's unique cardiovascular morbidity and mortality effects.

The findings of survey studies strongly suggest that there is no consensus around the dosing and use of metformin based on glycemic control or comorbidities. This confusion drives prescribers to other classes of drugs when targets for glucose control are not achieved and minimize consideration of diet and lifestyle in favor of the easy answer of writing another prescription. Optimizing the use of metformin, in combination with diet and exercise, is an effort that would pay great dividends in the management of T2DM.

7.5.4 Meal Replacements as a Tool for Planning Weight Management Diets

Partial meal replacement diets using protein-enriched shakes as meal substitutes are a viable strategy for weight reduction in patients with T2DM, resulting in beneficial changes in measures of glycemic control and a reduction of medications (Li et al. 2005). Structured meal replacements provide a defined amount of energy (usually 200–300 calories), often as a prepackaged meal, snack bar, or formula product. Most of the energy is derived from protein and carbohydrates. Vitamins, minerals, and fiber may also be included. Use of meal replacements once or twice daily to replace a usual meal can result in significant weight loss (Ditschuneit et al. 1999; Metz et al. 2000; Quinn Rothacker 2000; Ashley et al. 2001; Rothacker et al. 2001). Presumably, the meal replacement causes a reduction in energy intake by eliminating the choice of type and amount of food. Weight loss can be as much as 11% of starting weight at 2 years, but meal replacement therapy must be continued if weight loss is to be maintained; attrition may occur in about 33% of patients (Ditschuneit et al. 1999).

Studies including a meta-analysis of weight loss interventions in adults with T2DM showed that multidisciplinary interventions, including VLCDs, held promise for achieving weight loss (Amatruda et al. 1988; Henry and Gumbiner 1991; Wing et al. 1991; Capstick et al. 1997; Norris et al. 2005). A prospective, longitudinal study comprised three phases: a VLCD for 8 weeks, a stepped return to isocaloric intake of normal food over 2 weeks, and a structured, individualized weight maintenance program over 6 months achieved continuing remission of diabetes for at least 6 months in the 40% patients who responded to a VLCD by achieving an FPG of <7 mmol/L (Steven et al. 2016).

Abnormalities of protein metabolism are assumed to be less affected by insulin deficiency and insulin resistance than abnormalities of glucose metabolism (Henry 1994). However, moderate hyperglycemia may contribute to increased turnover of protein in T2DM subjects. During moderate hyperglycemia, obese subjects with T2DM, compared with nondiabetic obese subjects, demonstrate an increase in whole body nitrogen flux and a higher rate of protein synthesis and breakdown (Gougeon et al. 1997, 1998). A high-quality protein (95 g of protein/day), very low-energy diet capable of maintaining nitrogen balance in obese subjects without diabetes did not prevent negative nitrogen balance in diabetic subjects, despite weight loss and improved glycemic control (Gougeon et al. 1997). This increased protein turnover was restored to normal only with oral glucose-lowering agents or exogenous insulin sufficient to achieve euglycemia and with increased protein intake (Gougeon et al. 1998, 2000). These study results suggest that people with T2DM have an increased need for protein during moderate hyperglycemia and an altered adaptive mechanism for protein sparing during weight loss. Thus, with energy restriction, the protein requirements of people with diabetes are likely to be greater than the recommended dietary allowance (RDA) of 0.8 g of protein/kg of body weight, and increased amounts of protein may aid in weight management efforts through effects on satiety and maintenance of lean body mass (Flechtner-Mors et al. 2010). As detailed in Chapter 2, the use of protein-enriched meal replacements is safe and effective in patients with T2DM (Li et al. 2010).

In the remaining meals, as already discussed in Chapter 5, reducing dietary fat and hidden sugars restricts calorie intake, especially from processed foods. Spontaneous food consumption and total energy intake are increased when the diet is high in fat and decreased when the diet is low in fat (Lissner et al. 1987; Kendall et al. 1991). So, a minimal amount of olive and avocado oil should be used and high-glycemic-index (GI) foods avoided. There is no conflict between low-fat and reduced-GI foods. In the popular literature, there has been confusion over the idea that every low-fat diet is high in refined carbohydrates, while every high-protein diet is also high fat. It is possible, using meal replacements, to achieve a level of protein intake of 1 g/pound of lean body mass, which equates to 25–30% of total calories per day, in combination with good carbohydrates from fruits and vegetables, with limited amounts of whole grains. Fats should be used sparingly as needed, and overall processed food intake and restaurant eating should be minimized.

7.5.5 Physical Activity, Including Resistance Exercise, to Increase Muscle Mass

Exercise improves insulin sensitivity and lowers blood glucose in patients with diabetes. Exercise by itself has only a modest effect on weight loss, but it is the most efficient intervention for long-term weight maintenance and prevention of weight regain (Pavlou et al. 1989; Maggio and Pi-Sunyer 1997; Bouchard et al. 1993).

Aerobic exercise improves glucose control (Ronnemaa et al. 1986; Mourier et al. 1997; Boule et al. 2001) and insulin sensitivity (Ruderman et al. 1979; Dengel et al. 1996; Mourier et al. 1997).

It also reduces visceral adiposity (Mourier et al. 1997) and improves lipid profiles (Segal et al. 1991), arterial stiffness (Yokoyama et al. 2004), and endothelial function (Stewart 2002).

The ADA recommends that individuals with T2DM perform at least 150 minutes of moderate-intensity aerobic exercise and/or at least 90 minutes of vigorous aerobic exercise per week (Sigal et al. 2004). However only 28% of individuals with T2DM achieve these recommendations (Plotnikoff et al. 2006). Individuals with severe obesity, arthritis, physical disabilities, and/or diabetes complications may have difficulty walking for 30 minutes. Alternate forms of personalized physical activity recommendations that produce similar metabolic improvements are therefore vital to be integrated into the management of T2DM.

Resistance training has been used as a method to prevent and treat chronic diseases (Ghilarducci et al. 1989; Hare et al. 1999; Pu et al. 2001; Kongsgaard et al. 2004; Haykowsky et al. 2005). Its safety and efficacy have been demonstrated in the elderly (Singh et al. 1997, 1999) and obese (Cuff et al. 2003) individuals. Resistance training can increase muscle strength (Hunter et al. 2004; Ouellette et al. 2004), lean muscle mass (Ryan et al. 2001), and bone mineral density (Nelson et al. 1994; Hurley and Roth 2000), which could therefore enhance functional status and glycemic control and assist in the prevention of sarcopenia and osteoporosis. Resistance training was also demonstrated to improve insulin sensitivity (Miller et al. 1984; Eriksson et al. 1998; Poehlman et al. 2000), daily energy expenditure (Hunter et al. 2000; Ades et al. 2005), and quality of life (Kell et al. 2001). However, unlike aerobic exercise, resistance training is dependent on equipment and knowledge of exercise technique, and often requires some initial instruction. Therefore, research is needed to come up with practical, sustainable, safe, and cost-efficient ways to implement resistance training for individuals with T2DM.

7.5.6 Low-GI Foods, Fiber, and Resistant Starches in T1DM and T2DM

Low-GI foods include most fruits and vegetables, whole grains, and protein-rich and fat-rich foods. The acute effects of high-GI foods, such as rice, potatoes, and refined grain pasta, are established. However, the clinical utility of low-GI diets without any instructions on weight management is controversial (Pi-Sunyer 2002). Thomas and Elliott assessed randomized controlled trials (RCTs) with interventions greater than 4 weeks comparing a low-GI diet with a higher-GI diet for T1DM or T2DM (Thomas and Elliott 2010). Twelve RCTs with 612 participants were identified. There was a significantly greater decrease in glycated hemoglobin (HbA1c) with the low-GI diet than with the control diet, indicating improved glycemic control. Glycosylated albumin levels decreased significantly with the low-GI diet, but not with the high-GI diet, in the one study that reported this outcome. Therefore, lowering the GI of the diet in combination with other changes may contribute to improved glycemic control in diabetes.

In the Canadian Trial of Carbohydrates in Diabetes (CCD), a 1-year controlled trial of low-GI dietary carbohydrate in subjects with T2DM managed by diet alone with optimal glycemic control, the levels of HbA1c were not changed by altering the GI or the amount of dietary carbohydrate. Differences observed in the ratio of total cholesterol to high-density lipoprotein (HDL) cholesterol among diets had disappeared by 6 months. However, because of sustained reductions in postprandial glucose, a low-GI diet may be preferred for the dietary management of T2DM.

There is a positive effect of large amounts of fiber (>30 g/day) on glycemia in suboptimally controlled T1DM subjects, probably by changing intestinal transit times and the delivery of glucose into the bloodstream after meals (Vaaler et al. 1980; Chenon et al. 1984; Riccardi et al. 1984). In subjects being treated with two or more injections of insulin per day and HbA1c levels of 7–10% consuming either a high-fiber (50 g/day), low-GI diet or a low-fiber (15 g/day), high-GI diet for 24 weeks, the high-fiber diet significantly reduced the mean daily blood glucose concentration ($p < 0.05$), the number of hypoglycemic events ($p < 0.01$), and in the subgroup of patients compliant to the diet, HbA1c ($p < 0.05$). However, the diet had no beneficial effects on cholesterol, HDL cholesterol, or triglyceride concentrations (Giacco et al. 2000).

In T2DM, weight management has the greatest benefit. Since low-GI foods are also often high in fiber, the replacement of foods with a high-GI and/or low-fiber content for foods with a low-GI and/or high-fiber amount seems to be a practical alternative for the dietary management of patients with diabetes. However, this assumption needs to be confirmed in long-term clinical trials that factor in the effects of weight management.

Resistant starches, including nondigestible oligosaccharides and the starch amylose, are not digested and therefore not absorbed as glucose in the small intestine. They are almost completely fermented in the colon and produce about 2 kcal/g of energy (Carbohydrates in Human Nutrition 1998). It is estimated that resistant starch and unabsorbed starch represent <10 g/day of the total starch ingested in the average Western diet (Wursch 1989). Legumes are the major food source of resistant starch in the diet, containing 2–3 g of resistant starch per 100 g of cooked legumes. Uncooked cornstarch contains about 6 g of resistant starch per 100 g of dry weight (Englyst et al. 1996).

It has been suggested that ingestion of resistant starch produces a smaller increase in postprandial glucose than digestible starch, and correspondingly lower insulin levels. As a result, it has been proposed that food containing naturally occurring resistant starch, such as cornstarch, or food modified to contain more resistant starch with high-amylose cornstarch may modify postprandial glycemic response, prevent hypoglycemia, and reduce hyperglycemia. These effects may also explain differences in the GIs of some food (Brennan 2005).

There have been several one-meal (Raben et al. 1994; Granfeldt et al. 1995; Hoebler et al. 1999) and two-meal (Heijnen et al. 1995; Achour et al. 1997; Liljeberg et al. 1999) studies in nondiabetic subjects, comparing subjects' physical response to food high in resistant starch and their response to food with an equivalent amount of digestible starch. All studies found some reduction in postprandial glucose and insulin responses to the first meal, but observed mixed results after the second meal.

Long-term studies have not consistently confirmed these results (Behall and Howe 1995; Luo et al. 1996; Noakes et al. 1996; Jenkins et al. 1998; Axelsen et al. 1999). Published studies involving people with diabetes have focused on uncooked cornstarch and its potential to prevent nighttime hypoglycemia (Axelsen et al. 1997, 2000; Alles et al. 1999). In uncontrolled studies, evening cornstarch in specific dosages or dosages based on grams per kilogram of body weight resulted in less hypoglycemia around 2:00 a.m. in all groups (Kaufman et al. 1995; Axelsen et al. 1999). It has not been established that bedtime cornstarch snacks are more effective in preventing nocturnal hypoglycemia than other types of carbohydrates.

7.5.7 Monounsaturated Fats

Diets high in monounsaturated fat (MUFA) (Parillo et al. 1992; Rasmussen et al. 1993; Campbell et al. 1994; Walker et al. 1996) result in improvements in glucose tolerance and lipids compared with diets high in saturated fat. An important caveat is that adding fat to the diet adds calories, so added olive or avocado oil should be used to enhance taste by spraying them on fruits, vegetables, and whole grains, rather than liberally spooning these fats into recipes. A meta-analysis has found that high-MUFA diets reduce fasting glucose in patients with T2DM (Schwingshackl and Strasser 2012). Diets enriched with MUFA may also reduce insulin resistance (Parillo et al. 1992). There is, however, concern that when high-MUFA diets are eaten *ad libitum* outside of a controlled setting, they may result in increased energy intake and weight gain (Yu-Poth et al. 1999). A recent meta-analysis of nine randomized controlled intervention trials with a total of 1547 participants and a running time of at least 6 months compared high- and low-MUFA diets among adults with abnormal glucose metabolism (T2DM, impaired glucose tolerance, and insulin resistance), being overweight or obese. It was found that high-MUFA diets appear to be effective in reducing HbA1c, and therefore should be recommended in the dietary regimes of T2DM (Schwingshackl et al. 2011). More studies comparing diets high in MUFA with diets high in carbohydrate with *ad libitum* energy intake are needed to evaluate the efficacy of these diets and determine the effects of MUFA in reducing cardiovascular risk in diabetes.

7.5.8 Omega-3 Fatty Acids

The relationship between omega-3 polyunsaturated fatty acids (n-3 PUFAs) from seafood sources (eicosapentaenoic acid [EPA] and docosahexaenoic acid [DHA]) or plant sources (α-linolenic acid [ALA]) and risk of T2DM remains unclear. A meta-analysis that searched multiple literature databases through June 2011 did not support either major harms or benefits from fish and seafood or EPA and DHA on the development of diabetes mellitus, and suggested that ALA may be associated with a modestly lower risk (Wu et al. 2012).

A multicenter, randomized, double-blind, placebo-controlled study evaluated the possible worsening of glycemic control after a moderate daily intake of n-3 fatty acid ethyl esters in patients with hypertriglyceridemia with and without glucose intolerance or diabetes (Sirtori et al. 1997). Plasma triacylglycerol concentrations decreased significantly, up to 21.53% at 6 months compared with baseline (decreased 15% compared with placebo), with a tendency toward a progressive reduction with time. There was no evidence for a different response in patients with either non-insulin-dependent diabetes mellitus (NIDDM) or impaired glucose tolerance. Among NIDDM patients, the triacylglycerol reduction was greater in those with HDL cholesterol of ≤0.91 mmol/L. There was no alteration in the major GIs—fasting glucose, HbA1c, insulinemia, and oral glucose tolerance—in patients with impaired glucose tolerance or NIDDM after treatment with n-3 ethyl esters.

In a pooled analysis with 23 RCTs and 1075 participants, n-3 PUFA supplementation in T2DM lowered triglycerides and very low-density lipoprotein (VLDL) cholesterol, but it may raise LDL cholesterol (although results were nonsignificant in subgroups) and has no statistically significant effect on glycemic control or fasting insulin (Hartweg et al. 2008). Nonetheless, eating ocean-caught fish three times per week as a substitute for meats will reduce calories and provide some cardiovascular, eye, and brain benefits.

7.5.9 Spices and Glucose Control

Spices such as cinnamon (Ròu Guì, *Cinnamomum cassia*), red chili, cloves, black pepper, and ginger also exhibit effects in insulin resistance, and the most active of them is cinnamon (Hlebowicz et al. 2007; Aggarwal 2010). Cinnamon is commonly used as a spice across the world, and it is not toxic at culinary levels, where it has been shown to be beneficial. Several studies have been conducted to confirm the effect of cinnamon on decreasing the blood glucose of diabetic patients (Khan et al. 2003; Lu et al. 2012; Allen et al. 2013).

7.5.10 Micronutrients

Selected micronutrients may affect glucose and insulin metabolism, but the data are minimal and somewhat inconsistent for most trace minerals with this reputation, such as vanadium. On the other hand, the positive effects of chromium on glucose metabolism have been recognized since the observation that brewer's yeast improved glycemic control in the 1920s. In 1957, chromium was identified to be the active component of the glucose tolerance factor from brewer's yeast (Mertz 1998; Chowdhury et al. 2003). Two recent studies did not show an improvement in either glycemia or lipid parameters (Kleefstra et al. 2006; Ali et al. 2011). Western populations, which showed a negative result with chromium supplementation, were chromium sufficient, in contrast to Asian populations, such as the Chinese and Asian Indians, who tend to be chromium deficient. These differences, as well as ethnic variations, may account for the disparate results in different studies from various geographical and ethnic regions. Cefalu and coworkers conducted a comprehensive evaluation of chromium supplementation on metabolic parameters in a cohort of T2DM subjects representing a wide phenotype range to evaluate changes in "responders" and "nonresponders" (Cefalu et al. 2010). After preintervention testing to assess glycemia, insulin sensitivity (assessed by euglycemic clamps), chromium status, and body composition, subjects were randomized in a double-blind fashion to placebo or 1000 μg of chromium. There was not a consistent effect of chromium supplementation to improve insulin action across all phenotypes, but response to chromium was more likely in insulin-resistant individuals who had more elevated fasting glucose and A1c levels.

7.6 CONCLUSION

The nutritional approach to the adjunctive treatment of T1DM and T2DM patients is very different despite the common observation of increased glucose in both groups.

The type 1 patient must have insulin and may benefit from the effects of foods that minimize glucose excursions after meals, such as low-GI and high-fiber foods and foods rich in resistant starch. However, if a type 1 patient is also obese, they would benefit from weight management, which would also decrease the amount and complexity of their insulin regimen.

For type 2 patients, where obesity is almost universal, the primary goal is weight management. Metformin is the first-line therapy for this condition. When the additional drugs described in this chapter are added, it is important to question the adherence of the patient to dietary and exercise recommendations. Clearly, weight loss is possible in simply obese, prediabetic, and diabetic patients. To the degree that physicians and other caregivers communicate that weight management is futile or that pharmacology is preferable with agents beyond metformin, we do a disservice to diabetes patients. Recognizing that physicians alone cannot intervene effectively, we recommend that an integrated primary care program be utilized. Our experience in 2000 patients with obesity, prediabetes, or diabetes demonstrated clearly that significant weight loss can be achieved. Similarly, the Look AHEAD trial achieved weight losses using meal replacements, physical activity, and food logs. The treatment of T2DM can be revolutionized with the incorporation of these ideas into primary care practice.

REFERENCES

Achour, L., B. Flourie, F. Briet, C. Franchisseur, F. Bornet, M. Champ, J. C. Rambaud, and B. Messing. 1997. Metabolic effects of digestible and partially indigestible cornstarch: A study in the absorptive and postabsorptive periods in healthy humans. *Am J Clin Nutr* 66 (5):1151–1159.

ADA (American Diabetes Association). 2010. Diagnosis and classification of diabetes mellitus. *Diabetes Care* 33 (Suppl 1):S62–S69.

ADA (American Diabetes Association). 2015. Standards of medical care in diabetes. *Diabetes Care* 38 (Suppl 1):90.

Ades, P. A., P. D. Savage, M. Brochu, M. D. Tischler, N. M. Lee, and E. T. Poehlman. 2005. Resistance training increases total daily energy expenditure in disabled older women with coronary heart disease. *J Appl Physiol (1985)* 98 (4):1280–1285.

Aggarwal, B. B. 2010. Targeting inflammation-induced obesity and metabolic diseases by curcumin and other nutraceuticals. *Annu Rev Nutr* 30:173–199.

Alberti, K. G. M. M., P. Zimmet, and R. A. Defronzo. 1997. *International Textbook of Diabetes Mellitus*. 2nd ed. New York: John Wiley & Sons.

Albu, J., C. Konnarides, and F. X. Pi-Sunyer. 1995. Weight control: Metabolic and cardiovascular effects. *Diabetes Rev* 3:335–347.

Ali, A., Y. Ma, J. Reynolds, J. P. Wise Sr., S. E. Inzucchi, and D. L. Katz. 2011. Chromium effects on glucose tolerance and insulin sensitivity in persons at risk for diabetes mellitus. *Endocr Pract* 17 (1):16–25.

Allen, R. W., E. Schwartzman, W. L. Baker, C. I. Coleman, and O. J. Phung. 2013. Cinnamon use in type 2 diabetes: An updated systematic review and meta-analysis. *Ann Fam Med* 11 (5):452–459.

Alles, M. S., N. M. de Roos, J. C. Bakx, E. van de Lisdonk, P. L. Zock, and G. A. Hautvast. 1999. Consumption of fructooligosaccharides does not favorably affect blood glucose and serum lipid concentrations in patients with type 2 diabetes. *Am J Clin Nutr* 69 (1):64–69.

Amatruda, J. M., J. F. Richeson, S. L. Welle, R. G. Brodows, and D. H. Lockwood. 1988. The safety and efficacy of a controlled low-energy ("very-low-calorie") diet in the treatment of non-insulin-dependent diabetes and obesity. *Arch Intern Med* 148 (4):873–877.

Ashley, J. M., S. T. St. Jeor, J. P. Schrage, S. E. Perumean-Chaney, M. C. Gilbertson, N. L. McCall, and V. Bovee. 2001. Weight control in the physician's office. *Arch Intern Med* 161 (13):1599–1604.

Axelsen, M., P. Lonnroth, R. Arvidsson Lenner, and U. Smith. 1997. Suppression of the nocturnal free fatty acid levels by bedtime cornstarch in NIDDM subjects. *Eur J Clin Invest* 27 (2):157–163.

Axelsen, M., P. Lonnroth, R. Arvidsson Lenner, M. R. Taskinen, and U. Smith. 2000. Suppression of nocturnal fatty acid concentrations by bedtime carbohydrate supplement in type 2 diabetes: Effects on insulin sensitivity, lipids, and glycemic control. *Am J Clin Nutr* 71 (5):1108–1114.

Axelsen, M., C. Wesslau, P. Lonnroth, R. Arvidsson Lenner, and U. Smith. 1999. Bedtime uncooked cornstarch supplement prevents nocturnal hypoglycaemia in intensively treated type 1 diabetes subjects. *J Intern Med* 245 (3):229–236.

Behall, K. M., and J. C. Howe. 1995. Effect of long-term consumption of amylose vs amylopectin starch on metabolic variables in human subjects. *Am J Clin Nutr* 61 (2):334–340.

Berkowitz, S. A., A. A. Krumme, J. Avorn, T. Brennan, O. S. Matlin, C. M. Spettell, E. J. Pezalla, G. Brill, W. H. Shrank, and N. K. Choudhry. 2014. Initial choice of oral glucose-lowering medication for diabetes mellitus: A patient-centered comparative effectiveness study. *JAMA Intern Med* 174 (12):1955–1962.

Bouchard, C., J. P. Depres, and A. Tremblay. 1993. Exercise and obesity. *Obes Res* 1 (2):133–147.

Boule, N. G., E. Haddad, G. P. Kenny, G. A. Wells, and R. J. Sigal. 2001. Effects of exercise on glycemic control and body mass in type 2 diabetes mellitus: A meta-analysis of controlled clinical trials. *JAMA* 286 (10):1218–1227.

Brennan, C. S. 2005. Dietary fibre, glycaemic response, and diabetes. *Mol Nutr Food Res* 49 (6):560–570.

Bristol Myers Squibb. 2009. Glucophage [package insert]. Princeton, NJ: Bristol Myers Squibb.

Calabrese, A. T., K. C. Coley, S. V. DaPos, D. Swanson, and R. H. Rao. 2002. Evaluation of prescribing practices: Risk of lactic acidosis with metformin therapy. *Arch Intern Med* 162 (4):434–437.

Campbell, L. V., P. E. Marmot, J. A. Dyer, M. Borkman, and L. H. Storlien. 1994. The high-monounsaturated fat diet as a practical alternative for NIDDM. *Diabetes Care* 17 (3):177–182.

Campbell, P. J., and J. E. Gerich. 1990. Impact of obesity on insulin action in volunteers with normal glucose tolerance: Demonstration of a threshold for the adverse effect of obesity. *J Clin Endocrinol Metab* 70 (4):1114–1118.

Capstick, F., B. A. Brooks, C. M. Burns, R. R. Zilkens, K. S. Steinbeck, and D. K. Yue. 1997. Very low calorie diet (VLCD): A useful alternative in the treatment of the obese NIDDM patient. *Diabetes Res Clin Pract* 36 (2):105–111.

Carbohydrates in human nutrition. Report of a Joint FAO/WHO Expert Consultation. 1998. *FAO Food Nutr Pap* 66:1–140.

Cefalu, W. T., J. Rood, P. Pinsonat, J. Qin, O. Sereda, L. Levitan, R. A. Anderson et al. 2010. Characterization of the metabolic and physiologic response to chromium supplementation in subjects with type 2 diabetes mellitus. *Metabolism* 59 (5):755–762.

Chadban, S., M. Howell, S. Twigg, M. Thomas, G. Jerums, A. Cass, D. Campbell et al. 2010. The CARI guidelines. Assessment of kidney function in type 2 diabetes. *Nephrology (Carlton)* 15 (Suppl 1): S146–S161.

Chenon, D., M. Phaka, L. H. Monnier, C. Colette, A. Orsetti, and J. Mirouze. 1984. Effects of dietary fiber on postprandial glycemic profiles in diabetic patients submitted to continuous programmed insulin infusion. *Am J Clin Nutr* 40 (1):58–65.

Chowdhury, S., K. Pandit, P. Roychowdury, and B. Bhattacharya. 2003. Role of chromium in human metabolism, with special reference to type 2 diabetes. *J Assoc Physicians India* 51:701–705.

Claesen, M., P. Gillard, F. De Smet, M. Callens, B. De Moor, and C. Mathieu. 2016. Mortality in individuals treated with glucose-lowering agents: A large, controlled cohort study. *J Clin Endocrinol Metab* 101 (2):461–469.

Cowie, C. C., M. I. Harris, and M. S. Eberhardt. 1994. Frequency and determinants of screening for diabetes in the U.S. *Diabetes Care* 17 (10):1158–1163.

Cuff, D. J., G. S. Meneilly, A. Martin, A. Ignaszewski, H. D. Tildesley, and J. J. Frohlich. 2003. Effective exercise modality to reduce insulin resistance in women with type 2 diabetes. *Diabetes Care* 26 (11):2977–2982.

Delahanty, L. M., R. W. Grant, E. Wittenberg, J. L. Bosch, D. J. Wexler, E. Cagliero, and J. B. Meigs. 2007. Association of diabetes-related emotional distress with diabetes treatment in primary care patients with type 2 diabetes. *Diabet Med* 24 (1):48–54.

Del Prato, S., and N. Pulizzi. 2006. The place of sulfonylureas in the therapy for type 2 diabetes mellitus. *Metabolism* 55 (5 Suppl 1):S20–S27.

Dengel, D. R., R. E. Pratley, J. M. Hagberg, E. M. Rogus, and A. P. Goldberg. 1996. Distinct effects of aerobic exercise training and weight loss on glucose homeostasis in obese sedentary men. *J Appl Physiol (1985)* 81 (1):318–325.

Desai, N. R., W. H. Shrank, M. A. Fischer, J. Avorn, J. N. Liberman, S. Schneeweiss, J. Pakes, T. A. Brennan, and N. K. Choudhry. 2012. Patterns of medication initiation in newly diagnosed diabetes mellitus: Quality and cost implications. *Am J Med* 125 (3):302.e1–e7.

The Diabetes Control and Complications Trial (DCCT) Research Group. 1993. The effect of intensive treatment of diabetes on the development and progression of long-term complications in insulin-dependent diabetes mellitus. *N Engl J Med* 329 (14):977–986.

Ditschuneit, H. H., M. Flechtner-Mors, T. D. Johnson, and G. Adler. 1999. Metabolic and weight-loss effects of a long-term dietary intervention in obese patients. *Am J Clin Nutr* 69 (2):198–204.

DPP (Diabetes Prevention Program). 1999. Design and methods for a clinical trial in the prevention of type 2 diabetes. *Diabetes Care* 22 (4):623–634.

Duckworth, W., C. Abraira, T. Moritz, D. Reda, N. Emanuele, P. D. Reaven, F. J. Zieve et al. 2009. Glucose control and vascular complications in veterans with type 2 diabetes. *N Engl J Med* 360 (2):129–139.

Englyst, H. N., J. Veenstra, and G. J. Hudson. 1996. Measurement of rapidly available glucose (RAG) in plant foods: A potential in vitro predictor of the glycaemic response. *Br J Nutr* 75 (3):327–337.

Eriksson, J., J. Tuominen, T. Valle, S. Sundberg, A. Sovijarvi, H. Lindholm, J. Tuomilehto, and V. Koivisto. 1998. Aerobic endurance exercise or circuit-type resistance training for individuals with impaired glucose tolerance? *Horm Metab Res* 30 (1):37–41.

Eurich, D. T., D. L. Weir, S. R. Majumdar, R. T. Tsuyuki, J. A. Johnson, L. Tjosvold, S. E. Vanderloo, and F. A. McAlister. 2013. Comparative safety and effectiveness of metformin in patients with diabetes mellitus and heart failure: Systematic review of observational studies involving 34,000 patients. *Circ Heart Fail* 6 (3):395–402.

Flechtner-Mors, M., B. O. Boehm, R. Wittmann, U. Thoma, and H. H. Ditschuneit. 2010. Enhanced weight loss with protein-enriched meal replacements in subjects with the metabolic syndrome. *Diabetes Metab Res Rev* 26 (5):393–405.

Fonseca, V. 2003. Effect of thiazolidinediones on body weight in patients with diabetes mellitus. *Am J Med* 115 (Suppl 8A):42S–48S.

Frank, E., M. Nothnamm, and A. Wagner. 1926. Über synthetische dargestellte Korper mit Insulinartiger Wirkung auf den normallen und diabetisched Organismus. *Klin Wchnschr* 5.

Galloway, J. A. 1988. *Diabetes Mellitus*. 9th ed. Indianapolis: Eli Lilly and Company.

Gerstein, H. C., M. E. Miller, R. P. Byington, D. C. Goff Jr., J. T. Bigger, J. B. Buse, W. C. Cushman et al. 2008. Effects of intensive glucose lowering in type 2 diabetes. *N Engl J Med* 358 (24):2545–2559.

Gerstein, H. C., M. E. Miller, F. Ismail-Beigi, J. Largay, C. McDonald, H. A. Lochnan, and G. L. Booth. 2014. Effects of intensive glycaemic control on ischaemic heart disease: Analysis of data from the randomised, controlled ACCORD trial. *Lancet* 384 (9958):1936–1941.

Ghilarducci, L. E., R. G. Holly, and E. A. Amsterdam. 1989. Effects of high resistance training in coronary artery disease. *Am J Cardiol* 64 (14):866–870.

Giacco, R., M. Parillo, A. A. Rivellese, G. Lasorella, A. Giacco, L. D'Episcopo, and G. Riccardi. 2000. Long-term dietary treatment with increased amounts of fiber-rich low-glycemic index natural foods improves blood glucose control and reduces the number of hypoglycemic events in type 1 diabetic patients. *Diabetes Care* 23 (10):1461–1466.

Goldberg, T., M. E. Kroehl, K. H. Suddarth, and K. E. Trinkley. 2015. Variations in metformin prescribing for type 2 diabetes. *J Am Board Fam Med* 28 (6):777–784.

Gougeon, R., E. B. Marliss, P. J. Jones, P. B. Pencharz, and J. A. Morais. 1998. Effect of exogenous insulin on protein metabolism with differing nonprotein energy intakes in type 2 diabetes mellitus. *Int J Obes Relat Metab Disord* 22 (3):250–261.

Gougeon, R., P. B. Pencharz, and R. J. Sigal. 1997. Effect of glycemic control on the kinetics of whole-body protein metabolism in obese subjects with non-insulin-dependent diabetes mellitus during iso- and hypoenergetic feeding. *Am J Clin Nutr* 65 (3):861–870.

Gougeon, R., K. Styhler, J. A. Morais, P. J. Jones, and E. B. Marliss. 2000. Effects of oral hypoglycemic agents and diet on protein metabolism in type 2 diabetes. *Diabetes Care* 23 (1):1–8.

Granfeldt, Y., A. Drews, and I. Bjorck. 1995. Arepas made from high amylose corn flour produce favorably low glucose and insulin responses in healthy humans. *J Nutr* 125 (3):459–465.

Hahr, A. J., and M. E. Molitch. 2008. Optimizing insulin therapy in patients with type 1 and type 2 diabetes mellitus: Optimal dosing and timing in the outpatient setting. *Am J Ther* 15 (6):543–550.

Hare, D. L., T. M. Ryan, S. E. Selig, A. M. Pellizzer, T. V. Wrigley, and H. Krum. 1999. Resistance exercise training increases muscle strength, endurance, and blood flow in patients with chronic heart failure. *Am J Cardiol* 83 (12):1674–1677, A7.

Hartweg, J., R. Perera, V. Montori, S. Dinneen, H. A. Neil, and A. Farmer. 2008. Omega-3 polyunsaturated fatty acids (PUFA) for type 2 diabetes mellitus. *Cochrane Database Syst Rev* (1):CD003205.

Haykowsky, M., N. Eves, L. Figgures, A. McLean, M. Koller, D. Taylor, and W. Tymchak. 2005. Effect of exercise training on VO2peak and left ventricular systolic function in recent cardiac transplant recipients. *Am J Cardiol* 95 (8):1002–1004.

Hayward, R. A., P. D. Reaven, W. L. Wiitala, G. D. Bahn, D. J. Reda, L. Ge, M. McCarren, W. C. Duckworth, and N. V. Emanuele. 2015. Follow-up of glycemic control and cardiovascular outcomes in type 2 diabetes. *N Engl J Med* 372 (23):2197–2206.

Heijnen, M. L., P. Deurenberg, J. M. van Amelsvoort, and A. C. Beynen. 1995. Replacement of digestible by resistant starch lowers diet-induced thermogenesis in healthy men. *Br J Nutr* 73 (3):423–432.

Heller, S. 2004. Weight gain during insulin therapy in patients with type 2 diabetes mellitus. *Diabetes Res Clin Pract* 65 (Suppl 1):S23–S27.

Henry, R. R. 1994. Protein content of the diabetic diet. *Diabetes Care* 17 (12):1502–1513.

Henry, R. R., and B. Gumbiner. 1991. Benefits and limitations of very-low-calorie diet therapy in obese NIDDM. *Diabetes Care* 14 (9):802–823.

Henry, R. R., T. A. Wiest-Kent, L. Scheaffer, O. G. Kolterman, and J. M. Olefsky. 1986. Metabolic consequences of very-low-calorie diet therapy in obese non-insulin-dependent diabetic and nondiabetic subjects. *Diabetes* 35 (2):155–164.

Hlebowicz, J., G. Darwiche, O. Bjorgell, and L. O. Almer. 2007. Effect of cinnamon on postprandial blood glucose, gastric emptying, and satiety in healthy subjects. *Am J Clin Nutr* 85 (6):1552–1556.

Hoebler, C., A. Karinthi, H. Chiron, M. Champ, and J. L. Barry. 1999. Bioavailability of starch in bread rich in amylose: Metabolic responses in healthy subjects and starch structure. *Eur J Clin Nutr* 53 (5):360–366.

Hughes, T. A., J. T. Gwynne, B. R. Switzer, C. Herbst, and G. White. 1984. Effects of caloric restriction and weight loss on glycemic control, insulin release and resistance, and atherosclerotic risk in obese patients with type II diabetes mellitus. *Am J Med* 77 (1):7–17.

Hunter, G. R., J. P. McCarthy, and M. M. Bamman. 2004. Effects of resistance training on older adults. *Sports Med* 34 (5):329–348.

Hunter, G. R., C. J. Wetzstein, D. A. Fields, A. Brown, and M. M. Bamman. 2000. Resistance training increases total energy expenditure and free-living physical activity in older adults. *J Appl Physiol (1985)* 89 (3):977–984.

Hurley, B. F., and S. M. Roth. 2000. Strength training in the elderly: Effects on risk factors for age-related diseases. *Sports Med* 30 (4):249–268.

Inzucchi, S. E., R. M. Bergenstal, J. B. Buse, M. Diamant, E. Ferrannini, M. Nauck, A. L. Peters et al. 2012. Management of hyperglycemia in type 2 diabetes: A patient-centered approach: Position statement of the American Diabetes Association (ADA) and the European Association for the Study of Diabetes (EASD). *Diabetes Care* 35 (6):1364–1379.

Jenkins, D. J., V. Vuksan, C. W. Kendall, P. Wursch, R. Jeffcoat, S. Waring, C. C. Mehling, E. Vidgen, L. S. Augustin, and E. Wong. 1998. Physiological effects of resistant starches on fecal bulk, short chain fatty acids, blood lipids and glycemic index. *J Am Coll Nutr* 17 (6):609–616.

Kahn, C. R., and J. Roth. 2004. Berson, Yalow, and the JCI: The agony and the ecstasy. *J Clin Invest* 114 (8):1051–1054.

Kaufman, F. R., M. Halvorson, and N. D. Kaufman. 1995. A randomized, blinded trial of uncooked cornstarch to diminish nocturnal hypoglycemia at diabetes camp. *Diabetes Res Clin Pract* 30 (3):205–209.

Kell, R. T., G. Bell, and A. Quinney. 2001. Musculoskeletal fitness, health outcomes and quality of life. *Sports Med* 31 (12):863–873.

Kendall, A., D. A. Levitsky, B. J. Strupp, and L. Lissner. 1991. Weight loss on a low-fat diet: Consequence of the imprecision of the control of food intake in humans. *Am J Clin Nutr* 53 (5):1124–1129.

Khan, A., M. Safdar, M. M. Ali Khan, K. N. Khattak, and R. A. Anderson. 2003. Cinnamon improves glucose and lipids of people with type 2 diabetes. *Diabetes Care* 26 (12):3215–3218.

Kissebah, A. H., N. Vydelingum, R. Murray, D. J. Evans, A. J. Hartz, R. K. Kalkhoff, and P. W. Adams. 1982. Relation of body fat distribution to metabolic complications of obesity. *J Clin Endocrinol Metab* 54 (2):254–260.

Kleefstra, N., S. T. Houweling, F. G. Jansman, K. H. Groenier, R. O. Gans, B. Meyboom-de Jong, S. J. Bakker, and H. J. Bilo. 2006. Chromium treatment has no effect in patients with poorly controlled, insulin-treated type 2 diabetes in an obese Western population: A randomized, double-blind, placebo-controlled trial. *Diabetes Care* 29 (3):521–525.

Kongsgaard, M., V. Backer, K. Jorgensen, M. Kjaer, and N. Beyer. 2004. Heavy resistance training increases muscle size, strength and physical function in elderly male COPD-patients—A pilot study. *Respir Med* 98 (10):1000–1007.

Lapidus, L., C. Bengtsson, B. Larsson, K. Pennert, E. Rybo, and L. Sjostrom. 1984. Distribution of adipose tissue and risk of cardiovascular disease and death: A 12 year follow up of participants in the population study of women in Gothenburg, Sweden. *Br Med J (Clin Res Ed)* 289 (6454):1257–1261.

Larsson, B., K. Svardsudd, L. Welin, L. Wilhelmsen, P. Bjorntorp, and G. Tibblin. 1984. Abdominal adipose tissue distribution, obesity, and risk of cardiovascular disease and death: 13 year follow up of participants in the study of men born in 1913. *Br Med J (Clin Res Ed)* 288 (6428):1401–1404.

Li, Z., K. Hong, P. Saltsman, S. DeShields, M. Bellman, G. Thames, Y. Liu, H. J. Wang, R. Elashoff, and D. Heber. 2005. Long-term efficacy of soy-based meal replacements vs an individualized diet plan in obese type II DM patients: Relative effects on weight loss, metabolic parameters, and C-reactive protein. *Eur J Clin Nutr* 59 (3):411–418.

Li, Z., L. Treyzon, S. Chen, E. Yan, G. Thames, and C. L. Carpenter. 2010. Protein-enriched meal replacements do not adversely affect liver, kidney or bone density: An outpatient randomized controlled trial. *Nutr J* 9:72.

Li, Z., C. H. Tseng, Q. Li, M. L. Deng, M. Wang, and D. Heber. 2014. Clinical efficacy of a medically supervised outpatient high-protein, low-calorie diet program is equivalent in prediabetic, diabetic and normoglycemic obese patients. *Nutr Diabetes* 4:e105.

Liljeberg, H. G., A. K. Akerberg, and I. M. Bjorck. 1999. Effect of the glycemic index and content of indigestible carbohydrates of cereal-based breakfast meals on glucose tolerance at lunch in healthy subjects. *Am J Clin Nutr* 69 (4):647–655.

Lipska, K. J., C. J. Bailey, and S. E. Inzucchi. 2011. Use of metformin in the setting of mild-to-moderate renal insufficiency. *Diabetes Care* 34 (6):1431–1437.

Lissner, L., D. A. Levitsky, B. J. Strupp, H. J. Kalkwarf, and D. A. Roe. 1987. Dietary fat and the regulation of energy intake in human subjects. *Am J Clin Nutr* 46 (6):886–892.

Lu, T., H. Sheng, J. Wu, Y. Cheng, J. Zhu, and Y. Chen. 2012. Cinnamon extract improves fasting blood glucose and glycosylated hemoglobin level in Chinese patients with type 2 diabetes. *Nutr Res* 32 (6):408–412.

Luo, J., S. W. Rizkalla, C. Alamowitch, A. Boussairi, A. Blayo, J. L. Barry, A. Laffitte, F. Guyon, F. R. Bornet, and G. Slama. 1996. Chronic consumption of short-chain fructooligosaccharides by healthy subjects decreased basal hepatic glucose production but had no effect on insulin-stimulated glucose metabolism. *Am J Clin Nutr* 63 (6):939–945.

Maggio, C. A., and F. X. Pi-Sunyer. 1997. The prevention and treatment of obesity. Application to type 2 diabetes. *Diabetes Care* 20 (11):1744–1766.

Mertz, W. 1998. Chromium research from a distance: From 1959 to 1980. *J Am Coll Nutr* 17 (6):544–547.

Metz, J. A., J. S. Stern, P. Kris-Etherton, M. E. Reusser, C. D. Morris, D. C. Hatton, S. Oparil et al. 2000. A randomized trial of improved weight loss with a prepared meal plan in overweight and obese patients: Impact on cardiovascular risk reduction. *Arch Intern Med* 160 (14):2150–2158.

Miller, W. J., W. M. Sherman, and J. L. Ivy. 1984. Effect of strength training on glucose tolerance and post-glucose insulin response. *Med Sci Sports Exerc* 16 (6):539–543.

Milne, R. M., J. I. Mann, A. W. Chisholm, and S. M. Williams. 1994. Long-term comparison of three dietary prescriptions in the treatment of NIDDM. *Diabetes Care* 17 (1):74–80.

Monami, M., C. Nardini, and E. Mannucci. 2014. Efficacy and safety of sodium glucose co-transport-2 inhibitors in type 2 diabetes: A meta-analysis of randomized clinical trials. *Diabetes Obes Metab* 16 (5):457–466.

Mori, Y., Y. Murakawa, K. Okada, H. Horikoshi, J. Yokoyama, N. Tajima, and Y. Ikeda. 1999. Effect of troglitazone on body fat distribution in type 2 diabetic patients. *Diabetes Care* 22 (6):908–912.

Mourier, A., J. F. Gautier, E. De Kerviler, A. X. Bigard, J. M. Villette, J. P. Garnier, A. Duvallet, C. Y. Guezennec, and G. Cathelineau. 1997. Mobilization of visceral adipose tissue related to the improvement in insulin sensitivity in response to physical training in NIDDM. Effects of branched-chain amino acid supplements. *Diabetes Care* 20 (3):385–391.

Nelson, M. E., M. A. Fiatarone, C. M. Morganti, I. Trice, R. A. Greenberg, and W. J. Evans. 1994. Effects of high-intensity strength training on multiple risk factors for osteoporotic fractures. A randomized controlled trial. *JAMA* 272 (24):1909–1914.

Noakes, M., P. M. Clifton, P. J. Nestel, R. Le Leu, and G. McIntosh. 1996. Effect of high-amylose starch and oat bran on metabolic variables and bowel function in subjects with hypertriglyceridemia. *Am J Clin Nutr* 64 (6):944–951.

Norris, S. L., X. Zhang, A. Avenell, E. Gregg, T. J. Brown, C. H. Schmid, and J. Lau. 2005. Long-term non-pharmacologic weight loss interventions for adults with type 2 diabetes. *Cochrane Database Syst Rev* (2):CD004095.

Norwood, D. K., A. A. Chilipko, S. M. Amin, D. Macharia, and K. L. Still. 2013. Evaluating the potential benefits of metformin in patients with cardiovascular disease and heart failure. *Consult Pharm* 28 (9):579–583.

Ohlson, L. O., B. Larsson, K. Svardsudd, L. Welin, H. Eriksson, L. Wilhelmsen, P. Bjorntorp, and G. Tibblin. 1985. The influence of body fat distribution on the incidence of diabetes mellitus. 13.5 years of follow-up of the participants in the study of men born in 1913. *Diabetes* 34 (10):1055–1058.

Olefsky, J. M., O. G. Kolterman, and J. A. Scarlett. 1982. Insulin action and resistance in obesity and noninsulin-dependent type II diabetes mellitus. *Am J Physiol* 243 (1):E15–E30.

Ouellette, M. M., N. K. LeBrasseur, J. F. Bean, E. Phillips, J. Stein, W. R. Frontera, and R. A. Fielding. 2004. High-intensity resistance training improves muscle strength, self-reported function, and disability in long-term stroke survivors. *Stroke* 35 (6):1404–1409.

Parillo, M., A. A. Rivellese, A. V. Ciardullo, B. Capaldo, A. Giacco, S. Genovese, and G. Riccardi. 1992. A high-monounsaturated-fat/low-carbohydrate diet improves peripheral insulin sensitivity in non-insulin-dependent diabetic patients. *Metabolism* 41 (12):1373–1378.

Patel, J., R. J. Anderson, and E. B. Rappaport. 1999. Rosiglitazone monotherapy improves glycaemic control in patients with type 2 diabetes: A twelve-week, randomized, placebo-controlled study. *Diabetes Obes Metab* 1 (3):165–172.

Pavlou, K. N., S. Krey, and W. P. Steffee. 1989. Exercise as an adjunct to weight loss and maintenance in moderately obese subjects. *Am J Clin Nutr* 49 (5 Suppl):1115–1123.

Pi-Sunyer, F. X. 2002. Glycemic index and disease. *Am J Clin Nutr* 76 (1):290S–298S.

Pi-Sunyer, F. X. 2005. Weight loss in type 2 diabetic patients. *Diabetes Care* 28 (6):1526–1527.

Plotnikoff, R. C., L. M. Taylor, P. M. Wilson, K. S. Courneya, R. J. Sigal, N. Birkett, K. Raine, and L. W. Svenson. 2006. Factors associated with physical activity in Canadian adults with diabetes. *Med Sci Sports Exerc* 38 (8):1526–1534.

Poehlman, E. T., R. V. Dvorak, W. F. DeNino, M. Brochu, and P. A. Ades. 2000. Effects of resistance training and endurance training on insulin sensitivity in nonobese, young women: A controlled randomized trial. *J Clin Endocrinol Metab* 85 (7):2463–2468.

Pu, C. T., M. T. Johnson, D. E. Forman, J. M. Hausdorff, R. Roubenoff, M. Foldvari, R. A. Fielding, and M. A. Singh. 2001. Randomized trial of progressive resistance training to counteract the myopathy of chronic heart failure. *J Appl Physiol (1985)* 90 (6):2341–2350.

Quianzon, C. C., and I. E. Cheikh. 2012. History of current non-insulin medications for diabetes mellitus. *J Community Hosp Intern Med Perspect* 2 (3).

Quinn Rothacker, D. 2000. Five-year self-management of weight using meal replacements: Comparison with matched controls in rural Wisconsin. *Nutrition* 16 (5):344–348.

Raben, A., A. Tagliabue, N. J. Christensen, J. Madsen, J. J. Holst, and A. Astrup. 1994. Resistant starch: The effect on postprandial glycemia, hormonal response, and satiety. *Am J Clin Nutr* 60 (4):544–551.

Rasmussen, O. W., C. Thomsen, K. W. Hansen, M. Vesterlund, E. Winther, and K. Hermansen. 1993. Effects on blood pressure, glucose, and lipid levels of a high-monounsaturated fat diet compared with a high-carbohydrate diet in NIDDM subjects. *Diabetes Care* 16 (12):1565–1571.

Redmon, J. B., K. P. Reck, S. K. Raatz, J. E. Swanson, C. A. Kwong, H. Ji, W. Thomas, and J. P. Bantle. 2005. Two-year outcome of a combination of weight loss therapies for type 2 diabetes. *Diabetes Care* 28 (6):1311–1315.

Riccardi, G., A. Rivellese, D. Pacioni, S. Genovese, P. Mastranzo, and M. Mancini. 1984. Separate influence of dietary carbohydrate and fibre on the metabolic control in diabetes. *Diabetologia* 26 (2):116–121.

Richy, F. F., M. Sabido-Espin, S. Guedes, F. A. Corvino, and U. Gottwald-Hostalek. 2014. Incidence of lactic acidosis in patients with type 2 diabetes with and without renal impairment treated with metformin: A retrospective cohort study. *Diabetes Care* 37 (8):2291–2295.

Ronnemaa, T., K. Mattila, A. Lehtonen, and V. Kallio. 1986. A controlled randomized study on the effect of long-term physical exercise on the metabolic control in type 2 diabetic patients. *Acta Med Scand* 220 (3):219–224.

Rothacker, D. Q., B. A. Staniszewski, and P. K. Ellis. 2001. Liquid meal replacement vs traditional food: A potential model for women who cannot maintain eating habit change. *J Am Diet Assoc* 101 (3):345–347.

Ruderman, N. B., O. P. Ganda, and K. Johansen. 1979. The effect of physical training on glucose tolerance and plasma lipids in maturity-onset diabetes. *Diabetes* 28 (Suppl 1):89–92.

Ryan, A. S., D. E. Hurlbut, M. E. Lott, F. M. Ivey, J. Fleg, B. F. Hurley, and A. P. Goldberg. 2001. Insulin action after resistive training in insulin resistant older men and women. *J Am Geriatr Soc* 49 (3):247–253.

Salpeter, S. R., E. Greyber, G. A. Pasternak, and E. E. Salpeter. 2010. Risk of fatal and nonfatal lactic acidosis with metformin use in type 2 diabetes mellitus. *Cochrane Database Syst Rev* (4):CD002967.

Sanders, L. J. 2002. From Thebes to Toronto and the 21st century: An incredible journey. *Diabetes Spectrum* 15:56–60.

Schwingshackl, L., and B. Strasser. 2012. High-MUFA diets reduce fasting glucose in patients with type 2 diabetes. *Ann Nutr Metab* 60 (1):33–34.

Schwingshackl, L., B. Strasser, and G. Hoffmann. 2011. Effects of monounsaturated fatty acids on glycaemic control in patients with abnormal glucose metabolism: A systematic review and meta-analysis. *Ann Nutr Metab* 58 (4):290–296.

Segal, K. R., A. Edano, A. Abalos, J. Albu, L. Blando, M. B. Tomas, and F. X. Pi-Sunyer. 1991. Effect of exercise training on insulin sensitivity and glucose metabolism in lean, obese, and diabetic men. *J Appl Physiol (1985)* 71 (6):2402–2411.

Sigal, R. J., G. P. Kenny, D. H. Wasserman, and C. Castaneda-Sceppa. 2004. Physical activity/exercise and type 2 diabetes. *Diabetes Care* 27 (10):2518–2539.

Singh, M. A., W. Ding, T. J. Manfredi, G. S. Solares, E. F. O'Neill, K. M. Clements, N. D. Ryan, J. J. Kehayias, R. A. Fielding, and W. J. Evans. 1999. Insulin-like growth factor I in skeletal muscle after weight-lifting exercise in frail elders. *Am J Physiol* 277 (1 Pt 1):E135–E143.

Singh, N. A., K. M. Clements, and M. A. Fiatarone. 1997. A randomized controlled trial of progressive resistance training in depressed elders. *J Gerontol A Biol Sci Med Sci* 52 (1):M27–M35.

Sirtori, C. R., R. Paoletti, M. Mancini, G. Crepaldi, E. Manzato, A. Rivellese, F. Pamparana, and E. Stragliotto. 1997. N-3 fatty acids do not lead to an increased diabetic risk in patients with hyperlipidemia and abnormal glucose tolerance. Italian Fish Oil Multicenter Study. *Am J Clin Nutr* 65 (6):1874–1881.

Steven, S., K. G. Hollingsworth, A. Al-Mrabeh, L. Avery, B. Aribisala, M. Caslake, and R. Taylor. 2016. Very low-calorie diet and 6 months of weight stability in type 2 diabetes: Pathophysiological changes in responders and nonresponders. *Diabetes Care* 39 (5):808–815.

Stewart, K. J. 2002. Exercise training and the cardiovascular consequences of type 2 diabetes and hypertension: Plausible mechanisms for improving cardiovascular health. *JAMA* 288 (13):1622–1631.

Thomas, D. E., and E. J. Elliott. 2010. The use of low-glycaemic index diets in diabetes control. *Br J Nutr* 104 (6):797–802.

Trinkley, K. E., S. M. Nikels, R. L. Page 2nd, and M. S. Joy. 2014. Automating and estimating glomerular filtration rate for dosing medications and staging chronic kidney disease. *Int J Gen Med* 7:211–218.

Tuomilehto, J., J. Lindstrom, J. G. Eriksson, T. T. Valle, H. Hamalainen, P. Ilanne-Parikka, S. Keinanen-Kiukaanniemi et al. 2001. Prevention of type 2 diabetes mellitus by changes in lifestyle among subjects with impaired glucose tolerance. *N Engl J Med* 344 (18):1343–1350.

Turner, R. C., C. A. Cull, V. Frighi, and R. R. Holman. 1999. Glycemic control with diet, sulfonylurea, metformin, or insulin in patients with type 2 diabetes mellitus: Progressive requirement for multiple therapies (UKPDS 49). UK Prospective Diabetes Study (UKPDS) Group. *JAMA* 281 (21):2005–2012.

UK Prospective Diabetes Study (UKPDS) Group. 1998a. Effect of intensive blood-glucose control with metformin on complications in overweight patients with type 2 diabetes (UKPDS 34). Lancet 352: 854–865.

UK Prospective Diabetes Study (UKPDS) Group. 1998b. Intensive blood-glucose control with sulphonylureas or insulin compared with conventional treatment and risk of complications in patients with type 2 diabetes (UKPDS 33). *Lancet* 352 (9131):837–853.

Vaaler, S., K. F. Hanssen, and O. Aagenaes. 1980. Effect of different kinds of fibre on postprandial blood glucose in insulin-dependent diabetics. *Acta Med Scand* 208 (5):389–391.

Vague, J. 1996a. The degree of masculine differentiation of obesities: A factor determining predisposition to diabetes, atherosclerosis, gout, and uric calculous disease. 1956. *Obes Res* 4 (2):204–212.

Vague, J. 1996b. Sexual differentiation. A determinant factor of the forms of obesity. 1947. *Obes Res* 4 (2):201–203.

Wadden, T. A., D. S. West, R. H. Neiberg, R. R. Wing, D. H. Ryan, K. C. Johnson, J. P. Foreyt, J. O. Hill, D. L. Trence, and M. Z. Vitolins. 2009. One-year weight losses in the Look AHEAD study: Factors associated with success. *Obesity (Silver Spring)* 17 (4):713–722.

Walker, K. Z., K. O'Dea, L. Johnson, A. J. Sinclair, L. S. Piers, G. C. Nicholson, and J. G. Muir. 1996. Body fat distribution and non-insulin-dependent diabetes: Comparison of a fiber-rich, high-carbohydrate, low-fat (23%) diet and a 35% fat diet high in monounsaturated fat. *Am J Clin Nutr* 63 (2):254–260.
White, J. R., Jr. 2010. Apple trees to sodium glucose co-transporter inhibitors: A review of SGLT-2 inhibition. *Clin Diabetes* 28:6.
White, J. R., Jr. 2014. A brief history of the development of diabetes medications. *Diabetes Spectr* 27 (2):82–86.
White, J. R., Jr., and K. Campbell. 2008. *ADA/PDR Medications for the Treatment of Diabetes*. New York: Thomson Reuters.
Wing, R. R., M. D. Marcus, R. Salata, L. H. Epstein, S. Miaskiewicz, and E. H. Blair. 1991. Effects of a very-low-calorie diet on long-term glycemic control in obese type 2 diabetic subjects. *Arch Intern Med* 151 (7):1334–1340.
Wing, R. R., E. Venditti, J. M. Jakicic, B. A. Polley, and W. Lang. 1998. Lifestyle intervention in overweight individuals with a family history of diabetes. *Diabetes Care* 21 (3):350–359.
Wu, J. H., R. Micha, F. Imamura, A. Pan, M. L. Biggs, O. Ajaz, L. Djousse, F. B. Hu, and D. Mozaffarian. 2012. Omega-3 fatty acids and incident type 2 diabetes: A systematic review and meta-analysis. *Br J Nutr* 107 (Suppl 2):S214–S227.
Wursch, P. 1989. Starch in human nutrition. *World Rev Nutr Diet* 60:199–256.
Wycherley, T. P., M. Noakes, P. M. Clifton, X. Cleanthous, J. B. Keogh, and G. D. Brinkworth. 2010. A high-protein diet with resistance exercise training improves weight loss and body composition in overweight and obese patients with type 2 diabetes. *Diabetes Care* 33 (5):969–976.
Yokoyama, H., M. Emoto, S. Fujiwara, K. Motoyama, T. Morioka, H. Koyama, T. Shoji, M. Inaba, and Y. Nishizawa. 2004. Short-term aerobic exercise improves arterial stiffness in type 2 diabetes. *Diabetes Res Clin Pract* 65 (2):85–93.
Yu-Poth, S., G. Zhao, T. Etherton, M. Naglak, S. Jonnalagadda, and P. M. Kris-Etherton. 1999. Effects of the National Cholesterol Education Program's Step I and Step II dietary intervention programs on cardiovascular disease risk factors: A meta-analysis. *Am J Clin Nutr* 69 (4):632–646.
Zoungas, S., J. Chalmers, B. Neal, L. Billot, Q. Li, Y. Hirakawa, H. Arima et al. 2014. Follow-up of blood-pressure lowering and glucose control in type 2 diabetes. *N Engl J Med* 371 (15):1392–1406.

8 Fatty Liver Disease

8.1 INTRODUCTION

Nonalcoholic fatty liver disease (NAFLD) is the most common cause of liver disease and the third most common reason for liver transplantation. Other common liver diseases, including alcoholic liver disease and viral hepatitis, often occur in obese patients who also have NAFLD.

Among patients over 50 years of age with diabetes or obesity, two-thirds are estimated to have nonalcoholic steatohepatitis (NASH) with advanced fibrosis (Rinella 2015). The ability to identify the NASH subtype within those with nonalcoholic fatty liver requires liver biopsy. Weight management, diet, exercise, and lifestyle modification are the foundation of treatment for patients with nonalcoholic steatosis. The association between NASH and cardiovascular disease is likely related to the overlap with metabolic syndrome. The incidence of NAFLD-related hepatocellular carcinoma (HCC) is increasing.

This common nutrition-related disorder occurs in between 75 million and 100 million individuals in the United States alone, and it has clear influences on systemic diseases, including cardiovascular disease, when associated with metabolic syndrome (Rinella 2015). Current estimates suggest that NAFLD and its progressive subtype NASH affect 30% and 5%, respectively, of the current U.S. population. Fatty liver is found in 10–15% of normal-weight individuals and 70% of obese subjects (Vernon et al. 2011).

The most common causes of death in patients with NASH are cardiovascular disease and malignancy, and it is the most rapidly increasing indication for liver transplantation. Liver failure is often associated with malnutrition and a clinical presentation that is common with jaundice, ascites, and esophageal varices. Many of these patients require nutritional support, but there is no evidence that it affects outcomes significantly at this late stage of disease.

It is important that primary care physicians and other health care providers be aware of the commonality and the long-term health effects of NAFLD in association with obesity and diabetes. Identification of patients with NASH at an early stage may help improve patient outcome through lifestyle change.

8.2 PATHOPHYSIOLOGY OF NAFLD

The presence of liver fat deposition or steatosis is necessary but not sufficient for NASH to develop. Fat accumulation of at least 5% of liver weight in the absence of significant alcohol intake is the standard for diagnosing NAFLD (Vernon et al. 2011). The prevalence of NAFLD is approximately 20–30% in developed societies, but reaches up to 70–90% among subjects with obesity or diabetes (Targher et al. 2010). The evidence that NAFLD is an independent risk factor for cardiovascular diseases (Bhatia et al. 2012; Lonardo et al. 2015b; Hazlehurst et al. 2016), as well as for type 2 diabetes mellitus (Kotronen et al. 2007; Anstee et al. 2013; Yki-Jarvinen 2014), is solid. Moreover, the presence of both NAFLD and diabetes increases the likelihood of the development of complications of diabetes and more severe adverse outcomes of NAFLD.

The mechanisms leading one patient to develop NASH and another to only have steatosis without inflammation are not known. It is known that abdominal visceral fat is a limited depot for fat storage, and that fat is stored in the liver as well. In animal models, fat moves into the liver once apoptosis of abdominal fat cells occurs. Visceral adipose tissue secretes adipokines under these circumstances, which have been proposed to affect lipid and glucose metabolism, leading to hepatic fat deposition and establishing inflammatory microenvironments in the liver that trigger cellular injury. Oxidative stress, lipotoxic fatty acids, and apoptotic pathways contribute to liver damage. As part of the injury response, fibrosis develops and can lead to cirrhosis. Inflammation can also lead to the development of hepatocellular cancer in some patients (Figure 8.1).

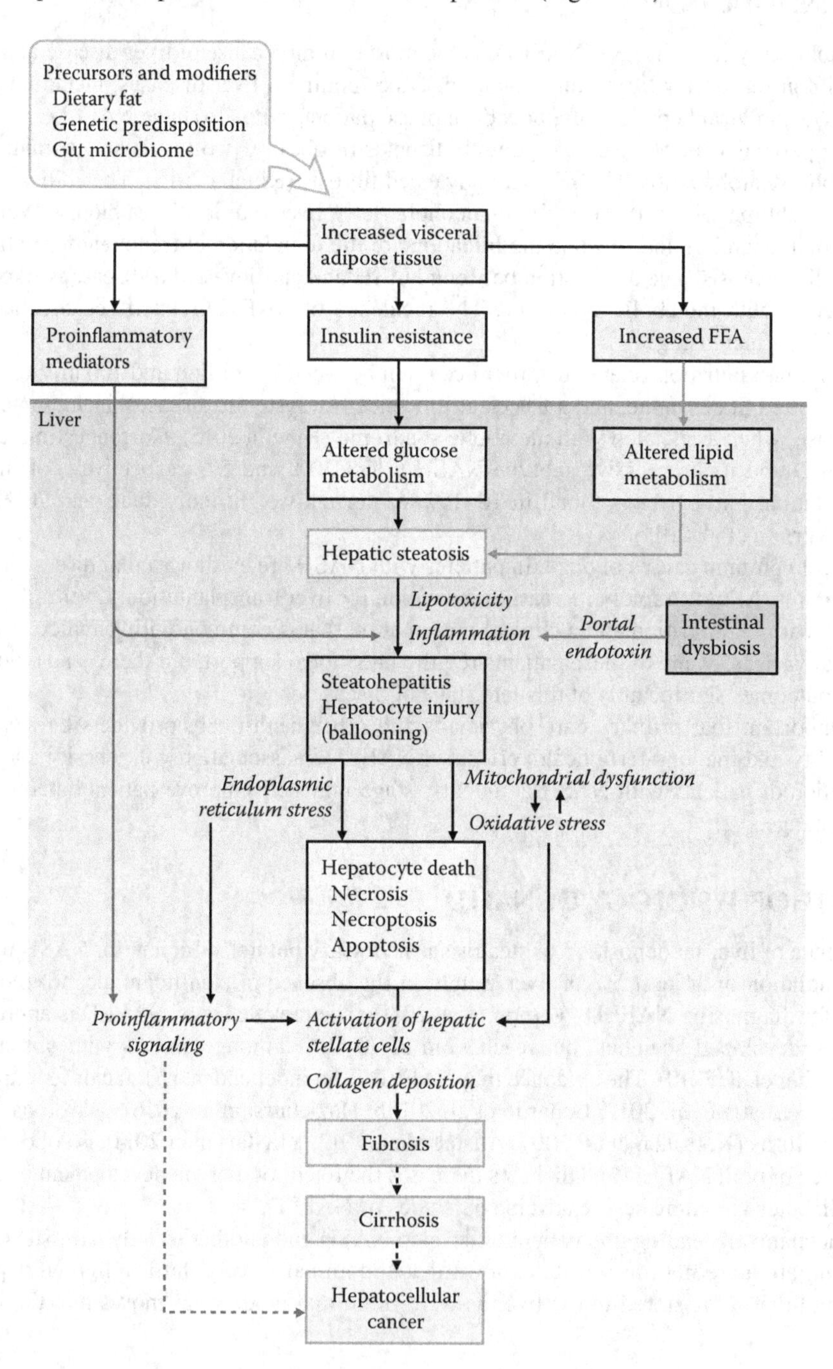

FIGURE 8.1 Mechanisms involved in the pathophysiology of fatty liver disease. FFA: Free fatty acids. (Reprinted from Rinella, M. E., *JAMA*, 313(22), 2263–2273, 2015.)

8.3 NAFLD AND METABOLIC SYNDROME

The overlap between NAFLD and metabolic syndrome is significant due to the common risk factors and pathophysiological mechanisms involved in both conditions (Kotronen et al. 2007; Stefan et al. 2008; Fabbrini et al. 2010; Anstee et al. 2013; Machado and Cortez-Pinto 2014; Yki-Jarvinen 2014; Lonardo et al. 2015a). There are also population studies demonstrating the association of metabolic syndrome and NAFLD (Ballestri et al. 2016). Insulin resistance, low adiponectin levels, subclinical inflammation, endothelial dysfunction, and a prothrombotic state with impaired fibrinolysis are all linked to NAFLD and cardiovascular diseases, and the more aggressive forms of NAFLD confer greater cardiovascular risk (Targher et al. 2010; Bhatia et al. 2012; Anstee et al. 2013; Liu and Lu 2014).

It has been proposed that in those who have NAFLD without concomitant metabolic syndrome, the condition may originate from genetic susceptibility, while in those who have both NAFLD and metabolic syndrome, the conditions are due to a Western lifestyle and its consequences, obesity and insulin resistance. In the absence of metabolic syndrome, NAFLD does not increase the risk for developing type 2 diabetes mellitus in comparison with healthy subjects. The perception that there are different phenotypes of NAFLD and that the major division between the phenotypes is whether the NAFLD is combined with insulin resistance is founded on numerous studies, including genetic studies, some on a polymorphism of the PNPLA3 gene that is associated with NAFLD without metabolic syndrome (Speliotes et al. 2010; Shen et al. 2014; Lonardo et al. 2015a; Park et al. 2015; Petaja and Yki-Jarvinen 2016).

8.4 NAFLD AND CIRRHOSIS

Cryptogenic cirrhosis is unexplained by any other etiologies, including chronic viral hepatitis, alcohol abuse, toxin exposure, autoimmune disease, congenital disorders, vascular outflow obstruction, or biliary tract disease. NAFLD is the most common cause of cryptogenic cirrhosis. A cause–effect relationship between NAFLD and cryptogenic cirrhosis was first suggested (Caldwell et al. 1999) when patients with cryptogenic cirrhosis typically presented one decade older with a high prevalence of obesity and diabetes, and similar in all other respects to patients with NASH. The relationship between NASH and cryptogenic cirrhosis was also supported by a subsequent case-controlled study (Poonawala et al. 2000). In one series, 27 of 37 (73%) patients presenting with cryptogenic cirrhosis were overweight, and among the overweight group, 88% had diabetes, 56% had hypertriglyceridemia, and 90% had a family history of obesity or diabetes (Ratziu et al. 2002). The observed rates were significantly increased in this overweight group compared with the lean patients with cryptogenic cirrhosis and obese or lean patients with hepatitis C cirrhosis. The latter findings lend additional credence to the concept that NAFLD is a common antecedent condition in many patients with cryptogenic cirrhosis.

8.5 NAFLD AND HEPATOCELLULAR CANCER

In 2008, primary liver cancer was estimated to be the fourth most often diagnosed cancer in males and the seventh in females (Jemal et al. 2011); moreover, it represented the second and fifth causes of cancer deaths in males and females, respectively. The estimate in 2012 was even more alarming, as liver cancer represented the overall second cause of cancer death in the world (IARC 2012). These statistics reflect the poor prognosis of liver cancer worldwide.

The prevalent histological subtype of primary liver malignancies is HCC, which accounts for 70–85% of cases (El-Serag 2011). The major risk factor for HCC is cirrhosis, and the underlying etiologies are viral infections (Tsukuma et al. 1993; Velazquez et al. 2003), alcohol, and metabolic factors. While the epidemiological data concerning HCC in viral hepatitis and alcoholic hepatitis are consistent, there is a lack of strong epidemiological data concerning the incidence and prevalence of HCC in NAFLD.

A few longitudinal outcome studies explored the prevalence of HCC in NAFL and NASH, reporting a prevalence varying from 0% to 3% on a follow-up period between 5.6 and 21 years (White et al. 2012). The percentage was increased if the incidence of HCC in NAFLD cirrhosis was considered, with a cumulative HCC incidence ranging between 2.4%, with a median follow-up of 7.2 years, and 12.8%, with a 3.2-year median follow-up (White et al. 2012).

Obesity is associated with an increased relative risk of dying of cancer. It has been associated with colorectal, breast, endometrial, and kidney cancer and esophageal adenocarcinoma (Calle and Kaaks 2004). This association has also been established for HCC in a population perspective study in the United States. More than 900,000 people were enrolled and stratified according to their body mass index (BMI).

When matched with normal-weight individuals, the relative risk of dying from HCC was about 4.5-fold greater in patients with obesity (Calle et al. 2003). Another study, from Korea, which followed 700,000 men for almost 10 years, confirmed the same strong association between HCC and obesity (Oh et al. 2005). A higher relative risk for HCC in obese patients has also been described in a Swedish population study of 362,552 subjects (Samanic et al. 2006). An article collecting data from Norway, Austria, and Sweden found a 1.5-fold increased risk for HCC in obese subjects when adjusted to the alcohol consumption in order to avoid confounding factors (Borena et al. 2012). In a European prospective cohort study, general and abdominal obesity correlated with the risk of HCC, and this was confirmed in a subanalysis that excluded hepatitis C virus (HCV)- and hepatitis B virus (HBV)-positive subjects (Schlesinger et al. 2013). Also, in an Italian study the correlation of obesity and HCC was confirmed; the correlation increased if the patients also had metabolic syndrome (Turati et al. 2013).

In between about 7% and 50% of HCC in different series, the underlying etiology of liver disease could not be determined (Marrero et al. 2002; Bosch et al. 2005; Bugianesi 2007). In 641 cases of HCC, 44 patients, or 6.9%, were categorized as having cryptogenic cirrhosis. The prevalence of diabetes and obesity was significantly higher in these subjects if compared with patients with viral and alcoholic etiologies for their cirrhosis.

Obesity and diabetes are also two recognized risk factors of NASH, and the authors suggest that NASH might represent the missing link between cryptogenic cirrhosis and HCC (Bugianesi et al. 2002). The pathological features typical of NASH may not be present in the late stages of liver disease (Powell et al. 1990; Caldwell et al. 1999; Poonawala et al. 2000), and in decompensated cirrhosis, the typical clinical characteristics of NAFLD may be missing. In another study, cryptogenic cirrhosis accounted for up to 29% of the cases of HCC. Half of these patients expressed histological or clinical features of NAFLD, and at least 13% had histologically confirmed NAFLD (Marrero et al. 2002). These data suggest that the role of NAFLD in HCC might be underestimated by the current epidemiological data, and that NAFLD could account for part of the cryptogenic-related HCC. Based on these studies, the incidence of HCC can be expected to grow globally, along with the increasing incidence of obesity and diabetes (Calle and Kaaks 2004). This observation is further supported by the fact that up to 70% of patients with type 2 diabetes and up to 90% of obese patients might have some degree of fatty liver disease (Siegel and Zhu 2009; Michelotti et al. 2013).

The emergence of HCC in chronic liver disease occurs slowly over decades, with a transition through dysplasia, precancer, and carcinoma (Thorgeirsson and Grisham 2002). There are many known tumorigenic mechanisms that may contribute to genomic instability, including telomere erosion, chromosome segregation defects, and alterations in the DNA damage repair pathways (Farazi and DePinho 2006). When NAFLD is present, mechanisms related to obesity and diabetes are also involved in the development of HCC (Karagozian et al. 2014; Margini and Dufour 2016) (Figure 8.2).

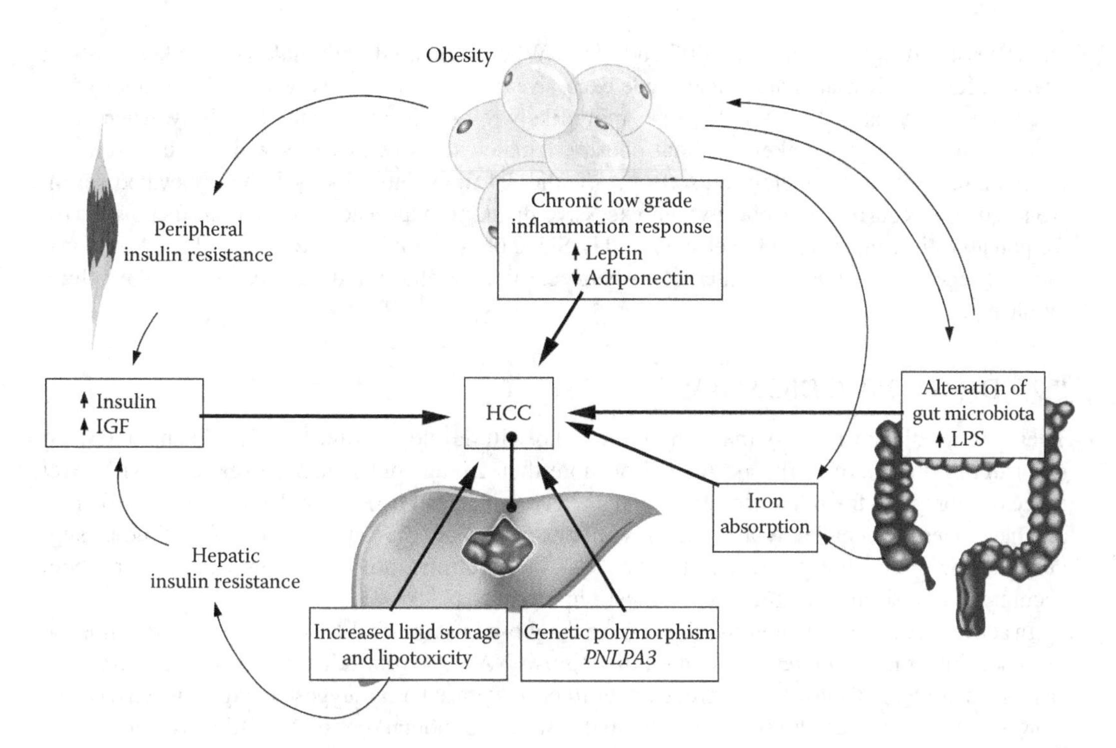

FIGURE 8.2 **(See color insert.)** The development of HCC in NAFLD is most likely multifactorial and involves obesity-mediated mechanisms, including low-grade chronic inflammatory response, increased lipid storage and lipotoxicity, alteration of gut microbiota with increased levels of lipopolysaccharide (LPS), and insulin resistance with hyperinsulinemia and increased insulin-like growth factor (IGF) levels. Genetic polymorphisms might also contribute to the development of HCC in NASH. Increased iron absorption in NASH has also been reported recently; although the mechanisms are at present still being investigated, a contribution of iron in the development of HCC has been suggested. All these mechanisms are, at least partially, independent from fibrosis, and this might explain the epidemiology of HCC in NASH, where noncirrhotic HCC is more than a sporadic event. (Reprinted from Margini, C., and Dufour, J. F., *Liver Int.*, 36(3), 317–324, 2016.)

8.6 FATTY LIVER INTERACTIONS WITH ALCOHOLIC AND VIRAL HEPATITIS

Fatty liver interacts with both alcohol and hepatitis C in increasing the risk of cirrhosis. The most common causes of liver injury include acute and chronic viral infections (hepatitis A, B, and C), alcohol damage, fatty liver, cirrhosis, and cancer. Much less common are drug-induced liver injuries due to direct toxicity or less well-defined immunoallergic reactions.

Alcohol abuse remains one of the most common causes of both acute and chronic liver disease in the United States and must be excluded in diagnosing NAFLD (Sofair et al. 2010). Up to 50% of cases of end-stage liver disease are related primarily to alcohol, but alcoholic liver disease and fatty liver due to obesity and diabetes can coexist and interact to promote the more rapid development of liver failure (Orholm et al. 1985).

The association of obesity (i.e., BMI ≥30.0 kg/m^2 or waist circumference ≥102 cm in men and ≥88 cm in women) and specific patterns of alcohol use (i.e., nondrinkers, nonexcessive drinkers, and excessive drinkers) as a predictor of elevations in serum alanine aminotransferase (ALT) and aspartate aminotransferase (AST) was studied in 8373 adults aged ≥20 years who participated in the 2005–2008 National Health and Nutrition Examination Survey (Kochanek et al. 2011). The survey revealed that 34.7% of adult men and 38.6% of adult women in the United States had both obesity and any alcohol use, including 16.4% of men and 9.8% of women who had both obesity and excessive drinking, between 2005 and 2008. When compared with male nondrinkers without obesity after multivariate adjustment, male excessive drinkers with obesity were three times more likely to have elevated ALT and 2.4 times more likely to have elevated AST. Similarly, when compared with female nondrinkers without obesity, female excessive drinkers with obesity were 2.4 times more likely to have elevated serum ALT and 3.4 times more likely to have elevated serum AST. The co-occurrence of obesity and excessive drinking may place adults at an increased risk for potential liver injury (Kochanek et al. 2011). Since obese individuals commonly have fatty liver, these observations support an interaction between alcohol abuse and obesity in promoting liver damage.

8.7 DIAGNOSTIC DILEMMAS

There are no diagnostic tests that can predict who will develop advanced NAFLD characterized by bridging fibrosis or cirrhosis. A BMI of more than 27, age older than 50 years, an ALT level twice or more than the reference range, and a triglyceride level of 1.7 mmol/L or higher (≥151 mg/dL) have been independently associated with advanced disease (Ratziu et al. 2002). Studies suggest that there are some clinical factors that can be used to identify high-risk patients for whom accurate diagnosis and staging may be most important.

In addition, there are no noninvasive tests to diagnose or stage NAFLD. Liver biopsy remains the most sensitive diagnostic test but cannot distinguish NAFLD from other causes of fatty liver disease, such as alcohol abuse. Elevated serum aminotransferase levels suggest a diagnosis of NAFLD. However, these tests are both nonspecific and insensitive biomarkers of NAFLD-associated liver damage. The degree of liver enzyme elevation does not correlate with the level of histologic cellular damage. Liver function tests cannot reliably distinguish steatosis from steatohepatitis or cirrhosis. Serum aminotransferase levels may be normal or only slightly elevated even though liver disease is advanced.

Imaging studies, such as abdominal ultrasound, computed tomography (CT), or MRI, are useful in demonstrating hepatic steatosis when fat accumulation is moderate to severe. However, these tests cannot separate steatosis from NASH. Portal hypertension as evidenced by splenomegaly, ascites, and varices indicates the presence of cirrhosis, which can occur without much liver fat being present at the time of diagnosis. Thus, imaging tests for fat are most useful for detecting earlier stages of the disease, when hepatic steatosis predominates.

Therefore, the diagnosis of NAFLD remains one of exclusion after other causes of chronic liver disease have been excluded. Operationally, therefore, NAFLD percolates to the top of the list of potential diagnoses in individuals whose liver disease remains cryptogenic after the standard, noninvasive clinical and laboratory evaluation for liver disease has been completed. Diagnostic confidence is increased considerably when overweight, obesity, and type 2 diabetes mellitus are present as well. In one study of asymptomatic patients who were referred for diagnosis of mild, cryptogenic liver enzyme elevations, histological proof of steatosis or steatohepatitis was found in approximately 70% of individuals (Skelly et al. 2001).

A presumptive diagnosis can be made when the following are present: (1) elevated serum liver enzyme levels (AST, ALT, or γ-glutamyltransferase), (2) imaging studies with evidence of fat, (3) minimal or no alcohol intake, and (4) negative test results for viral hepatitis, autoimmune disease (primary biliary cirrhosis), and congenital liver diseases such as Wilson's disease.

8.8 CLINICAL PRESENTATION OF SIGNIFICANT LIVER DAMAGE

Once advanced liver disease results in a significant breakdown of hepatic reserve for repair and regeneration, jaundice occurs secondary to increased levels of bilirubin in the blood and in tissues. The increased bilirubin results from the breakup of the hemoglobin of dead red blood cells. Normally, the liver removes bilirubin from the blood and excretes it through the bile. Diseases that interfere with liver function will lead to derangement of these processes. However, the liver has a great capacity to regenerate and has a large reserve capacity. In most cases, the liver only produces symptoms after extensive damage.

The classic symptoms of liver damage include the following:

1. Pale stools, when stercobilin, a brown pigment, is absent from the stool. Stercobilin is derived from bilirubin metabolites produced in the liver.
2. Dark urine, when bilirubin mixes with urine.
3. Jaundice, which is a yellowing of the skin and whites of the eyes due to bilirubin deposits, and pruritus, which is a common presenting complaint with liver failure, even in patients without jaundice. Often, this pruritus cannot be relieved by drugs.
4. Swelling of the abdomen, ankles, and feet, because the liver fails to make albumin, leading to osmotic flow of fluids into extracellular space and peritoneal fluid.
5. Fatigue, as a result of malnutrition associated with nausea and anorexia.
6. Bruising and easy bleeding, from reduced liver synthesis of clotting proteins.

Liver diseases can be diagnosed by physical examination, imaging, and liver-associated laboratory tests. The term *liver function tests* is commonly used for AST, ALT, bilirubin, alkaline phosphatase, and lactate dehydrogenase (LDH) measurements. These tests are not measures of liver function, but rather reflect biochemical functions of the liver or the release of liver enzymes into the bloodstream due to damage to liver cells. These liver-associated tests can be used in the overall evaluation of liver function, but sometimes can be normal even in the face of liver cirrhosis or liver failure. When infections are suspected, serologic studies can be informative, and when trace minerals are suspected, chemical testing can be informative.

8.9 NUTRITIONAL APPROACHES TO LIVER DISEASE

There are currently no approved proven treatments for NAFLD. Some options under study are (1) lifestyle modifications to induce weight loss through caloric restriction and physical activity; (2) insulin-sensitizing agents, including biguanide (metformin) and thiazolidinediones (rosiglitazone and pioglitazone); (3) antioxidants, including but not limited to vitamin E, betaine, and N-acetylcysteine; (4) ursodeoxycholic acid; and (5) lipid-lowering agents.

Lifestyle modifications, including smoking cessation and weight loss, if applicable, are crucial to improving the outcome of those suffering from NAFLD complicated by obesity, alcoholic liver disease, and viral hepatitis. Smoking is an independent risk factor for the advancement of hepatic fibrosis, which can lead to more rapid progression of liver disease, and may be linked to the development of HCC (Armstrong 1992; Corrao et al. 1994). Obesity, which can also cause fatty liver, NASH, and cirrhosis, may be an independent risk factor for the progression of alcoholic liver disease (Naveau et al. 1997).

8.9.1 Fructose and Fatty Liver

Fructose is an isomer of glucose (Stanhope and Havel 2010) but is metabolized very differently from glucose. Recent decades have witnessed an enormous rise in fructose consumption. Studies on ancient diets have shown that at the dawn of agriculture 8500 years ago, the intake of fructose per capita was around 2 kg/year from fruits and vegetables. The industrialization of sugar production from plantations in the seventeenth century converted a rare spice from the Orient into an expensive staple item used in baked goods and candies. Significant increases in consumption occurred following the abolition of sugar taxes in the 1870s. By 1950, annual consumption had increased to 45 kg/person/year, and by 1997, nearly 20 years after the introduction of high-fructose corn syrup into the food supply, consumption had risen to 69 kg/year (Lim et al. 2010; Lustig 2010). Fructose is used in a wide variety of food products due to its sweeter taste and its lack of inhibition of satiety compared with other sugars (Lustig 2010). From a metabolic standpoint, fructose is absorbed by the small intestine and is transported across the epithelial barrier into cells and the bloodstream by the fructose-specific GLUT5 transporter (Tappy et al. 2010). Entry of fructose into cells is not insulin dependent and does not promote insulin secretion, unlike glucose. Absorbed fructose is transported in plasma via the hepatic portal vein to the liver, where fructose is predominantly metabolized via its phosphorylation; only a small amount of fructose is metabolized by hexokinase in muscle and adipose tissue (Lim et al. 2010; Lustig 2010).

Starting in the 1960s, a number of animal and human studies have reported associations between excessive fructose consumption and adverse metabolic effects, which may have important hepatic consequences (including the development of NAFLD). The potential role of fructose in the pathogenesis of NAFLD has recently gained increased attention (Lim et al. 2010; Lustig 2010; Nseir et al. 2010; Stanhope and Havel 2010; Tappy et al. 2010; Alisi et al. 2011; Anania 2011; Castro et al. 2011; Nomura and Yamanouchi 2012). Fructose can lead to NAFLD by promoting an increase in fasting and postprandial triglycerides, which can in turn result in liver fat deposition (Teff et al. 2004; Ackerman et al. 2005; D'Angelo et al. 2005; Lê and Tappy 2006; Koo et al. 2008; Zhu et al. 2008; Gallagher et al. 2010, 2011; Moore 2010; Sanyal et al. 2010; Huang et al. 2011; McCullough 2011). In addition, hypertriglyceridemia secondary to excess fructose consumption under conditions of positive calorie balance has been shown to promote insulin resistance (Gallagher et al. 2010; Huang et al. 2011). Chronic fructose consumption causes hyperinsulinemia due to insulin resistance (Gallagher et al. 2010).

Continuous fructose ingestion may impose a metabolic burden on the liver through the induction of fructokinase and fatty acid synthase. In the liver, fructose is metabolized to fructose-1-phosphate by fructokinase, which consumes ATP (Lim et al. 2010; Lustig 2010). As a consequence, a massive incorporation of fructose into liver metabolism can lead to high levels of metabolic stress via ATP depletion. In an experimental study in the rat (Koo et al. 2008), it was shown that fructose-induced fructokinase hyperexpression in the liver can be reduced (by 0.6-fold) by the hydroxymethylglutaryl-coenzyme A reductase inhibitor atorvastatin. Of note, clinical studies have shown that atorvastatin can improve liver injury in NAFLD patients with hyperlipidemia (Teff et al. 2004; Lê and Tappy 2006). Fatty acid synthase catalyzes the last step in the fatty acid biosynthetic pathway and is a key determinant of the maximal capacity of the liver to synthesize fatty acids by *de novo* lipogenesis (D'Angelo et al. 2005). In a clinical study, increased fructose consumption in patients with NAFLD was associated with hyperexpression of hepatic mRNA for fatty acid synthase, suggesting that this molecular derangement could play a crucial role in fructose-induced fatty liver infiltration (Ackerman et al. 2005).

8.9.2 Vitamin E, Fish Oils, Phytonutrients, and Overall Nutrition for Liver Disease

In fatty liver disease, some evidence exists supporting the use of vitamin E. Vitamin E was studied in 167 adult patients with NASH and without diabetes who received either vitamin E at a dose of 800 IU daily (84 subjects) or placebo (83 subjects) for 96 weeks (Sanyal et al. 2010). The primary outcome was an improvement in histologic features of NASH, as assessed with the use of a composite of standardized scores for steatosis, lobular inflammation, hepatocellular ballooning, and fibrosis. There was an improvement in histologic features in 43% of those who received vitamin E compared with 19% of those receiving placebo. Additional studies are necessary to confirm these findings.

Omega-3 fatty acids are approved in the United States to treat hypertriglyceridemia. They are also available over the counter as dietary supplements. There has been significant interest in exploring the effects of omega-3 fatty acids in animal models of fatty liver, as well as in humans with NAFLD. Many of the human trials have been in small numbers of individuals treated for varying times. In one study of 144 NAFLD patients with dyslipidemia given either 2 g of omega-3 fatty acids from seal oils or placebo for 24 weeks, omega-3 fatty acid supplementation was associated with significant improvement in serum aminotransferases, serum triglycerides, and hepatic steatosis at 24 weeks (Zhu et al. 2008). There is an ongoing phase 3, multicenter, randomized controlled trial of eicosapentaenoic acid (EPA) in patients with biopsy-proven NASH in the United States, and its results are expected to shed further light on the role of omega-3 fatty acids in the management of NAFLD (ClinicalTrials.gov identifier: NCT01154985).

Coffee consumption has been associated with benefits in liver disease for unclear reasons, with some proposing that aromatic extracts isolated from coffee beans may be beneficial (Huber et al. 2002). Coffee oils, called diterpenes, have been evaluated. The diterpenes kahweol and cafestol have been shown to have beneficial effects on glutathione metabolism (Scharf et al. 2001). However, the idea of diterprene effects on liver health may be mitigated by the fact that most of these fats are trapped by the filter paper used to make traditional American coffee by the drip method. They survive in coffee made by the French press method. Nonetheless, it is also possible that caffeine itself may have antioxidant activity providing a beneficial effect (Lee 2000).

Lecithin, a mixture of phospholipids from plant sources, may have a role to play in liver disease, but to date, the human studies have not demonstrated clear benefits. Lecithin has been demonstrated to prevent alcoholic liver cirrhosis in baboons (Lieber et al. 1994) and appears to have anti-inflammatory, antiapoptotic, and antifibrotic effects (Cao et al. 2002; Okiyama et al. 2009). However, a Veterans Affairs Cooperative Study evaluating lecithin in humans with early alcoholic liver disease (Lieber et al. 2003b) failed to show definitive benefits. It has been proposed that the results were compromised by patients decreasing their alcohol use markedly during the trial.

Milk thistle (*Silybum marianum*) is a popular dietary supplement for patients wishing to maintain liver health. The active ingredient on which studies have been performed is silymarin, and supplements recommended should be standardized for silymarin content. In animal models, hepatoprotective effects of milk thistle in several forms of liver injury (toxic hepatitis, fatty liver, cirrhosis, ischemic injury, radiation toxicity, and viral hepatitis) have been shown. Mechanisms including anti-inflammatory, antioxidative, antifibrotic, and immunomodulating effects are thought to explain the benefit of silymarin in liver disease (Lieber et al. 2003a). A randomized, double-blind control evaluating placebo versus silymarin in alcohol- and non-alcohol-induced cirrhosis showed a 39% versus 58% 4-year survival, respectively (Ferenci et al. 1989). However, similar trials have failed to show outcome benefit (Parés et al. 1998; Lucena et al. 2002). Meta-analyses have failed to demonstrate a benefit for silymarin, but as is often the case in meta-analyses, the trials analyzed had numerous flaws, making any interpretation difficult (Rambaldi and Gluud 2006).

In hepatitis and cirrhosis, abnormal hepatic gene expression of methyl donor metabolism, specifically in methionine and glutathione metabolism, occurs and often contributes to decreased hepatic S-adenosylmethionine (SAM), cysteine, and glutathione levels (Lee et al. 2004). Rodent and primate studies demonstrate that SAM depletion occurs in the early stages of fatty liver infiltration, and decreased SAM concentration, liver injury, and mitochondrial damage can be reversed with SAM supplementation (Lieber 2002). SAM appears to attenuate oxidative stress and hepatic stellate cell activation in an ethanol-LPS-induced fibrotic rat model (Karaa et al. 2008). Clinical trial evidence is lacking.

Betaine (trimethylglycine) is a key nutrient for humans that is similar in function to choline and can be obtained from a variety of foods and nutritional supplements (Purohit et al. 2007). In the liver, betaine can transfer one methyl group to homocysteine to form methionine. This process removes toxic metabolites (homocysteine and S-adenosylhomocysteine), restores SAM levels, reverses steatosis, prevents apoptosis, and reduces both damaged protein accumulation and oxidative stress (Kharbanda et al. 2007; Kharbanda 2009). Betaine also appears to attenuate alcoholic steatosis by restoring phosphatidylcholine generation via the phosphatidylethanolamine methyltransferase pathway (Kharbanda et al. 2007). Studies suggest that betaine offers hepatic protection against ethanol-induced oxidative stress by decreasing sulfur-containing amino acid breakdown as well (Kim et al. 2008). Betaine supplementation is promising, but there are further clinical studies needed.

8.9.3 Management of Protein Malnutrition in Advanced Liver Disease

It has long been established that patients with liver disease can be malnourished, with the degree of malnutrition correlating with disease severity (Prijatmoko et al. 1993; Halsted 2004). In addition, complications of liver disease (e.g., infections, encephalopathy, ascites, and variceal bleeding) have been shown to be strongly associated with protein–calorie malnutrition (PCM) (Nielsen et al. 1993; Prijatmoko et al. 1993). Micronutrient deficiencies of folate, vitamin B6, vitamin A, and thiamin are among the most commonly encountered. Mineral and element (e.g., selenium, zinc, copper, and magnesium) levels are often altered in alcoholic liver disease and, in some instances, are thought to be involved in its pathogenesis (Halsted 2004). In particular, zinc is decreased in patients with liver disease. In animal models, zinc supplementation has been shown to improve, attenuate, and/or prevent alcoholic liver disease through a variety of mechanisms (Kang and Zhou 2005).

Patients with liver disease can have varying nutritional status, from morbid obesity to profound underweight and malnutrition. Given the high-caloric content of alcohol (7.1 kilocalories/g), patients with both alcoholic liver disease and fatty liver due to obesity can expect to have more rapid progression of underlying liver damage, such as that associated with alcoholic liver disease (Nielsen et al. 1993; Raynard et al. 2002). Given similar mechanisms of pathogenesis, including oxidative stress and inflammation, patients with the metabolic syndrome or insulin resistance and concomitant alcoholic liver disease or viral liver disease would be expected to have more severe disease with a quicker progression to fibrosis (Griffith and Schenker 2006).

At the other end of the nutritional spectrum, several mechanisms are hypothesized to contribute to advanced liver disease-associated malnutrition. Decreased caloric intake (secondary to anorexia and reduced intake of nonalcohol calories), decreased intestinal absorption and digestion of nutrients (secondary to altered gut integrity, pancreatic insufficiency, decreased bile excretion, and a decrease in intestinal enzymes), and decreased processing and storage of nutrients (secondary to decreased functional liver mass, abnormal oxidation of fat, and preferential metabolism of alcohol) are all thought to be involved in the malnutrition associated with alcoholic liver disease (Griffith and Schenker 2006). Increased catabolism of skeletal muscle and visceral proteins leading to a hypermetabolic state in alcoholic hepatitis is also a key component in the development of PCM in alcoholic liver disease (John et al. 1989).

With so many mechanisms at play, the diagnosis and treatment of malnutrition in patients with liver disease is sometimes difficult. The laboratory tests most commonly used to assess nutritional status (e.g., anthropometry and serum albumin concentration) are often affected by concomitant liver disease. In order to obtain valid data on the prevalence and degree of malnutrition among alcoholics with alcoholic liver disease, reliable and sensitive methods to assess nutritional status are required. Easily applicable techniques include anthropometric measurements, such as BMI, triceps skinfold thickness, and midarm muscle area. Other approaches include bioelectric impedance analysis for assessing body composition, and the determination of resting energy expenditure by indirect calorimetry. Each technique has limitations and may give erroneous results in patients with alcohol-related cirrhosis. For metabolic studies, direct measurements are needed. In a recent study, different methods for the assessment of body composition in patients with liver cirrhosis were compared (Prijatmoko et al. 1993). All applied techniques, including bioelectric impedance analysis, total body nitrogen content, dual x-ray absorptiometry, and four-site skin-fold measurements, could detect advanced protein malnutrition, but differed significantly in patients with high volumes of extracellular fluid, such as ascites and peripheral edema. Although these mistakes may be avoided with more precise approaches, such as *in vivo* neutron activation analysis and isotope dilution techniques (Nielsen et al. 1993), application of these methods is time-consuming and restricted to the research setting. Patients with severe forms of liver disease should simply be considered malnourished and treated as such.

Nutritional support for these patients depends on the severity of liver disease, concomitant factors leading to malnutrition (e.g., anorexia and pancreatic insufficiency), and the presence of obesity.

Obese patients with less severe liver injury should be referred to a dietician and advised concerning dietary restriction and regular exercise. In outpatient therapy for patients with liver disease, nutritional support in patients with cirrhosis improves nutritional status and cell-mediated immunity, as well as decreases infectious complications and consequent hospitalizations (Hirsch et al. 1993, 1999). Another study of patients with cirrhosis demonstrated that a late-evening nutritional supplement over a 12-month period improved body protein stores (Plank et al. 2008). While more study is warranted, our general practice is to encourage bedtime nutritional supplements in outpatients with severe liver disease or cirrhosis.

The Veterans Administration Cooperative Studies Program (Mendenhall et al. 1984, 1985, 1986, 1993, 1995; Prijatmoko et al. 1993) included more than 600 patients hospitalized with alcoholic liver cirrhosis. PCM was present in nearly all patients. The degree of malnutrition correlated with the development of serious complications, such as encephalopathy, ascites, and hepatorenal syndrome. Moreover, nutritional support improved nutritional and metabolic parameters, severity of liver injury, and most importantly, mortality in patients with moderate malnutrition and alcoholic liver disease. A major multicenter study demonstrated that enteral nutrition, when compared with corticosteroids, has similar short-term mortality rates, improved 1-year mortality rates, and reduced infectious complications (Cabré et al. 2000). An additional study demonstrated the benefit of tube-fed nutrition (improved clinical status, bilirubin, and markers of liver function based on drug clearance) compared with a regular diet (Kearns et al. 1992). Parenteral nutrition for patients with liver disease is rarely indicated but appears to improve liver function and nitrogen balance. However, it fails to convey a survival benefit over standard therapy (Simon and Galambos 1988; Cabré et al. 2000).

The American College of Gastroenterology (ACG) and the American Association for the Study of Liver Diseases (AASLD) guidelines recommend 1.2–1.5 g/kg of protein and 35–40 kilocalories/kg of body weight/day in patients with advanced liver disease (McCullough and O'Connor 1998). The available clinical trials vary considerably regarding the composition of the nutritional support utilized (Griffith and Schenker 2006). In patients with advanced cirrhosis, supplementation with oral branched-chain amino acids (BCAA) was compared to lactalbumin or maltodextrin. BCAA supplementation by comparison to lactalbumin or maltodextrin led to improved perceived health status, improved biomarkers, and reduced hospital stays (Marchesini et al. 2003). Another study demonstrated that long-term BCAA supplementation is associated with decreased frequency of hepatic failure and overall complication frequency (Charlton 2006). Other studies have not been as clear in establishing a benefit (Calvey et al. 1985).

While some studies have failed to demonstrate a clear survival benefit for all patients with severe liver disease receiving enteral nutrition (Cabré et al. 2000; Griffith and Schenker 2006), the implementation of aggressive nutritional support in these patients is generally performed since at a minimum, nutritional support will improve metabolic status.

8.10 CONCLUSION

The majority of patients with NAFLD are overweight and obese, lead relatively sedentary lifestyles, and have underlying insulin resistance. Treatment aimed at improving body weight and activity should be the basis of approaches to combating this disease. Evidence suggests that diets low in processed carbohydrates and saturated fats with a goal to achieve a 500–1000 calorie/day deficit improve insulin sensitivity, reduce serum aminotransferases, and decrease hepatic steatosis. Improvements are seen with as little as a 5% reduction in body weight. Weight loss through total caloric restriction results in improved parameters of insulin sensitivity and regression of hepatic steatosis (Petersen et al. 2005). Data regarding the utility of specific dietary regimens may be debated, but it appears that diets consisting of a reduction in processed carbohydrates and saturated fats to effect a caloric deficit of 500–1000 calories/day may be beneficial and can be recommended in overweight or obese patients with NAFLD (Paredes et al. 2012). Histopathologic parameters of steatohepatitis also appear to improve with weight loss. Antioxidant supplementation, specifically with vitamin E, may be considered as adjunctive therapy. Larger confirmatory studies are needed to ensure they are safe and beneficial in patients with NASH. For patients failing to achieve weight loss goals, future approaches are likely to consist of combination therapy targeting insulin resistance, oxidative stress, and fibrogenesis.

REFERENCES

Ackerman, Z., M. Oron-Herman, M. Grozovski, T. Rosenthal, O. Pappo, G. Link, and B.-A. Sela. 2005. Fructose-induced fatty liver disease hepatic effects of blood pressure and plasma triglyceride reduction. *Hypertension* 45 (5):1012–1018.

Alisi, A., M. Manco, M. Pezzullo, and V. Nobili. 2011. Fructose at the center of necroinflammation and fibrosis in nonalcoholic steatohepatitis. *Hepatology* 53 (1):372–373.

Anania, F. A. 2011. Non-alcoholic fatty liver disease and fructose: Bad for us, better for mice. *J Hepatol* 55 (1):218–220.

Anstee, Q. M., G. Targher, and C. P. Day. 2013. Progression of NAFLD to diabetes mellitus, cardiovascular disease or cirrhosis. *Nat Rev Gastroenterol Hepatol* 10 (6):330–344.

Armstrong, M. A. 1992. Alcohol, smoking, coffee, and cirrhosis. *Am J Epidemiol* 136 (10):1248–1257.

Ballestri, S., S. Zona, G. Targher, D. Romagnoli, E. Baldelli, F. Nascimbeni, A. Roverato, G. Guaraldi, and A. Lonardo. 2016. Nonalcoholic fatty liver disease is associated with an almost twofold increased risk of incident type 2 diabetes and metabolic syndrome. Evidence from a systematic review and meta-analysis. *J Gastroenterol Hepatol* 31 (5):936–944.

Bhatia, L. S., N. P. Curzen, P. C. Calder, and C. D. Byrne. 2012. Non-alcoholic fatty liver disease: A new and important cardiovascular risk factor? *Eur Heart J* 33 (10):1190–1200.

Borena, W., S. Strohmaier, A. Lukanova, T. Bjorge, B. Lindkvist, G. Hallmans, M. Edlinger et al. 2012. Metabolic risk factors and primary liver cancer in a prospective study of 578,700 adults. *Int J Cancer* 131 (1):193–200.

Bosch, F. X., J. Ribes, R. Cléries, and M. Díaz. 2005. Epidemiology of hepatocellular carcinoma. *Clin Liver Dis* 9 (2):191–211.

Bugianesi, E. 2007. Non-alcoholic steatohepatitis and cancer. *Clin Liver Dis* 11 (1):191–207.

Bugianesi, E., N. Leone, E. Vanni, G. Marchesini, F. Brunello, P. Carucci, A. Musso, P. De Paolis, L. Capussotti, M. Salizzoni, and M. Rizzetto. 2002. Expanding the natural history of nonalcoholic steatohepatitis: From cryptogenic cirrhosis to hepatocellular carcinoma. *Gastroenterology* 123 (1):134–140.

Cabré, E., P. Rodríguez-Iglesias, J. Caballería, J. C. Quer, J. L. Sánchez-Lombraña, A. Parés, M. Papo, R. Planas, and M. A. Gassull. 2000. Short- and long-term outcome of severe alcohol-induced hepatitis treated with steroids or enteral nutrition: A multicenter randomized trial. *Hepatology* 32 (1):36–42.

Caldwell, S. H., D. H. Oelsner, J. C. Iezzoni, E. E. Hespenheide, E. H. Battle, and C. J. Driscoll. 1999. Cryptogenic cirrhosis: Clinical characterization and risk factors for underlying disease. *Hepatology* 29 (3):664–669.

Calle, E. E., and R. Kaaks. 2004. Overweight, obesity and cancer: Epidemiological evidence and proposed mechanisms. *Nat Rev Cancer* 4 (8):579–591.

Calle, E. E., C. Rodriguez, K. Walker-Thurmond, and M. J. Thun. 2003. Overweight, obesity, and mortality from cancer in a prospectively studied cohort of U.S. adults. *N Engl J Med* 348 (17):1625–1638.

Calvey, H., M. Davis, and R. Williams. 1985. Controlled trial of nutritional supplementation, with and without branched chain amino acid enrichment, in treatment of acute alcoholic hepatitis. *J Hepatol* 1 (2):141–151.

Cao, Q., K. M. Mak, and C. S. Lieber. 2002. Dilinoleoylphosphatidylcholine prevents transforming growth factor-β1-mediated collagen accumulation in cultured rat hepatic stellate cells. *J Lab Clin Med* 139 (4):202–210.

Castro, G. S. F., J. F. R. Cardoso, H. Vannucchi, S. Zucoloto, and A. A. Jordão. 2011. Fructose and NAFLD: Metabolic implications and models of induction in rats. *Acta Cir Bras* 26:45–50.

Charlton, M. 2006. Branched-chain amino acid enriched supplements as therapy for liver disease. *J Nutr* 136 (1):295S–298S.

Corrao, G., A. R. Lepore, P. Torchio, M. Valenti, G. Galatola, A. D'amicis, S. Arico, F. Di Orio, and Provincial Group for the Study of Chronic Liver Disease. 1994. The effect of drinking coffee and smoking cigarettes on the risk of cirrhosis associated with alcohol consumption. *Eur J Epidemiol* 10 (6):657–664.

D'Angelo, G., A. A. Elmarakby, D. M. Pollock, and D. W. Stepp. 2005. Fructose feeding increases insulin resistance but not blood pressure in Sprague-Dawley rats. *Hypertension* 46 (4):806–811.

El-Serag, H. B. 2011. Hepatocellular carcinoma. *N Engl J Med* 365 (12):1118–1127.

Fabbrini, E., S. Sullivan, and S. Klein. 2010. Obesity and nonalcoholic fatty liver disease: Biochemical, metabolic, and clinical implications. *Hepatology* 51 (2):679–689.

Farazi, P. A., and R. A. DePinho. 2006. Hepatocellular carcinoma pathogenesis: From genes to environment. *Nat Rev Cancer* 6 (9):674–687.

Ferenci, P., B. Dragosics, H. Dittrich, H. Frank, L. Benda, H. Lochs, S. Meryn, W. Base, and B. Schneider. 1989. Randomized controlled trial of silymarin treatment in patients with cirrhosis of the liver. *J Hepatol* 9 (1):105–113.

Gallagher, E. J., D. LeRoith, and E. Karnieli. 2010. Insulin resistance in obesity as the underlying cause for the metabolic syndrome. *Mt Sinai J Med* 77 (5):511–523.

Gallagher, E. J., D. LeRoith, and E. Karnieli. 2011. The metabolic syndrome—From insulin resistance to obesity and diabetes. *Med Clin North Am* 95 (5):855–873.

Griffith, C. M., and S. Schenker. 2006. The role of nutritional therapy in alcoholic liver disease. *Alcohol Res Health* 29 (4):296.

Halsted, C. H. 2004. Nutrition and alcoholic liver disease. *Semin Liver Dis* 24 (3):289–304.

Hazlehurst, J. M., C. Woods, T. Marjot, J. F. Cobbold, and J. W. Tomlinson. 2016. Non-alcoholic fatty liver disease and diabetes. *Metabolism* 65 (8):1096–1108.

Hirsch, S., D. Bunout, P. De La Maza, H. Iturriaga, M. Petermann, G. Icazar, V. Gattas, and G. Ugarte. 1993. Controlled trial on nutrition supplementation in outpatients with symptomatic alcoholic cirrhosis. *JPEN J Parenter Enteral Nutr* 17 (2):119–124.

Hirsch, S., M. P. de la Maza, V. Gattás, G. Barrera, M. Petermann, M. Gotteland, C. Muñoz, M. Lopez, and D. Bunout. 1999. Nutritional support in alcoholic cirrhotic patients improves host defenses. *J Am Coll Nutr* 18 (5):434–441.

Huang, D., T. Dhawan, S. Young, W. H. Yong, L. G. Boros, and A. P. Heaney. 2011. Fructose impairs glucose-induced hepatic triglyceride synthesis. *Lipids Health Dis* 10 (1):1.

Huber, W. W., G. Scharf, W. Rossmanith, S. Prustomersky, B. Grasl-Kraupp, B. Peter, R. J. Turesky, and R. Schulte-Hermann. 2002. The coffee components kahweol and cafestol induce γ-glutamylcysteine synthetase, the rate limiting enzyme of chemoprotective glutathione synthesis, in several organs of the rat. *Arch Toxicol* 75 (11–12):685–694.

IARC (International Agency for Research on Cancer). 2012. GLOBOCAN 2012: Estimated cancer incidence, mortality and prevalence worldwide in 2012. http://globocan.iarc.fr/Pages/fact_sheets_population.aspx.

Jemal, A., F. Bray, M. M. Center, J. Ferlay, E. Ward, and D. Forman. 2011. Global cancer statistics. *CA Cancer J Clin* 61 (2):69–90.

John, W. J., R. Phillips, L. Ott, L. J. Adams, and C. J. McClain. 1989. Resting energy expenditure in patients with alcoholic hepatitis. *JPEN J Parenter Enteral Nutr* 13 (2):124–127.

Kang, Y. J., and Z. Zhou. 2005. Zinc prevention and treatment of alcoholic liver disease. *Mol Aspects Med* 26 (4):391–404.

Karaa, A., K. J. Thompson, I. H. McKillop, M. G. Clemens, and L. W. Schrum. 2008. S-adenosyl-L-methionine attenuates oxidative stress and hepatic stellate cell activation in an ethanol-LPS-induced fibrotic rat model. *Shock* 30 (2):197–205.

Karagozian, R., Z. Derdak, and G. Baffy. 2014. Obesity-associated mechanisms of hepatocarcinogenesis. *Metabolism* 63 (5):607–617.

Kearns, P. J., H. Young, G. Garcia, T. Blaschke, G. O'Hanlon, M. Rinki, K. Sucher, and P. Gregory. 1992. Accelerated improvement of alcoholic liver disease with enteral nutrition. *Gastroenterology* 102 (1):200–205.

Kharbanda, K. K. 2009. Alcoholic liver disease and methionine metabolism. *Semin Liver Dis* 29 (2):155–165.

Kharbanda, K. K., M. E. Mailliard, C. R. Baldwin, H. C. Beckenhauer, M. F. Sorrell, and D. J. Tuma. 2007. Betaine attenuates alcoholic steatosis by restoring phosphatidylcholine generation via the phosphatidylethanolamine methyltransferase pathway. *J Hepatol* 46 (2):314–321.

Kim, S. J., Y. S. Jung, D. Y. Kwon, and Y. C. Kim. 2008. Alleviation of acute ethanol-induced liver injury and impaired metabolomics of S-containing substances by betaine supplementation. *Biochem Biophys Res Commun* 368 (4):893–898.

Kochanek, K. D., J. Xu, S. L. Murphy, A. M. Miniño, and H.-C. Kung. 2011. National vital statistics reports. *Natl Vital Stat Rep* 59 (4):1.

Koo, H.-Y., M. A. Wallig, B. H. Chung, T. Y. Nara, B. H. S. Cho, and M. T. Nakamura. 2008. Dietary fructose induces a wide range of genes with distinct shift in carbohydrate and lipid metabolism in fed and fasted rat liver. *Biochim Biophys Acta* 1782 (5):341–348.

Kotronen, A., J. Westerbacka, R. Bergholm, K. H. Pietilainen, and H. Yki-Jarvinen. 2007. Liver fat in the metabolic syndrome. *J Clin Endocrinol Metab* 92 (9):3490–3497.

Lê, K.-A., and L. Tappy. 2006. Metabolic effects of fructose. *Curr Opin Clin Nutr Metab Care* 9 (4):469–475.

Lee, C. 2000. Antioxidant ability of caffeine and its metabolites based on the study of oxygen radical absorbing capacity and inhibition of LDL peroxidation. *Clin Chim Acta* 295 (1):141–154.

Lee, T. D., M. R. Sadda, M. H. Mendler, T. Bottiglieri, G. Kanel, J. M. Mato, and S. C. Lu. 2004. Abnormal hepatic methionine and glutathione metabolism in patients with alcoholic hepatitis. *Alcohol Clin Exp Res* 28 (1):173–181.

Lieber, C. S. 2002. S-Adenosyl-L-methionine and alcoholic liver disease in animal models: Implications for early intervention in human beings. *Alcohol* 27 (3):173–177.

Lieber, C. S., M. A. Leo, Q. Cao, C. Ren, and L. M. DeCarli. 2003a. Silymarin retards the progression of alcohol-induced hepatic fibrosis in baboons. *J Clin Gastroenterol* 37 (4):336–339.

Lieber, C. S., S. J. Robins, J. Li, L. M. DeCarli, K. M. Mak, J. M. Fasulo, and M. A. Leo. 1994. Phosphatidylcholine protects against fibrosis and cirrhosis in the baboon. *Gastroenterology* 106:152.

Lieber, C. S., D. G. Weiss, R. Groszmann, F. Paronetto, and S. Schenker. 2003b. II. Veterans Affairs Cooperative Study of polyenylphosphatidylcholine in alcoholic liver disease. *Alcohol Clin Exp Res* 27 (11):1765–1772.

Lim, J. S., M. Mietus-Snyder, A. Valente, J.-M. Schwarz, and R. H. Lustig. 2010. The role of fructose in the pathogenesis of NAFLD and the metabolic syndrome. *Nat Rev Gastroenterol Hepatol* 7 (5):251–264.

Liu, H., and H. Y. Lu. 2014. Nonalcoholic fatty liver disease and cardiovascular disease. *World J Gastroenterol* 20 (26):8407–8415.

Lonardo, A., S. Ballestri, G. Marchesini, P. Angulo, and P. Loria. 2015a. Nonalcoholic fatty liver disease: A precursor of the metabolic syndrome. *Dig Liver Dis* 47 (3):181–190.

Lonardo, A., S. Ballestri, G. Targher, and P. Loria. 2015b. Diagnosis and management of cardiovascular risk in nonalcoholic fatty liver disease. *Expert Rev Gastroenterol Hepatol* 9 (5):629–650.

Lucena, M. I., R. J. Andrade, J. P. De la Cruz, M. Rodriguez-Mendizabal, E. Blanco, and F. Sánchez de la Cuesta. 2002. Effects of silymarin MZ-80 on oxidative stress in patients with alcoholic cirrhosis. Results of a randomized, double-blind, placebo-controlled clinical study. *Int J Clin Pharmacol Ther* 40 (1):2–8.

Lustig, R. H. 2010. Fructose: Metabolic, hedonic, and societal parallels with ethanol. *J Am Diet Assoc* 110 (9):1307–1321.

Machado, M. V., and H. Cortez-Pinto. 2014. Non-alcoholic fatty liver disease: What the clinician needs to know. *World J Gastroenterol* 20 (36):12956–12980.

Marchesini, G., G. Bianchi, M. Merli, P. Amodio, C. Panella, C. Loguercio, F. R. Fanelli, R. Abbiati, and Italian BCAA Study Group. 2003. Nutritional supplementation with branched-chain amino acids in advanced cirrhosis: A double-blind, randomized trial. *Gastroenterology* 124 (7):1792–1801.

Margini, C., and J. F. Dufour. 2016. The story of HCC in NAFLD: From epidemiology, across pathogenesis, to prevention and treatment. *Liver Int* 36 (3):317–324.

Marrero, J. A., R. J. Fontana, G. L. Su, H. S. Conjeevaram, D. M. Emick, and A. S. Lok. 2002. NAFLD may be a common underlying liver disease in patients with hepatocellular carcinoma in the United States. *Hepatology* 36 (6):1349–1354.

McCullough, A. J. 2011. Epidemiology of the metabolic syndrome in the USA. *J Dig Dis* 12 (5):333–340.

McCullough, A. J., and J. F. B. O'Connor. 1998. Alcoholic liver disease: Proposed recommendations for the American College of Gastroenterology. *Am J Gastroenterol* 93 (11):2022–2036.

Mendenhall, C. L., S. Anderson, R. E. Weesner, S. J. Goldberg, and K. A. Crolic. 1984. Protein-calorie malnutrition associated with alcoholic hepatitis: Veterans Administration Cooperative Study Group on Alcoholic Hepatitis. *Am J Med* 76 (2):211–222.

Mendenhall, C. L., G. Bongiovanni, S. J. Goldberg, B. Miller, J. Moore, S. Rouster, D. Schneider, C. Tamburro, T. Tosch, and R. E. Weesner. 1985. VA Cooperative Study on Alcoholic Hepatitis III: Changes in protein-calorie malnutrition associated with 30 days of hospitalization with and without enteral nutritional therapy. *JPEN J Parenter Enteral Nutr* 9 (5):590–596.

Mendenhall, C. L., T. E. Moritz, G. A. Roselle, T. R. Morgan, B. A. Nemchausky, C. H. Tamburro, E. R. Schiff, C. J. McClain, L. S. Marsano, and J. I. Allen. 1993. A study of oral nutritional support with oxandrolone in malnourished patients with alcoholic hepatitis: Results of a Department of Veterans Affairs Cooperative Study. *Hepatology* 17 (4):564–576.

Mendenhall, C. L., T. E. Moritz, G. A. Roselle, T. R. Morgan, B. A. Nemchausky, C. H. Tamburro, E. R. Schiff, C. J. McClain, L. S. Marsano, and J. I. Allen. 1995. Protein energy malnutrition in severe alcoholic hepatitis: Diagnosis and response to treatment. *JPEN J Parenter Enteral Nutr* 19 (4):258–265.

Mendenhall, C. L., T. Tosch, R. E. Weesner, P. Garcia-Pont, S. J. Goldberg, T. Kiernan, L. B. Seeff, M. Sorell, C. Tamburro, and R. Zetterman. 1986. VA Cooperative Study on Alcoholic Hepatitis. II. Prognostic significance of protein-calorie malnutrition. *Am J Clin Nutr* 43 (2):213–218.

Michelotti, G. A., M. V. Machado, and A. M. Diehl. 2013. NAFLD, NASH and liver cancer. *Nat Rev Gastroenterol Hepatol* 10 (11):656–665.

Moore, J. B. 2010. Non-alcoholic fatty liver disease: The hepatic consequence of obesity and the metabolic syndrome. *Proc Nutr Soc* 69 (2):211–220.

Naveau, S., V. Giraud, E. Borotto, A. Aubert, F. Capron, and J. Chaput. 1997. Excess weight risk factor for alcoholic liver disease. *Hepatology* 25 (1):108–111.

Nielsen, K., J. Kondrup, L. Martinsen, B. Stilling, and B. Wikman. 1993. Nutritional assessment and adequacy of dietary intake in hospitalized patients with alcoholic liver cirrhosis. *Br J Nutr* 69 (3):665–679.

Nomura, K., and T. Yamanouchi. 2012. The role of fructose-enriched diets in mechanisms of nonalcoholic fatty liver disease. *J Nutr Biochem* 23 (3):203–208.

Nseir, W., F. Nassar, and N. Assy. 2010. Soft drinks consumption and nonalcoholic fatty liver. *World J Gastroenterol* 16 (21):2579–2588.

Oh, S. W., Y. S. Yoon, and S. A. Shin. 2005. Effects of excess weight on cancer incidences depending on cancer sites and histologic findings among men: Korea National Health Insurance Corporation Study. *J Clin Oncol* 23 (21):4742–4754.

Okiyama, W., N. Tanaka, T. Nakajima, E. Tanaka, K. Kiyosawa, F. J. Gonzalez, and T. Aoyama. 2009. Polyenephosphatidylcholine prevents alcoholic liver disease in PPARα-null mice through attenuation of increases in oxidative stress. *J Hepatol* 50 (6):1236–1246.

Orholm, M., T. I. Sorensen, K. Bentsen, G. Hoybye, K. Eghoje, and P. Christoffersen. 1985. Mortality of alcohol abusing men prospectively assessed in relation to history of abuse and degree of liver injury. *Liver* 5 (5):253–260.

Paredes, A. H., D. M. Torres, and S. A. Harrison. 2012. Nonalcoholic fatty liver disease. *Clin Liver Dis* 16 (2):397–419.

Parés, A., R. Planas, M. Torres, J. Caballería, J. M. Viver, D. Acero, J. Panés, J. Rigau, J. Santos, and J. Rodés. 1998. Effects of silymarin in alcoholic patients with cirrhosis of the liver: Results of a controlled, double-blind, randomized and multicenter trial. *J Hepatol* 28 (4):615–621.

Park, J. H., B. Cho, H. Kwon, D. Prilutsky, J. M. Yun, H. C. Choi, K. B. Hwang, I. H. Lee, J. I. Kim, and S. W. Kong. 2015. I148M variant in PNPLA3 reduces central adiposity and metabolic disease risks while increasing nonalcoholic fatty liver disease. *Liver Int* 35 (12):2537–2546.

Petaja, E. M., and H. Yki-Jarvinen. 2016. Definitions of normal liver fat and the association of insulin sensitivity with acquired and genetic NAFLD—A systematic review. *Int J Mol Sci* 17 (5):633.

Petersen, K. F., S. Dufour, D. Befroy, M. Lehrke, R. E. Hendler, and G. I. Shulman. 2005. Reversal of nonalcoholic hepatic steatosis, hepatic insulin resistance, and hyperglycemia by moderate weight reduction in patients with type 2 diabetes. *Diabetes* 54 (3):603–608.

Plank, L. D., E. J. Gane, S. Peng, C. Muthu, S. Mathur, L. Gillanders, K. McIlroy, A. J. Donaghy, and J. L. McCall. 2008. Nocturnal nutritional supplementation improves total body protein status of patients with liver cirrhosis: A randomized 12-month trial. *Hepatology* 48 (2):557–566.

Poonawala, A., S. P. Nair, and P. J. Thuluvath. 2000. Prevalence of obesity and diabetes in patients with cryptogenic cirrhosis: A case-control study. *Hepatology* 32 (4 Pt 1):689–692.

Powell, E. E., W. G. Cooksley, R. Hanson, J. Searle, J. W. Halliday, and L. W. Powell. 1990. The natural history of nonalcoholic steatohepatitis: A follow-up study of forty-two patients for up to 21 years. *Hepatology* 11 (1):74–80.

Prijatmoko, D. W. I., B. J. Strauss, J. R. Lambert, W. Sievert, D. B. Stroud, M. L. Wahlqvist, B. Katz, J. Colman, P. Jones, and M. G. Korman. 1993. Early detection of protein depletion in alcoholic cirrhosis: Role of body composition analysis. *Gastroenterology* 105 (6):1839–1845.

Purohit, V., M. F. Abdelmalek, S. Barve, N. J. Benevenga, C. H. Halsted, N. Kaplowitz, K. K. Kharbanda, Q.-Y. Liu, S. C. Lu, and C. J. McClain. 2007. Role of S-adenosylmethionine, folate, and betaine in the treatment of alcoholic liver disease: Summary of a symposium. *Am J Clin Nutr* 86 (1):14–24.

Rambaldi, A., and C. Gluud. 2006. S-Adenosyl-L-methionine for alcoholic liver diseases. *Cochrane Database Syst Rev* 2:CD002235.

Ratziu, V., L. Bonyhay, V. Di Martino, F. Charlotte, L. Cavallaro, M. H. Sayegh-Tainturier, P. Giral, A. Grimaldi, P. Opolon, and T. Poynard. 2002. Survival, liver failure, and hepatocellular carcinoma in obesity-related cryptogenic cirrhosis. *Hepatology* 35 (6):1485–1493.

Raynard, B., A. Balian, D. Fallik, F. Capron, P. Bedossa, J.-C. Chaput, and S. Naveau. 2002. Risk factors of fibrosis in alcohol-induced liver disease. *Hepatology* 35 (3):635–638.

Rinella, M. E. 2015. Nonalcoholic fatty liver disease: A systematic review. *JAMA* 313 (22):2263–2273.

Samanic, C., W. H. Chow, G. Gridley, B. Jarvholm, and J. F. Fraumeni Jr. 2006. Relation of body mass index to cancer risk in 362,552 Swedish men. *Cancer Causes Control* 17 (7):901–909.

Sanyal, A. J., N. Chalasani, K. V. Kowdley, A. McCullough, A. M. Diehl, N. M. Bass, B. A. Neuschwander-Tetri, J. E. Lavine, J. Tonascia, and A. Unalp. 2010. Pioglitazone, vitamin E, or placebo for nonalcoholic steatohepatitis. *N Engl J Med* 362 (18):1675–1685.

Scharf, G., S. Prustomersky, and W. W. Huber. 2001. Elevation of glutathione levels by coffee components and its potential mechanisms. In *Biological Reactive Intermediates VI*, ed. P. M. Dansette, R. Snyder, M. Delaforge, G. G. Gibson, H. Greim, D. J. Jollow, T. J. Monks, and I. G. Sipes, 535–539. Vol. 500. Berlin: Springer.

Schlesinger, S., K. Aleksandrova, T. Pischon, V. Fedirko, M. Jenab, E. Trepo, P. Boffetta et al. 2013. Abdominal obesity, weight gain during adulthood and risk of liver and biliary tract cancer in a European cohort. *Int J Cancer* 132 (3):645–657.

Shen, J., G. L. Wong, H. L. Chan, H. Y. Chan, D. K. Yeung, R. S. Chan, A. M. Chim et al. 2014. PNPLA3 gene polymorphism accounts for fatty liver in community subjects without metabolic syndrome. *Aliment Pharmacol Ther* 39 (5):532–539.

Siegel, A. B., and A. X. Zhu. 2009. Metabolic syndrome and hepatocellular carcinoma: Two growing epidemics with a potential link. *Cancer* 115 (24):5651–5661.

Simon, D., and J. T. Galambos. 1988. A randomized controlled study of peripheral parenteral nutrition in moderate and severe alcoholic hepatitis. *J Hepatol* 7 (2):200–207.

Skelly, M. M., P. D. James, and S. D. Ryder. 2001. Findings on liver biopsy to investigate abnormal liver function tests in the absence of diagnostic serology. *J Hepatol* 35 (2):195–199.

Sofair, A. N., V. Barry, M. M. Manos, A. Thomas, A. Zaman, N. A. Terrault, R. C. Murphy et al. 2010. The epidemiology and clinical characteristics of patients with newly diagnosed alcohol-related liver disease: Results from population-based surveillance. *J Clin Gastroenterol* 44 (4):301–307.

Speliotes, E. K., J. L. Butler, C. D. Palmer, B. F. Voight, GIANT Consortium, MIGen Consortium, NASH CRN, and J. N. Hirschhorn. 2010. PNPLA3 variants specifically confer increased risk for histologic nonalcoholic fatty liver disease but not metabolic disease. *Hepatology* 52 (3):904–912.

Stanhope, K. L., and P. J. Havel. 2010. Fructose consumption: Recent results and their potential implications. *Ann NY Acad Sci* 1190 (1):15–24.

Stefan, N., K. Kantartzis, and H. U. Haring. 2008. Causes and metabolic consequences of fatty liver. *Endocr Rev* 29 (7):939–960.

Tappy, L., K. A. Lê, C. Tran, and N. Paquot. 2010. Fructose and metabolic diseases: New findings, new questions. *Nutrition* 26 (11):1044–1049.

Targher, G., C. P. Day, and E. Bonora. 2010. Risk of cardiovascular disease in patients with nonalcoholic fatty liver disease. *N Engl J Med* 363 (14):1341–1350.

Teff, K. L., S. S. Elliott, M. Tschöp, T. J. Kieffer, D. Rader, M. Heiman, R. R. Townsend, N. L. Keim, D. D'Alessio, and P. J. Havel. 2004. Dietary fructose reduces circulating insulin and leptin, attenuates postprandial suppression of ghrelin, and increases triglycerides in women. *J Clin Endocrinol Metab* 89 (6):2963–2972.

Thorgeirsson, S. S., and J. W. Grisham. 2002. Molecular pathogenesis of human hepatocellular carcinoma. *Nat Genet* 31 (4):339–346.

Tsukuma, H., T. Hiyama, S. Tanaka, M. Nakao, T. Yabuuchi, T. Kitamura, K. Nakanishi, I. Fujimoto, A. Inoue, and H. Yamazaki. 1993. Risk factors for hepatocellular carcinoma among patients with chronic liver disease. *N Engl J Med* 328 (25):1797–1801.

Turati, F., R. Talamini, C. Pelucchi, J. Polesel, S. Franceschi, A. Crispo, F. Izzo, C. La Vecchia, P. Boffetta, and M. Montella. 2013. Metabolic syndrome and hepatocellular carcinoma risk. *Br J Cancer* 108 (1):222–228.

Velazquez, R. F., M. Rodriguez, C. A. Navascues, A. Linares, R. Perez, N. G. Sotorrios, I. Martinez, and L. Rodrigo. 2003. Prospective analysis of risk factors for hepatocellular carcinoma in patients with liver cirrhosis. *Hepatology* 37 (3):520–527.

Vernon, G., A. Baranova, and Z. M. Younossi. 2011. Systematic review: The epidemiology and natural history of non-alcoholic fatty liver disease and non-alcoholic steatohepatitis in adults. *Aliment Pharmacol Ther* 34 (3):274–285.

White, D. L., F. Kanwal, and H. B. El-Serag. 2012. Association between nonalcoholic fatty liver disease and risk for hepatocellular cancer, based on systematic review. *Clin Gastroenterol Hepatol* 10 (12):1342–1359.e2.

Yki-Jarvinen, H. 2014. Non-alcoholic fatty liver disease as a cause and a consequence of metabolic syndrome. *Lancet Diabetes Endocrinol* 2 (11):901–910.

Zhu, F.-S., S. Liu, X.-M. Chen, Z.-G. Huang, and D.-W. Zhang. 2008. Effects of n-3 polyunsaturated fatty acids from seal oils on nonalcoholic fatty liver disease associated with hyperlipidemia. *World J Gastroenterol* 14 (41):6395–6400.

9 Lipid Disorders and Management

9.1 INTRODUCTION

This chapter examines and discusses the issues around lipid disorders and primary care management, integrating nutrition and lifestyle intervention, which is not the traditional educational paradigm. Education on lipid metabolism in primary care has traditionally centered on the pharmacological treatment of elevated blood cholesterol levels in order to prevent atherosclerosis and cardiovascular (CV) events and mortality (Berliner et al. 1995; Levine et al. 1995).

In the 1980s, statins were being strongly credited as a singular way to prevent heart disease.

When cholesterol-lowering drugs were first marketed, it was already evident that the etiology of atherosclerosis was a complex of factors at the cellular level involving oxidation, inflammation, and genetics (Berliner et al. 1995). Beyond simply cholesterol, the differing dietary responsiveness of lipid levels among individuals with different lipid disorders is stressed in this chapter, along with the role of nutrition in these processes. While official guidelines always mentioned that dietary intervention should be the first step in treating lipid disorders, this was always followed by the statement that if diet failed, as was frequently expected, one should use pharmacological treatment.

The most common dyslipidemias have elevations of both triglycerides and cholesterol and respond to weight reduction and the inclusion of nutrients that lower blood cholesterol levels. Patients with isolated hypercholesterolemia (Fredrickson type IIa) have minimal responses to dietary changes. However, these unrepresentative patients with isolated hypercholesterolemia were studied in some of the most widely read publications, incidentally supported by the drug industry. To balance the emphasis in primary care education, the effects of dietary changes on lipids need to be emphasized, along with the importance of a healthy diet and lifestyle for overall health. Therefore, this chapter concentrates on nutritional effects in more common lipid disorders, with a brief review of current drug therapies and clinical guidelines on pharmacotherapy in lipid management.

Familial hypercholesterolemia (FH) of the most common type, which includes both elevated triglycerides and cholesterol, demonstrated greater effects of statin in lowering cholesterol levels when statins were used together with low-fat diets than when they were used with high-fat diets under metabolic ward conditions (Cobb et al. 1991).

The observations on the interactions of diet and lipid-lowering therapy have not made it into the consciousness of many primary care practitioners. As a result, some patients believe that they can eat whatever they want as long as they are taking cholesterol-lowering drugs, without fear of developing heart disease.

While there has been a somewhat consistent but evolving message on cholesterol-lowering pharmacotherapy and heart disease, which is reviewed later in this chapter, changes over the past few decades in dietary advice to the public have been filled with controversies, such as the one on the effects of saturated fats and dietary cholesterol on blood lipid levels and the general cacophony of controversies on the importance of nutrition altogether in lipid management. These controversies have led many primary care health care providers to simply give lip service to nutrition while relying on drug therapy to manage lipid disorders. Starting from basic physiology and metabolism and describing the most common lipid disorders, this chapter redirects your attention to the important role of nutrition.

9.2 LIPOPROTEINS AND LIPID METABOLISM

Lipoproteins consist of both lipids and protein, as the term implies. Since lipids are not soluble in the aqueous phase of the circulation, lipoproteins, with a polar surface and lipophilic core, enable the movement of lipids around the circulation for delivery to cells for synthesis of various hormones and other lipid metabolites. In addition, lipoproteins have proteins embedded in their outer core that signal the identity of the particular lipoprotein to enzymes that mediate their metabolism.

Lipoproteins are classified based on their behavior in sucrose gradient centrifugation so that they are characterized as high density if they deposit lower in the gradient (e.g., high-density lipoproteins [HDLs]) or low density (e.g., low-density lipoproteins [LDLs] and very low-density lipoproteins [VLDLs]), which float at higher levels. In addition, LDLs exist in small, dense and large, fluffy fractions with different atherogenic potentials.

This chapter is a discussion of lipid disorders and management. While disorders of cholesterol metabolism and transport are important, the numerous implications of maintaining lipid levels beyond just cholesterol in a healthy range are also important. For example, triglycerides and HDL cholesterol (HDL-C) can serve as important biomarkers of metabolic syndrome, insulin resistance, and prediabetes, among other disorders. Small, dense LDLs are associated with visceral obesity and hypertriglyceridemia. Moreover, it is important to understand the important role of nutrition and how recommendations such at the step I and step II diets by the American Heart Association (AHA) have evolved over the last decade to incorporate modern nutritional concepts.

9.3 DISORDERS OF CHOLESTEROL METABOLISM AND TRANSPORT

Cholesterol is carried into vessel walls by several types of lipoproteins to different extents, including VLDL (Knopp et al. 1994), remnant lipoprotein (Coresh and Kwiterovich 1996), LDL, and the small, dense form of LDL found in association with abdominal obesity (Coresh and Kwiterovich 1996). Conversely, cholesterol is carried away from the arterial wall by HDL (Fielding and Fielding 1995; Oram and Yokoyama 1996).

In healthy persons, these lipoproteins function to distribute and recycle cholesterol, triglycerides, and other lipid-soluble substances, including phytonutrients (Knopp 1989). Cholesterol is absorbed from the intestine and transported to the liver by chylomicron remnants, which are

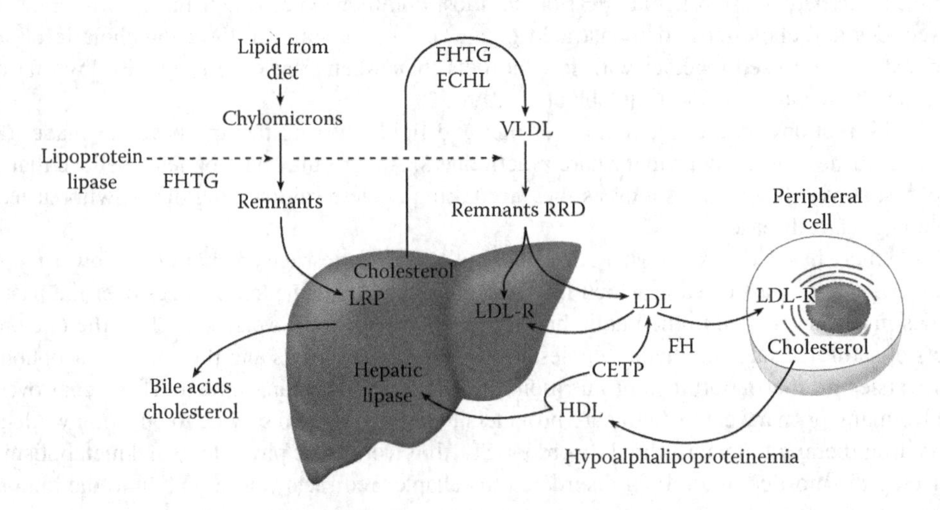

FIGURE 9.1 **(See color insert.)** Pathways of lipid transport. (Reprinted from Knopp, R. H., *N. Engl. J. Med.*, 341(7), 498–511, 1999.)

taken up by the LDL receptor-related protein (LRP). Hepatic cholesterol enters the circulation as VLDL and is metabolized to remnant lipoproteins after lipoprotein lipase removes triglyceride. The remnant lipoproteins are removed by LDL receptors (LDL-Rs) or further metabolized to LDL and then removed by these receptors. Cholesterol is transported from peripheral cells to the liver by HDL. Cholesterol is recycled to LDL and VLDL by the cholesterol-ester transport protein (CETP) or is taken up in the liver by hepatic lipase. Cholesterol is then excreted in bile.

The points in the processes of cholesterol transport in Figure 9.1 can be affected by five primary lipoprotein disorders, including (1) familial hypertriglyceridemia (FHTG), (2) familial combined hyperlipidemia (FCHL), (3) remnant removal disease (RRD) (also known as familial dysbetalipoproteinemia), (4) FH, and (5) hypoalphalipoproteinemia.

9.4 DIFFERENTIATING COMMON AND RARE LIPID DISORDERS

9.4.1 Familial Hypertriglyceridemia and Secondary Hypertriglyceridemia

Hypertriglyceridemia is one of the most commonly encountered lipid abnormalities. Elevations of fasting triglycerides above 150 mg/dL are found in a significant percentage of populations diagnosed with the metabolic syndrome and are extremely common. On the other hand, only 1.7% of a sample of 5680 subjects participating in the National Health and Nutrition Examination Survey from 2001 and 2006 had severe hypertriglyceridemia, defined as levels between 500 and 2000 mg/dL. These individuals were more likely to be men (75.3%), non-Hispanic whites (70.1%), and ages 40–59 years (58.5%). More than 14% of those with severe hypertriglyceridemia reported having diabetes mellitus, and 31.3% reported having hypertension. Only 14% of the subjects reported using statins, and 4.0% reported using fibrates. The factors significantly associated with having severe hypertriglyceridemia included HDL of <40 mg/dL, non-HDL of 160–189 mg/dL, diabetes mellitus, and chronic renal disease (Christian et al. 2011).

Evidence of fasting hypertriglyceridemia should prompt an investigation for secondary causes, such as high-fat diet, uncontrolled carbohydrate intake, excessive alcohol intake, certain medications, and medical conditions, such as type 2 diabetes mellitus and hypothyroidism. Patients should also be evaluated for other components of the metabolic syndrome, including abdominal obesity, fasting hyperglycemia, reduced HDL levels, and hypertension.

Hypertriglyceridemias are classified as primary FHTG when there are no secondary causes found. The two most common familial dyslipidemias are Fredrickson type IIb (FCHL) and type IV (FHTG). Together, these two dyslipidemias account for 85% of familial dyslipidemias. Primary hypertriglyceridemia is the result of various genetic defects leading to disordered triglyceride metabolism. It is important to treat severe hypertriglyceridemia in order to prevent pancreatitis by reducing triglyceride levels to <500 mg/dL. Severe hypertriglyceridemia accounts for 1–4% of cases of acute pancreatitis. Although a few patients can develop pancreatitis with triglyceride levels of >500 mg/dL, the risk for pancreatitis does not become clinically significant until levels are >1000 mg/dL (Athyros et al. 2002; DiMagno and Chari 2002).

Lifestyle changes are the first line of treatment for most patients with hypertriglyceridemia. These changes include a weight management plan incorporating a low-saturated-fat, carbohydrate-controlled diet, combined with alcohol reduction, smoking cessation, and regular aerobic and resistance exercise. High doses of omega-3 fatty acids on the order of 2–4 g/day from fish and fish oil supplements will lower triglyceride levels significantly. When patients do not reach their goals by lifestyle and nutritional interventions, then drug therapy should be started. In cases of isolated hypertriglyceridemia, fibrates are indicated. In patients with low HDL levels and hypertriglyceridemia, extended-release niacin can be considered.

While cholesterol has been the focus of preventive cardiology for decades, there is an increased interest in triglycerides for two reasons. First, hypertriglyceridemia is the most common lipid disorder, as it is associated with dyslipidemias and insulin resistance, both of which are components of the metabolic syndrome. Second, despite aggressive statin therapy, residual risk remains a problem for patients with this disorder, especially those with mixed hyperlipidemia (Christian et al. 2011). They have increased triglyceride-rich lipoproteins and small, dense LDL particles that easily penetrate the endothelium of coronary arteries and arterioles throughout the body.

Although triglyceride is not directly found in atheromas, high triglyceride levels are found in excess atherogenic remnants, such as VLDL and small, dense LDL. Insulin resistance can contribute to hypertriglyceridemia by increasing free fatty acid delivery to the liver, which can either increase lipoprotein production or promote hepatic lipogenesis. Triglycerides are the most sensitive index of the metabolic syndrome (Li et al. 2013).

Despite triglyceride levels being cardiovascular disease (CVD) risk predictors based on epidemiologic studies, clinical studies have thus far not examined the direct effects of triglyceride lowering. A triglyceride-to-HDL ratio of >3.5 is a good predictor of insulin resistance and can thus be used as a target for treatment with diet and lifestyle or drug therapy. A triglyceride level of <150 mg/dL is considered an achievable target; if the level is below 150 mg/dL, further reductions can raise HDL. In addition to dietary changes and drugs, increased exercise by increasing the insulin sensitivity and fatty acid oxidation capacity of muscle can further reduce triglyceride levels.

Combination therapy aimed at lowering triglyceride levels can be used, along with aggressive statin therapy in individuals at high risk of CVD (Davidson 2007). Potential combinations include niacin and fibrates. The addition of omega-3 fatty acid supplements to simvastatin (40 mg) further lowers non-HDL-C, triglycerides, and VLDL (Harris 2007). Omega-3 fatty acids work as well as fenofibric acid and do not have some of the potentially negative effects of fenofibrate, such as increased creatinine and homocysteine levels. Omega-3 fatty acids reduce triglyceride levels by inhibiting hepatic lipogenesis and increasing hepatic fatty acid oxidation, while also increasing peroxisome proliferator-activated receptor (PPAR) α.

Tissue triglyceride stores are a balance among uptake, oxidation, and storage. Although the release of stored triglyceride from adipocytes was thought to depend on the actions of hormone-sensitive lipase (HSL), creation of HSL knockout mice failed to show this and led to the discovery

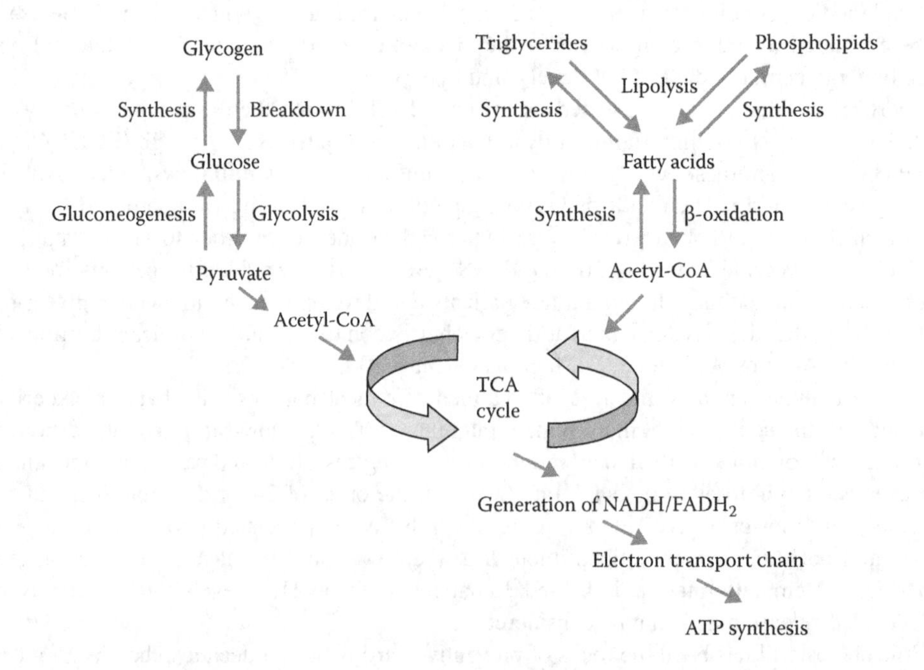

FIGURE 9.2 Mobilization of stored triglycerides is initiated by lipolytic enzymes. Liberated fatty acids are then activated to their respective acetyl-CoA metabolites. Breakdown of fatty acyl-CoA to acetyl-CoA occurs in peroxisomes or mitochondria via β-oxidation enzymes. TCA, tricarboxylic acid.

of a new enzyme, adipose triglyceride lipase (ATGL). Genetic deletion of ATGL in mice leads to a marked increase in triglyceride storage in tissues (Zechner 2007). Intricate metabolic networks tightly coordinate the flow of sugars and triglycerides through synthesis, storage, and breakdown pathways (Figure 9.2).

9.4.2 Hypercholesterolemia and Familial Hypercholesterolemia

FH is due to genetic mutations in either the *LDLR* gene that encodes the LRP, which normally removes LDL from the circulation, or apolipoprotein B (apoB), which is the part of LDL that binds with the receptor. Mutations in other genes are rare. People who have one abnormal copy of the *LDLR* gene may develop CVD prematurely at the age of 30–40. Having two abnormal copies may cause severe CVD in childhood. Heterozygous FH is a common genetic disorder, inherited in an autosomal dominant pattern, occurring in 1 in 500 people in most countries. Homozygous FH is much rarer, occurring in 1 in 1 million births (Rader et al. 2003).

Heterozygous FH is normally treated with statins that lower cholesterol levels. New cases are generally offered genetic counseling. Homozygous FH often does not respond to medical therapy and may require other treatments, including LDL apheresis (removal of LDL in a method similar to dialysis) and occasionally liver transplantation (Rader et al. 2003).

Hypercholesterolemia is typically due to a combination of environmental and genetic factors (Rader et al. 2003). Environmental factors include obesity, diet, and stress. A number of secondary causes of hypercholesterolemia include diabetes mellitus type 2, obesity, alcohol, monoclonal gammopathy, dialysis, nephrotic syndrome, hypothyroidism, Cushing's syndrome, anorexia nervosa, and medications (thiazide diuretics, ciclosporin, glucocorticoids, β-blockers, and retinoic acid) (Bhatnagar et al. 2008).

9.5 HYPERTRIGLYCERIDEMIA AND THE UNRECOGNIZED IMPACT OF VISCERAL FAT

As already discussed, a large body of evidence supports the reduction of LDL cholesterol (LDL-C) as the primary objective of dyslipidemia management, and the administration of statins is considered the most effective regimen for achieving this. Consequently, statins have become the treatment of choice in the majority of patients, including those with type 2 diabetes mellitus, with the overwhelming majority of these patients having concomitant excess internal body fat or obvious obesity (Graham et al. 2007).

The Cholesterol Treatment Trialists' (CTT) meta-analysis of 27 large statin trials, with almost 175,000 participants with five categories of CVD risk, demonstrated that statin treatment is beneficial in all categories (Mihaylova et al. 2012). However, it is also clear that many patients remain at high risk despite reaching recommended LDL-C targets using statins. The "residual risk" identified with these observations is due to hypertriglyceridemia and reduced levels of HDL-C (Fruchart et al. 2008). It is likely that HDL-C is an integrated biomarker of several metabolic processes, including insulin resistance and inflammation. HDL-C has multiple targets, and both the amount of HDL-C and functions of HDL lipoprotein are associated with CVD risk in a complex fashion (Voight et al. 2012). Hypertriglyceridemia is also associated with an increased CVD risk, but the association is weakened by adjustment for other risk factors, including HDL-C, so that some studies find no association with CVD risk (Emerging Risk Factors Collaboration et al. 2009). The poor understanding among physicians and patients of the importance of hypertriglyceridemia in association with low HDL-C as a risk factor is one of the reasons for inadequate treatment of residual CVD risk (Reiner et al. 2010a,b). Another major reason is that this lipid pattern is associated with the metabolic syndrome, obesity, and type 2 diabetes, all these requiring a combined diet and lifestyle change program, as well as pharmacotherapy.

Fibrates are the most efficient drugs for treating hypertriglyceridemia, in addition to diet and lifestyle (Rubins et al. 1999; Bezafibrate Infarction Prevention Study 2000; Keech et al. 2005). Gemfibrozil monotherapy has been shown to decrease rates of CVD events in subjects with elevated non-HDL-C or low HDL-C (Rubins et al. 1999; Fruchart et al. 2008), including men with type 2 diabetes (Rubins et al. 2002; Voight et al. 2012). However, gemfibrozil is not recommended for addition to a statin (Oram and Yokoyama 1996; Zechner 2007; European Association for Cardiovascular Prevention & Rehabilitation et al. 2011; Perk et al. 2012) because of its association with an elevated risk of myopathy and/or rhabdomyolysis. The randomized Action to Control Cardiovascular Risk in Diabetes (ACCORD) lipid study investigated whether fenofibrate reduced the risk of CVD when added to simvastatin in patients with type 2 diabetes mellitus (ACCORD Study Group et al. 2010). The primary outcome, the annual rate of first occurrence of nonfatal MI, nonfatal stroke, or CVD mortality, was not significantly different between treatments. Heterogeneity in the patient population was thought to contribute to the lack of a statistically significant result, while subgroup analysis suggested a benefit in patients who at baseline had elevated triglycerides and low HDL-C. Data from ACCORD were included in a meta-analysis of five trials, which was published as a letter (Sacks et al. 2010). These data suggest that fibrates reduced the risk of CVD events by 35% in subjects with low HDL-C and high triglycerides, but not in those without this dyslipidemia.

9.6 CONTROL OF LDL CHOLESTEROL FOR PREVENTION OF ATHEROSCLEROTIC CARDIOVASCULAR DISEASES

In 1985, the National Heart, Lung, and Blood Institute of the National Institutes of Health created the National Cholesterol Education Program (NCEP) in order to educate the medical profession and the general public on the need to identify and treat high blood cholesterol in reducing coronary heart disease (CHD) risk (Warnick et al. 2002). Most experts agree that there is clear evidence of benefit, but the natural history of atherosclerosis goes beyond cholesterol in millions of individuals. Therefore, the clinical guidelines have evolved under the guidance of the Adult Treatment Panel (ATP), a panel of experts from major medical and health professional associations, voluntary health organizations, community programs, and governmental agencies. The ATP was formed to develop guidelines for the detection, evaluation, and treatment of high blood cholesterol in adults.

The ATP guidelines remain the most accepted reference guideline for clinical management of high blood cholesterol. With continual clinical advances in the science of cholesterol management, these guidelines have been updated several times. The first ATP guideline (ATP-I) published in 1988, outlined a strategy for the primary prevention of CHD in individuals with high LDL-C (>160 mg/dL) or borderline-high LDL-C (130–159 mg/dL) and more than two risk factors (Report of the National Cholesterol Education Program 1988; Expert Panel on Detection, Evaluation, and Treatment of High Blood Cholesterol in Adults 2001). In 1993, ATP-II, the second ATP guideline, supported the approach of ATP-I and added a new feature of intensive management of LDL-C in patients with established CHD (secondary prevention) and fixed a new, lower LDL-C goal of <100 mg/dL in CHD patients (Anon 1993; Ansell et al. 1999). In 2001, the third ATP guideline, ATP-III (Report of the National Cholesterol Education Program 1988; Expert Panel on Detection, Evaluation, and Treatment of High Blood Cholesterol in Adults 2001; National Cholesterol Education Program Expert Panel on Detection, Evaluation, and Treatment of High Blood Cholesterol in Adults 2002), updated the recommendations for clinical management of high blood cholesterol and related abnormalities. The key features of ATP-III included consideration of LDL-C of <100 mg/dL as an optimal level and the introduction of the Framingham risk score (10-year CHD risk) to calculate treatment intensity. It also, for the first time, introduced a diet and lifestyle program called "therapeutic lifestyle modification," or TLC. Also for the first time, secondary targets in ATP-III included non-HDL-C in patients with a triglyceride value of ≥200 mg/dL and metabolic syndrome.

Since ATP-III, five major clinical trials involving statins have been completed. In 2004, a further updated ATP-III based on the results of these five clinical trials was published (Grundy et al. 2004;

Stone et al. 2005). These trials addressed important issues that were not included in ATP-III. For patients at extremely high risk, a new LDL-C goal of <70 mg/dL was added.

This gradual evolution of NCEP guidelines in the form of ATP guidelines (ATP-I through ATP-III) has had a significant impact on cholesterol management (Conti 2002). The 2013 American College of Cardiology/American Heart Association (ACC/AHA) Guideline on the Treatment of Blood Cholesterol to Reduce Atherosclerotic Cardiovascular Risk in Adults: A Report of the ACC/AHA Task Force on Practice Guidelines in November 2013 (Warnick et al. 2002). The final document now serves as the most current U.S. guidelines for management of blood cholesterol for CVD risk reduction (Gibbons et al. 2013).

For primary prevention, the recommended risk assessment tool in the ACC/AHA guidelines is the new CV risk calculator based on the pooled cohort equations, as described in the 2013 ACC/AHA Guideline on the Assessment of Cardiovascular Risk (Goff et al. 2014). The equations are derived from large, diverse, community-based cohorts that are generally representative of the U.S. population of whites and African Americans (Dawber et al. 1963; Kannel et al. 1979; Friedman et al. 1988; Atherosclerosis Risk in Communities 1989; Fried et al. 1991). The calculator provides race- and sex-specific estimates of the 10-year risk of first hard atherosclerotic cardiovascular disease (ASCVD) event (nonfatal myocardial infarction, CHD death, and fatal or nonfatal stroke) and should be used in non-Hispanic African Americans and non-Hispanic whites between 40 and 79 years of age.

Lifetime or 30-year risk is also provided for individuals age 20–59 years who are not at high short-term risk. Recommended optional variables and/or screening tests that may be considered to refine risk assessment include family history of premature ASCVD; high-sensitivity C-reactive protein (hsCRP) of >2 mg/L; coronary artery calcium score of >300 Agatston units, or >75th percentile for age, sex, and ethnicity; and ankle brachial index. Based on expert opinion, the presence of any of these screening abnormalities supports revising the patient's risk assessment to a higher level of risk.

In addition to a new risk calculator for CVD risk assessment, the ACC/AHA guidelines also recommend a novel strategy for the management of LDL-related risk. Guidelines from multiple organizations have previously focused on the fasting lipid panel as the initial evaluation of lipid-related CVD risk. Within each category of ASCVD risk, targets of treatment are then specified in these recommendations.

Upon systematic review of the evidence, authors of the new ACC/AHA guidelines determined that current clinical trial data did not support this approach. Also, the data are inadequate to indicate specific lipoprotein goals of therapy. Therefore, the panel made no recommendation for or against specific targets (LDL-C or non-HDL-C) for primary or secondary ASCVD prevention. Instead, these experts identified four groups of patients in which there is the most extensive evidence of the benefit of statin therapy for the prevention of ASCVD:

1. Individuals with clinical ASCVD
2. Individuals with primary elevations of LDL-C of >190 mg/dL
3. Individuals 40–75 years of age with diabetes and LDL-C of 70–189 mg/dL
4. Individuals without clinical ASCVD or diabetes who are 40–75 years of age with LDL-C of 70–189 mg/dL and an estimated 10-year ASCVD risk of >7.5% by the pooled risk equations

For each risk group, the guidelines recommend an intensity of statin therapy, either moderate or high intensity. Low-intensity statins are recommended only in patients who have experienced or are at risk for adverse effects of treatment. The guidelines do not support dose titration to achieve optimal levels of LDL-C, non-HDL-C, or apoB, as recommended in previous guidelines. Also, in a significant departure from previous guidelines, the 2013 ACC/AHA guidelines recommend measurement of on-therapy LDL-C only as an assessment of adherence and response to therapy.

Application of the new risk assessment tool in the National Health and Nutrition Examination Surveys of 2005 and 2010 resulted in a substantial increase in adults eligible for statin therapy (12.8 million), particularly in older adults (Pencina et al. 2014). In a European cohort, investigators determined that application of the new CV risk calculator would recommend that all men and 65% of women older than age 55 years would be candidates for treatment with a statin (Kavousi et al. 2014). In the study populations of the Multi-Ethnic Study of Atherosclerosis, the Women's Health Study, the Physicians' Health Study, and the Women's Health Initiative Observational Study, authors compared the observed and predicted event rates by the CV risk calculator, finding that the new algorithm overestimated observed risks by approximately 75–150% (Ridker and Cook 2013). However, in the Reasons for Geographic and Racial Differences in Stroke study, the observed and predicted 5-year ASCVD risks were similar when patients with diabetes, LDL-C of <40 or >189 mg/dL, and current statin therapy were excluded, and in Medicare participants (Muntner et al. 2014). Certainly, validation of the CV risk calculator in other data sets will address these concerns and determine its applicability in persons at varying levels of ASCVD risk and in more ethnically diverse populations. Finally, the risk calculator also provides 30-year or lifetime risk for patients who are age 20–59 years, but the guidelines provide limited specific information on treatment recommendations for individuals with high lifetime risk.

It is no surprise that a revolutionary change from decades of emphasis on LDL-C goals of therapy in dyslipidemia would generate considerable controversy and confusion among health care providers, the media, and patients. It is important to note that although there are significant changes in the new 2013 ACC/AHA guidelines, there are recommendations that are consistent with those of the NCEP ATP-III, ATP-III update panels, and other organizations. LDL remains the lipoprotein of interest, as recommended in the previous guidelines of the ATP-III and current recommendations of the International Atherosclerosis Society (IAS), American Association of Clinical Endocrinologists (AACE), Kidney Disease: Improving Global Outcomes (KDIGO), and others not reviewed here. Very high-risk patients with manifest ASCVD or FH and/or LDL-C of >190 mg/dL continue to be candidates for high-intensity statin therapy. Also, in patients with FH, combination therapy with high-intensity statins and cholesterol absorption inhibitors, bile acid sequestrants, LDL apheresis, or newer therapies is considered for additional reduction of LDL-C levels, even in the absence of a specific LDL-C target. As in previous guidelines, the new ACC/AHA recommendations consider diabetic patients as a high-risk group; however, the intensity of therapy is now based on the 10-year estimate of risk of a hard ASCVD event by the pooled risk equations.

Overall, adherence to all doses of statin therapy in at-risk patients is poor in both primary prevention and high-risk populations (Anon 1997; Jackevicius et al. 2008; Kumbhani et al. 2013). As the new ACC/AHA guidelines recommend initiation of only high- and moderate-intensity statins in high-risk patients, there is concern for even further reductions in compliance with prescribed statin or appropriate statin intensity. Although a newly validated risk assessment algorithm is recommended by the ACC/AHA in primary prevention patients and diabetics without ASCVD, the intensity of statin therapy is still closely related to the intensity of risk, as recommended by other guidelines.

In summary, all these guidelines now recognize the heterogeneity of the populations with elevated cholesterol and are working around the edges of what is clearly a multifactorial disease in which statins are not the total solution. Personalized nutrition therapy, in conjunction with pharmacotherapy as needed, with an emphasis on compliance, should do much to rationalize the overuse of statins, as recommended in the most recent guidelines.

9.7 IMPACT OF NUTRITION ON LIPID DISORDERS

Diet has an effect on blood cholesterol, but the size of this effect varies substantially between individuals. Reductions in the dietary intake of cholesterol lead to increased production of the cholesterol principally by the liver. As the cholesterol pool is reduced through binding and excretion, the rate of cholesterol synthesis increases in the liver so that net reductions in blood levels of cholesterol are modest (Howell et al. 1997). As recognized in the latest U.S. dietary guidelines, eating high-cholesterol foods is not prohibited in cholesterol-lowering diets, including shellfish, which were on the avoidance list of the American Heart Association for decades. Foods rich in saturated fats and calories are also rich in omega-6 fatty acids, so lean meats should be recommended for occasional intake, while ocean-caught fish, plant proteins, and low-fat poultry, such as chicken breast and turkey breast meats, are consistent with a nutritional plan intended to help manage lipid levels.

A number of dietary interventions have been developed with an emphasis on lipid management. Meta-analyses and randomized controlled trials published in English and including data on the effect on blood lipid levels were reviewed to establish an evidence-based recommendation on these diets (Huang et al. 2011). Randomized controlled trials were included if they were at least 4 weeks in duration and had a minimum of 50 participants. A total of 22 different dietary interventions and 136 studies published between January 1990 and December 2009 were reviewed that met specific inclusion criteria. In this broad-based approach, the Pritikin, Ornish, Mediterranean, and portfolio diets, discussed below, were found to have beneficial effects on lipids.

Special dietary patterns beyond the low-fat diets of Nathan Pritikin (Barnard et al. 1982; Pritikin 1984) and Dean Ornish (Ornish et al. 1990) have been recommended to reduce cholesterol levels and prevent heart disease. In fact, both the Ornish and Pritikin diets were approved by Medicare to be included in cardiac rehabilitation programs (Anon 2010). The original composition of these very low-fat diets included only about 15% of calories from fat and 15% of calories from low-fat protein from plant and animal sources. As a result, the balance of calories often came from refined carbohydrates, which at calorie balance led to increased triglycerides in about half of patients treated.

The Atkins high-fat diet, originally a weight loss diet as a result of severely restricted refined carbohydrates, has been shown to help control triglycerides, especially in patients with diabetes or prediabetes (Dr. Atkins' 1973). However, the initial benefits on weight loss and lipids by comparison with a low-fat diet seen over 6 months disappear at 1 year. Compliance with the recommended high-fat proteins is especially difficult for women, and men tend to introduce carbohydrates after a few months on this strict diet (Foster et al. 2003). The Mediterranean diet emphasized using omega-9 fat from olives and avocados, together with a diet based on Italian and Greek cuisine (de Lorgeril 2013), with no particular emphasis on calorie restriction. The portfolio, developed by Dr. David Jenkins in Canada, emphasized monounsaturated fats from nuts and seeds (Ramprasath et al. 2014).

In addition to the above dietary patterns, a number of individual foods and nutrient have been used for lipid management. Soy protein substituted for animal protein led to a reduction in cholesterol levels and an approved health claim in the United States for soy protein when used with a low-fat diet (Anderson and Bush 2011). Soluble fibers, such as guar and pectin, have been shown to lower cholesterol modestly (Gunness and Gidley 2010). Plants do not synthesize cholesterol, but they do make phytosterols, which are structurally similar to cholesterol (Malina et al. 2015). As a result, phytosterols are able compete for uptake in the ileum with cholesterol, resulting in a modest drop in cholesterol levels (Malina et al. 2015). β-Glucan, found in oatmeal and whole grain foods, can also lower cholesterol (Ho et al. 2016). While omega-3 fatty acid supplementation primarily lowers triglyceride levels, it also finds its way into general recommendations for lipid management.

Chinese red yeast rice is derived from a yeast called *Monascus purpureus*, which was fermented on white rice in traditional Chinese medicine. The yeast synthesizes a family of polyketide antibiotics called monacolins. One of these, monacolin K, is structurally identical to lovastatin, sold as Mevacor by Merck and approved by the Food and Drug Administration (FDA) in 1987 for the control of cholesterol The Dietary Supplement Health and Education Act (DSHEA) was approved in 1994 and had within it a paragraph stating that any substance previously approved as a drug could not be considered a dietary supplement. It was originally marketed in the United States following a clinical study at the University of California, Los Angeles (UCLA) showing that 6 mg of monacolin K within a 1200 mg capsule containing rice and yeast led to a 20% reduction in cholesterol levels over 12 weeks, comparable to the effects of 20 mg of lovastatin (Heber et al. 1999). It was proposed that the other monacolins and bioactive substances in the red yeast rice contributed to the cholesterol-lowering activity. The clearance by the liver of Chinese red yeast rice is greater than the clearance of lovastatin, likely due to the multiple compounds activating liver clearance mechanisms (Heber et al. 1999). In any case, the FDA sued the manufacturer and based on the DSHEA law, Chinese red yeast rice was declared an unapproved drug from China. It is legal in most other countries, and in 2010, it was the subject of a positive opinion by the European Food Safety Authority.

Suffice it to say that used in the way that drugs are used without regard to diet, none of the above supplements will provide adequate lipid control. The basis of all efforts to control lipids must be to exercise regularly and eat a diet low in fat, high in fiber, and using low-fat plant and animal protein. Beyond those guidelines, patients should be given discretion to choose supplements that are safely manufactured and shown to be effective in clinical studies.

REFERENCES

ACCORD Study Group, H. N. Ginsberg, M. B. Elam, L. C. Lovato, J. R. Crouse 3rd, L. A. Leiter, P. Linz et al. 2010. Effects of combination lipid therapy in type 2 diabetes mellitus. *N Engl J Med* 362 (17):1563–1574.

Anderson, J. W., and H. M. Bush. 2011. Soy protein effects on serum lipoproteins: A quality assessment and meta-analysis of randomized, controlled studies. *J Am Coll Nutr* 30 (2):79–91.

Anon. 1993. Summary of the second report of the National Cholesterol Education Program (NCEP) Expert Panel on Detection, Evaluation, and Treatment of High Blood Cholesterol in Adults (Adult Treatment Panel II). *JAMA* 269 (23):3015–3023.

Anon. 1997. Compliance and adverse event withdrawal: Their impact on the West of Scotland Coronary Prevention *Study. Eur Heart J* 18 (11):1718–1724.

Anon. 2010. Ornish, Pritikin get Medicare okay for cardiac rehab. *Harv Heart Lett* 21 (4):7.

Ansell, B. J., K. E. Watson, and A. M. Fogelman. 1999. An evidence-based assessment of the NCEP Adult Treatment Panel II guidelines. National Cholesterol Education Program. *JAMA* 282 (21):2051–2057.

The Atherosclerosis Risk in Communities (ARIC) Study: Design and objectives. The ARIC investigators. 1989. *Am J Epidemiol* 129 (4):687–702.

Athyros, V. G., O. I. Giouleme, N. L. Nikolaidis, T. V. Vasiliadis, V. I. Bouloukos, A. G. Kontopoulos, and N. P. Eugenidis. 2002. Long-term follow-up of patients with acute hypertriglyceridemia-induced pancreatitis. *J Clin Gastroenterol* 34 (4):472–475.

Barnard, R. J., L. Lattimore, R. G. Holly, S. Cherny, and N. Pritikin. 1982. Response of non-insulin-dependent diabetic patients to an intensive program of diet and exercise. *Diabetes Care* 5 (4):370–374.

Berliner, J. A., M. Navab, A. M. Fogelman, J. S. Frank, L. L. Demer, P. A. Edwards, A. D. Watson, and A. J. Lusis. 1995. Atherosclerosis: Basic mechanisms. Oxidation, inflammation, and genetics. *Circulation* 91 (9):2488–2496.

Bezafibrate Infarction Prevention Study. 2000. Secondary prevention by raising HDL cholesterol and reducing triglycerides in patients with coronary artery disease. *Circulation* 102 (1):21–27.

Bhatnagar, D., H. Soran, and P. N. Durrington. 2008. Hypercholesterolaemia and its management. *BMJ* 337:a993.

Christian, J. B., N. Bourgeois, R. Snipes, and K. A. Lowe. 2011. Prevalence of severe (500 to 2,000 mg/dl) hypertriglyceridemia in United States adults. *Am J Cardiol* 107 (6):891–897.

Cobb, M. M., H. S. Teitelbaum, and J. L. Breslow. 1991. Lovastatin efficacy in reducing low-density lipoprotein cholesterol levels on high- vs low-fat diets. *JAMA* 265 (8):997–1001.

Conti, C. R. 2002. Evolution of NCEP guidelines: ATP1-ATPIII risk estimation for coronary heart disease in 2002. National Cholesterol Education Program. *Clin Cardiol* 25 (3):89–90.

Coresh, J., and P. O. Kwiterovich Jr. 1996. Small, dense low-density lipoprotein particles and coronary heart disease risk: A clear association with uncertain implications. *JAMA* 276 (11):914–915.

Davidson, M. H. 2007. Weighing the evidence for adding a second drug to statin in the patient with mixed hyperlipidemia. Program and abstracts of the XVI International Symposium on Drugs Affecting Lipid Metabolism, New York.

Dawber, T. R., W. B. Kannel, and L. P. Lyell. 1963. An approach to longitudinal studies in a community: The Framingham Study. *Ann NY Acad Sci* 107:539–556.

de Lorgeril, M. 2013. Mediterranean diet and cardiovascular disease: Historical perspective and latest evidence. *Curr Atheroscler Rep* 15 (12):370.

DiMagno, E. P., and S. Chari. 2002. Acute pancreatitis. In *Sleisenger & Fordtran's Gastrointestinal and Liver Disease*, ed. L. S. Friedman, M. Feldman, and L. H. Sleisenger, 913–942. St. Louis, MO: W.B. Saunders.
Dr. Atkins' diet revolution. 1973. *Med Lett Drugs Ther* 15 (10):41–42.
Emerging Risk Factors Collaboration, E. Di Angelantonio, N. Sarwar, P. Perry, S. Kaptoge, K. K. Ray, A. Thompson et al. 2009. Major lipids, apolipoproteins, and risk of vascular disease. *JAMA* 302 (18):1993–2000.
European Association for Cardiovascular Prevention & Rehabilitation, Z. Reiner, A. L. Catapano, G. De Backer, I. Graham, M. R. Taskinen, O. Wiklund et al. 2011. ESC/EAS guidelines for the management of dyslipidaemias: The Task Force for the Management of Dyslipidaemias of the European Society of Cardiology (ESC) and the European Atherosclerosis Society (EAS). *Eur Heart J* 32 (14):1769–1818.
Expert Panel on Detection, Evaluation, and Treatment of High Blood Cholesterol in Adults. 2001. Executive summary of the third report of the National Cholesterol Education Program (NCEP) Expert Panel on Detection, Evaluation, and Treatment of High Blood Cholesterol in Adults (Adult Treatment Panel III). *JAMA* 285 (19):2486–2497.
Fielding, C. J., and P. E. Fielding. 1995. Molecular physiology of reverse cholesterol transport. *J Lipid Res* 36 (2):211–228.
Foster, G. D., H. R. Wyatt, J. O. Hill, B. G. McGuckin, C. Brill, B. S. Mohammed, P. O. Szapary, D. J. Rader, J. S. Edman, and S. Klein. 2003. A randomized trial of a low-carbohydrate diet for obesity. *N Engl J Med* 348 (21):2082–2090.
Fried, L. P., N. O. Borhani, P. Enright, C. D. Furberg, J. M. Gardin, R. A. Kronmal, L. H. Kuller et al. 1991. The Cardiovascular Health Study: Design and rationale. *Ann Epidemiol* 1 (3):263–276.
Friedman, G. D., G. R. Cutter, R. P. Donahue, G. H. Hughes, S. B. Hulley, D. R. Jacobs Jr., K. Liu, and P. J. Savage. 1988. CARDIA: Study design, recruitment, and some characteristics of the examined subjects. *J Clin Epidemiol* 41 (11):1105–1116.
Fruchart, J. C., F. Sacks, M. P. Hermans, G. Assmann, W. V. Brown, R. Ceska, M. J. Chapman et al. 2008. The Residual Risk Reduction Initiative: A call to action to reduce residual vascular risk in patients with dyslipidemia. *Am J Cardiol* 102 (10a):1k–34k.
Gibbons, G. H., S. B. Shurin, G. A. Mensah, and M. S. Lauer. 2013. Refocusing the agenda on cardiovascular guidelines: An announcement from the National Heart, Lung, and Blood Institute. *Circulation* 128 (15):1713–1715.
Goff, D. C., Jr., D. M. Lloyd-Jones, G. Bennett, S. Coady, R. B. D'Agostino Sr., R. Gibbons, P. Greenland et al. 2014. 2013 ACC/AHA Guideline on the Assessment of Cardiovascular Risk: A report of the American College of Cardiology/American Heart Association Task Force on Practice Guidelines. *J Am Coll Cardiol* 63 (25 Pt B):2935–2959.
Graham, I., D. Atar, K. Borch-Johnsen, G. Boysen, G. Burell, R. Cifkova, J. Dallongeville et al. 2007. European guidelines on cardiovascular disease prevention in clinical practice: Executive summary. Fourth Joint Task Force of the European Society of Cardiology and Other Societies on Cardiovascular Disease Prevention in Clinical Practice (constituted by representatives of nine societies and by invited experts). *Eur J Cardiovasc Prev Rehabil* 14 (Suppl 2):E1–E40.
Grundy, S. M., J. I. Cleeman, C. N. Merz, H. B. Brewer Jr., L. T. Clark, D. B. Hunninghake, R. C. Pasternak et al. 2004. Implications of recent clinical trials for the National Cholesterol Education Program Adult Treatment Panel III guidelines. *Circulation* 110 (2):227–239.
Gunness, P., and M. J. Gidley. 2010. Mechanisms underlying the cholesterol-lowering properties of soluble dietary fibre polysaccharides. *Food Funct* 1 (2):149–155.
Harris, W. S. 2007. Omega-3 fatty acids for treatment of hyperlipidemia: Mechanisms and evidence. Program and abstracts of the XVI International Symposium on Drugs Affecting Lipid Metabolism, New York.
Heber, D., I. Yip, J. M. Ashley, D. A. Elashoff, R. M. Elashoff, and V. L. Go. 1999. Cholesterol-lowering effects of a proprietary Chinese red-yeast-rice dietary supplement. *Am J Clin Nutr* 69 (2):231–236.
Ho, H. V., J. L. Sievenpiper, A. Zurbau, S. B. Mejia, E. Jovanovski, F. Au-Yeung, A. L. Jenkins, and V. Vuksan. 2016. A systematic review and meta-analysis of randomized controlled trials of the effect of barley beta-glucan on LDL-C, non-HDL-C and apoB for cardiovascular disease risk reduction[i-iv]. *Eur J Clin Nutr* 70 (11):1239–1245.
Howell, W. H., D. J. McNamara, M. A. Tosca, B. T. Smith, and J. A. Gaines. 1997. Plasma lipid and lipoprotein responses to dietary fat and cholesterol: A meta-analysis. *Am J Clin Nutr* 65 (6):1747–1764.
Huang, J., J. Frohlich, and A. P. Ignaszewski. 2011. The impact of dietary changes and dietary supplements on lipid profile. *Can J Cardiol* 27 (4):488–505.
Jackevicius, C. A., P. Li, and J. V. Tu. 2008. Prevalence, predictors, and outcomes of primary nonadherence after acute myocardial infarction. *Circulation* 117 (8):1028–1036.

Kannel, W. B., M. Feinleib, P. M. McNamara, R. J. Garrison, and W. P. Castelli. 1979. An investigation of coronary heart disease in families. The Framingham Offspring Study. *Am J Epidemiol* 110 (3):281–290.

Kavousi, M., M. J. Leening, D. Nanchen, P. Greenland, I. M. Graham, E. W. Steyerberg, M. A. Ikram, B. H. Stricker, A. Hofman, and O. H. Franco. 2014. Comparison of application of the ACC/AHA guidelines, Adult Treatment Panel III guidelines, and European Society of Cardiology guidelines for cardiovascular disease prevention in a European cohort. *JAMA* 311 (14):1416–1423.

Keech, A., R. J. Simes, P. Barter, J. Best, R. Scott, M. R. Taskinen, P. Forder, et al. 2005. Effects of long-term fenofibrate therapy on cardiovascular events in 9795 people with type 2 diabetes mellitus (the FIELD study): Randomised controlled trial. *Lancet* 366 (9500):1849–1861.

Knopp, R. H. 1989. The effects of oral contraceptives and postmenopausal estrogens on lipoprotein physiology and atherosclerosis. In *Oral Contraception into the 1990s*, ed. H. Rekers and H. W. Halbe, 31–45 Carnforth, UK: Parthenon Publishing.

Knopp, R. H. 1999. Drug treatment of lipid disorders. *N Engl J Med* 341 (7):498–511.

Knopp, R. H., X. Zhu, and B. Bonet. 1994. Effects of estrogens on lipoprotein metabolism and cardiovascular disease in women. *Atherosclerosis* 110 (Suppl):S83–S91.

Kumbhani, D. J., P. G. Steg, C. P. Cannon, K. A. Eagle, S. C. Smith Jr., E. Hoffman, S. Goto, E. M. Ohman, D. L. Bhatt, and Reduction of Atherothrombosis for Continued Health Registry Investigators. 2013. Adherence to secondary prevention medications and four-year outcomes in outpatients with atherosclerosis. *Am J Med* 126 (8):693.e1–700.e1.

Levine, G. N., J. F. Keaney Jr., and J. A. Vita. 1995. Cholesterol reduction in cardiovascular disease. Clinical benefits and possible mechanisms. *N Engl J Med* 332 (8):512–521.

Li, Z. P., M. L. Deng, C. H. Tseng, and D. Heber. 2013. Hypertriglyceridemia is a practical biomarker of metabolic syndrome in individuals with abdominal obesity. *Metab Syndr Relat Disord* 11 (2):87–91.

Malina, D. M., F. A. Fonseca, S. A. Barbosa, S. H. Kasmas, V. A. Machado, C. N. Franca, N. C. Borges, R. A. Moreno, and M. C. Izar. 2015. Additive effects of plant sterols supplementation in addition to different lipid-lowering regimens. *J Clin Lipidol* 9 (4):542–552.

Mihaylova, B., J. Emberson, L. Blackwell, A. Keech, J. Simes, E. H. Barnes, M. Voyseys et al. 2012. The effects of lowering LDL cholesterol with statin therapy in people at low risk of vascular disease: Meta-analysis of individual data from 27 randomised trials. *Lancet* 380 (9841):581–590.

Muntner, P., L. D. Colantonio, M. Cushman, D. C. Goff Jr., G. Howard, V. J. Howard, B. Kissela, E. B. Levitan, D. M. Lloyd-Jones, and M. M. Safford. 2014. Validation of the atherosclerotic cardiovascular disease pooled cohort risk equations. *JAMA* 311 (14):1406–1415.

National Cholesterol Education Program Expert Panel on Detection, Evaluation, and Treatment of High Blood Cholesterol in Adults. 2002. Third Report of the National Cholesterol Education Program (NCEP) Expert Panel on Detection, Evaluation, and Treatment of High Blood Cholesterol in Adults (Adult Treatment Panel III) final report. *Circulation* 106 (25):3143–3421.

Oram, J. F., and S. Yokoyama. 1996. Apolipoprotein-mediated removal of cellular cholesterol and phospholipids. *J Lipid Res* 37 (12):2473–2491.

Ornish, D., S. E. Brown, L. W. Scherwitz, J. H. Billings, W. T. Armstrong, T. A. Ports, S. M. McLanahan, R. L. Kirkeeide, R. J. Brand, and K. L. Gould. 1990. Can lifestyle changes reverse coronary heart disease? The Lifestyle Heart Trial. *Lancet* 336 (8708):129–133.

Pencina, M. J., A. M. Navar-Boggan, R. B. D'Agostino Sr., K. Williams, B. Neely, A. D. Sniderman, and E. D. Peterson. 2014. Application of new cholesterol guidelines to a population-based sample. *N Engl J Med* 370 (15):1422–1431.

Perk, J., G. De Backer, H. Gohlke, I. Graham, Z. Reiner, W. M. M. Verschuren, C. Albus et al. 2012. The Fifth Joint Task Force of the European Society of Cardiology and Other Societies on Cardiovascular Disease Prevention in Clinical Practice (constituted by representatives of nine societies and by invited experts) developed with the special contribution of the European Association for Cardiovascular Prevention & Rehabilitation (EACPR) (vol 33, pg 1635, 2012). *Eur Heart J* 33 (17):2126.

Pritikin, N. 1984. The Pritikin diet. *JAMA* 251 (9):1160–1161.

Rader, D. J., J. Cohen, and H. H. Hobbs. 2003. Monogenic hypercholesterolemia: New insights in pathogenesis and treatment. *J Clin Invest* 111 (12):1795–1803.

Ramprasath, V. R., D. J. A. Jenkins, B. Lamarche, C. W. C. Kendall, D. Faulkner, L. Cermakova, P. Couture et al. 2014. Consumption of a dietary portfolio of cholesterol lowering foods improves blood lipids without affecting concentrations of fat soluble compounds. *Nutr J* 13:101.

Reiner, Z., Z. Sonicki, and E. Tedeschi-Reiner. 2010a. Physicians' perception, knowledge and awareness of cardiovascular risk factors and adherence to prevention guidelines: The PERCRO-DOC survey. *Atherosclerosis* 213 (2):598–603.

Reiner, Z., Z. Sonicki, and E. Tedeschi-Reiner. 2010b. Public perceptions of cardiovascular risk factors in Croatia: The PERCRO survey. *Prev Med* 51 (6):494–496.

Report of the National Cholesterol Education Program Expert Panel on Detection, Evaluation, and Treatment of High Blood Cholesterol in Adults. The Expert Panel. 1988. *Arch Intern Med* 148 (1):36–69.

Ridker, P. M., and N. R. Cook. 2013. Statins: New American guidelines for prevention of cardiovascular disease. *Lancet* 382 (9907):1762–1765.

Rubins, H. B., S. J. Robins, D. Collins, C. L. Fye, J. W. Anderson, M. B. Elam, F. H. Faas et al. 1999. Gemfibrozil for the secondary prevention of coronary heart disease in men with low levels of high-density lipoprotein cholesterol. Veterans Affairs High-Density Lipoprotein Cholesterol Intervention Trial Study Group. *N Engl J Med* 341 (6):410–418.

Rubins, H. B., S. J. Robins, D. Collins, D. B. Nelson, M. B. Elam, E. J. Schaefer, F. H. Faas, and J. W. Anderson. 2002. Diabetes, plasma insulin, and cardiovascular disease: Subgroup analysis from the Department of Veterans Affairs high-density lipoprotein intervention trial (VA-HIT). *Arch Intern Med* 162 (22):2597–2604.

Sacks, F. M., V. J. Carey, and J. C. Fruchart. 2010. Combination lipid therapy in type 2 diabetes. *N Engl J Med* 363 (7):692–694.

Stone, N. J., S. Bilek, and S. Rosenbaum. 2005. Recent National Cholesterol Education Program Adult Treatment Panel III update: Adjustments and options. *Am J Cardiol* 96 (4A):53E–59E.

Voight, B. F., G. M. Peloso, M. Orho-Melander, R. Frikke-Schmidt, M. Barbalic, M. K. Jensen, G. Hindy et al. 2012. Plasma HDL cholesterol and risk of myocardial infarction: A Mendelian randomisation study. *Lancet* 380 (9841):572–580.

Warnick, G. R., G. L. Myers, G. R. Cooper, and N. Rifai. 2002. Impact of the third cholesterol report from the Adult Treatment Panel of the National Cholesterol Education Program on the clinical laboratory. *Clin Chem* 48 (1):11–17.

Zechner, R. 2007. Lipolysis: Effects on lipid- and energy-homeostasis. Program and abstracts of the XVI International Symposium on Drugs Affecting Lipid Metabolism, New York.

10 Nutrition and Coronary Artery Disease

10.1 INTRODUCTION

Over the past 30 years, the cellular and molecular basis of coronary artery disease (CAD) has been demonstrated to be linked to inflammation promoted by unbalanced nutrition, hypertension, diabetes, stress, sedentary lifestyle, obesity, and poor-quality diets. The reduction of the progression of atherosclerosis through modulation of inflammatory, immune, and vascular factors reinforces a nutritional approach to secondary prevention in individuals with diagnosed CAD. For patients who have yet to develop disease of the coronary arteries, the concept of heart disease is theoretical and focused on a reduction in cholesterol and other lipid levels for some preventive benefit, as discussed in Chapter 9. The emphasis of that chapter was to move patients away from a sole focus on cholesterol by discussing lipid disorders and metabolism broadly, while stressing the importance of triglycerides, dyslipidemia, and the metabolic syndrome as the most common lipid disorders.

In this chapter, the emphasis is on patients who have suffered a cardiac event and have diagnosed CAD. These patients are likely to be concerned with secondary prevention and, much like a cancer survivor, are likely to be interested in detailed discussions of how to prevent a recurrence of their cardiovascular event and death. According to the World Health Organization, cardiovascular disease is the leading cause of mortality worldwide, leading to an estimated 18 million deaths each year (Murray et al. 2012). CAD is considered the main cardiovascular disorder, causing 46% of the cardiovascular mortality in men and 38% in women (Wong 2014). It is estimated that about 80% of all mortality from cardiovascular disorders could be prevented with the elimination of obesity, sedentary lifestyles, and poor-quality diets (World Health Organization 2011).

It has been demonstrated repeatedly that adherence to a higher-quality diet is associated with decreased mortality risk (Jankovic et al. 2014). In common with the state of primary care education on other age-related chronic diseases reviewed in this book, nutrition and lifestyle changes are not the focus of primary care education in the treatment of CAD and secondary prevention. In addition to the treatment of CAD with drugs, primary care education focuses on the availability of modern interventional cardiology procedures, such as stenting, percutaneous aortic valve replacement, and cardiac surgery. While these advances in procedures have a central role in cardiology practice, the primary care practice can contribute to better patient outcomes by adding an emphasis on dietary and lifestyle factors that can delay, reduce, or reverse the progression of CAD to an unstable plaque that bursts and causes a cardiac event that may be fatal.

CAD shares many features of the age-related chronic diseases reviewed in other chapters and involves a critical role for elevated blood lipids, but also involves multiple cellular and molecular events, providing an opportunity for diet and lifestyle changes to reduce the progression of atherosclerosis in patients with diagnosed CAD until the very late stages of the disease.

Inflammation has a significant role at all stages of atherosclerosis, including initiation, progression, and plaque formation. Secondary prevention is possible even after a cardiac event occurs or when atherosclerosis is advanced based on imaging evidence, such as coronary arterial calcification by computed tomography (CT) scan, or evidence of cardiac muscle dysfunction by electrocardiogram (EKG) stress treadmill or cardiac angiograms. The progression of atherosclerosis is not an inevitable forward process. Not only does elevated cholesterol from the circulation settle in the space below the endothelium of the coronary arteries as oxidized cholesterol, but there is also reverse cholesterol transport mediated by high-density lipoprotein (HDL) cholesterol particles.

In addition, there are other healing processes, such as angiogenesis and nitric oxide (NO) production, that can be augmented through nutrition and exercise.

Therefore, the role of inflammation and oxidative stress in atherosclerosis, which has been established over the past 30 years, will be the central emphasis of this chapter, with dietary recommendations that augment those already provided with regard to the control of lipid metabolism and lipid disorders in Chapter 9.

10.2 CORONARY ARTERY DISEASE, UNSTABLE PLAQUES, AND MYOCARDIAL INFARCTION

The heart is the only organ that provides its own blood supply via branches from the major coronary arteries, including the main coronary artery, the left anterior descending artery, the right coronary artery, and the circumflex artery. From each of these major arteries, there are smaller branches providing oxygen and nutrients to a region of the heart muscle. Most regions of the heart muscle are supplied by two coronary arteries. In the regions between zones of coronary artery blood supply, there are areas of the heart muscle that are particularly vulnerable to hypoxic injury.

The coronary arteries supply blood flow to the heart, and when functioning normally, they ensure adequate oxygenation of the myocardium at all levels of cardiac activity. Constriction and dilation of the coronary arteries, governed primarily by local regulatory mechanisms, regulate the amount of blood flow to the myocardium in a manner that matches the amount of oxygen delivered to the myocardium with the myocardial demand for oxygen.

Gradual hypoxia stimulates angiogenesis in the heart, providing additional oxygen as needed in areas where blood flow may be diminished due to CAD. Angiogenesis during cardiac rehabilitation from a myocardial infarction can play a major role in protecting the heart. However, a sudden blockage of a large or medium-sized coronary artery can trigger hypoxic injury of large amounts of heart muscle, leading to sudden death or congestive heart failure. Such sudden blockages result from the formation of blood clots when an unstable atherosclerotic plaque bursts suddenly. The transition of atherosclerotic plaques with necrotic cores, calcified regions, accumulated modified lipids, inflamed smooth muscle cells, endothelial cells, leukocytes, and foam cells from stable lesions to unstable plaques that rupture or erode suddenly is responsible for the sudden blockage of a coronary artery (Figure 10.1), leading to a myocardial infarction (Murray et al. 2012).

Intracoronary imaging studies have revealed that unstable plaques that are vulnerable to rupture have a number of typical features, including increased plaque volume, a necrotic core, increased lipid and inflammatory cell content, thin fibrous caps, and neovascularization and hemorrhage within the plaque (Virmani et al. 2002). Many unstable plaques often coexist in the coronary arteries of individuals with CAD. Clinical trials have demonstrated the benefits of primary and secondary prevention therapies targeted against CAD risk, and progress has been made in reducing some risk factors, such as dyslipidemia (Cholesterol Treatment Trialists Collaboration et al. 2010) and hypertension (blood pressure) (Turnbull and Blood Pressure Lowering Treatment Trialists Collaboration 2003), while both diabetes and obesity are increasingly common, so that the prevalence of plaque rupture or erosion leading to initial or recurrent myocardial infarctions remains high (Libby 2005).

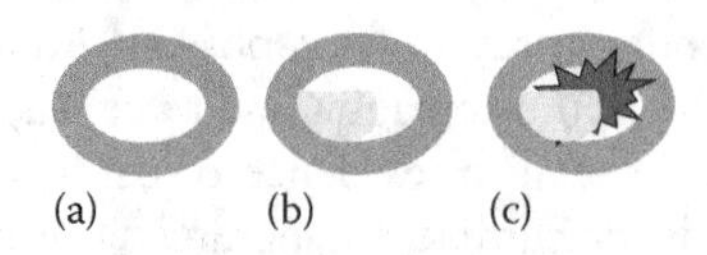

FIGURE 10.1 Schematic representation of (a) normal coronary artery with normal blood flow, (b) partially blocked coronary artery with stable plaque, and (c) acutely ruptured unstable plaque leading to blockage and myocardial infarction.

The realization that unstable plaques are the cause of heart attacks, rather than some uniform and gradual accumulation of cholesterol that completely blocks a coronary artery, led to a major shift in preventive cardiology, from the idea of simply lowering cholesterol levels to stabilizing or reversing the process of atherosclerosis so that unstable plaques would be stabilized and some stable plaques reduced in size.

10.2.1 Cellular Basis of Atherosclerosis and Inflammation

Atherosclerosis is the most common pathological process that leads to CAD, a disease of large- and medium-sized arteries of the heart. Atherosclerosis has been called hardening of the arteries due to calcification in the walls of the vessels, first noted by Rudolf Virchow in the early twentieth century, as he noticed a loud click as he passed a scalpel through a coronary artery vessel during an autopsy. For much of the nineteenth and early twentieth centuries, it was believed that atherosclerosis was simply a lipid storage disorder that gradually narrowed blood flow through the coronary arteries, ultimately blocking them. Low-density lipoprotein (LDL) cholesterol that enters the endothelial space and is oxidized remains the most important risk factor for atherosclerosis, and has been the focus of most pharmacological research on CAD. However, immune and inflammatory mechanisms of atherosclerosis have come to be understood as important mechanisms for the development of CAD over the past 30 years (Ross 1999; Hansson and Libby 2006; Mayerl et al. 2006; Methe and Weis 2007; Weber et al. 2008). Inflammation plays a vital role in all stages of the disease, from plaque initiation and lesion progression up to ultimate complications, such as plaque rupture, intraplaque hemorrhage, and thromboembolism (Ross 1999). The many components of atherosclerotic plaques demonstrate that the vascular, metabolic, and immune systems are involved in this process.

The term *arteriosclerosis* was first introduced in 1829 (Mayerl et al. 2006). Within a few years, the associated cellular immune alterations within the arteries were described by two different schools of pathology, resulting in two theories of atherosclerosis. Rudolf Virchow postulated an initial role for aortic cellular conglomerates, emphasizing that cellular actions were critical to the progression of atherosclerosis. In contrast, Carl von Rokitansky suggested that initial injury of the vessel wall owing to mechanical injury and toxins led to endothelial dysfunction and further inflammation (Methe and Weis 2007). As with many competing theories in medicine, both ideas came to be accepted as part of the pathogenesis of atherosclerosis.

In the 1970s, the response-to-injury model was described (Ross 1999). However, a large number of recent papers have emphasized that the chronic inflammatory response also has an immune component (Hansson and Libby 2006). Arterial samples from Rokitansky's collection of vessels obtained at autopsy were analyzed and showed T-cell accumulation present in early lesions, suggesting that lymphocytes play an essential role in atherosclerosis. The detailed mechanisms whereby endothelial cell function, lipid metabolism, and lipid retention become unbalanced and disturbed within the plaque have not been determined, but it appears that atherosclerosis entails immune responses locally mediated through complex cellular interactions within the endothelium, and that, in addition, injury to the wall of the blood vessel may trigger an innate immune response.

There are multiple factors involved in the formation and progression of established atherosclerotic plaques. Most of the research on atherosclerotic plaque formation, progression, and instability has been conducted on tissues obtained at autopsy and surgery or from studies on experimental animals, since it is difficult to acquire atherosclerotic tissue from living patients (Ludewig et al. 2000; Libby et al. 2002). The presence of active inflammation with resident T-lymphocytes or macrophages within plaque is one of the criteria that make these arterial wall lesions vulnerable to rupture (Gerrity et al. 1979). White blood cells within atherosclerotic lesions were first found in the early 1980s (Gerrity et al. 1979), including neutrophils, macrophages, and lymphocytes (van der Wal and Becker 1999; Galkina and Ley 2007a). Blood monocytes enter different tissues and differentiate into tissue-resident macrophages or dendritic cells.

Atherosclerotic plaques are formed in very specific regions of the aortic tree in mice, where flow is disturbed. On the other hand, very little inflammation or atherosclerosis is found in portions of the aorta in mice where there is smooth laminar flow (Jongstra-Bilen et al. 2006). Activated by disturbed flow, endothelial cells increase their expression of adhesion molecules and chemokines, which accelerate leukocyte recruitment to the vessel wall. Rolling and firm adhesion of monocytes to aortic endothelium was documented in an *ex vivo* model of the carotid artery and *in vivo* (Galkina and Ley 2007b) as the first step in monocyte entry into the subendothelial space.

Macrophages within plaques can assume different phenotypes (Byrne and Kalayoglu 1999; Stoneman et al. 2007). M1 macrophages are characterized by high local production of NO and reactive oxygen intermediates. The production of NO in this context is a pro-inflammatory event mediated by the inducible nitric oxide synthase (NOS) in macrophages, similar to events documented in tumor tissue. This reaction should not be confused with the production of NO from nitrite in cardiac muscle under conditions of hypoxia, which is a beneficial event discussed later in this chapter. M1 macrophages typically participate in the resistance against intracellular parasites and tumor development (Mantovani et al. 2009). M2 macrophages are mainly functional in tissue remodeling, angiogenesis, and tumor progression. M2 macrophages are also involved in the regulation of immune function and allergic reactions (Mantovani et al. 2004; Adamson and Leitinger 2011). There is further complexity of macrophage phenotype beyond simply M1 and M2. According to the stimulus they receive, alternative M2 macrophages can be classified into at least four distinct phenotypes (Adamson and Leitinger 2011). Human atherosclerotic lesions have highly heterogeneous macrophage phenotypes. Many factors in the microenvironment can modulate the macrophage phenotype, including various cytokines and bioactive lipids, such as cholesterol crystals, oxidized lipoproteins, fatty acids, and immune complexes (Adamson and Leitinger 2011).

Dendritic cells of the immune system get their name from their similarity to neurons in having thin branches extending out from the cell body to gather information for transmission to B-cells and T-cells in the immune system. These cells leave the atherosclerotic lesions within a few days of entering the subendothelial space and migrate back to lymph nodes and the spleen through the lymphatic vessels. The number of dendritic cells is significantly elevated in atherosclerosis-prone arteries, demonstrating the involvement of the immune system in atherosclerosis (Stoneman et al. 2007). Atherosclerosis is a dynamic process, and the inflammation that accompanies atherosclerosis progresses through different stages.

During regression of plaques, monocytes leave the plaque, but during progression, they remain in the plaque. The inflammation mediated by lymphocytes is tightly controlled by regulatory T-lymphocytes, which are critical in maintaining immunological tolerance (Sakaguchi et al. 2006). Atherosclerosis has some aspects of an autoimmune disease, as significant evidence shows a response to self-antigens such as HSP-60 and oxidized LDL during atherosclerosis. Many autoimmune diseases, such as systemic lupus erythematosus and diabetes, accelerate atherosclerosis development, probably through the defective clearance of apoptotic cells.

Platelets also play a major role in plaque thrombus formation upon injury and form the acute clot that leads to a myocardial infarction when an unstable plaque ruptures. They also secrete inflammatory mediators that modulate the recruitment of white blood cells into inflamed tissues (Lundberg and Govoni 2004; von Hundelshausen and Weber 2007).

There is a large body of evidence supporting the notion that obesity, diabetes, and atherosclerosis are connected via their effects on immune function and inflammation (Katagiri et al. 2007). Visceral adipocytes secrete cytokines, resulting in modulation of inflammation, including adiponectin, leptin, resistin, visfatin, tumor necrosis factor α (TNF-α), interleukin 6 (IL-6), IL-1, and CCL2 (Tilg and Moschen 2006). Serum levels of adiponectin are markedly decreased in obesity, insulin resistance, type 2 diabetes, and atherosclerosis (Arita et al. 1999). Basic science studies in animals demonstrate that adiponectin counteracts both atherosclerosis progression and thrombosis by reducing lipid accumulation in macrophage-derived foam cells (Tian et al. 2009) and suppressing the production of chemokines, including CXCL10, CXCL11, and CXCL9, leading to reduced

T-cell homing into atherosclerosis-prone aortic regions (Okamoto et al. 2008). Adiponectin can also reduce the inflammatory phenotype of endothelial cells and smooth muscle cells (Tilg and Moschen 2006) and reduce platelet aggregation (Kato et al. 2006).

On the other hand, leptin, which is increased in the circulation of individuals with visceral obesity, promotes inflammation and atherosclerosis. Leptin increases the secretion of the chemokine, CCL2, and initiates proliferation and oxidative stress in endothelial cells. Leptin also promotes migration and proliferation of smooth muscle cells (Yang and Barouch 2007) and promotes thrombosis by increasing platelet aggregation (Maruyama et al. 2000). The discovery of adipokines has spawned the concept of an association between atherosclerosis and inflammation mediated systemically by distant visceral fat and locally by fat associated with the pericardium, which is a visceral fat depot increased in obesity.

10.2.2 Endothelial Dysfunction and Nitric Oxide in CAD

NO is an important protective mediator that helps to control blood flow in the heart by modulating the amount of dilation of very small blood vessels in the myocardium. This function is mediated by the endothelial cell lining of these blood vessels, which produces NO as a gas that is short-lived but functions to relax smooth muscle in myocardial arterioles, increasing vessel diameter and blood flow. Abnormalities in NO generation play an important role in the pathophysiology of CAD (Kugiyama et al. 1996). NO is synthesized from L-arginine by the action of NOS. There are at least three isoenzymes of NOS: inducible NOS, neuronal NOS, and endothelial NOS (eNOS) (Nathan and Xie 1994). The inducible NOS, as already mentioned, is found in macrophages and is part of an inflammatory response that should not be confused with the vascular roles described here.

NOS enzymes produce NO by catalyzing a five-electron oxidation of the guanidine nitrogen of arginine that requires the binding of five cofactors: flavin adenine dinucleotide, flavin mononucleotide, heme iron, tetrahydrobiopterin, and calcium–calmodulin (Bredt and Snyder 1990). If any of these cofactors is deficient or limiting, NO production from NOS is restricted and NOS produces superoxide instead, which is a pro-oxidant. This mechanism has been termed "NOS uncoupling" (Landmesser et al. 2003). Therefore, both adequate oxygen and sufficient substrate supply are necessary for proper NOS function, and in the absence of these factors, NOS becomes harmful.

NO is involved in a wide variety of regulatory mechanisms of the cardiovascular system, beyond endothelium-dependent vasodilatation. NO also inhibits smooth muscle cell proliferation, platelet adhesion and aggregation, and monocyte adhesion. Cardiovascular disease risk factors, including hypercholesterolemia, hypertension, diabetes mellitus, and cigarette smoking, lead to a reduction in the ability of the endothelium to produce NO (Galle et al. 1991; Makimattila et al. 1996; Busse and Fleming 1999). *Endothelial dysfunction* is the term used to refer to a decrease of endothelial NO formation due to insufficient oxygen and cofactor supply or inactivation by reactive oxygen species.

In a healthy heart, the vascular endothelium plays an important role in maintaining homeostasis, and it functions to promote vasodilation, inhibit luminal and vascular wall coagulation, and prevent the proliferation of smooth muscle and foam cells. However, these functions may be perturbed, particularly when the bioavailability of NO is low, leading to a state favoring vasoconstriction, thrombosis, vascular smooth muscle cell proliferation, and the generation of atherosclerotic plaque (Cooke and Dzau 1997).

Endothelial dysfunction is a key element facilitating the development of atherosclerosis. Lack of NO also promotes aggregation and invasion of inflammatory cells in the vessel wall and promotes the calcification of arteries. There is a vicious cycle in which progressive deprivation of blood supply with hypoxia of tissues and organs leads to less NO production. Despite the growth of new vessels as the result of angiogenesis, the resulting blood vessels often do a poor job of providing adequate oxygen to damaged areas of cardiac muscle, and there is reduction in cardiac output, which in extreme cases leads to heart failure. A damaged heart is also more susceptible to sudden and sometimes fatal ventricular arrhythmias.

10.2.3 Coronary Artery Calcification

Coronary artery calcification (CAC) is an easily detected biomarker of atherosclerosis, often occurring as calcified atheroma or spotty calcification within a lipid core. Its measurement by rapid CT scan of the chest is commonly used clinically to avoid an invasive angiogram or as a marker for atherosclerosis in studies (Rumberger et al. 1995). Cardiovascular risk factors and the presence and extent of CAC are predictive of coronary event risk (National Cholesterol Education Program Expert Panel on Detection, Evaluation, and Treatment of High Blood Cholesterol in Adults 2002; Zeb and Budoff 2015), and are used as a decision point in whether to begin statin therapy in men over 65 years of age. There is currently no specific treatment for arterial calcification, with both statins and vasodilators having little effect (Henein and Owen 2010).

Arterial calcification represents segmental bone formation, which is known to be progressive even after controlling risk factors. Calcification of the coronary arteries results from some biochemical or other pathological effect associated with CAD risk factors, and it cannot be reduced through optimum control of risk factors (McCullough and Chinnaiyan 2009; Henein and Owen 2011; Zhao et al. 2016). Nonetheless, dyslipidemia, smoking, obesity, and family history of CAD have been shown to be predictive of CAC presence and progression in large population studies, such as the Multi-Ethnic Study of Atherosclerosis and Heinz Nixdorf Recall (Kronmal et al. 2007; Schmermund et al. 2007).

10.3 TYPE 2 DIABETES AND CAD

Type 2 diabetes mellitus is associated with a markedly increased incidence of cardiovascular diseases, accounting for ~70% of diabetic mortality (Grundy et al. 2005; Tziomalos et al. 2010). In the background of cardiovascular complications, disorders of microcirculation and endothelial dysfunction associated with type 2 diabetes precede atherosclerosis and critically alter the functions of the healthy endothelium and its production of factors that regulate vascular tone, smooth muscle cell proliferation, and vessel wall inflammation (Berwick et al. 2012). Advanced glycation end products (AGEs) produced in type 2 diabetes affect nearly every type of cell and molecule in the body and are thought to be one factor in aging and some age-related chronic diseases (Glenn and Stitt 2009; Semba et al. 2009a,b). In diabetes-associated CAD, modification of proteins by reducing sugars leads to the formation of AGEs *in vivo*, and there is evidence that dietary AGEs (called dAGEs) can be absorbed into the circulation and add to the burden of AGEs promoting disease (Uribarri et al. 2010).

These nonenzymatic glycation reactions continue progressively during aging and substantially accelerate with type 2 diabetes and atherosclerosis, providing a rationale for the effects of sustained hyperglycemia on chronic disease progression (Basta et al. 2004). Alterations in glucose and lipid metabolism likely lead to the production of excess aldehydes and formation of AGEs, although the exact mechanisms have not been established. AGEs act directly or via receptors and participate in the cross-linking proteins of extracellular matrix (Basta et al. 2004).

The receptor for AGE (RAGE) is a member of the immunoglobulin superfamily and is expressed by endothelial cells, smooth muscle cells, monocytes, and lymphocytes with enhanced expression in atherosclerotic lesions. The AGE-RAGE interaction leads to oxidative stress, increased endothelial dysfunction, increased production of inflammatory cytokines and tissue factors, elevated expression of adhesion molecules, and accelerated development and progression of atherosclerosis (Basta et al. 2004).

10.4 EFFECTS OF STATIN DRUGS IN CAD BEYOND LIPID LOWERING

Statins are produced naturally by 39 species of fungi and yeast as polyketides which act as antibiotics against bacteria attacking these species. Through a serendipitous investigation of *Aspergillus* species of fungi, Japanese researchers discovered monacolins in the 1970s. The drug isolated from these fungi is mevinolin, which is converted to the active drug mevalonic acid in the body. This compound inhibits 3-hydroxy-3-methylglutaryl coenzyme A reductase and increases the hepatic expression of the LDL receptor, which decreases LDL levels in the circulation (Le et al. 2013; Hennessy et al. 2015). In addition to these cholesterol-lowering effects, which have led to a multi-billion-dollar global bonanza for the pharmaceutical industry, statins also provide protection against cardiovascular diseases by other effects, such as antioxidation, anti-inflammation, and increased bioavailability of NO (Kureishi et al. 2000; Wolfrum et al. 2003; Thanassoulis et al. 2014). Since the lipid-lowering effects are the most widely known and publicized effects of statins, these other effects are called pleiotropic effects of statins.

At the cellular and molecular level, statins can increase eNOS activity and NO production in endothelial cells through a kinase-dependent pathway and protein–protein interactions (Sun et al. 2006; Su et al. 2014). Despite the many heralded advances of statins in preventing cardiac events, statin treatment is not uniformly effective in improving endothelial cell function and inflammation in patients with CAD (Kureishi et al. 2000; Walsh and Pignone 2004; Artom et al. 2014; Drapala et al. 2014; Goldstein and Brown 2015).

It is a well-founded community standard to prescribe statins for all patients leaving the hospital after a coronary event, which is a good idea given the effects reviewed above beyond simply lowering LDL cholesterol. However, given that other cardiovascular disease risk factors related to lifestyle, such as smoking, obesity, diabetes, and sedentary lifestyle, are commonly present, these should also be addressed through diet and exercise prescriptions, which are the focus of this text.

10.5 DIETARY RECOMMENDATIONS FOR PATIENTS WITH CORONARY ARTERY DISEASE

Patients with CAD who have suffered angina or a cardiac event are motivated to obtain any advice that can prevent another cardiac event or improve their quality of life. The fear of death that pervades the interaction with patients who have CAD is similar to that encountered with cancer survivors and may push individuals to consider invasive procedures for cure while also minimizing their confidence in the role of nutrition and exercise.

Given the multifactorial etiology of the progression of atherosclerosis, diet and lifestyle intervention has an advantage over drugs in targeting multiple pathways simultaneously. While dietary and lifestyle changes are not as potent as drug therapy, they have the advantage of an improved quality of life.

10.6 WEIGHT MANAGEMENT THROUGH NUTRITION AND EXERCISE TO REDUCE VISCERAL FAT

Chief among the various recommendations is to achieve and maintain optimum personal body composition, especially as it concerns visceral adiposity. Obesity was only identified as an independent risk factor in the 1990s, and evidence for the impact of excess visceral fat on atherosclerosis progression has already been reviewed above. Excess visceral adiposity promotes diabetes, hypertension, and dyslipidemia and has other effects that could affect progression of atherosclerosis (Figure 10.2).

These dietary recommendations are adjunctive in that patients with established CAD are typically treated with statins to lower cholesterol and drugs for hypertension and diabetes as needed. Statin treatment is a standard of care after discharge from the hospital with a coronary event.

10.6.1 Dietary Pattern and CAD

The idea that nutrition was important for established CAD only became accepted in the late 1950s due to the efforts of Nathan Pritikin, a successful inventor who was not a doctor.

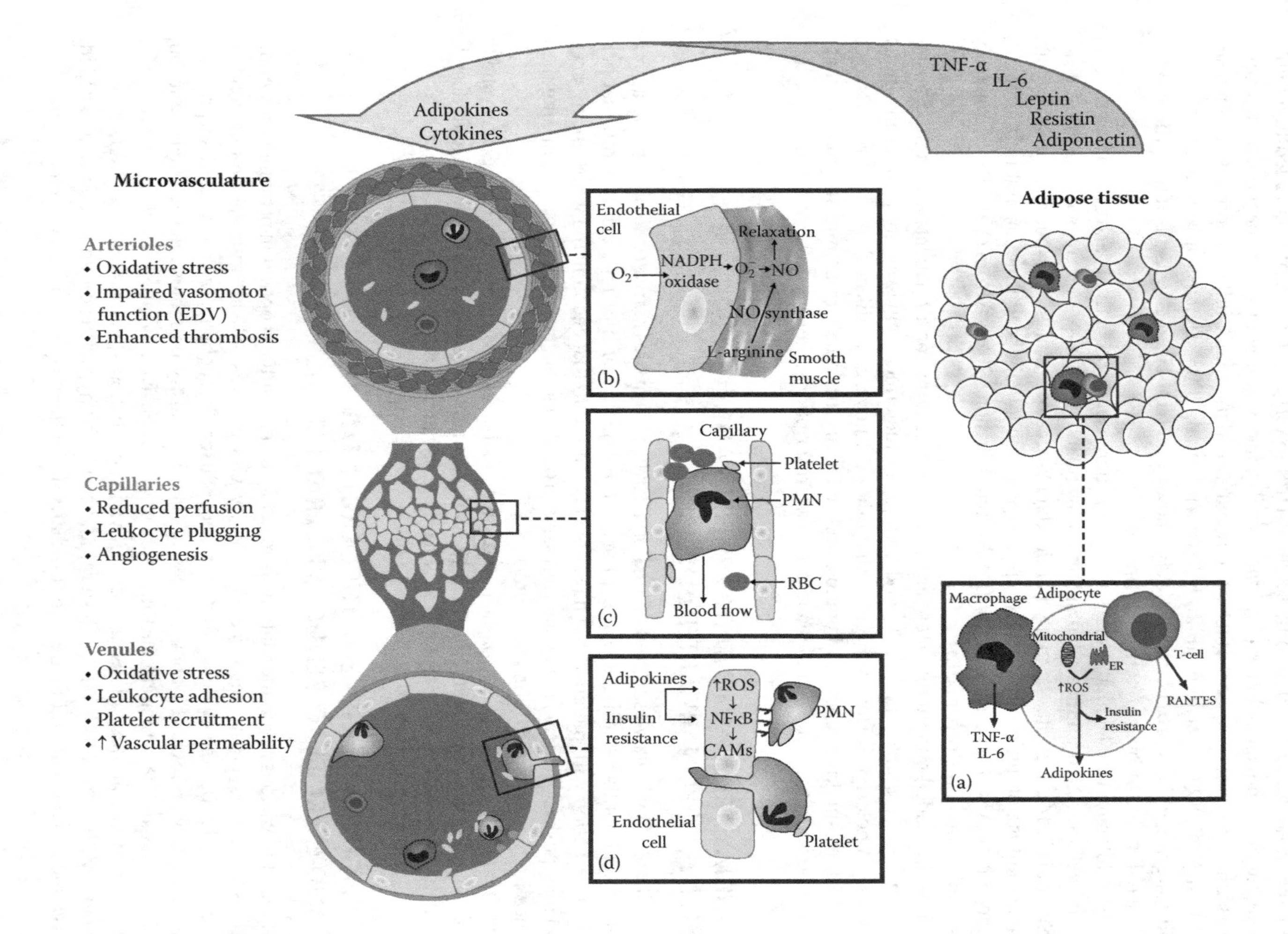

FIGURE 10.2 **(See color insert.)** Interaction of excess visceral fat with cellular and molecular mechanisms promoting the progression of atherosclerosis. EDV, end-diastolic volume; NADPH, nicotinamide adenine dinucleotide phosphate; PMN, polymorphonuclear; RBC, red blood cell; ROS, reactive oxygen species; NFκB, nuclear factor κB; CAMs, cell adhesion molecules. (Reprinted from Vachharajani, V., and Granger, D. N., *IUBMB Life*, 61(4), 424–430, 2009.)

After being diagnosed with heart disease in 1957, he was told he needed open-heart surgery. Based on studies indicating that people in primitive cultures with primarily vegetarian lifestyles had little history of heart disease, he developed a low-fat diet high in unrefined carbohydrates, including vegetables, fruits, beans, and whole grains, along with a modest aerobic exercise regime. The Pritikin diet has been called one of the "gold standards of American dieting success." He established the Pritikin Longevity Center in 1976 and served as its director. In the early 1980s, he began to suffer severe pain and complications related to hairy cell leukemia. He committed suicide on February 21, 1985, in Albany, New York, registered in a hospital under an assumed name so that no one would think his diet played a role in the leukemia that killed him. While many people lost weight and improved their endurance on the Pritikin diet, it was not a weight loss diet.

His major competitor was Dr. Robert Atkins, whose primary focus was a high-fat, high-protein diet for weight management, which contrasted with the low-fat diet of Pritikin. During the early years of his medical practice, stress and poor eating habits led Atkins to gain a considerable amount of weight. In 1963, at a weight of 224 pounds, he decided to go on a restrictive diet based on the research of Dr. Alfred W. Pennington, who recommended removing all starch and sugar from meals. He advocated for the complete elimination of sugar from the diet and a marked increase in both fat and protein. Atkins found immediate and lasting success on the plan, and began advertising its effects to his patients. Atkins suffered cardiac arrest in April 2002, leading many of his critics to point to this episode as proof of the inherent dangers in the consumption of high levels of saturated fat associated with the Atkins diet. A medical report issued by the New York medical examiner's office a year after his death showed that Atkins had a history of heart attack, congestive heart failure, and hypertension. It also noted that he weighed 258 pounds at his death.

There has continued to be a debate on whether restricting carbohydrates and lowering triglycerides or reducing fats without concern over whether carbohydrates were refined or unrefined would reduce cardiac deaths. For men, the Atkins diet promised that they could lose weight while still eating red meat and other high-fat foods, and so would not have to give up on tasty treats, as was required with the Pritikin diet.

Dr. Dean Ornish embraced many of Nathan Pritikin's ideas, with a strong focus on heart disease. Ornish is known for his lifestyle-driven approach to the control of CAD. He promotes lifestyle changes, including whole foods, plant-based diet, smoking cessation, moderate exercise, and stress management techniques, including yoga and meditation. His program has a strong element of psychosocial support. He has acknowledged Swami Satchidananda for helping him develop his holistic perspective on prevention.

Medicare reviewed six studies of the Pritikin program and nine on the Ornish version appearing in peer-reviewed publications. Most of these were conducted or sponsored by the Ornish and Pritikin programs. For example, eight of the nine Ornish studies include Ornish as the lead or senior author. Nevertheless, Medicare accepted the reported data as valid and adequate to demonstrate the effectiveness of the programs under the agency's statutory and regulatory requirements. The agency's review of published data on the Ornish and Pritikin intensive cardiac rehabilitation programs found that they effectively slowed or reversed progression of coronary heart disease and reduced the need for coronary artery bypass graft surgeries and percutaneous interventions. These programs are considered medically appropriate alternatives to standard intensive cardiac rehabilitation for persons who meet medical necessity criteria for intensive cardiac rehabilitation. However, they are considered experimental and investigational as a treatment for diabetes, hyperlipidemia, prostate cancer, metabolic syndrome, and all other indications.

Elements of the Pritikin and Ornish approach include (1) smoking cessation; (2) a vegetarian diet with less than 10% of calories from fat and minimal amounts of saturated fat; (3) group support and psychological counseling to identify sources of stress and develop tools that help manage stress more effectively; (4) moderate exercise, usually a treadmill and walking program; and (5) reliance on the daily use of stress management techniques, including various stretching, breathing, meditation, yoga, and relaxation exercises. The greatest advantage of this program over usual cardiac rehabilitation programs is the emotional reassurance provided to patients frightened about the possibility of a sudden heart attack and death.

Using the Ornish program, the Lifestyle Heart Trial found that 82% of patients diagnosed with heart disease who followed this plant-based diet program had some level of regression of atherosclerosis, and 91% had a reduction in the frequency of angina episodes, whereas 53% of the control group, fed the American Heart Association diet, had progression of atherosclerosis (Ornish et al. 1998). In addition, the study showed a reduction in LDL (37.2%) that is similar to results achieved with lipid-lowering medications. Similarly, other researchers showed that compared with a control group, the plant-based diet group had a 73% decrease in coronary events and a 70% decrease in all-cause mortality (de Lorgeril et al. 1999). In 1998, a collaborative analysis using original data from five prospective studies was reviewed and showed that, compared with nonvegetarians, vegetarians had a 24% reduction in ischemic heart disease death rates (Key et al. 1998).

There are several varieties of vegetarian diets. The so-called semivegetarians eat chicken and fish but not red meat. The strict vegetarians eat eggs and milk, as well as fruits and vegetables, and vegans eat no meat, fish, eggs, or dairy. The moderate position in this spectrum is the plant-based diet, which is followed by many who are semivegetarian or vegetarian.

A plant-based diet is increasingly becoming recognized as a healthier alternative to a diet dominated by meat fat and refined carbohydrates. A plant-based diet has significant health benefits, and studies have shown that a plant-based diet can be an effective treatment for obesity (Berkow and Barnard 2006; Rosell et al. 2006; Tonstad et al. 2009; Farmer et al. 2011), diabetes (Snowdon and Phillips 1985; Campbell 2004; Barnard et al. 2006; Rosell et al. 2006; Vang et al. 2008), hypertension (de Lorgeril et al. 1999), hyperlipidemia (Appleby et al. 1995), and heart disease (Ornish et al. 1998; Esselstyn 2001).

While the Pritikin and Ornish programs were clearly directed at CAD, many other diets that promote wellness have documented some benefits for heart disease. The basic message here is that eating a healthy diet according to general criteria set forth by the U.S. Department of Agriculture (USDA) is beneficial for heart health. The Healthy Eating Index 2010 (HEI-2010), the Alternative Healthy Eating Index 2010 (AHEI-2010), the Alternate Mediterranean Diet Score (aMED), and the Dietary Approaches to Stop Hypertension (DASH) have all been associated with a lower risk of all-cause mortality, cardiovascular disease, cancer, cognitive impairment, Alzheimer's disease, type 2 diabetes, and obesity in both adults and children (Boggs et al. 2013; Singh et al. 2014; Harmon et al. 2015; Perry et al. 2015; Jacobs et al. 2016).

The components and scoring of these healthy dietary patterns vary somewhat, but overall, they emphasize a diet containing a variety of fruits and vegetables, along with whole grains, lean protein (including legumes, nuts, and fish), and a higher ratio of unsaturated fats to saturated fat. In addition, most recommend limiting red and processed meat, sugar-sweetened beverages (SSBs) and fruit juice, *trans* fats, added sugars, sodium, and refined carbohydrates (Harmon et al. 2015). The AHEI-2010 and aMED favor the consumption of limited quantities of alcohol (Harmon et al. 2015).

10.6.2 Nitrate-Rich Foods Defend Endothelial Health under Hypoxic Conditions

Among the benefits of a plant-based diet are an increased intake of nitrates, especially from dark green leafy vegetables. While nitrate levels were controlled in agriculture by the USDA with the idea that they promoted formation of carcinogenic nitrosamines in the stomach of humans, this has turned out to be a phenomenon restricted to rodents (Katan 2009). Nitrates ingested in vegetables such as spinach are converted to nitrite by anaerobic bacteria in the mouth (Lundberg et al. 1994, 2004; Duncan et al. 1995; Lundberg and Govoni 2004). This is a reaction humans do not carry out, but one that has been proven to be critical through experiments in which mouthwash was administered to kill the anaerobic bacteria with the result that NO was not formed (Lundberg et al. 2004). The nitrite then is converted to nitrous acid in the stomach, and NO diffuses into the bloodstream acutely. It is then converted to nitrite again and stored in the muscle, including

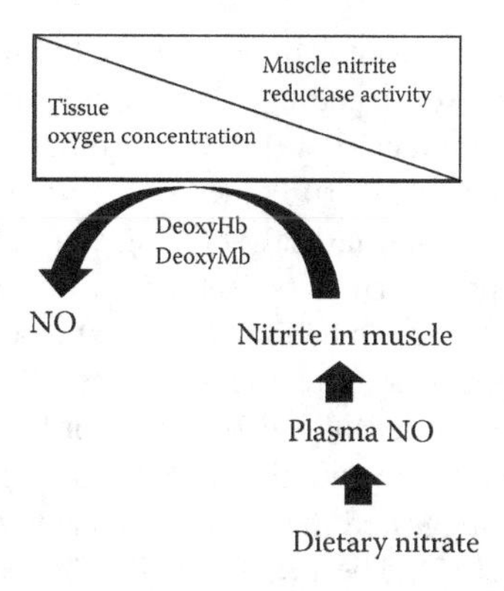

FIGURE 10.3 Nonenzymatic NO formation occurs through one electron reduction of nitrite to NO by ferrous heme proteins like deoxyhemoglobin in the blood or deoxymyoglobin in the heart. This occurs under conditions of low oxygen, shown in the two triangles in the figure. The nitrite reductase activity of these proteins increases as oxygen tension in the tissues decreases with hypoxia.

cardiac muscle. NO can also stimulate angiogenesis beneficial to heart tissue that has been damaged (Kumar et al. 2008).

NO can be obtained from nitrites stored in muscle under conditions of low oxygen (Figure 10.3). In recent years, it could be demonstrated that NO can be formed independently of its enzymatic synthesis in the endothelium by reduction of inorganic nitrite under hypoxic conditions. This nitrite stored in muscle awaits hypoxia and comes to the rescue when low-oxygen conditions occur in skeletal or myocardial muscle.

A diet rich in vegetables, such as the Mediterranean or the traditional Japanese diets, contains more nitrate than the recommended acceptable daily intake recommended by the World Health Organization (Katan 2009). Even a portion of spinach consumed in one serving of salad can exceed the acceptable daily intake for nitrate (Lundberg and Govoni 2004). However, scientific evidence supports the conclusion of the European Food Safety Authority that benefits of vegetable and fruit consumption outweigh any perceived risk of developing cancer from the consumption of nitrate and nitrite in these foods. Observational epidemiologic and human clinical studies support the hypothesis that nitrates and nitrites of plant origin play essential physiologic roles in supporting cardiovascular health.

10.6.3 Refined Carbohydrates and Sugar versus Fruits and Vegetables in Low-Glycemic-Index Diets

Carbohydrates are arguably the most misunderstood of the macronutrients, as they exist in a vast array of foods, ranging from fiber-rich fruits, vegetables, low-fat dairy, and whole grains (all of which are generally underconsumed) to sugar-sweetened beverages (SSBs), processed foods with added sugar, refined "white" carbohydrates, and baked goods (which are generally overconsumed) (U.S. Department of Health and Human Services 2015).

The view on carbohydrates has shifted somewhat in the past decade due to research showing that refined starch and sugar may actually increase cardiometabolic risk, while increased intakes of carbohydrate-containing vegetables and fruits decreased cardiometabolic risk (Malik et al. 2010; Burger et al. 2012; Ley et al. 2014; Yang et al. 2014).

Sugar intake has increased dramatically over the past century. More than 70% of U.S. adults consume at least 10% of their total daily calories from added sugar, and 10% consume 25% or more of their calories from sugar according to recent data (Yang et al. 2014). Approximately 75% of all foods and beverages contain some form of added sugar (Bray and Popkin 2014), and the association of added versus total sugar is far more robust in terms of both diet quality and disease risk (Louie and Tapsell 2015). Added sugar intake exceeding 10% not only displaces healthy nutrients, leading to micronutrient dilution (Moshtaghian et al. 2016), but also has been associated with an increased risk of overweight and obesity (Wang et al. 2013), metabolic syndrome, type 2 diabetes (Malik et al. 2010; Ley et al. 2014), and cardiovascular mortality (Yang et al. 2014).

SSBs, including soft drinks, sports drinks, sweetened milk, water, teas, and juices, are major sources of added sugar, but added sugar can be found in unexpected products, including salad dressing, bread, sauces, and baked beans, in addition to foods generally perceived as healthful, including yogurt and whole grain cereals (Chun et al. 2010). A number of prospective cohort studies have investigated the associations between consumption of SSBs and the risk of CAD.

A meta-analysis of six studies suggested that a higher consumption of SSB was associated with a higher risk of CAD (Xi et al. 2015). The PREDIMED (PREvención con DIeta MEDiterránea) study prospectively examined 1868 participants and found that consumption of >5 servings/week of all types of beverages, including artificially sweetened beverages, was associated with an increased risk of metabolic syndrome in elderly individuals at high risk of CAD (Ferreira-Pêgo et al. 2016). Cohort studies have consistently shown a dose–response relationship between SSB consumption, weight gain, and diabetes, and a recent meta-analysis showed a 55% higher risk of being overweight or obese in adulthood with high versus low intake (Hu 2013).

The *2015–2020 Dietary Guidelines for Americans* (DGAs) recommend limiting added sugar to less than 10% of total calories (U.S. Department of Health and Human Services 2015), and the American Heart Association has even more stringent criteria, limiting added sugar to 6 teaspoons daily for women (24 g) and 9 teaspoons daily for men (36 g) (Johnson et al. 2009). The Food and Drug Administration (FDA) recently finalized new labeling changes that included listing "added sugar" in both grams and percent daily value to the label, which will make it much easier to choose a more healthful dietary pattern that includes packaged foods (U.S. Food and Drug Administration 2016).

Many foods that do not contain sugar, such as white potatoes and rice, have a high glycemic index (GI) and increase blood sugar rapidly after they are consumed. The clinical application of the GI to the prevention and treatment of heart disease is controversial. No evidence exists for the implementation of low-GI diets for a reduction in coronary heart disease mortality, events, or morbidity.

10.6.4 Phytonutrients, Potential Role in Stabilizing Atherosclerotic Plaques

Atherosclerotic lesions become unstable and prone to rupture due to the formation of reactive oxygen species that are produced by the inflammatory milieu in the atherosclerotic plaque. The carotenoids are a group of red, orange, or yellow pigmented polyisoprenoid hydrocarbons synthesized by prokaryotes and higher plants. Lycopene, lutein, and other carotenoids have antioxidant activity that attenuates the inflammatory atherosclerotic process and delays vascular aging. This ability improves endothelial function due to the increase in bioavailability of NO. Carotenoid consumption also improves the metabolic profile, decreasing the incidence of diabetes, lowering LDL levels, and improving blood pressure control. The beneficial metabolic effect is translated to improvement in atherosclerosis, which is characterized by a decrease in carotid intima-media thickness (IMT). The favorable antiatherosclerotic effect of carotenoids was also demonstrated in cross-sectional population studies showing a positive correlation between low carotenoid levels and adverse cardiovascular outcome.

In particular, the impact of the oxygenated carotenoid lutein, a pigment found in dark green leafy vegetables, egg yolks, and other foods, has been studied in the Los Angeles Atherosclerosis Study. Progression of IMT of the common carotid arteries over 18 months was determined ultrasonographically and was related to plasma lutein among a randomly sampled cohort of 480 utility employees age 40–60 years (Figure 10.4).

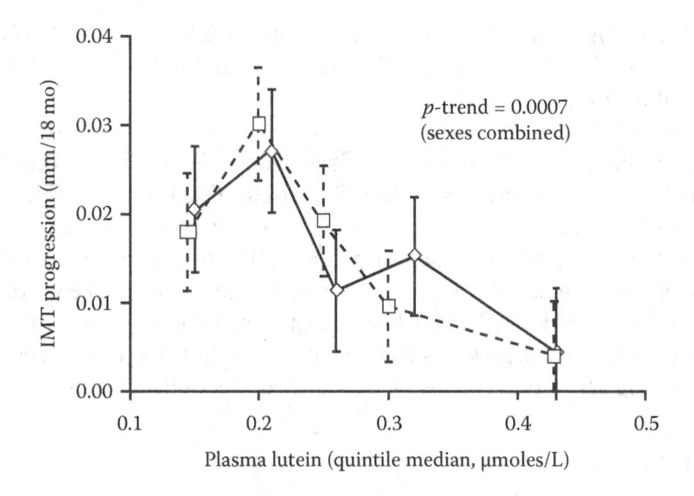

FIGURE 10.4 Inverse relation between change in carotid IMT and quintiles of plasma lutein. Graph depicts IMT means within lutein quintiles (median) for women (n = 5214) and men (n = 5248) adjusted for cardiovascular risk factors. Ranges of plasma lutein concentrations (mmol/L) for consecutive quintiles were 0.070–0.182, 0.184–0.240, 0.244–0.296, 0.297–0.360, and 0.367–0.805 for women and 0.019–0.180, 0.184–0.230, 0.231–0.279, 0.280–0.347, and 0.350–0.790 for men. Error bars indicate the standard error of the mean (SEM). Serum lutein was measured by high-performance liquid chromatography (HPLC) at the University of California, Los Angeles (UCLA) Center for Human Nutrition. (Reprinted from Dwyer, J. H. et al., *Circulation*, 103(24), 2922–2927, 2001.)

In vitro, lutein was highly effective in a dose-dependent manner in reducing the attraction of monocytes in the coculture model of lipoprotein oxidation in the artery wall. A dramatic inhibitory effect of lutein on chemotaxis was observed with pretreatment of cultured cells. The impact of lutein supplementation on atherosclerotic lesion formation was assessed *in vivo* by assigning apoE null mice to chow or chow plus lutein (0.2% by weight) and LDL receptor null mice to Western diet or Western diet plus lutein. IMT progression declined with increasing quintile of plasma lutein. Lutein supplementation reduced lesion size by 44% in apoE null mice ($p < 0.009$) and 43% in LDL receptor null mice ($p < 0.02$) by comparison with mice fed the control diets.

According to the latest dietary guidelines report, less than 20% of Americans meet the daily recommendations for vegetable intake, and just over 20% meet the recommended intake for fruit, while most Americans exceed the recommendations for added sugar, saturated fat, and sodium (U.S. Department of Health and Human Services 2015). A significant percentage of Americans do not consume daily recommended micronutrient intakes from food alone (Fulgoni et al. 2011), despite consuming adequate or, in many cases, excess calories. We are in the midst of an obesity epidemic, with more than one-third of adults and 17% of youth in the United States classified as obese, and yet much of our population is inadequately nourished from a nutrient, not calorie, perspective (Ogden et al. 2014).

Dietary fiber is defined by the Institute of Medicine (IOM) as nondigestible carbohydrates and lignins that are intrinsic and intact in plants (Dahl and Stewart 2015). The recommended daily intake for fiber is 14 g/1000 kilocalories/day, or 25 g for women and 38 g for men. The health benefits of dietary fiber continue to be an area of great interest and represent a tremendous opportunity for improving diet quality, particularly with the emerging research on the essential role of the gut microbiome in improving health and preventing disease (Zhernakova et al. 2016).

There are established benefits of dietary fiber in reducing the risk of CAD (Threapleton et al. 2013). A recent prospective study that included 367,442 participants followed over 14 years found an inverse association between whole grain and cereal fiber intake and all-cause mortality, including death from cancer, cardiovascular disease, diabetes, respiratory disease, and infections (Huang et al. 2015). A pooled analysis with 23 randomized controlled trials (RCTs) for CAD risk factors suggested reductions in total cholesterol and LDL cholesterol, and reductions in diastolic blood pressure with increased fiber intake.

Whole grains as dietary fiber have been associated with a lower risk for CAD since 1977 (Trowell 1972). Fruits and vegetables are a great source of fibers with added nutritional benefits. A prospective study done in the Netherlands found a 34% decreased risk of CAD in those with high fruit and vegetable intake compared with those with lower intake. The association was especially strong with deep-orange-colored fruits and vegetables (Oude Griep et al. 2011). A meta-analysis of prospective cohort studies found a significantly reduced risk of type 2 diabetes with higher intake of fruit and green leafy vegetables (Li et al. 2014). Berries, rich in the bioactive phytonutrient polyphenols, have been associated with better cardiovascular outcomes (Pribis and Shukitt-Hale 2014). The most prudent dietary patterns should include much greater amounts of a variety of fiber-rich foods than we are currently consuming.

10.7 CONCLUSION

The primary role of cholesterol and oxidized lipids in promoting atherosclerosis is well established. However, the advent of new science on the cellular and molecular basis of atherosclerosis has opened new avenues of investigation into multiple aspects of diet and lifestyle that can impact cardiac events and CAD-associated mortality.

While controversial areas continue to exist in nutrition science, there are far more areas of agreement among nutrition experts. The benefits of consuming a healthy diet rich in minimally processed fruits, vegetables, whole grains, lean protein, and healthful fats, along with reducing sugar and limiting or eliminating processed red meat, are convincing. Debate will undoubtedly continue surrounding specific recommendations within individual food and nutrient groups, but focusing on an overall healthful dietary pattern gives the individual a great deal of flexibility in developing a healthful, enjoyable and sustainable approach to eating. For the CAD patient, it is important to provide social and emotional support, as well as exercise therapy.

Whether intensive cardiac rehabilitation as practiced by Ornish is superior to more individualized approaches has not been established.

Offering each patient an overview of what is known about atherosclerosis and emphasizing that it can be slowed or reversed with diet and lifestyle should increase adherence to healthy dietary patterns as adjuncts to medical treatment, including statins and antihypertensive drugs, as needed.

REFERENCES

Adamson, S., and N. Leitinger. 2011. Phenotypic modulation of macrophages in response to plaque lipids. *Curr Opin Lipidol* 22 (5):335–342.

Appleby, P. N., M. Thorogood, K. McPherson, and J. I. Mann. 1995. Associations between plasma lipid concentrations and dietary, lifestyle and physical factors in the Oxford Vegetarian Study. *J Hum Nutr Diet* 8 (5):305–314.

Arita, Y., S. Kihara, N. Ouchi, M. Takahashi, K. Maeda, J. Miyagawa, K. Hotta et al. 1999. Paradoxical decrease of an adipose-specific protein, adiponectin, in obesity. *Biochem Biophys Res Commun* 257 (1):79–83.

Artom, N., F. Montecucco, F. Dallegri, and A. Pende. 2014. Carotid atherosclerotic plaque stenosis: The stabilizing role of statins. *Eur J Clin Invest* 44 (11):1122–1134.

Barnard, N. D., J. Cohen, D. J. A. Jenkins, G. Turner-McGrievy, L. Gloede, B. Jaster, K. Seidl, A. A. Green, and S. Talpers. 2006. A low-fat vegan diet improves glycemic control and cardiovascular risk factors in a randomized clinical trial in individuals with type 2 diabetes. *Diabetes Care* 29 (8):1777–1783.

Basta, G., A. M. Schmidt, and R. De Caterina. 2004. Advanced glycation end products and vascular inflammation: Implications for accelerated atherosclerosis in diabetes. *Cardiovasc Res* 63 (4):582–592.

Berkow, S. E., and N. Barnard. 2006. Vegetarian diets and weight status. *Nutr Rev* 64 (4):175–188.

Berwick, Z. C., G. M. Dick, and J. D. Tune. 2012. Heart of the matter: Coronary dysfunction in metabolic syndrome. *J Mol Cell Cardiol* 52 (4):848–856.

Boggs, D. A., L. Rosenberg, C. L. Rodríguez-Bernal, and J. R. Palmer. 2013. Long-term diet quality is associated with lower obesity risk in young African American women with normal BMI at baseline. *J Nutr* 143 (10):1636–1641.

Bray, G. A., and B. M. Popkin. 2014. Dietary sugar and body weight: Have we reached a crisis in the epidemic of obesity and diabetes? Health be damned! Pour on the sugar. *Diabetes Care* 37 (4):950–956.

Bredt, D. S., and S. H. Snyder. 1990. Isolation of nitric oxide synthetase, a calmodulin-requiring enzyme. *Proc Natl Acad Sci USA* 87 (2):682–685.

Burger, K. N., J. W. Beulens, Y. T. van der Schouw, I. Sluijs, A. M. Spijkerman, D. Sluik, H. Boeing et al. 2012. Dietary fiber, carbohydrate quality and quantity, and mortality risk of individuals with diabetes mellitus. *PLoS One* 7 (8):e43127.

Busse, R., and I. Fleming. 1999. Nitric oxide, nitric oxide synthase, and hypertensive vascular disease. *Curr Hypertens Rep* 1 (1):88–95.

Byrne, G. I., and M. V. Kalayoglu. 1999. *Chlamydia pneumoniae* and atherosclerosis: Links to the disease process. *Am Heart J* 138 (5 Pt 2):S488–S490.

Campbell, T. M. 2004. *The China Study: The Most Comprehensive Study of Nutrition Ever Conducted and the Startling Implications for Diet, Weight Loss and Long-Term Health.* Dallas, TX: BenBella Books.

Cholesterol Treatment Trialists Collaboration, C. Baigent, L. Blackwell, J. Emberson, L. E. Holland, C. Reith, N. Bhala et al. 2010. Efficacy and safety of more intensive lowering of LDL cholesterol: A meta-analysis of data from 170,000 participants in 26 randomised trials. *Lancet* 376 (9753):1670–1681.

Chun, O. K., C. E. Chung, Y. Wang, A. Padgitt, and W. O. Song. 2010. Changes in intakes of total and added sugar and their contribution to energy intake in the U.S. *Nutrients* 2 (8):834–854.

Cooke, J. P., and V. J. Dzau. 1997. Nitric oxide synthase: Role in the genesis of vascular disease. *Annu Rev Med* 48:489–509.

Dahl, W. J., and M. L. Stewart. 2015. Position of the Academy of Nutrition and Dietetics: Health implications of dietary fiber. *J Acad Nutr Diet* 115 (11):1861–1870.

de Lorgeril, M., P. Salen, J. L. Martin, I. Monjaud, J. Delaye, and N. Mamelle. 1999. Mediterranean diet, traditional risk factors, and the rate of cardiovascular complications after myocardial infarction: Final report of the Lyon Diet Heart Study. *Circulation* 99 (6):779–785.

Drapala, A., M. Sikora, and M. Ufnal. 2014. Statins, the renin-angiotensin-aldosterone system and hypertension—A tale of another beneficial effect of statins. *J Renin Angiotensin Aldosterone Syst* 15 (3):250–258.

Duncan, C., H. Dougall, P. Johnston, S. Green, R. Brogan, C. Leifert, L. Smith, M. Golden, and N. Benjamin. 1995. Chemical generation of nitric oxide in the mouth from the enterosalivary circulation of dietary nitrate. *Nat Med* 1 (6):546–551.

Dwyer, J. H., M. Navab, K. M. Dwyer, K. Hassan, P. Sun, A. Shircore, S. Hama-Levy, G. Hough, X. Wang, and T. Drake. 2001. Oxygenated carotenoid lutein and progression of early atherosclerosis: The Los Angeles Atherosclerosis Study. *Circulation* 103 (24):2922–2927.

Esselstyn, C. B., Jr. 2001. Resolving the coronary artery disease epidemic through plant-based nutrition. *Prev Cardiol* 4 (4):171–177.

Farmer, B., B. T. Larson, V. L. Fulgoni, A. J. Rainville, and G. U. Liepa. 2011. A vegetarian dietary pattern as a nutrient-dense approach to weight management: An analysis of the National Health and Nutrition Examination Survey 1999–2004. *J Am Diet Assoc* 111 (6):819–827.

Ferreira-Pêgo, C., N. Babio, M. Bes-Rastrollo, D. Corella, R. Estruch, E. Ros, M. Fitó, L. Serra-Majem, F. Arós, and M. Fiol. 2016. Frequent consumption of sugar- and artificially sweetened beverages and natural and bottled fruit juices is associated with an increased risk of metabolic syndrome in a Mediterranean population at high cardiovascular disease risk. *J Nutr* 146 (8):1528–1536.

Fulgoni, V. L., 3rd, D. R. Keast, R. L. Bailey, and J. Dwyer. 2011. Foods, fortificants, and supplements: Where do Americans get their nutrients? *J Nutr* 141 (10):1847–1854.

Galkina, E., and K. Ley. 2007a. Leukocyte influx in atherosclerosis. *Curr Drug Targets* 8 (12):1239–1248.

Galkina, E., and K. Ley. 2007b. Vascular adhesion molecules in atherosclerosis. *Arterioscler Thromb Vasc Biol* 27 (11):2292–2301.

Galle, J., A. Mulsch, R. Busse, and E. Bassenge. 1991. Effects of native and oxidized low density lipoproteins on formation and inactivation of endothelium-derived relaxing factor. *Arterioscler Thromb* 11 (1):198–203.

Gerrity, R. G., H. K. Naito, M. Richardson, and C. J. Schwartz. 1979. Dietary induced atherogenesis in swine. Morphology of the intima in prelesion stages. *Am J Pathol* 95 (3):775–792.

Glenn, J. V., and A. W. Stitt. 2009. The role of advanced glycation end products in retinal ageing and disease. *Biochim Biophys Acta* 1790 (10):1109–1116.

Goldstein, J. L., and M. S. Brown. 2015. A century of cholesterol and coronaries: From plaques to genes to statins. *Cell* 161 (1):161–172.

Grundy, S. M., J. I. Cleeman, S. R. Daniels, K. A. Donato, R. H. Eckel, B. A. Franklin, D. J. Gordon et al. 2005. Diagnosis and management of the metabolic syndrome: An American Heart Association/National Heart, Lung, and Blood Institute Scientific Statement. *Circulation* 112 (17):2735–2752.

Hansson, G. K., and P. Libby. 2006. The immune response in atherosclerosis: A double-edged sword. *Nat Rev Immunol* 6 (7):508–519.

Harmon, B. E., C. J. Boushey, Y. B. Shvetsov, R. Ettienne, J. Reedy, L. R. Wilkens, L. Le Marchand, B. E. Henderson, and L. N. Kolonel. 2015. Associations of key diet-quality indexes with mortality in the multiethnic cohort: The Dietary Patterns Methods Project. *Am J Clin Nutr* 101 (3):587–597.

Henein, M., and A. Owen. 2010. Statins moderate coronary atheroma but not coronary calcification: Results from meta-analyses. *Scand Cardiovasc J* 44:3.

Henein, M. Y., and A. Owen. 2011. Statins moderate coronary stenoses but not coronary calcification: Results from meta-analyses. *Int J Cardiol* 153 (1):31–35.

Hennessy, D. A., T. Bushnik, D. G. Manuel, and T. J. Anderson. 2015. Comparing guidelines for statin treatment in Canada and the United States. *J Am Heart Assoc* 4 (7):e001758.

Hu, F. B. 2013. Resolved: There is sufficient scientific evidence that decreasing sugar-sweetened beverage consumption will reduce the prevalence of obesity and obesity-related diseases. *Obes Rev* 14 (8):606–619.

Huang, T., M. Xu, A. Lee, S. Cho, and L. Qi. 2015. Consumption of whole grains and cereal fiber and total and cause-specific mortality: Prospective analysis of 367,442 individuals. *BMC Med* 13:59.

Jacobs, S., B. E. Harmon, N. J. Ollberding, L. R. Wilkens, K. R. Monroe, L. N. Kolonel, L. Le Marchand, C. J. Boushey, and G. Maskarinec. 2016. Among 4 diet quality indexes, only the alternate Mediterranean diet score is associated with better colorectal cancer survival and only in African American women in the multiethnic cohort. *J Nutr* 146 (9):1746–1755.

Jankovic, N., A. Geelen, M. T. Streppel, L. C. de Groot, P. Orfanos, E. H. van den Hooven, H. Pikhart et al. 2014. Adherence to a healthy diet according to the World Health Organization guidelines and all-cause mortality in elderly adults from Europe and the United States. *Am J Epidemiol* 180 (10):978–988.

Johnson, R. K., L. J. Appel, M. Brands, B. V. Howard, M. Lefevre, R. H. Lustig, F. Sacks, L. M. Steffen, J. Wylie-Rosett, American Heart Association Nutrition Committee of the Council on Nutrition, Physical Activity, and Metabolism, and the Council on Epidemiology and Prevention. 2009. Dietary sugars intake and cardiovascular health: A scientific statement from the American Heart Association. *Circulation* 120 (11):1011–1020.

Jongstra-Bilen, J., M. Haidari, S. N. Zhu, M. Chen, D. Guha, and M. I. Cybulsky. 2006. Low-grade chronic inflammation in regions of the normal mouse arterial intima predisposed to atherosclerosis. *J Exp Med* 203 (9):2073–2083.

Katagiri, H., T. Yamada, and Y. Oka. 2007. Adiposity and cardiovascular disorders: Disturbance of the regulatory system consisting of humoral and neuronal signals. *Circ Res* 101 (1):27–39.

Katan, M. B. 2009. Nitrate in foods: Harmful or healthy? *Am J Clin Nutr* 90 (1):11–12.

Kato, H., H. Kashiwagi, M. Shiraga, S. Tadokoro, T. Kamae, H. Ujiie, S. Honda et al. 2006. Adiponectin acts as an endogenous antithrombotic factor. *Arterioscler Thromb Vasc Biol* 26 (1):224–230.

Key, T. J., G. E. Fraser, M. Thorogood, P. N. Appleby, V. Beral, G. Reeves, M. L. Burr et al. 1998. Mortality in vegetarians and non-vegetarians: A collaborative analysis of 8300 deaths among 76,000 men and women in five prospective studies. *Public Health Nutr* 1 (1):33–41.

Kronmal, R. A., R. L. McClelland, R. Detrano, S. Shea, J. A. Lima, M. Cushman, D. E. Bild, and G. L. Burke. 2007. Risk factors for the progression of coronary artery calcification in asymptomatic subjects: Results from the Multi-Ethnic Study of Atherosclerosis (MESA). *Circulation* 115 (21):2722–2730.

Kugiyama, K., H. Yasue, K. Okumura, H. Ogawa, K. Fujimoto, K. Nakao, M. Yoshimura, T. Motoyama, Y. Inobe, and H. Kawano. 1996. Nitric oxide activity is deficient in spasm arteries of patients with coronary spastic angina. *Circulation* 94 (3):266–271.

Kumar, D., B. G. Branch, C. B. Pattillo, J. Hood, S. Thoma, S. Simpson, S. Illum et al. 2008. Chronic sodium nitrite therapy augments ischemia-induced angiogenesis and arteriogenesis. *Proc Natl Acad Sci USA* 105 (21):7540–7545.

Kureishi, Y., Z. Luo, I. Shiojima, A. Bialik, D. Fulton, D. J. Lefer, W. C. Sessa, and K. Walsh. 2000. The HMG-CoA reductase inhibitor simvastatin activates the protein kinase Akt and promotes angiogenesis in normocholesterolemic animals. *Nat Med* 6 (9):1004–1010.

Landmesser, U., S. Dikalov, S. R. Price, L. McCann, T. Fukai, S. M. Holland, W. E. Mitch, and D. G. Harrison. 2003. Oxidation of tetrahydrobiopterin leads to uncoupling of endothelial cell nitric oxide synthase in hypertension. *J Clin Invest* 111 (8):1201–1209.

Le, N. A., R. Jin, J. E. Tomassini, A. M. Tershakovec, D. R. Neff, and P. W. Wilson. 2013. Changes in lipoprotein particle number with ezetimibe/simvastatin coadministered with extended-release niacin in hyperlipidemic patients. *J Am Heart Assoc* 2 (4):e000037.

Ley, S. H., O. Hamdy, V. Mohan, and F. B. Hu. 2014. Prevention and management of type 2 diabetes: Dietary components and nutritional strategies. *Lancet* 383 (9933):1999–2007.

Li, M., Y. Fan, X. Zhang, W. Hou, and Z. Tang. 2014. Fruit and vegetable intake and risk of type 2 diabetes mellitus: Meta-analysis of prospective cohort studies. *BMJ Open* 4 (11):e005497.

Libby, P. 2005. The forgotten majority: Unfinished business in cardiovascular risk reduction. *J Am Coll Cardiol* 46 (7):1225–1228.

Libby, P., P. M. Ridker, and A. Maseri. 2002. Inflammation and atherosclerosis. *Circulation* 105 (9): 1135–1143.

Louie, J. C. Y., and L. C. Tapsell. 2015. Association between intake of total vs added sugar on diet quality: A systematic review. *Nutr Rev* 73 (12):837–857.

Ludewig, B., S. Freigang, M. Jaggi, M. O. Kurrer, Y. C. Pei, L. Vlk, B. Odermatt, R. M. Zinkernagel, and H. Hengartner. 2000. Linking immune-mediated arterial inflammation and cholesterol-induced atherosclerosis in a transgenic mouse model. *Proc Natl Acad Sci USA* 97 (23):12752–12757.

Lundberg, J. O., and M. Govoni. 2004. Inorganic nitrate is a possible source for systemic generation of nitric oxide. *Free Radic Biol Med* 37 (3):395–400.

Lundberg, J. O., E. Weitzberg, J. A. Cole, and N. Benjamin. 2004. Nitrate, bacteria and human health. *Nat Rev Microbiol* 2 (7):593–602.

Lundberg, J. O., E. Weitzberg, J. M. Lundberg, and K. Alving. 1994. Intragastric nitric oxide production in humans: Measurements in expelled air. *Gut* 35 (11):1543–1546.

Makimattila, S., A. Virkamaki, P. H. Groop, J. Cockcroft, T. Utriainen, J. Fagerudd, and H. Yki-Jarvinen. 1996. Chronic hyperglycemia impairs endothelial function and insulin sensitivity via different mechanisms in insulin-dependent diabetes mellitus. *Circulation* 94 (6):1276–1282.

Malik, V. S., B. M. Popkin, G. A. Bray, J. P. Despres, W. C. Willett, and F. B. Hu. 2010. Sugar-sweetened beverages and risk of metabolic syndrome and type 2 diabetes: A meta-analysis. *Diabetes Care* 33 (11):2477–2483.

Mantovani, A., C. Garlanda, and M. Locati. 2009. Macrophage diversity and polarization in atherosclerosis: A question of balance. *Arterioscler Thromb Vasc Biol* 29 (10):1419–1423.

Mantovani, A., A. Sica, S. Sozzani, P. Allavena, A. Vecchi, and M. Locati. 2004. The chemokine system in diverse forms of macrophage activation and polarization. *Trends Immunol* 25 (12):677–686.

Maruyama, I., M. Nakata, and K. Yamaji. 2000. Effect of leptin in platelet and endothelial cells. Obesity and arterial thrombosis. *Ann NY Acad Sci* 902:315–319.

Mayerl, C., M. Lukasser, R. Sedivy, H. Niederegger, R. Seiler, and G. Wick. 2006. Atherosclerosis research from past to present—On the track of two pathologists with opposing views, Carl von Rokitansky and Rudolf Virchow. *Virchows Arch* 449 (1):96–103.

McCullough, P. A., and K. M. Chinnaiyan. 2009. Annual progression of coronary calcification in trials of preventive therapies: A systematic review. *Arch Intern Med* 169 (22):2064–2070.

Methe, H., and M. Weis. 2007. Atherogenesis and inflammation—Was Virchow right? *Nephrol Dial Transplant* 22 (7):1823–1827.

Moshtaghian, H., J. C. Y. Louie, K. E. Charlton, Y. C. Probst, B. Gopinath, P. Mitchell, and V. M. Flood. 2016. Added sugar intake that exceeds current recommendations is associated with nutrient dilution in older Australians. *Nutrition* 32 (9):937–942.

Murray, C. J., T. Vos, R. Lozano, M. Naghavi, A. D. Flaxman, C. Michaud, M. Ezzati et al. 2012. Disability-adjusted life years (DALYs) for 291 diseases and injuries in 21 regions, 1990–2010: A systematic analysis for the Global Burden of Disease Study 2010. *Lancet* 380 (9859):2197–2223.

Nathan, C., and Q. W. Xie. 1994. Nitric oxide synthases: Roles, tolls, and controls. *Cell* 78 (6):915–918.

National Cholesterol Education Program Expert Panel on Detection, Evaluation, and Treatment of High Blood Cholesterol in Adults. 2002. Third Report of the National Cholesterol Education Program (NCEP) Expert Panel on Detection, Evaluation, and Treatment of High Blood Cholesterol in Adults (Adult Treatment Panel III) final report. *Circulation* 106 (25):3143–3421.

Ogden, C. L., M. D. Carroll, B. K. Kit, and K. M. Flegal. 2014. Prevalence of childhood and adult obesity in the United States, 2011–2012. *JAMA* 311 (8):806–814.

Okamoto, Y., E. J. Folco, M. Minami, A. K. Wara, M. W. Feinberg, G. K. Sukhova, R. A. Colvin, S. Kihara, T. Funahashi, A. D. Luster, and P. Libby. 2008. Adiponectin inhibits the production of CXC receptor 3 chemokine ligands in macrophages and reduces T-lymphocyte recruitment in atherogenesis. *Circ Res* 102 (2):218–225.

Ornish, D., L. W. Scherwitz, J. H. Billings, S. E. Brown, K. L. Gould, T. A. Merritt, S. Sparler et al. 1998. Intensive lifestyle changes for reversal of coronary heart disease. *JAMA* 280 (23):2001–2007.

Oude Griep, L. M., W. M. Verschuren, D. Kromhout, M. C. Ocke, and J. M. Geleijnse. 2011. Colours of fruit and vegetables and 10-year incidence of CHD. *Br J Nutr* 106 (10):1562–1569.

Perry, C. P., E. Keane, R. Layte, A. P. Fitzgerald, I. J. Perry, and J. M. Harrington. 2015. The use of a dietary quality score as a predictor of childhood overweight and obesity. *BMC Public Health* 15 (1):1.

Pribis, P., and B. Shukitt-Hale. 2014. Cognition: The new frontier for nuts and berries. *Am J Clin Nutr* 100 (Suppl 1):347S–352S.

Rosell, M., P. Appleby, E. Spencer, and T. Key. 2006. Weight gain over 5 years in 21 966 meat-eating, fish-eating, vegetarian, and vegan men and women in EPIC-Oxford. *Int J Obes* 30 (9):1389–1396.

Ross, R. 1999. Atherosclerosis—An inflammatory disease. *N Engl J Med* 340 (2):115–126.

Rumberger, J. A., D. B. Simons, L. A. Fitzpatrick, P. F. Sheedy, and R. S. Schwartz. 1995. Coronary artery calcium area by electron-beam computed tomography and coronary atherosclerotic plaque area. A histopathologic correlative study. *Circulation* 92 (8):2157–2162.

Sakaguchi, S., M. Ono, R. Setoguchi, H. Yagi, S. Hori, Z. Fehervari, J. Shimizu, T. Takahashi, and T. Nomura. 2006. Foxp3+ CD25+ CD4+ natural regulatory T cells in dominant self-tolerance and autoimmune disease. *Immunol Rev* 212:8–27.

Schmermund, A., N. Lehmann, L. F. Bielak, P. Yu, P. F. Sheedy 2nd, A. E. Cassidy-Bushrow, S. T. Turner et al. 2007. Comparison of subclinical coronary atherosclerosis and risk factors in unselected populations in Germany and US-America. *Atherosclerosis* 195 (1):e207–e216.

Semba, R. D., L. Ferrucci, K. Sun, J. Beck, M. Dalal, R. Varadhan, J. Walston, J. M. Guralnik, and L. P. Fried. 2009a. Advanced glycation end products and their circulating receptors predict cardiovascular disease mortality in older community-dwelling women. *Aging Clin Exp Res* 21 (2):182–190.

Semba, R. D., S. S. Najjar, K. Sun, E. G. Lakatta, and L. Ferrucci. 2009b. Serum carboxymethyl-lysine, an advanced glycation end product, is associated with increased aortic pulse wave velocity in adults. *Am J Hypertens* 22 (1):74–79.

Singh, B., M. M. Mielke, A. K. Parsaik, R. H. Cha, R. O. Roberts, P. D. Scanlon, Y. E. Geda, T. J. Christianson, V. S. Pankratz, and R. C. Petersen. 2014. A prospective study of chronic obstructive pulmonary disease and the risk for mild cognitive impairment. *JAMA Neurol* 71 (5):581–588.

Snowdon, D. A., and R. L. Phillips. 1985. Does a vegetarian diet reduce the occurrence of diabetes? *Am J Public Health* 75 (5):507–512.

Stoneman, V., D. Braganza, N. Figg, J. Mercer, R. Lang, M. Goddard, and M. Bennett. 2007. Monocyte/macrophage suppression in CD11b diphtheria toxin receptor transgenic mice differentially affects atherogenesis and established plaques. *Circ Res* 100 (6):884–893.

Su, K. H., S. J. Lin, J. Wei, K. I. Lee, J. F. Zhao, S. K. Shyue, and T. S. Lee. 2014. The essential role of transient receptor potential vanilloid 1 in simvastatin-induced activation of endothelial nitric oxide synthase and angiogenesis. *Acta Physiol (Oxf)* 212 (3):191–204.

Sun, W., T. S. Lee, M. Zhu, C. Gu, Y. Wang, Y. Zhu, and J. Y. Shyy. 2006. Statins activate AMP-activated protein kinase in vitro and in vivo. *Circulation* 114 (24):2655–2662.

Thanassoulis, G., K. Williams, K. Ye, R. Brook, P. Couture, P. R. Lawler, J. de Graaf, C. D. Furberg, and A. Sniderman. 2014. Relations of change in plasma levels of LDL-C, non-HDL-C and apoB with risk reduction from statin therapy: A meta-analysis of randomized trials. *J Am Heart Assoc* 3 (2):e000759.

Threapleton, D. E., D. C. Greenwood, C. E. L. Evans, C. L. Cleghorn, C. Nykjaer, C. Woodhead, J. E. Cade, C. P. Gale, and V. J. Burley. 2013. Dietary fibre intake and risk of cardiovascular disease: Systematic review and meta-analysis. *BMJ* 347:f6879.

Tian, L., N. Luo, R. L. Klein, B. H. Chung, W. T. Garvey, and Y. Fu. 2009. Adiponectin reduces lipid accumulation in macrophage foam cells. *Atherosclerosis* 202 (1):152–161.

Tilg, H., and A. R. Moschen. 2006. Adipocytokines: Mediators linking adipose tissue, inflammation and immunity. *Nat Rev Immunol* 6 (10):772–783.

Tonstad, S., T. Butler, R. Yan, and G. E. Fraser. 2009. Type of vegetarian diet, body weight, and prevalence of type 2 diabetes. *Diabetes Care* 32 (5):791–796.

Trowell, H. 1972. Ischemic heart disease and dietary fiber. *Am J Clin Nutr* 25 (9):926–932.

Turnbull, F., and Blood Pressure Lowering Treatment Trialists Collaboration. 2003. Effects of different blood-pressure-lowering regimens on major cardiovascular events: Results of prospectively-designed overviews of randomised trials. *Lancet* 362 (9395):1527–1535.

Tziomalos, K., V. G. Athyros, A. Karagiannis, and D. P. Mikhailidis. 2010. Endothelial dysfunction in metabolic syndrome: Prevalence, pathogenesis and management. *Nutr Metab Cardiovasc Dis* 20 (2):140–146.

Uribarri, J., S. Woodruff, S. Goodman, W. Cai, X. Chen, R. Pyzik, A. Yong, G. E. Striker, and H. Vlassara. 2010. Advanced glycation end products in foods and a practical guide to their reduction in the diet. *J Am Diet Assoc* 110 (6):911–916.e12.

U.S. Department of Health and Human Services. 2015. *2015–2020 Dietary Guidelines for Americans.* Washington, DC: U.S. Government Printing Office.

U.S. Food and Drug Administration. 2016. Changes to the Nutrition Facts label. Silver Spring, MD: U.S. Food and Drug Administration.

Vachharajani, V., and D. N. Granger. 2009. Adipose tissue: A motor for the inflammation associated with obesity. *IUBMB Life* 61 (4):424–430.

van der Wal, A. C., and A. E. Becker. 1999. Atherosclerotic plaque rupture—Pathologic basis of plaque stability and instability. *Cardiovasc Res* 41 (2):334–344.

Vang, A., P. N. Singh, J. W. Lee, E. H. Haddad, and C. H. Brinegar. 2008. Meats, processed meats, obesity, weight gain and occurrence of diabetes among adults: Findings from Adventist Health Studies. *Ann Nutr Metab* 52 (2):96–104.

Virmani, R., A. P. Burke, F. D. Kolodgie, and A. Farb. 2002. Vulnerable plaque: The pathology of unstable coronary lesions. *J Interv Cardiol* 15 (6):439–446.

von Hundelshausen, P., and C. Weber. 2007. Platelets as immune cells: Bridging inflammation and cardiovascular disease. *Circ Res* 100 (1):27–40.

Walsh, J. M., and M. Pignone. 2004. Drug treatment of hyperlipidemia in women. *JAMA* 291 (18):2243–2252.

Wang, H., L. M. Steffen, X. Zhou, L. Harnack, and R. V. Luepker. 2013. Consistency between increasing trends in added-sugar intake and body mass index among adults: The Minnesota Heart Survey, 1980–1982 to 2007–2009. *Am J Public Health* 103 (3):501–507.

Weber, C., A. Zernecke, and P. Libby. 2008. The multifaceted contributions of leukocyte subsets to atherosclerosis: Lessons from mouse models. *Nat Rev Immunol* 8 (10):802–815.

Wolfrum, S., K. S. Jensen, and J. K. Liao. 2003. Endothelium-dependent effects of statins. *Arterioscler Thromb Vasc Biol* 23 (5):729–736.

Wong, N. D. 2014. Epidemiological studies of CHD and the evolution of preventive cardiology. *Nat Rev Cardiol* 11 (5):276–289.

World Health Organization. 2011. *Global Atlas on Cardiovascular Disease Prevention and Control.* Geneva: World Heart Federation and World Stroke Organization, WHO Press.

Xi, B., Y. Huang, K. H. Reilly, S. Li, R. Zheng, M. T. Barrio-Lopez, M. A. Martinez-Gonzalez, and D. Zhou. 2015. Sugar-sweetened beverages and risk of hypertension and CVD: A dose–response meta-analysis. *Br J Nutr* 113 (5):709–717.

Yang, Q., Z. Zhang, E. W. Gregg, W. D. Flanders, R. Merritt, and F. B. Hu. 2014. Added sugar intake and cardiovascular diseases mortality among US adults. *JAMA Intern Med* 174 (4):516–524.

Yang, R., and L. A. Barouch. 2007. Leptin signaling and obesity: Cardiovascular consequences. *Circ Res* 101 (6):545–559.

Zeb, I., and M. Budoff. 2015. Coronary artery calcium screening: Does it perform better than other cardiovascular risk stratification tools? *Int J Mol Sci* 16 (3):6606–6620.

Zhao, Y., R. Nicoll, Y. H. He, and M. Y. Henein. 2016. The effect of statins on valve function and calcification in aortic stenosis: A meta-analysis. *Atherosclerosis* 246:318–324.

Zhernakova, A., A. Kurilshikov, M. J. Bonder, E. F. Tigchelaar, M. Schirmer, T. Vatanen, Z. Mujagic et al. 2016. Population-based metagenomics analysis reveals markers for gut microbiome composition and diversity. *Science* 352 (6285):565–569.

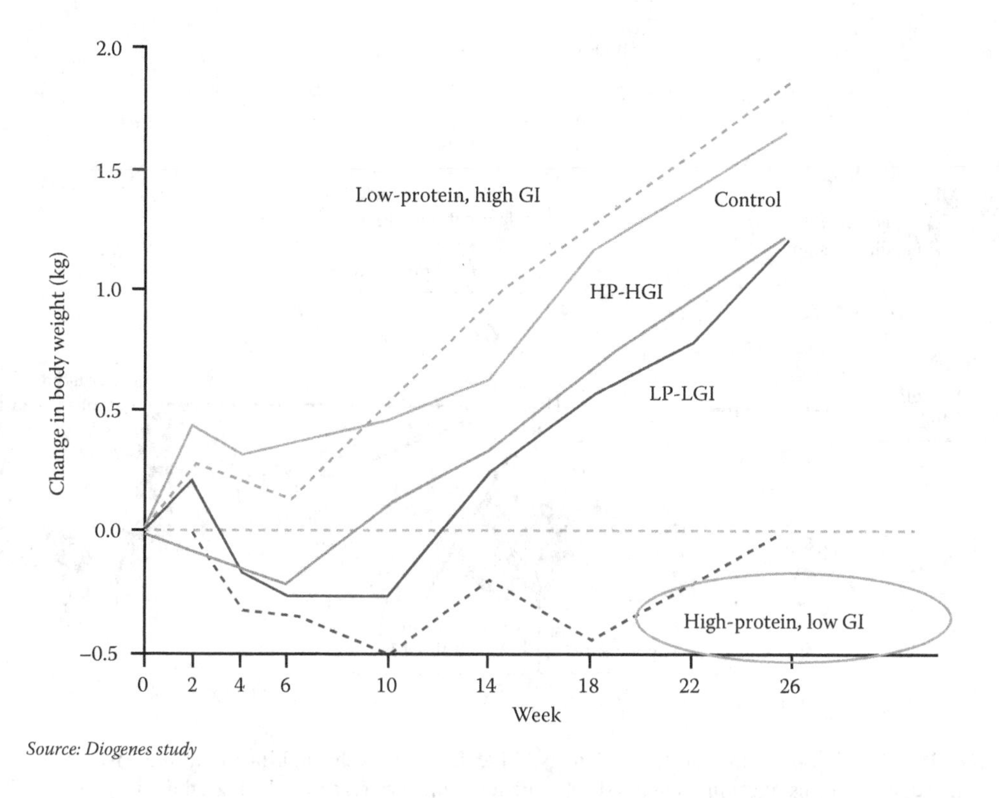

FIGURE 2.12 Science backs protein: change in body weight during the DIOGENES study. As the chart shows, the high-protein, low-GI diet produced the best weight loss results. HP, high protein; LP, low protein; HGI, high GI; LGI, low GI. (Reprinted from Larsen, T. M., *N. Engl. J. Med.*, 363(22), 2102–2113, 2010.)

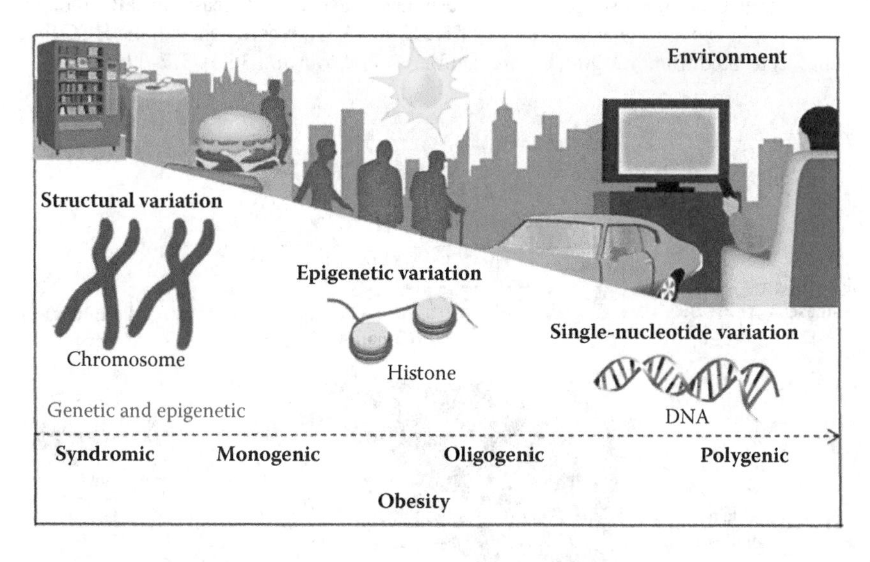

FIGURE 5.1 Contribution of genetic, epigenetic, and environmental stimuli to obesity. In monogenic and syndromic obesity, a single gene mutation could result in severe obesity, irrespective of environmental stimuli. However, in cases of oligogenic and polygenic obesity, environmental factors can exacerbate the progression of obesity if the individuals have a genetic predisposition to weight gain. (Reprinted from Pigeyre, M. et al., *Clin. Sci.*, 130, 943–986, 2016.)

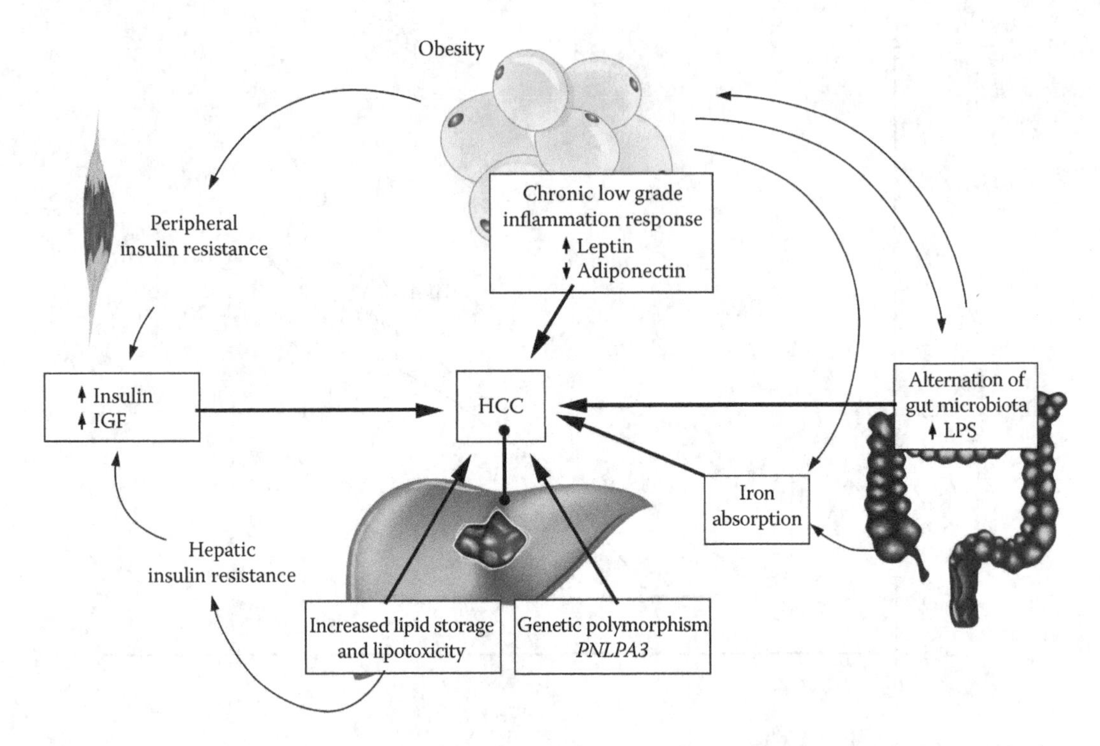

FIGURE 8.2 The development of HCC in NAFLD is most likely multifactorial and involves obesity-mediated mechanisms, including low-grade chronic inflammatory response, increased lipid storage and lipotoxicity, alteration of gut microbiota with increased levels of lipopolysaccharide (LPS), and insulin resistance with hyperinsulinemia and increased insulin-like growth factor (IGF) levels. Genetic polymorphisms might also contribute to the development of HCC in NASH. Increased iron absorption in NASH has also been reported recently; although the mechanisms are at present still being investigated, a contribution of iron in the development of HCC has been suggested. All these mechanisms are, at least partially, independent from fibrosis, and this might explain the epidemiology of HCC in NASH, where noncirrhotic HCC is more than a sporadic event. (Reprinted from Margini, C., and Dufour, J. F., *Liver Int.*, 36(3), 317–324, 2016.)

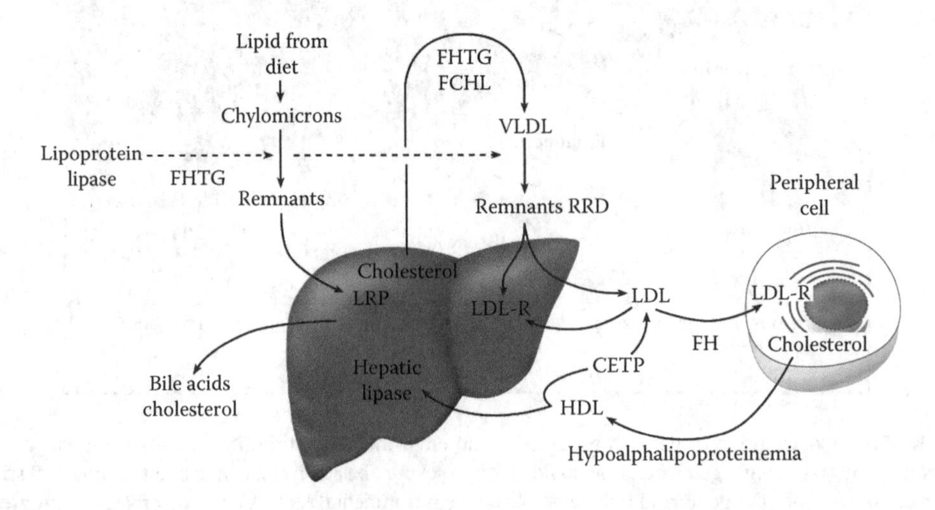

FIGURE 9.1 Pathways of lipid transport. (Reprinted from Knopp, R. H., *N. Engl. J. Med.*, 341(7), 498–511, 1999.)

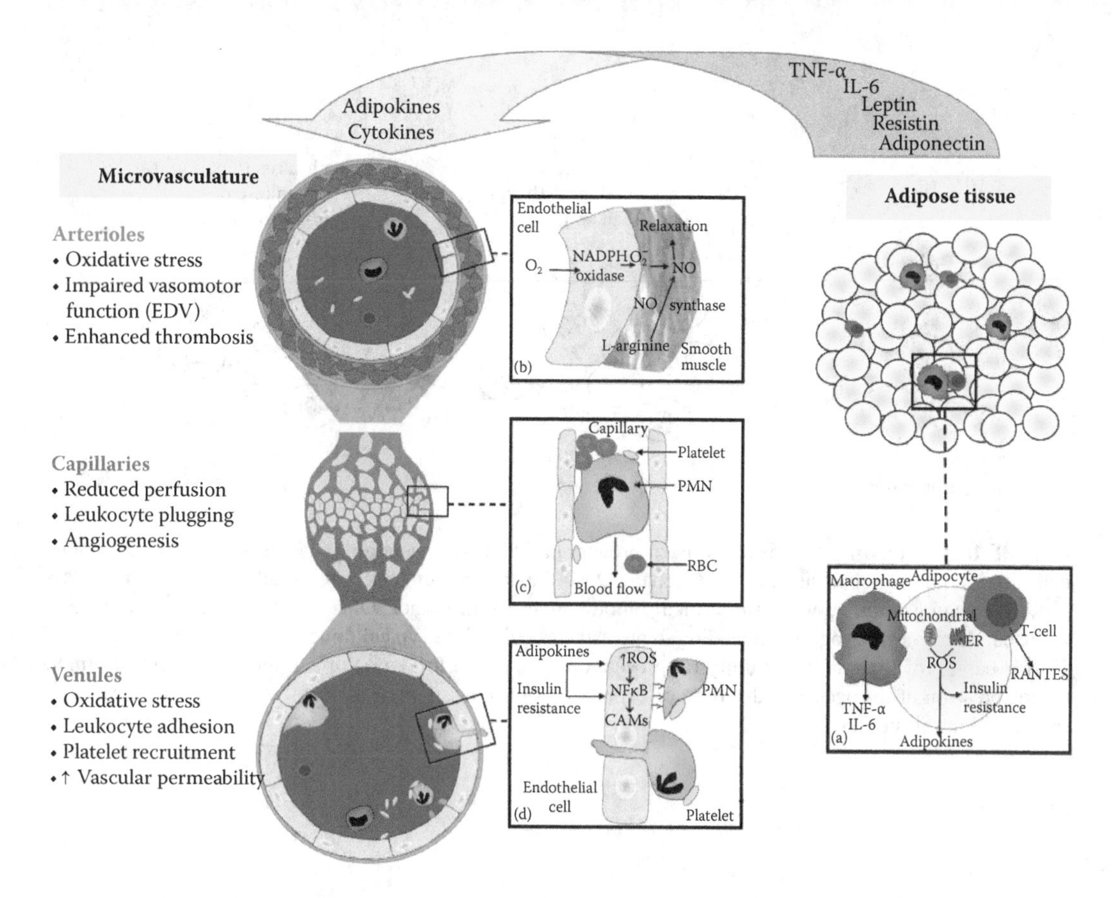

FIGURE 10.2 Interaction of excess visceral fat with cellular and molecular mechanisms promoting the progression of atherosclerosis. EDV, end-diastolic volume; NADPH, nicotinamide adenine dinucleotide phosphate; PMN, polymorphonuclear; RBC, red blood cell; ROS, reactive oxygen species; NFκB, nuclear factor κB; CAMs, cell adhesion molecules. (Reprinted from Vachharajani, V., and Granger, D. N., *IUBMB Life*, 61(4), 424–430, 2009.)

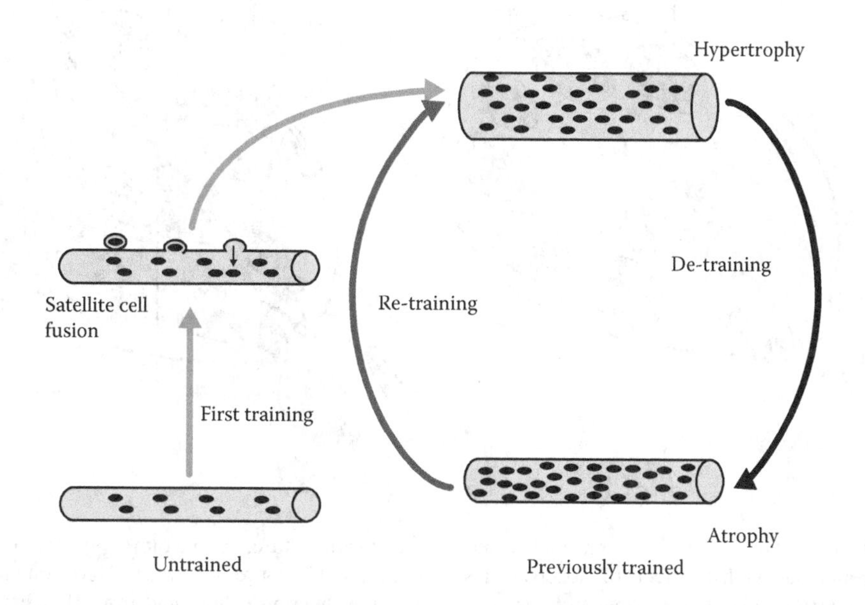

FIGURE 15.1 Model for the connection between muscle size and number of myonuclei. In this model, myonuclei are permanent. Previously untrained muscles acquire newly formed nuclei by fusion of satellite cells preceding the hypertrophy. Subsequent detraining leads to atrophy but no loss of myonuclei. The elevated number of nuclei in muscle fibers that had experienced a hypertrophic episode would provide a mechanism for muscle memory, explaining the long-lasting effects of training and the ease with which previously trained individuals are more easily retrained. (Reprinted from Egner, I. M. et al., *Development*, 143(16), 2898–2906, 2016.)

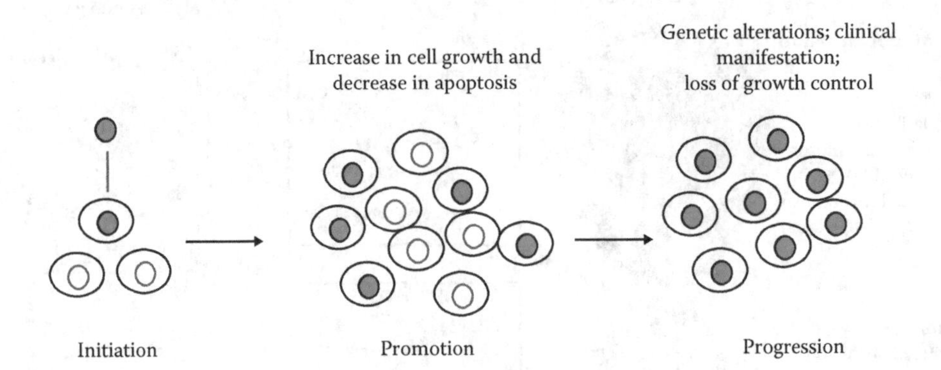

FIGURE 18.1 Tumorigenesis is a multistep process initiated with mutation of genes that control cell cycle, cell differentiation, apoptosis, and DNA repair. Once the cancer stem cells are established, the tumor mass grows as angiogenesis provides the critical blood supply to the tumor. Once the tumor mass is clinically detected, the phase of progression leading to metastasis begins. The typical tumor develops over a window of 10–15 years, providing an opportunity for prevention prior to the formation of a clinically detectable tumor. Overexpression of oncogenes and failure of expression of tumor suppressor genes in tumor cells have been implicated in this process.

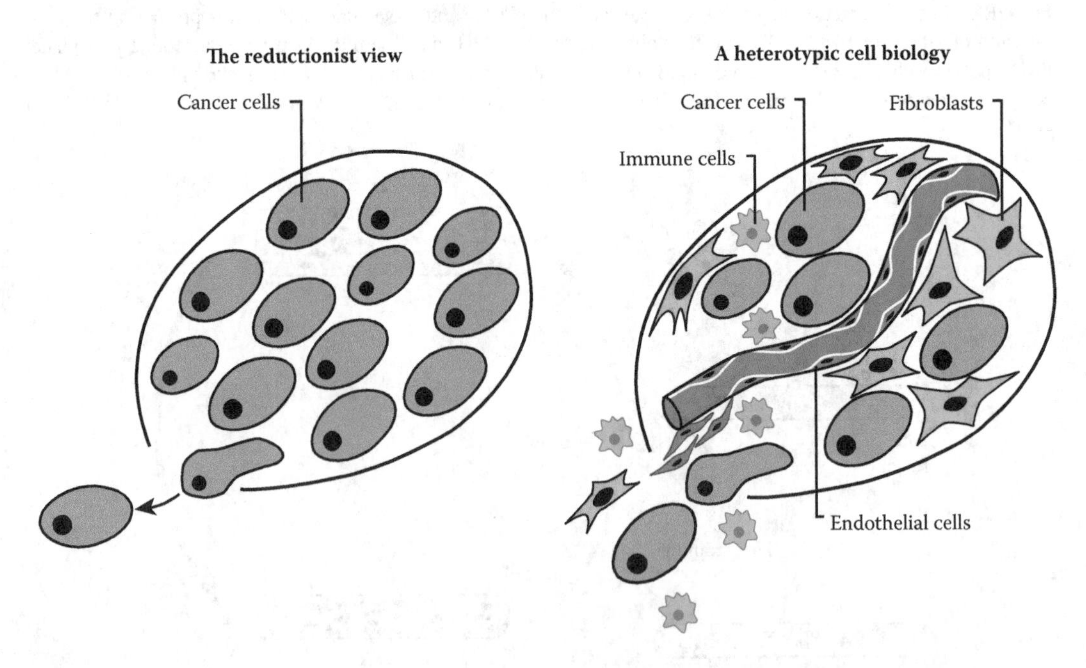

FIGURE 18.2 Much research is done on isolated cancer cells in culture, but the tumor microenvironment is complex and may mediate effects of bioactive substances not found in pure cell culture. Nutrition may impact tumor growth by inhibiting angiogenesis or altering immune function. (Reprinted from Hanahan, D., and Weinberg, R. A., *Cell*, 100(1), 57–70, 2000.)

11 Hypertension and Obesity

11.1 INTRODUCTION

In order to understand the common condition of obesity-associated hypertension, it is helpful to understand the regulation of body sodium and body water as an adaptation to ancient environments requiring exertion with the potential of limited or absent water and salt. On a natural plant-based diet, potassium would be plentiful and sodium would need to be conserved. Freshwater fish have a similar problem living in a sodium-poor environment. In addition, long days on the savannahs of Africa looking for food would create a need to maintain extracellular fluid volume in the face of water lost through sweat or the gastrointestinal tract. Just as modern humankind has flooded an obesogenic environment with sugar and fat, mostly hidden in processed foods, salt has also been introduced for its various benefits in food processing, including masking of off-tastes of meats and paradoxically enhancing the taste of some sweet and fat foods, such as salty chocolate bars. The key objectives for health in ancient environments would be to maintain adequate pressure and blood flow to nourish the organs and excrete toxins through the kidney in the face of water losses through sweat, diarrhea, or inadequate sources of water.

In discussing many of the issues around obesity, the concept that humankind is well adapted to starvation and poorly adapted to obesity resulting from changes in lifestyle and diet over the last few hundred years has been a key point of reference. The same notion applies to dehydration. If you stop all food intake and starve, within the first day, one of your major discomforts, in addition to hunger, will be thirst. A dinner at a restaurant with salty foods often leads to thirst a few hours later. While the body adapts to hunger through shifts in macronutrient metabolism, the drive to consume water and sodium continues unabated. The systems that are disordered in obesity and hypertension are the same ones that permitted survival under adverse conditions of salt or water restriction in ancient times.

Hypertension is extremely common, affecting one in three adult Americans and contributing to nearly half of all cardiovascular deaths in the United States (Egan et al. 2010). Obesity is by far the most common cause of essential hypertension. Although the diagnosis of hypertension is made at a sustained blood pressure (BP) level of 140/90 mmHg, the risk of cardiovascular death with elevated BP is actually a continuum of risk that doubles for every 20/10 mmHg rise in BP above 115/75 mmHg (Chobanian et al. 2003)—hence the creation of the new category of "prehypertension" in the hypertension classification scheme for BP (120–139/80–89 mmHg) to promote the adoption of lifestyle changes that have been shown to lower BP prior to the onset of hypertension.

As we have already discussed extensively in previous chapters, two-thirds of the U.S. population is either overweight or obese, and globally, for the first time in human history, there are more overweight than underweight individuals around the world. This chapter examines the overlap between these two common conditions, including the adaptive mechanisms underlying the influence of obesity on BP, and the role of nutrition and weight management in addressing this common and preventable condition that causes so much morbidity and mortality. Finally, we examine the controversies around sodium restriction as a primary means of nutritional prevention of hypertension, as well as the evidence for effective means of using potassium-rich, nitrate-rich vegetables; arginine-rich proteins; and antioxidant spices as strategies to enable the use of salt as a spice to retain the taste of foods while maintaining BP in the normal range.

11.2 EPIDEMIOLOGY OF OBESITY AND HYPERTENSION

BP varies in different populations and among individuals in the same population for a wide variety of reasons (Blackburn and Prineas 1982). Populations eating a vegetarian diet typically have lower BP than nonvegetarians, and plant-based dietary patterns in which whole grains, fruits, and vegetables are eaten regularly have been associated with lower BPs (Ascherio et al. 1996). As we discuss the mechanisms underlying BP elevation in association with obesity, the reasons for better BP maintenance as the result of eating a plant-based diet will become clear. BP typically increases with age, but the changes can be lessened by a high intake of fruits and vegetables in both men and women (Ascherio et al. 1992; Bazzano et al. 2002). The intake of as little as three or more servings of fruits and vegetables a day has been associated with a 42% lower stroke mortality and a 27% lower cardiovascular disease mortality in one cohort over 19 years after adjustment for established cardiovascular disease risk factors (Appel et al. 1997).

As a consequence of being overweight or obese, individuals have a higher prevalence of hypertension and of associated metabolic disorders. Studies in diverse populations throughout the world have shown that the relationship between body mass index (BMI) and systolic and diastolic BP is nearly linear (Jones et al. 1994; Hall 2003). Risk estimates from the Framingham Heart Study, for example, suggest that 78% of primary or essential hypertension in men and 65% in women can be ascribed to excess weight gain (Garrison et al. 1987). Clinical studies indicate that maintenance of a BMI of <25 kg/m^2 is effective in the primary prevention of hypertension, and that weight loss reduces BP in most hypertensive subjects (Jones et al. 1999; Stevens et al. 2001).

The distribution of fat is another important consideration. Most population studies that have investigated the relationship between obesity and BP have measured BMI rather than visceral or retroperitoneal fat, which appear to be better predictors of increased BP than subcutaneous fat (Tchernof and Després 2013). Although the importance of obesity, especially when associated with increased visceral or retroperitoneal fat, is well established as a cause of hypertension, the pathophysiological mechanisms involved, which are reviewed in the next sections, are complex and interacting. Therefore, in thinking about hypertension and obesity, it is important not to look for the single factor promoting this disorder and the drug that can reverse it. This goes against the grain of primary care education. Despite the availability of very sophisticated and targeted drugs, hypertension remains poorly addressed from a public health standpoint.

11.3 DIET IN OBESITY AND HYPERTENSION

The undesirable dietary changes in the United States contributing to both obesity and hypertension during the past 50 years include fructose, fat, and sodium. The introduction of high-fructose corn syrup (HFCS) and its dramatic increase in consumption compared with other carbohydrates after 1990 has been implicated in the observed increases in obesity, renal disease, and diabetes mellitus over the last few decades (Bray et al. 2004; Johnson et al. 2013; Khitan and Kim 2013). Fructose is found in sucrose, a disaccharide of fructose and glucose, as well as sugar cane, beets, and HFCS. In excess, all these sugars increase the circulating levels of triglycerides, insulin, glucose, and LDL cholesterol (Hallfrisch 1990). It is not that HFCS is a toxin, but rather that its widespread use in colas, cakes, pastries, and even pizza and ketchup has increased overall sugar and fructose consumption in the setting of an obesogenic environment. As fructose is phosphorylated initially without regard to energy status, the process continues unabated even in the face of excess calories from fructose. The need for phosphate to continue this process results in the stripping of phosphate consecutively from ATP, then ADP, then AMP and IMP leading to the formation of excess blood levels of uric acid with can cause gout or deposit in the kidney leading to kidney failure (Hallfrisch 1990) (Figure 11.1). Emerging evidence supports a role for uric acid in the development of hypertension, renal failure, and heart disease by decreasing nitric oxide (NO) (Nguyen et al. 2009; Johnson et al. 2013).

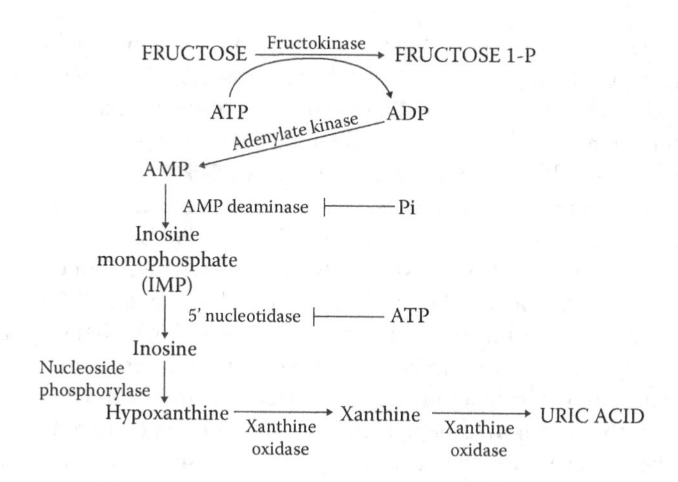

FIGURE 11.1 Fructose metabolism when excess in the liver leads to formation of uric acid, which is implicated in the metabolic syndrome. (Reprinted from Pillinger, M. H., and Keenan, R. T., *Bull. NYU Hosp. Jt. Dis.*, 66(3), 231–239, 2008.)

Another undesirable change in the Western diet has been an increase in the intake of omega-6 fatty acid-rich fats and oils, many hidden in processed food products (see Chapter 2 for a more detailed discussion). The excess of omega-6 from processed foods in the Western diet relative to a lack of intake of omega-3-rich fats from ocean-caught fish, seafood, and fish oil supplements has created an imbalance in the immune system favoring chronic low-grade inflammation. Omega-3 and omega-6 fatty acids must be obtained from the diet, and humans evolved on plant-based diets that contained fairly equal amounts of omega-6 and omega-3 fatty acids. However, in the past 50 years, the U.S. diet has become overloaded with omega-6 fatty acids, with a ratio of omega-6 to omega-3 of greater than 15 to 1. This increase in omega-6 intake reflected in blood and tissue content resulted from increased consumption of plant-derived oils such as corn oil, which have had the omega-3 removed to extend shelf life, as well as red meat from grain-fed animals, which are rich in omega-6 but not omega-3 fatty acids (Simopoulos 2002). Clinical studies demonstrate that fish oil supplements can lower BP in patients with hypertension (Appel et al. 1993; Morris et al. 1993).

The Dietary Approaches to Stop Hypertension (DASH) diet (Appel et al. 1997), which is rich in nutrients from fruits, vegetables, and dairy, with modest levels of sodium and omega-3 and omega-6 fatty acids, has emerged as a balanced dietary strategy for the management of hypertension. Approaches such as the DASH diet include green leafy (e.g., cabbages, spinach, and lettuces) and root (carrots and beets) vegetables that are rich in inorganic nitrate (Hord et al. 2009). Beetroot juice, which also contains high levels of inorganic nitrate, can also lower BP (Coles and Clifton 2012; Siervo et al. 2013). The nitrate content of these foods is likely to contribute to increased NO bioavailability, which has multiple beneficial pleiotropic effects in the vasculature, such as vasodilation (Moncada et al. 1991).

However, the DASH study also revealed another interesting finding. Subjects consuming the DASH diet with a similar sodium intake had even lower BPs than the low-sodium diet alone. This raised the question of how the DASH diet differed from the control diet, accounting for this added antihypertensive effect. The DASH diet contained more protein than the control diet (17.9% vs. 13.8%). To date, the majority of studies conducted on hypertensive patients to determine whether dietary protein intake has an effect on BP have suggested that a moderate increase in protein intake will indeed lower BP. For instance, a study conducted using the 10,020 participants from the International Study of Electrolyte Excretion and Blood Pressure (INTERSALT) investigated the relationship of BP and dietary protein. The study demonstrated an inverse relationship between BP and dietary protein intake (Stamler et al. 1996b). Similar results were found during other population-based studies, such as the Multiple Risk Factor Intervention Trial (MRFIT) (Stamler et al. 1996a), OmniHeart randomized trial (Bramlage et al. 2004), and Caerphilly Heart Study (Yach et al. 2006). Typically, human studies use data from 24-hour dietary recall, food frequency questionnaires, and common methods of BP measurement to determine whether an inverse relationship between protein intake and BP exists. However, human studies that used data from biochemical methods such as urinary markers of protein intake have also confirmed the existence of an inverse relationship between BP and protein intake (Krotkiewski et al. 1983).

One component of protein that may explain its antihypertensive properties is arginine. Soy protein, a protein rich in arginine, is effective in lowering BP (He et al. 2005). Dietary L-arginine can improve serum nitrate and nitrite levels, an index of NO bioavailability, in obese subjects (Mirmiran et al. 2016). The relationship between L-arginine and serum nitrate and nitrite levels is greater in obese normotensives than in obese hypertensives (Sledzinski et al. 2010). Therefore, it has been proposed that L-arginine-dependent NO formation is compromised in obese hypertensive subjects when compared with obese nonhypertensive subjects. Plasma nitrate and nitrite levels are lower in obese hypertensive subjects than in obese subjects without hypertension (Rajapakse et al. 2014).

Weight reduction in obese patients not only results in the expected decrease in BP but also was demonstrated to be associated with increased plasma nitrate and nitrite levels and reduced plasma L-arginine levels (Sledzinski et al. 2010). These findings are consistent with the concept that weight reduction improves L-arginine-dependent NO formation while also leading to normalization of BP.

L-Arginine is the main substrate for NO formation, and extracellular L-arginine concentration can affect NO bioavailability (Chin-Dusting et al. 2007; Rajapakse et al. 2014). Within the endothelial cell, L-arginine concentrations far exceed the amount needed for endothelial NO synthase, suggesting that transport of arginine into the cell is critical to the generation of NO (Chin-Dusting et al. 2007). In normal rats, the reduced expression or deletion of the gene for the L-arginine transporter protein, found in endothelial cells and in the kidney, results in the development of hypertension in otherwise normal rats (Kakoki et al. 2002). In experimentally induced obesity with hypertension animals, expression of the renal transporter for L-arginine is reduced (Rajapakse et al. 2014). Increasing endothelial-specific L-arginine transport, including that within the kidney, abolished obesity-induced hypertension in mice (Rajapakse et al. 2014). In addition, it has been demonstrated that arginase expression and activity are greater in obese hypertensive rats than in lean controls (Johnson et al. 2015). Arginase inhibition normalized BP in these rats, suggesting that augmented arginase activity and subsequent reductions in L-arginine levels can contribute to obesity-induced hypertension (Johnson et al. 2015). Augmented arginase activity has also been documented in morbidly obese humans (El Assar et al. 2016).

Increased dietary L-arginine can improve NO bioavailability in obese normotensive subjects, and this association is weakened in obese hypertensives (Mirmiran et al. 2016). Therefore, the association between the L-arginine-NO pathway and obesity-related hypertension holds true beyond the experimental setting. Further studies are required to determine the mechanisms underlying augmented arginase activity, impaired L-arginine transport, and reduced NO bioavailability in the setting of obesity.

These experimental and human observations raise an important question as to whether reductions in NO bioavailability are central to the development of obesity-associated hypertension (Giam et al. 2016). Support for this notion comes from findings that indicate that reduced NO levels can induce and maintain hypertension via multiple mechanisms (Rajapakse et al. 2014). Further experimental and, in particular, clinical studies are required to assess whether interventional strategies aimed at augmenting L-arginine transport and/or NO bioavailability can halt or reverse obesity-related hypertension in man and nitrite levels (Kakoki et al. 2002), and as expected, weight reduction also leads to reduced arterial pressure (Sledzinski et al. 2010).

11.4 MECHANISMS MEDIATING OBESITY-RELATED HYPERTENSION

This adaptation to dehydration starts in the hypothalamus with the secretion from hypothalamic nerve cells of arginine vasopression (AVP), also known as antidiuretic hormone (ADH). Secretion results from the shrinkage of specific nerve cells in the hypothalamus as the result of dehydration or other losses of perfusion. Dehydration leads to changes in membrane structure and physical effects on microtubules and ion channels. These changes are highly sensitive to osmolality dependent on sodium concentration related to hydration status (Figure 11.2). The end product of this interaction is the extracellular fluid volume that perfuses the kidney. This system works perfectly in healthy individuals when they lose fluid volume due to strenuous exercise, water deprivation, or increased water intake. Given that ancient man was dependent on running to find food or escape predators, being able to survive while losing fluid volume through sweating was a critical body function. Today, long-distance runners continue to be fascinated by the issue of water balance and hotly debate the best hydration for athletic performance.

The global epidemic of obesity and the concomitant increase in hypertension have led to numerous investigations over the past few decades into the role of obesity in the pathogenesis of hypertension. Overweight and obesity, especially when associated with increased visceral adiposity, increase the risk of hypertension, accounting for 65–75% of the risk for human primary or essential hypertension. Increased renal sodium retention impairs pressure-induced sodium excretion in renal tubules, playing a key role in the development of obesity-associated hypertension.

The mechanisms underlying abnormal kidney function and increased BP during the development of obesity-associated hypertension include activation of the renin–angiotensin–aldosterone system (RAAS), increased sympathetic nervous system (SNS) activity, and physical compression of the kidneys by fat in and around the kidneys. Other than physical compression of the kidneys by fat and secondary changes in fatty kidney promoting chronic kidney disease and renal failure,

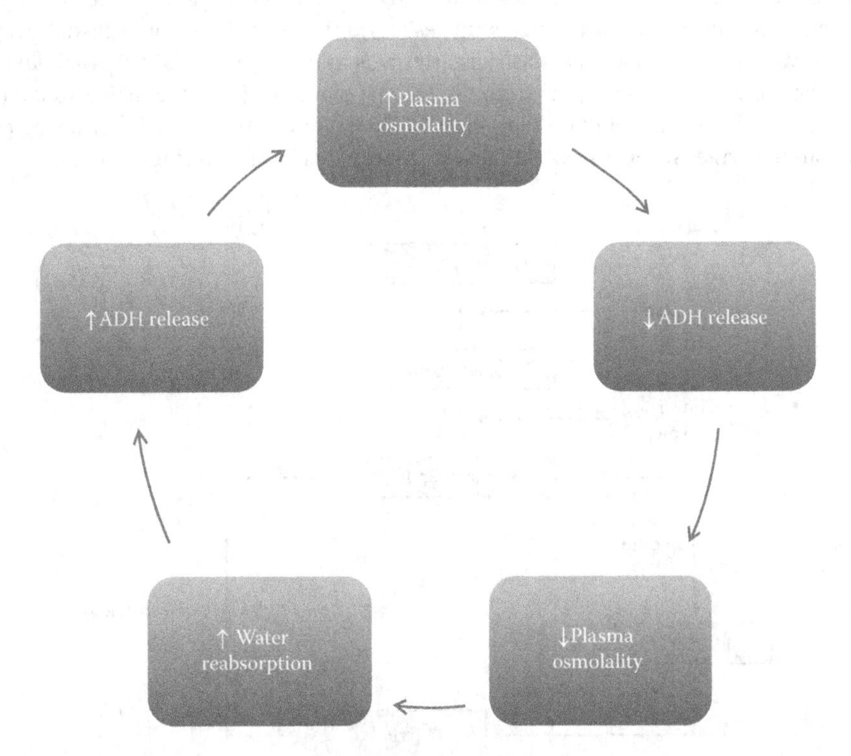

FIGURE 11.2 Plasma osmolality is tightly regulated between 275 and 295 mOsm/L by release of ADH, which prompts water reabsorption by the kidney. Similarly, a decrease in osmolality triggers a decrease in ADH secretion and greater water excretion by the kidneys.

the activation of the RAAS and the associated hormonal and SNS changes can be understood as a maladaptation of the normal mechanisms maintaining fluid and sodium homeostasis.

In order to understand the impact of obesity on hypertension at the level of the kidneys, it is useful to review some basic physiology principles. In 1989, Arthur C. Guyton was recognized for stating the hypothesis that sustained hypertension can occur only when the relationship between arterial pressure and sodium excretion in the urine is abnormal. If a normal relationship between BP and renal sodium excretion exists, then increased pressure results in increased sodium excretion and lowering of BP (Laragh 1989). In fact, the amount of sodium excreted in the urine reflects sodium intake and has been used in epidemiological studies to assess the impact of salt intake on BP and disease outcomes.

The hormone aldosterone, by increasing renal tubular sodium reabsorption, causes hypertension when present in excess due to endocrine disorders even in patients with normal renal function. Obesity is associated with increased blood flow, vasodilatation, cardiac output, and hypertension. Although cardiac index (cardiac output divided by body weight) does not increase, cardiac output and glomerular filtration are increased. Renal sodium reabsorption also increases, leading to hypertension (Hall 2000; Frohlich 2002; Hall et al. 2002).

The RAAS is a hormone system that acts to regulate the plasma sodium concentration and arterial BP, among other functions. The RAAS is activated whenever blood flow through the kidneys is reduced, and when there are sodium losses in conditions such as diarrhea, vomiting, or excessive sweating. These losses reduce extracellular fluid volume, and this in turn reduces arterial BP, which triggers the RAAS through several different mechanisms.

Whenever plasma sodium concentration is reduced or renal blood flow is reduced, juxtaglomerular cells in the kidneys convert prorenin into the enzyme renin, which is then secreted directly into the circulation. Plasma renin then removes a decapeptide from angiotensinogen, forming angiotensin I. Angiotensin I is then converted to angiotensin II, by the enzyme angiotensin-converting enzyme (ACE) found in the lung capillaries, which removes two amino acids from angiotensin I. Angiotensin II is a potent vasoactive peptide that constricts arterioles to increase arterial BP. Angiotensin II also stimulates the secretion of aldosterone from the adrenal gland. Aldosterone increases the reabsorption of sodium ions from the tubular fluid into the blood, while at the same time causing potassium excretion into the urine. When the RAAS is overactive, BP is increased (Figure 11.3).

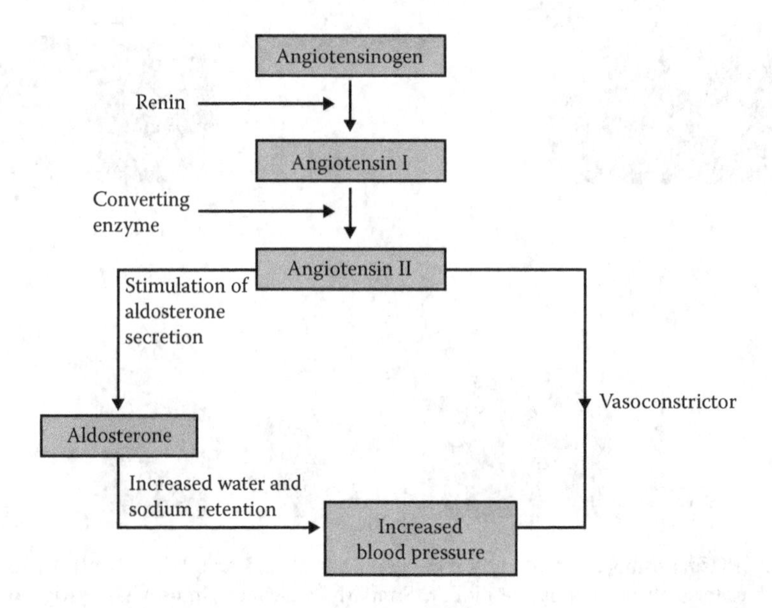

FIGURE 11.3 The RAAS maintains BP in the face of varying sodium and vascular volume challenges.

The RAAS also functions as a hormonal system that is able to act directly in many tissues in an autocrine and paracrine way (Paul et al. 2006). White adipose tissue (WAT) plays a central role in the pathophysiology of the metabolic syndrome not only through the secretion of angiotensinogen, but also because it accounts for the increased oxidative stress and the low-grade inflammatory state observed in obesity, which in turn favors insulin resistance (Paul et al. 2006).

RAAS blockade improves glucose homeostasis and prevents diabetes in patients suffering from the metabolic syndrome (Dream Trial Investigators et al. 2006; Andraws and Brown 2007; Navigator Study Group et al. 2010). Modulation of RAAS components leads to changes in body WAT content and function (Engeli et al. 2003; Giacchetti et al. 2005; Jandeleit-Dahm et al. 2005; Henriksen 2007; Luther and Brown 2011; Putnam et al. 2012; Underwood and Adler 2013). For example, RAAS in the WAT of lean subjects regulates adipogenesis, triglyceride storage, or release in a homeostatic fashion, while in obesity, RAAS increases oxidative stress and inflammation in WAT.

RAAS components are not only present in WAT but also produced in the skeletal muscle, the liver, and the pancreatic islets, where they modulate insulin production from β-cells. In these key tissues for blood glucose control, RAAS governs a dual axis with opposing effects on glucose homeostasis. The angiotensin II receptor type 1 (AT1R) and aldosterone favor hyperglycemia and generate an increased diabetes risk. On the flip side, the angiotensin II receptor type 2 (AT2R) tends to lower blood glucose and protect against the risk of developing diabetes.

Adipocytes in obese patients, especially those located in the visceral fat, contribute to vascular and systemic insulin resistance and stimulation of the SNS and RAAS (Kurukulasuriya et al. 2011; Sowers 2013). Structural and functional changes in the kidney, including activation of intrarenal angiotensin II, are also important in the development of obesity-associated hypertension (Sharma 2004). Arterial hypertension in obesity is mediated, in part, by increased intravascular volume, cardiac output (Messerli et al. 1981), and proximal tubule sodium absorption in the kidney (Strazzullo et al. 2001). However, cross talk between components of the intravascular RAAS, specifically angiotensin II and aldosterone, can also regulate vasoconstriction independently of renal control (McCurley et al. 2012; Bender et al. 2013).

Accumulating evidence suggests that endothelial dysfunction also contributes to vascular stiffness, which is in turn strongly associated with insulin resistance (Sandoo et al. 2010; Aroor et al. 2013). Impaired vascular reactivity to insulin before the onset of hypertension is seen in spontaneously hypertensive rats (Li et al. 2010), suggesting that insulin resistance is an early event in hypertension development.

Endothelial dysfunction and arterial stiffness are thought to be the earliest manifestations of vascular dysfunction in obesity and precede the development of prehypertension and hypertension (Liao et al. 1999; Femia et al. 2007; Cavalcante et al. 2011; Aroor et al. 2013). Increased arterial stiffness is seen in patients who are normotensive but have obesity and who are predisposed to develop hypertension; moreover, incident hypertension is more robustly predicted in patients who are in the highest quartile of arterial stiffness (Liao et al. 1999; Femia et al. 2007; Cavalcante et al. 2011; Aroor et al. 2013).

Effects on sodium and pressure natriuresis can be caused by an increase in adipose tissue mass and extracellular matrix accumulation, which compress the renal medulla. Renal vascular remodeling, characterized by inflammation, endothelial dysfunction, and vascular smooth muscle proliferation, is found in individuals with hypertension and ultimately contributes to progression to renal failure (Montecucco et al. 2011). Tubulointerstitial inflammation owing to a systemic immune and inflammatory response, elevated uric acid levels, tubulointestinal infiltration of immune cells, circulating pro-inflammatory immune cells and enhanced inflammation, oxidative stress, and fibrosis collectively contribute to renal damage (Kurukulasuriya et al. 2011; Harrison et al. 2012; Johnson et al. 2013; Khitan and Kim 2013).

In obesity, other systems interact with the normal control mechanisms. For example, activation of the RAAS is likely due, in part, to renal compression, as well as SNS activation. Obesity also causes mineralocorticoid receptor activation independent of aldosterone or angiotensin II.

SNS activation in obesity appears to require leptin and activation of the brain melanocortin system. With prolonged obesity and development of target organ injury, especially renal injury, obesity-associated hypertension often requires multiple antihypertensive drugs and treatment of other risk factors, including dyslipidemia, insulin resistance and diabetes, and inflammation. Obesity is a risk factor for so-called treatment-resistant hypertension, as these associated factors related to obesity and the metabolic syndrome are often not remedied in the setting of drug therapy for hypertension.

Other factors generally considered responsible for obesity-related alterations in the relationship between pressure and sodium excretion include enhanced sympathetic tone, activation of the RAAS, hyperinsulinemia, structural changes in the kidney, and visceral fat-associated adipokines.

11.5 NUTRITION APPROACHES TO OBESITY-ASSOCIATED HYPERTENSION AND THE METABOLIC SYNDROME

The morbidity and mortality of hypertension stem in part from the tendency of elevated BP to occur, together with other cardiovascular disease risk factors and a cluster of metabolic disorders known as metabolic syndrome. Since the risk of cardiovascular death at any given level of BP depends on the number of concurrent cardiovascular disease risk factors, a comprehensive clinical and laboratory cardiovascular risk assessment is needed to establish the cardiovascular disease burden and determine the scope of lifestyle changes and/or need for pharmaceutical intervention in patients with hypertension.

Many of the cardiovascular disease risk factors are behavioral and modifiable by lifestyle changes. Although the potential therapeutic impact of established lifestyle changes on BP varies across the spectrum, they have all been shown to lower BP and/or mitigate the risk of cardiovascular death in a dose- and time-dependent fashion.

11.5.1 Sodium Restriction in Therapy of Hypertension and Obesity

There is no disagreement that weight management is an essential component of treating obesity-associated hypertension based on the well-documented effects of weight reduction on BP (The Trials of Hypertension Prevention Collaborative Research Group 1997). Salt restriction as a recommendation to the general public has encountered significant controversy. Based on the discussions in this chapter, it should be clear that there is a difference in sodium regulation in obese and lean individuals. In the obese patient, insulin acts to retain sodium and water, which could increase BP. In the first week of a hypocaloric diet, a sodium chloride and water diuresis leads to weight loss and a decrease in BP. So if weight management is successful, sodium restriction becomes a secondary consideration. Sodium reduction will have some minor effects on BP, especially when vascular dysfunction is present.

The key recommendation to obese patients for sodium reduction should be to replace high-salt, high-fat, and high-sugar processed snack foods with fruits and vegetables. This has the dual effect of decreasing calorie intake and increasing both water and potassium intakes, which counteracts effects of dietary sodium. Salt used as a spice, together with other spices, can reduce excessive amounts of salt found in some snack foods, such as potato chips and processed meats. However, salt-free foods often sacrifice taste, leading to noncompliance. Spices can help maintain taste in the face of reduced salt, which properly used should be a spice to enhance taste and not an adulterant to cover up off-tastes or enhance the habituation of high sugar consumption. While the sodium consumed is generally excreted in normal individuals, in obese patients resistant to weight management, there is an argument that sodium increases BP and should be reduced.

Here are some tips that you can transmit to obese patients with hypertension:

1. Check nutrition labels on prepared and packaged foods, because up to 75% of the sodium consumed is hidden in processed foods. Watch for the words *soda* and *sodium* and the symbol Na on labels, which means sodium compounds are present.

2. Cook fresh, skinless poultry that is not enhanced with sodium solution, instead of fried or processed chicken.
3. Choose lower-sodium varieties of soups and enhance tastes with herbs and spices, such as cilantro, garlic, or chili powders.
4. Make sandwiches with lower-sodium meats and low-fat, low-sodium cheeses.
5. Eat more fruits and vegetables in preference to starchy salted side dishes. Fruits and vegetables have little sodium and lots of potassium, which can counter the effects of sodium.

During weight maintenance, the general guidelines for healthy individuals pertain. While no one argues with the kind of commonsense advice about healthy diets given above, there is a significant disagreement among scientists with regard to the 2300 mg/day and even stricter 1500 mg/day recommendations of government advisory groups.

Public health guidelines for the general public have recommended that adults consume less salt, but the relationship of salt intake to hypertension remains controversial (Institute of Medicine 2004, 2006, 2013). The need to define more precisely the efficacy of reduction in salt intake for the general population has been particularly controversial given conflicting Institute of Medicine (IOM) reports (Institute of Medicine 2004, 2006, 2013). One report defined a recommended upper sodium intake amount of 2300 mg/day or 100 mmol/day (Institute of Medicine 2004). However, the most recent IOM report concluded that "science was insufficient and inadequate to establish whether reducing sodium intake below 2300 mg/day either decreases or increases cardiovascular disease risk in the general population" (Institute of Medicine 2013). Furthermore, the 2300 mg/day recommendation is in conflict with the IOM's own rules on how to define adequate intake for a nutrient, which is "the approximate intake found in apparently healthy populations" (Institute of Medicine 2006). This is much higher than 2300 mg/day (McCarron et al. 2013).

When typical sodium intakes around the world based on urinary sodium excretion are estimated, the recommended levels are much lower than the usual levels of intake globally, which are in the range of 3000–5000 mg/day of sodium. Opponents of the government efforts to reduce sodium have stated, "If a 'normal' range of sodium intake exists that is consistent with the optimal function of established peripheral and central nervous system (CNS) mechanisms, that fact should be the sole basis of national nutrition guidelines for dietary sodium intake. To attempt to use public policy to abrogate human physiology would be futile and possibly harmful to human health" (McCarron et al. 2009).

The justification for the 2300 mg/day recommendation is based on the controversial association between sodium intake and BP (Graudal et al. 1998; Sacks et al. 2001; He and MacGregor 2002; Graudal et al. 2011) and on modeling studies (Bibbins-Domingo et al. 2010; Mozaffarian et al. 2014). These use selected cross-sectional sodium intake data and BP data to create a sodium dose–BP response relation and successively apply this dose–response relation to BP mortality data. Disregarding side effects, these models predict millions of lives saved through salt restriction (Bibbins-Domingo et al. 2010; Mozaffarian et al. 2014). However, these artificial data are in contrast to the outcome of real data from population studies, which indicate that both low and excessive sodium intake are associated with increased mortality, thus demonstrating a J-shape relation between sodium intake and outcome (Graudal et al. 2014).

Based on measures of urinary sodium excretion, which are the research standard, opponents of the guidelines to reduce salt intake see 2300 mg/day or 100 mmol/day as being below a physiological minimum of 117 mmol/day, where sodium appetite is increased, and doubt that such a reduction could be practically achieved.

11.5.2 Pharmacological Adjunctive Treatment May Be Necessary

Lifestyle modifications that include dietary changes, weight reduction, and exercise are the cornerstones in the prevention and treatment of obesity-associated prehypertension and hypertension.

However, adherence to this approach often meets with failure in clinical practice; therefore, drug therapy should not be delayed when hypertension is diagnosed.

This chapter, however, has approached the prevention and treatment of hypertension in obesity from a nutritional rather than the typical drug treatment vantage point. Changing diet and lifestyle can lead to a reduced need for medication, but careful follow-up is required to properly integrate nutrition and lifestyle changes with pharmacological treatment. A detailed discussion of the various pharmacological approaches to hypertension and the weaning of patients off of antihypertensive drugs as they lose weight is outside the scope of this chapter.

A practical issue in writing about pharmacological treatment is the variety of different drugs targeting sodium and fluid balance, the SNS, and different parts of the RAAS. Theoretically, the ideal pharmacological antihypertensive regimen should target the underlying mechanisms involved in this syndrome in obese patients, including sympathetic activation, increased renal tubular sodium reabsorption, and overexpression of the RAAS by the adipocyte. Few prospective trials have been conducted in the search for the ideal antihypertensive regimen in patients with obesity and hypertension. It is safe to say that the optimal antihypertensive drug therapy in these patients has not been defined and an individualized tailored approach should be taken based on efficacy and side effects.

Although caution exists regarding the use of thiazide diuretics due to potential metabolic derangements, there is insufficient data to show worsened cardiovascular or renal outcomes in patients treated with these drugs. In regard to β-blockers, the risk of accelerating conversion to diabetes and worsening of inflammatory mediators described in patients treated with traditional β-blockers appears much less pronounced or absent when using the vasodilating β-blockers. RAAS inhibition with an ACE or an angiotensin receptor blocker (ARB) and treatment with calcium channel blockers appear safe and well tolerated in obesity-related hypertension and in patients with metabolic syndrome.

Future prospective pharmacological studies in this population are needed.

11.6 SUMMARY AND OVERALL TREATMENT RECOMMENDATIONS

Hypertension, like obesity, remains a very common and significant risk factor for cardiovascular and renal diseases, including stroke, coronary heart disease, heart failure, and kidney failure, and obesity-associated hypertension is the most common form of essential hypertension. According to recent National Health and Nutrition Examination Survey (NHANES) surveys (1999–2000), 27% of adult Americans have hypertension (systolic BP of ≥140 mmHg, diastolic of BP ≥90 mmHg, or use of antihypertensive medication), and another 31% have prehypertension (systolic BP of 120–139 mmHg or diastolic BP of 80–89 mmHg, not on medication) (Wang and Wang 2004).

Prehypertensive individuals have a high probability of developing hypertension and carry an excess risk of cardiovascular disease compared with those with a normal BP (systolic BP of <120 mmHg and diastolic BP of <80 mmHg) (Vasan et al. 2001). It has been estimated that among adults over 50 years of age, the lifetime risk of developing hypertension approaches 90% (Vasan et al. 2002).

Notably, no evidence of a BP threshold exists. The risk of cardiovascular disease increases progressively throughout a range of increased BP, including for those in the prehypertensive range (Lewington et al. 2002). It has been estimated that almost a third of BP-related deaths from coronary heart disease occur in individuals with BP in the nonhypertensive range (Stamler et al. 1993).

Nutrition and lifestyle factors have a predominant role in BP regulation. In nonhypertensive individuals, including those with prehypertension, dietary changes that lower BP have the potential to prevent hypertension and, more broadly, reduce BP and thereby lower the risk of BP-related clinical complications. Indeed, even an apparently small reduction in BP, if applied to an entire population, could have an enormous beneficial impact. For instance, it has been estimated that a 3 mmHg reduction in systolic BP could lead to an 8% reduction in stroke mortality and a 5% reduction in mortality from coronary heart disease (Stamler 1991).

In uncomplicated stage I hypertension (systolic BP of 140–159 mmHg or diastolic BP of 90–99 mmHg), dietary changes can serve as initial treatment before the start of drug therapy.

Among hypertensive individuals who are already on drug therapy, dietary changes, particularly a reduced salt intake, can further lower BP and facilitate medication step-down. In general, the extent of BP reduction from dietary therapies is greater in hypertensive than in nonhypertensive individuals.

Numerous clinical trials have documented that weight loss lowers BP before attainment of a desirable body weight. In a meta-analysis that combined results from 25 clinical trials, mean systolic and diastolic BP reductions from an average weight loss of 5.1 kg were 4.4 and 3.6 mmHg, respectively (Stamler 1991). Within-trial dose–response analyses (Stevens et al. 1993; Neter et al. 2003) and prospective observational studies (Stevens et al. 2001) document that greater weight loss leads to greater BP reduction. Additional trials have documented that modest weight loss, with or without sodium reduction, can prevent hypertension by about 20% among overweight, prehypertensive individuals (Huang et al. 1998) and can facilitate medication step-down and drug withdrawal (Langford et al. 1985). Lifestyle intervention trials have uniformly achieved short-term weight loss, primarily through a reduction in total caloric intake, with maintenance achieved through a sustained habit of daily physical activity. After all is said and done, this is the central principle of nutrition therapy for obesity and hypertension.

REFERENCES

Andraws, R., and D. L. Brown. 2007. Effect of inhibition of the renin-angiotensin system on development of type 2 diabetes mellitus (meta-analysis of randomized trials). *Am J Cardiol* 99 (7):1006–1012.

Appel, L. J., E. R. Miller 3rd, A. J. Seidler, and P. K. Whelton. 1993. Does supplementation of diet with "fish oil" reduce blood pressure? A meta-analysis of controlled clinical trials. *Arch Intern Med* 153 (12):1429–1438.

Appel, L. J., T. J. Moore, E. Obarzanek, W. M. Vollmer, L. P. Svetkey, F. M. Sacks, G. A. Bray et al. 1997. A clinical trial of the effects of dietary patterns on blood pressure. DASH Collaborative Research Group. *N Engl J Med* 336 (16):1117–1124.

Aroor, A. R., V. G. Demarco, G. Jia, Z. Sun, R. Nistala, G. A. Meininger, and J. R. Sowers. 2013. The role of tissue renin-angiotensin-aldosterone system in the development of endothelial dysfunction and arterial stiffness. *Front Endocrinol (Lausanne)* 4:161.

Ascherio, A., C. Hennekens, W. C. Willett, F. Sacks, B. Rosner, J. Manson, J. Witteman, and M. J. Stampfer. 1996. Prospective study of nutritional factors, blood pressure, and hypertension among US women. *Hypertension* 27 (5):1065–1072.

Ascherio, A., E. B. Rimm, E. L. Giovannucci, G. A. Colditz, B. Rosner, W. C. Willett, F. Sacks, and M. J. Stampfer. 1992. A prospective study of nutritional factors and hypertension among US men. *Circulation* 86 (5):1475–1484.

Bazzano, L. A., J. He, L. G. Ogden, C. M. Loria, S. Vupputuri, L. Myers, and P. K. Whelton. 2002. Fruit and vegetable intake and risk of cardiovascular disease in US adults: The first National Health and Nutrition Examination Survey Epidemiologic Follow-up Study. *Am J Clin Nutr* 76 (1):93–99.

Bender, S. B., A. P. McGraw, I. Z. Jaffe, and J. R. Sowers. 2013. Mineralocorticoid receptor-mediated vascular insulin resistance: An early contributor to diabetes-related vascular disease? *Diabetes* 62 (2):313–319.

Bibbins-Domingo, K., G. M. Chertow, P. G. Coxson, A. Moran, J. M. Lightwood, M. J. Pletcher, and L. Goldman. 2010. Projected effect of dietary salt reductions on future cardiovascular disease. *N Engl J Med* 362 (7):590–599.

Blackburn, H., and R. Prineas. 1982. Diet and hypertension: Anthropology, epidemiology, and public health implications. *Prog Biochem Pharmacol* 19:31–79.

Bramlage, P., D. Pittrow, H. U. Wittchen, W. Kirch, S. Boehler, H. Lehnert, M. Hoefler, T. Unger, and A. M. Sharma. 2004. Hypertension in overweight and obese primary care patients is highly prevalent and poorly controlled. *Am J Hypertens* 17 (10):904–910.

Bray, G. A., S. J. Nielsen, and B. M. Popkin. 2004. Consumption of high-fructose corn syrup in beverages may play a role in the epidemic of obesity. *Am J Clin Nutr* 79 (4):537–543.

Cavalcante, J. L., J. A. Lima, A. Redheuil, and M. H. Al-Mallah. 2011. Aortic stiffness: Current understanding and future directions. *J Am Coll Cardiol* 57 (14):1511–1522.

Chin-Dusting, J. P., L. Willems, and D. M. Kaye. 2007. L-Arginine transporters in cardiovascular disease: A novel therapeutic target. *Pharmacol Ther* 116 (3):428–436.

Chobanian, A. V., G. L. Bakris, H. R. Black, W. C. Cushman, L. A. Green, J. L. Izzo, D. W. Jones, B. J. Materson, S. Oparil, and J. T. Wright. 2003. Seventh report of the Joint National Committee on Prevention, Detection, Evaluation, and Treatment of High Blood Pressure. *Hypertension* 42 (6):1206–1252.

Coles, L. T., and P. M. Clifton. 2012. Effect of beetroot juice on lowering blood pressure in free-living, disease-free adults: A randomized, placebo-controlled trial. *Nutr J* 11:106.

Dream Trial Investigators, J. Bosch, S. Yusuf, H. C. Gerstein, J. Pogue, P. Sheridan, G. Dagenais et al. 2006. Effect of ramipril on the incidence of diabetes. *N Engl J Med* 355 (15):1551–1562.

Egan, B. M., Y. Zhao, and R. N. Axon. 2010. US trends in prevalence, awareness, treatment, and control of hypertension, 1988–2008. *JAMA* 303 (20):2043–2050.

El Assar, M., J. Angulo, M. Santos-Ruiz, J. C. Ruiz de Adana, M. L. Pindado, A. Sanchez-Ferrer, A. Hernandez, and L. Rodriguez-Manas. 2016. Asymmetric dimethylarginine (ADMA) elevation and arginase up-regulation contribute to endothelial dysfunction related to insulin resistance in rats and morbidly obese humans. *J Physiol* 594 (11):3045–3060.

Engeli, S., P. Schling, K. Gorzelniak, M. Boschmann, J. Janke, G. Ailhaud, M. Teboul, F. Massiera, and A. M. Sharma. 2003. The adipose-tissue renin-angiotensin-aldosterone system: Role in the metabolic syndrome? *Int J Biochem Cell Biol* 35 (6):807–825.

Femia, R., M. Kozakova, M. Nannipieri, C. Gonzales-Villalpando, M. P. Stern, S. M. Haffner, and E. Ferrannini. 2007. Carotid intima-media thickness in confirmed prehypertensive subjects: Predictors and progression. *Arterioscler Thromb Vasc Biol* 27 (10):2244–2249.

Frohlich, E. D. 2002. Clinical management of the obese hypertensive patient. *Cardiol Rev* 10 (3):127–138.

Garrison, R. J., W. B. Kannel, J. Stokes, and W. P. Castelli. 1987. Incidence and precursors of hypertension in young adults: The Framingham Offspring Study. *Prev Med* 16 (2):235–251.

Giacchetti, G., L. A. Sechi, S. Rilli, and R. M. Carey. 2005. The renin-angiotensin-aldosterone system, glucose metabolism and diabetes. *Trends Endocrinol Metab* 16 (3):120–126.

Giam, B., S. Kuruppu, G. A. Head, D. M. Kaye, and N. W. Rajapakse. 2016. Effects of dietary L-arginine on nitric oxide bioavailability in obese normotensive and obese hypertensive subjects. *Nutrients* 8 (6):E364.

Graudal, N. A., A. M. Galloe, and P. Garred. 1998. Effects of sodium restriction on blood pressure, renin, aldosterone, catecholamines, cholesterols, and triglyceride: A meta-analysis. *JAMA* 279 (17):1383–1391.

Graudal, N. A., T. Hubeck-Graudal, and G. Jurgens. 2011. Effects of low sodium diet versus high sodium diet on blood pressure, renin, aldosterone, catecholamines, cholesterol, and triglyceride. *Cochrane Database Syst Rev* (11):CD004022.

Graudal, N., G. Jurgens, B. Baslund, and M. H. Alderman. 2014. Compared with usual sodium intake, low- and excessive-sodium diets are associated with increased mortality: A meta-analysis. *Am J Hypertens* 27 (9):1129–1137.

Hall, J. E. 2000. Pathophysiology of obesity hypertension. *Curr Hypertens Rep* 2 (2):139–147.

Hall, J. E. 2003. The kidney, hypertension, and obesity. *Hypertension* 41 (3):625–633.

Hall, J. E., E. D. Crook, D. W. Jones, M. R. Wofford, and P. M. Dubbert. 2002. Mechanisms of obesity-associated cardiovascular and renal disease. *Am J Med Sci* 324 (3):127–137.

Hallfrisch, J. 1990. Metabolic effects of dietary fructose. *FASEB J* 4 (9):2652–2660.

Harrison, D. G., P. J. Marvar, and J. M. Titze. 2012. Vascular inflammatory cells in hypertension. *Front Physiol* 3:128.

He, F. J., and G. A. MacGregor. 2002. Effect of modest salt reduction on blood pressure: A meta-analysis of randomized trials. Implications for public health. *J Hum Hypertens* 16 (11):761–770.

He, J., D. Gu, X. Wu, J. Chen, X. Duan, J. Chen, and P. K. Whelton. 2005. Effect of soybean protein on blood pressure: A randomized, controlled trial. *Ann Intern Med* 143 (1):1–9.

Henriksen, E. J. 2007. Improvement of insulin sensitivity by antagonism of the renin-angiotensin system. *Am J Physiol Regul Integr Comp Physiol* 293 (3):R974–R980.

Hord, N. G., Y. Tang, and N. S. Bryan. 2009. Food sources of nitrates and nitrites: The physiologic context for potential health benefits. *Am J Clin Nutr* 90 (1):1–10.

Huang, Z., W. C. Willett, J. E. Manson, B. Rosner, M. J. Stampfer, F. E. Speizer, and G. A. Colditz. 1998. Body weight, weight change, and risk for hypertension in women. *Ann Intern Med* 128 (2):81–88.

Institute of Medicine. 2004. *Dietary reference intakes: Water, potassium, sodium, chloride, and sulfate.* Washington, DC: National Academies Press.

Institute of Medicine. 2006. *Dietary reference intakes: Essential guide to nutrient requirements.* Washington, DC: National Academies Press.

Institute of Medicine. 2013. *Sodium intake in populations: Assessment of evidence.* Washington, DC: National Academies Press.

Jandeleit-Dahm, K. A., C. Tikellis, C. M. Reid, C. I. Johnston, and M. E. Cooper. 2005. Why blockade of the renin-angiotensin system reduces the incidence of new-onset diabetes. *J Hypertens* 23 (3):463–473.

Johnson, F. K., K. J. Peyton, X. M. Liu, M. A. Azam, A. R. Shebib, R. A. Johnson, and W. Durante. 2015. Arginase promotes endothelial dysfunction and hypertension in obese rats. *Obesity (Silver Spring)* 23 (2):383–390.

Johnson, R. J., T. Nakagawa, L. G. Sanchez-Lozada, M. Shafiu, S. Sundaram, M. Le, T. Ishimoto, Y. Y. Sautin, and M. A. Lanaspa. 2013. Sugar, uric acid, and the etiology of diabetes and obesity. *Diabetes* 62 (10):3307–3315.

Jones, D. W., J. S. Kim, M. E. Andrew, S. J. Kim, and Y. P. Hong. 1994. Body mass index and blood pressure in Korean men and women: The Korean National Blood Pressure Survey. *J Hypertens* 12 (12):1433.

Jones, D. W., M. E. Miller, M. R. Wofford, D. C. Anderson, M. E. Cameron, D. L. Willoughby, C. T. Adair, and N. S. King. 1999. The effect of weight loss intervention on antihypertensive medication requirements in the Hypertension Optimal Treatment (HOT) study. *Am J Hypertens* 12 (12):1175–1180.

Kakoki, M., W. Wang, and D. L. Mattson. 2002. Cationic amino acid transport in the renal medulla and blood pressure regulation. *Hypertension* 39 (2):287–292.

Khitan, Z., and D. H. Kim. 2013. Fructose: A key factor in the development of metabolic syndrome and hypertension. *J Nutr Metab* 2013:682673.

Krotkiewski, M., P. Bjorntorp, L. Sjostrom, and U. Smith. 1983. Impact of obesity on metabolism in men and women. Importance of regional adipose tissue distribution. *J Clin Invest* 72 (3):1150–1162.

Kurukulasuriya, L. R., S. Stas, G. Lastra, C. Manrique, and J. R. Sowers. 2011. Hypertension in obesity. *Med Clin North Am* 95 (5):903–917.

Langford, H. G., M. D. Blaufox, A. Oberman, C. M. Hawkins, J. D. Curb, G. R. Cutter, S. Wassertheil-Smoller et al. 1985. Dietary therapy slows the return of hypertension after stopping prolonged medication. *JAMA* 253 (5):657–664.

Laragh, J. H. 1989. Presentation of the Harvey Award to Arthur C. Guyton. *Am J Hypertens* 2 (7):573–574.

Lewington, S., R. Clarke, N. Qizilbash, R. Peto, R. Collins, and Prospective Studies Collaboration. 2002. Age-specific relevance of usual blood pressure to vascular mortality: A meta-analysis of individual data for one million adults in 61 prospective studies. *Lancet* 360 (9349):1903–1913.

Li, R., H. Zhang, W. Wang, X. Wang, Y. Huang, C. Huang, and F. Gao. 2010. Vascular insulin resistance in prehypertensive rats: Role of PI3-kinase/Akt/eNOS signaling. *Eur J Pharmacol* 628 (1–3):140–147.

Liao, D., D. K. Arnett, H. A. Tyroler, W. A. Riley, L. E. Chambless, M. Szklo, and G. Heiss. 1999. Arterial stiffness and the development of hypertension. The ARIC study. *Hypertension* 34 (2):201–206.

Luther, J. M., and N. J. Brown. 2011. The renin-angiotensin-aldosterone system and glucose homeostasis. *Trends Pharmacol Sci* 32 (12):734–739.

McCarron, D. A., J. C. Geerling, A. G. Kazaks, and J. S. Stern. 2009. Can dietary sodium intake be modified by public policy? *Clin J Am Soc Nephrol* 4 (11):1878–1882.

McCarron, D. A., A. G. Kazaks, J. C. Geerling, J. S. Stern, and N. A. Graudal. 2013. Normal range of human dietary sodium intake: A perspective based on 24-hour urinary sodium excretion worldwide. *Am J Hypertens* 26 (10):1218–1223.

McCurley, A., P. W. Pires, S. B. Bender, M. Aronovitz, M. J. Zhao, D. Metzger, P. Chambon, M. A. Hill, A. M. Dorrance, M. E. Mendelsohn, and I. Z. Jaffe. 2012. Direct regulation of blood pressure by smooth muscle cell mineralocorticoid receptors. *Nat Med* 18 (9):1429–1433.

Messerli, F. H., B. Christie, J. G. DeCarvalho, G. G. Aristimuno, D. H. Suarez, G. R. Dreslinski, and E. D. Frohlich. 1981. Obesity and essential hypertension. Hemodynamics, intravascular volume, sodium excretion, and plasma renin activity. *Arch Intern Med* 141 (1):81–85.

Mirmiran, P., Z. Bahadoran, A. Ghasemi, and F. Azizi. 2016. The association of dietary l-arginine intake and serum nitric oxide metabolites in adults: A population-based study. *Nutrients* 8 (5):311.

Moncada, S., R. M. Palmer, and E. A. Higgs. 1991. Nitric oxide: Physiology, pathophysiology, and pharmacology. *Pharmacol Rev* 43 (2):109–142.

Montecucco, F., A. Pende, A. Quercioli, and F. Mach. 2011. Inflammation in the pathophysiology of essential hypertension. *J Nephrol* 24 (1):23–34.

Morris, M. C., F. Sacks, and B. Rosner. 1993. Does fish oil lower blood pressure? A meta-analysis of controlled trials. *Circulation* 88 (2):523–533.

Mozaffarian, D., S. Fahimi, G. M. Singh, R. Micha, S. Khatibzadeh, R. E. Engell, S. Lim, G. Danaei, M. Ezzati, J. Powles, and Global Burden of Diseases Nutrition and Chronic Diseases Expert Group. 2014. Global sodium consumption and death from cardiovascular causes. *N Engl J Med* 371 (7):624–634.

Navigator Study Group, J. J. McMurray, R. R. Holman, S. M. Haffner, M. A. Bethel, B. Holzhauer, T. A. Hua et al. 2010. Effect of valsartan on the incidence of diabetes and cardiovascular events. *N Engl J Med* 362 (16):1477–1490.

Neter, J. E., B. E. Stam, F. J. Kok, D. E. Grobbee, and J. M. Geleijnse. 2003. Influence of weight reduction on blood pressure: A meta-analysis of randomized controlled trials. *Hypertension* 42 (5):878–884.

Nguyen, S., H. K. Choi, R. H. Lustig, and C. Y. Hsu. 2009. Sugar-sweetened beverages, serum uric acid, and blood pressure in adolescents. *J Pediatr* 154 (6):807–813.

Paul, M., A. Poyan Mehr, and R. Kreutz. 2006. Physiology of local renin-angiotensin systems. *Physiol Rev* 86 (3):747–803.

Pillinger, M. H., and R. T. Keenan. 2008. Update on the management of hyperuricemia and gout. *Bull NYU Hosp Jt Dis* 66 (3):231–239.

Putnam, K., R. Shoemaker, F. Yiannikouris, and L. A. Cassis. 2012. The renin-angiotensin system: A target of and contributor to dyslipidemias, altered glucose homeostasis, and hypertension of the metabolic syndrome. *Am J Physiol Heart Circ Physiol* 302 (6):H1219–H1230.

Rajapakse, N. W., F. Karim, N. E. Straznicky, S. Fernandez, R. G. Evans, G. A. Head, and D. M. Kaye. 2014. Augmented endothelial-specific L-arginine transport prevents obesity-induced hypertension. *Acta Physiol (Oxf)* 212 (1):39–48.

Sacks, F. M., L. P. Svetkey, W. M. Vollmer, L. J. Appel, G. A. Bray, D. Harsha, E. Obarzanek et al. 2001. Effects on blood pressure of reduced dietary sodium and the Dietary Approaches to Stop Hypertension (DASH) diet. DASH-Sodium Collaborative Research Group. *N Engl J Med* 344 (1):3–10.

Sandoo, A., J. J. van Zanten, G. S. Metsios, D. Carroll, and G. D. Kitas. 2010. The endothelium and its role in regulating vascular tone. *Open Cardiovasc Med J* 4:302–312.

Sharma, A. M. 2004. Is there a rationale for angiotensin blockade in the management of obesity hypertension? *Hypertension* 44 (1):12–19.

Siervo, M., J. Lara, I. Ogbonmwan, and J. C. Mathers. 2013. Inorganic nitrate and beetroot juice supplementation reduces blood pressure in adults: A systematic review and meta-analysis. *J Nutr* 143 (6):818–826.

Simopoulos, A. P. 2002. The importance of the ratio of omega-6/omega-3 essential fatty acids. *Biomed Pharmacother* 56 (8):365–379.

Sledzinski, T., M. Sledzinski, R. T. Smolenski, and J. Swierczynski. 2010. Increased serum nitric oxide concentration after bariatric surgery—A potential mechanism for cardiovascular benefit. *Obes Surg* 20 (2):204–210.

Sowers, J. R. 2013. Diabetes mellitus and vascular disease. *Hypertension* 61 (5):943–947.

Stamler, J., A. Caggiula, G. A. Grandits, M. Kjelsberg, and J. A. Cutler. 1996a. Relationship to blood pressure of combinations of dietary macronutrients. Findings of the Multiple Risk Factor Intervention Trial (MRFIT). *Circulation* 94 (10):2417–2423.

Stamler, J., P. Elliott, H. Kesteloot, R. Nichols, G. Claeys, A. R. Dyer, and R. Stamler. 1996b. Inverse relation of dietary protein markers with blood pressure. Findings for 10,020 men and women in the INTERSALT study. INTERSALT Cooperative Research Group. INTERnational study of SALT and blood pressure. *Circulation* 94 (7):1629–1634.

Stamler, J., R. Stamler, and J. D. Neaton. 1993. Blood pressure, systolic and diastolic, and cardiovascular risks. US population data. *Arch Intern Med* 153 (5):598–615.

Stamler, R. 1991. Implications of the INTERSALT study. *Hypertension* 17 (1 Suppl):I16–I20.

Stevens, V. J., S. A. Corrigan, E. Obarzanek, E. Bernauer, N. R. Cook, P. Hebert, M. Mattfeldt-Beman et al. 1993. Weight loss intervention in phase 1 of the Trials of Hypertension Prevention. The TOHP Collaborative Research Group. *Arch Intern Med* 153 (7):849–858.

Stevens, V. J., E. Obarzanek, N. R. Cook, I. M. Lee, L. J. Appel, D. Smith West, N. C. Milas et al. 2001. Long-term weight loss and changes in blood pressure: Results of the Trials of Hypertension Prevention, phase II. *Ann Intern Med* 134 (1):1–11.

Strazzullo, P., G. Barba, F. P. Cappuccio, A. Siani, M. Trevisan, E. Farinaro, E. Pagano, A. Barbato, R. Iacone, and F. Galletti. 2001. Altered renal sodium handling in men with abdominal adiposity: A link to hypertension. *J Hypertens* 19 (12):2157–2164.

Tchernof, A., and J.-P. Després. 2013. Pathophysiology of human visceral obesity: An update. *Physiol Rev* 93 (1):359–404.

The Trials of Hypertension Prevention Collaborative Research Group. 1997. Effects of weight loss and sodium reduction intervention on blood pressure and hypertension incidence in overweight people with high-normal blood pressure. The Trials of Hypertension Prevention, phase II. *Arch Intern Med* 157 (6):657–667.

Underwood, P. C., and G. K. Adler. 2013. The renin angiotensin aldosterone system and insulin resistance in humans. *Curr Hypertens Rep* 15 (1):59–70.

Vasan, R. S., A. Beiser, S. Seshadri, M. G. Larson, W. B. Kannel, R. B. D'Agostino, and D. Levy. 2002. Residual lifetime risk for developing hypertension in middle-aged women and men: The Framingham Heart Study. *JAMA* 287 (8):1003–1010.

Vasan, R. S., M. G. Larson, E. P. Leip, J. C. Evans, C. J. O'Donnell, W. B. Kannel, and D. Levy. 2001. Impact of high-normal blood pressure on the risk of cardiovascular disease. *N Engl J Med* 345 (18):1291–1297.

Wang, Y., and Q. J. Wang. 2004. The prevalence of prehypertension and hypertension among US adults according to the new joint national committee guidelines: New challenges of the old problem. *Arch Intern Med* 164 (19):2126–2134.

Yach, D., D. Stuckler, and K. D. Brownell. 2006. Epidemiologic and economic consequences of the global epidemics of obesity and diabetes. *Nat Med* 12 (1):62–66.

12 Nutrition, Chronic Kidney Disease, and Kidney Failure

12.1 INTRODUCTION

Obesity is associated with an increase in the risk of a number of age-related chronic diseases, including chronic kidney disease (CKD), which often progresses to renal failure (Bray et al. 1998; Anon 2000; U.S. Department of Health and Human Services 2001). In the United States, obesity is now the second leading cause of preventable disease and death, surpassed only by smoking. These two common conditions are clearly connected by more than coincidence, as both the association and the pathogenic mechanisms involved are well established (Kambham et al. 2001; Fox et al. 2004). The concurrent rise in CKD with the dramatic rise in obesity has led to an increased prevalence of renal failure, doubling in the past decade (Hsu et al. 2006). The prevalence of CKD has held steady since the early 2000s, a reversal of the previous increasing trend from the 1990s, according to a report from the Centers for Disease Control and Prevention Chronic Kidney Disease Surveillance Team (Murphy et al. 2016).

The number of people with end-stage renal disease (ESRD) has been increasing over the past four decades, but recent studies have suggested a declining incidence of the disease. The crude prevalence of stage 3 and 4 CKD increased from 4.8% in 1988–1994 to 6.9% in 2003–2004, but remained stable thereafter, with a prevalence of 6.9% in 2011–2012 (Murphy et al. 2016). Non-Hispanic whites showed a prevalence trend similar to the overall trend, but the crude prevalence among non-Hispanic blacks increased progressively across the study period, from 3.7% in 1988–1994 to 4.9% in 2003–2004 to 6.2% by 2011–2012. The prevalence of CKD among individuals with diabetes was 19.1% in 2011–2012 (Murphy et al. 2016), pointing to the major role of diabetes in CKD, as discussed further in the next section. Awareness of kidney disease remains very low among the public, as CKD is an asymptomatic condition until the very end stage.

The definition of ESRD in the medical literature is chronic irreversible renal failure. Renal failure is also called CKD stage 6. Early diagnosis of renal dysfunction and prevention or delay of progression through treatment of comorbid conditions, including primarily hypertension, but also obesity, glucose intolerance, and type 2 diabetes mellitus, through diet, lifestyle, and adjunctive pharmacotherapy, are obviously preferable to treating diagnosed renal failure.

Once renal failure has been diagnosed, renal replacement therapy is needed, as either dialysis or transplant. Unfortunately, most individuals with CKD at earlier stages have no symptoms, which is why active screening for this condition through monitoring of estimated glomerular filtration rate (eGFR) in all at-risk patients and for microalbuminuria in some at-risk patients is so critical.

A retrospective survival analysis in 311 ESRD patients treated at a hospital in the Netherlands between 2004 and 2014 at ages over 70 demonstrated how little survival benefit, on average, is provided by renal dialysis. In the study, patients chose either conservative medical management using pharmacotherapy or dialysis (Verberne et al. 2016). A total of 107 patients chose conservative management and 204 chose dialysis. Comorbidity scores were similar for both groups. The median survival from the time they chose either course of action was only 3.1 years for patients treated with dialysis and 1.5 years for those who chose conservative management. This was statistically significant ($p < 0.001$), but neither group had very good survival on dialysis. Among patients 80 and older, median survival was 2.1 years for the dialysis group and 1.4 years for the conservative management group, a statistically nonsignificant difference ($p = 0.08$). These data and others demonstrate that dialysis is not a cure for renal failure. These median survival times emphasize the need for early detection and efforts in the prevention of progression of CKD to ESRD.

Because they generally are older and frequently have comorbidities, patients with type 2 diabetes mellitus and ESRD seldom are selected for renal transplantation. Thus, information on transplantation results from controlled studies in this high-risk category of patients is scarce. Patient survival after kidney transplant has been improving for all age ranges in comparison with dialysis therapy. The main causes of mortality after transplant are cardiovascular and cerebrovascular events, infections, and cancer. Therefore, renal transplantation is not the ultimate answer to reducing the morbidity and mortality of CKD, underlining again the importance of early detection and treatment of CKD.

If nutrition and weight management could prevent obesity-associated kidney disease and its progression to renal failure, many hundreds of thousands of lives would be saved and health care costs for dialysis and transplantation would be saved (Zandi-Nejad and Brenner 2005; Hallan et al. 2006b). Modifiable risk factors for kidney disease are closely associated with obesity, including hypertension and type 2 diabetes mellitus (Erdmann 2006; Hallan et al. 2006b; Kramer 2006; Keller 2006; Ram et al. 2006; Ritz 2006; Srivastava 2006).

The incidence of kidney disease outcomes varies in conjunction with the variation in obesity rates across different regions of the world, with the highest incidence in North America and the lowest incidences in Asia (Parkin 1998; Calle et al. 2003; Chalmers et al. 2006; Hallan et al. 2006a; Iseki 2006; Wang et al. 2006). Studying risk factors for kidney disease is difficult due to the low incidence and long latency period of many forms of kidney disease, but many studies suggest that obesity is a risk factor for CKD and renal failure (Perneger et al. 1995).

12.2 OBESITY, FATTY KIDNEY, AND CHRONIC KIDNEY DISEASE

Excess visceral fat is a major driving force for almost all the disorders associated with the metabolic syndrome, including CKD, through systemic effects on blood pressure (BP), lipids, and cytokines (Hall et al. 2004; Tchernof and Despres 2013). CKD rates have increased in parallel to increases in overweight and obesity (Hall et al. 2002, 2004). In the United States, more than 10% of people over 20 years of age, or about 200,000 individuals, are estimated to have some degree of CKD, and the prevalence of CKD in those over age 60 is approximately 25% (Centers for Disease Control and Prevention 2014). In 2009, almost 900,000 people in the United States were being treated for renal failure, with an estimated cost of nearly $40 billion (U.S. Department of Health and Human Services 2013). CKD is associated with increased morbidity and mortality, so that after adjusting for age, sex, race, comorbidity, and prior hospitalizations, CKD patients experience a 59% higher mortality rate than patients without CKD (National Institutes of Health 2012).

Overweight and obesity account for 65–75% of the risk for essential hypertension (Garrison et al. 1987). Type 2 diabetes, which accounts for more than 90% of diabetes, is uniformly accompanied by increased visceral adiposity. Hypertension and diabetes, along with other disorders associated with the metabolic syndrome, may interact synergistically to increase the risk of CKD and progression to renal failure. However, there is also evidence that obesity may damage the kidney and increase the risk for CKD independent of diabetes and hypertension (Hall et al. 2004; Ejerblad et al. 2006).

Abdominal visceral obesity is associated with CKD independently of overall adiposity or increased body mass index (BMI), although there is generally a good association between BMI and visceral obesity. In a study of almost 6500 nondiabetic participants, increasing BMI and waist circumference were associated with reduced eGFR and increased CKD (Burton et al. 2012). Abdominal obesity, defined as a waist circumference of >102 cm in men or >88 cm in women, was associated with a higher risk of renal insufficiency (odds ratio = 1.40), even after adjustment for other components of the metabolic syndrome, such as dyslipidemia, hyperglycemia, hypertension, and BMI, in patients with essential hypertension (Gomez et al. 2006).

Ectopic fat accumulation in and around the kidney may also have adverse consequences on renal function and has been called "fatty kidney." Renal sinus fat is associated with stage 2 hypertension and the number of antihypertensive medications required to control BP (Morales et al. 2003). Furthermore, in the Framingham Heart Study, individuals with fatty kidneys (high perinephric fat levels) had a higher risk for hypertension (odds ratio = 2.12), which persisted after adjustment for BMI and visceral fat (Navaneethan et al. 2009). Fatty kidney was also associated with increased risk for CKD (odds ratio = 2.30), even after adjustment for BMI and visceral adiposity.

Obesity can affect the kidneys directly through so-called obesity-related glomerulopathy. It is characterized histologically by enlargement of glomeruli, which can be accompanied by focal and segmental glomerulosclerosis observed in association with hypertrophied glomeruli (D'Agati et al. 2011). There are also lipid deposits in mesangial and tubular cells, along with changes similar to those seen in type 2 diabetes, including focal mesangial sclerosis. Focal thickening of glomerular and tubular basement membranes, a feature of diabetic nephropathy, is also seen in obese patients without diabetes.

Glomerular hyperfiltration accompanies obesity and has been implicated as one of the most important pathogenic mechanisms in producing the characteristic changes in fatty kidney (Chagnac et al. 2008). There is a linear correlation between different markers of obesity, including BMI, waist circumference, and waist-to-hip ratio, and GFR (Bosma et al. 2004). Increased glomerular blood flow in obesity results in glomerular hypertension, glomerular enlargement, and stretching of microvessels in the kidney.

Epidemiological studies provide insight into why some obese patients develop CKD, while others, with equal or greater degree of obesity, do not. Once again, it is not simply body weight or BMI, but the presence of each of the components of metabolic syndrome, including hypertension, hypertriglyceridemia, low HDL cholesterol, and elevated fasting serum glucose levels, that is significantly associated with the risk of developing CKD. The risk for developing CKD was higher in metabolically unhealthy nonobese subjects than in metabolically healthy obese ones (Hashimoto et al. 2015). These observations point the way toward effective prevention and secondary prevention strategies to reduce the rate of progression of CKD.

Fatty kidney typically presents with proteinuria in an obese patient with otherwise normal urinalysis. In about 70% of cases, proteinuria is below the nephrotic range of >3.5 g/day, while the remaining 30% have frank proteinuria without other signs of nephrotic syndrome, such as hypoalbuminemia, edema, and hyperlipidemia (Kambham et al. 2001; Praga et al. 2001). Another important consequence of this presentation is that obese people who develop proteinuria can go unnoticed for years, owing to the absence of clinical manifestations, and be detected at a stage when the renal function is already severely impaired. Besides proteinuria, hypertension and dyslipidemia are found in a majority of obese patients with fatty kidney characterized by large glomeruli secondary to increased blood flow, with secondary changes in the kidney including focal glomerular sclerosis.

Both observational studies and prospective randomized trials have shown that weight loss is associated with a significant reduction in proteinuria (Morales et al. 2003; Navaneethan et al. 2009) and is the preferred treatment. Blockade of the renin–angiotensin–aldosterone system (RAAS) with ACE inhibitors or angiotensin receptor blockers in observational studies has demonstrated significant reductions in proteinuria studies (Praga et al. 2001). Aldosterone antagonists can also reduce proteinuria in obese patients. In the REIN study, comparing an ACE inhibitor, ramipril, versus placebo in patients with chronic proteinuric nephropathies, obese patients were more sensitive to the effects of ramipril in protecting the kidney and reducing proteinuria than nonobese patients (Mallamaci et al. 2011).

12.3 RENAL INSUFFICIENCY AND CHRONIC KIDNEY DISEASE

Chronic renal insufficiency is the ninth leading cause of death in the United States, according to the Centers for Disease Control and Prevention (2012). In this disease, the kidneys are damaged and cannot filter blood effectively. This damage can cause wastes to build up in the body and lead to other health problems, including cardiovascular disease (CVD), anemia, and bone disease. People with early CKD tend not to feel any symptoms. The only ways to detect CKD are through a blood test to estimate kidney function, and a urine test to assess kidney damage. If left untreated, chronic renal insufficiency leads to renal failure.

The most common cause of chronic renal insufficiency is diabetes (Vallon and Thomson 2012). After 10–20 years of diabetes mellitus, approximately 20% of patients with either type 1 or type 2 diabetes mellitus develop diabetic nephropathy, making diabetes mellitus the leading cause of ESRD. Both genetic and environmental factors determine which patients eventually develop diabetic nephropathy, and there remains a need for research to better understand the pathophysiology and molecular pathways that lead from the onset of hyperglycemia to renal failure. Changes in the vasculature and the glomerulus, including those to mesangial cells, the filtration barrier, and podocytes, play important roles in the pathophysiology of the diabetic kidney.

High BP is the second most common cause of chronic renal insufficiency and is often associated with metabolic syndrome and obesity. However, the exact mechanism of the development of hypertension in obesity remains to be established (Hall et al. 1992). Patients with nondiabetic and diabetic CKD should have a target BP goal of <130/80 mmHg (National Kidney Foundation 2002; Chobanian et al. 2003; American Diabetes Association 2012). Ultimately, the rationale for lowering BP in all patients with CKD is to reduce both renal and cardiovascular morbidity and mortality. Maintaining BP control and minimizing proteinuria in patients with CKD and hypertension is essential for the prevention of the progression of kidney disease and the development or worsening of CVD (National Kidney Foundation 2002; Chobanian et al. 2003; American Diabetes Association 2012).

Recent literature suggests that BP targets in diabetic and nondiabetic CKD may need to be individualized based on the presence of proteinuria. Some trials have failed to show a reduction in cardiovascular or renal outcomes in diabetic and nondiabetic patients with CKD when a BP target of <130/80 mmHg is achieved compared with lowering BP to <140/90 mmHg (ACCORD Study Group et al. 2011; Upadhyay et al. 2011).

However, patients who have proteinuria are less likely to experience a decline in renal function, kidney failure, or death when the lower BP target is achieved (Brenner et al. 2001; Upadhyay et al. 2011). It is likely that future guidelines may include a lower BP goal, <130/80 mmHg, for patients with proteinuria, but maintain a goal of <140/90 mmHg for patients without proteinuria.

Polycystic kidney disease is the most common inherited kidney disease (Nishiura et al. 2009). It causes cyst formation in the kidneys. If the cysts are numerous and large enough, they may prevent the kidneys from carrying out their normal functions.

Kidney stones can also lead to chronic renal insufficiency. When kidney stones become too numerous and too big, they can interfere with normal kidney functions, causing chronic renal insufficiency (Nishiura et al. 2009). Having one kidney stone puts a patient at a 50% increased risk of having another within 5–7 years. Treatment of kidney stones is essential to preventing chronic renal insufficiency.

Urinary infections, if long lasting, can lead to chronic renal insufficiency (Heikkila et al. 2011). Urinary infections mostly affect the bladder but can also spread to the kidneys. If the glomeruli in the kidneys become infected, they can no longer eliminate excess fluid and waste at the rate that is necessary to keep the body healthy. Urinary infections, if treated successfully, can prevent chronic renal insufficiency. Once renal function declines so that metabolic derangements, including electrolyte balance and uremia, become prominent, protein restriction is used to increase the interval between dialysis sessions (Aparicio et al. 2012).

Cardiovascular disease is the leading cause of morbidity and mortality among people with CKD. CKD has increased over the past decade to become a worldwide public health problem. The definition of a biomarker is a characteristic objectively measured and evaluated as an indicator of normal biologic processes, pathogenic processes, or pharmacologic response to a therapeutic intervention. Thus, biomarkers of kidney function would include serum creatinine and, more recently, eGFR.

These biomarkers and microalbuminuria, a potential biomarker, predict cardiovascular events and mortality. Recent analyses of cross-sectional data indicate that eGFR is a much stronger predictor of cardiovascular events than microalbuminuria. While microalbuminuria indicates endothelial dysfunction and is associated with increased risk for cardiovascular events, its level is related more to the level of BP and glycemic control than directly to the pathophysiology of atherosclerosis. Hence, microalbuminuria could be viewed as a biomarker but not a risk factor for cardiovascular since risk factors must be an integral part of the disease pathophysiology. Conversely, while microalbuminuria is not of prognostic value to predict CKD outcomes, increases over time into the albuminuria range, >200 mg/day, clearly indicate the presence of kidney disease and are associated with a more rapid decline in kidney function. Thus, concomitant evaluation of both biomarkers eGFR and albuminuria is recommended to assess kidney function and cardiovascular risk thoroughly.

Since the risk of cardiovascular death at any given level of BP depends on the number of concurrent cardiovascular disease risk factors, a comprehensive clinical and laboratory cardiovascular risk assessment is needed to establish the cardiovascular disease burden and determine the scope of lifestyle changes and/or need for pharmaceutical intervention in patients with hypertension and renal insufficiency. Many of the cardiovascular disease risk factors are behavioral and modifiable by lifestyle changes. Although the potential therapeutic impact of established lifestyle changes on BP varies among individuals based on their adherence, lifestyle changes, when implemented, have all been shown to lower BP and/or mitigate the risk of cardiovascular death in a dose- and time-dependent fashion.

Damage to the glomeruli leads to an increase in protein filtration, resulting in abnormally increased amounts of protein in the urine (microalbuminuria or proteinuria) (Yoshioka et al. 1987; Keane and Eknoyan 1999). Microalbuminuria is the presentation of small amounts of albumin in the urine and is often the first sign of CKD. Proteinuria (protein-to-creatinine ratio ≥200 mg/g) develops as CKD progresses, and is associated with a poor prognosis for both kidney disease and CVD (Sarnak et al. 2003; Rashidi et al. 2008; Chronic Kidney Disease Prognosis Consortium et al. 2010).

The estimated GFR, which helps clinicians determine how well the kidneys are filtering waste, is used in the staging of CKD. The National Kidney Foundation defines CKD as either kidney damage, identified by markers in the urine or blood or by imaging, with or without changes in the GFR, or a GFR of <60 mL/minute/1.73 m^2 for a minimum of 3 months (National Kidney Foundation 2002). Table 12.1 depicts the staging criteria as determined by the Kidney Disease Outcomes Quality Initiative (K/DOQI) guidelines.

TABLE 12.1
Staging of Chronic Kidney Disease

Stage	Description	GFR[a] (mL/minute/1.73 m^2)
1	Kidney damage with normal or increased GFR	≥90
2	Kidney damage with mildly decreased GFR	60–90
3	Moderately decreased GFR	30–59
4	Severely decreased GFR	15–29
5	Kidney failure	<15 or on dialysis

[a] The GFRs are from Collins, A. J. et al., *Am. J. Kidney Dis.*, 59(1 Suppl. 1), A7.e1–e420, 2012.

12.4 NUTRITION AND PREVENTION OF CHRONIC KIDNEY DISEASE

Nutrition plays its most prominent role in the prevention of renal disease through the treatment of hypertension and diabetes. CKD has become more common over the last 20 years in association with increases in the prevalence of metabolic syndrome, hypertension, diabetes, and obesity. It was reported to affect more than 13% of the U.S. population in 2004 (Coresh et al. 2007). In 2010, it was reported by the Centers for Disease Control and Prevention that more than 35% of people aged 20 years or older with diabetes have CKD, and that more than 20% of people aged 20 years or older with hypertension have CKD (Collins et al. 2012). The rise in incidence of CKD has been attributed to an aging populace and increases in hypertension, diabetes, and obesity within the U.S. population, conditions affected by diet. CKD is associated with electrolyte imbalances, mineral and bone disorders, anemia, dyslipidemia, and hypertension. Furthermore, a reduced GFR and albuminuria are independently associated with an increase in cardiovascular and all-cause mortality (Rashidi et al. 2008; Chronic Kidney Disease Prognosis Consortium et al. 2010).

From another viewpoint, hypertension has been reported to occur in 85–95% of patients with CKD (stages 3–5) (Rao et al. 2008). The relationship between hypertension and CKD is cyclic in nature. Uncontrolled hypertension is a risk factor for developing CKD, and hypertension is associated with a more rapid progression of CKD, and is the second leading cause of ESRD in the United States (Botdorf et al. 2011; Segura and Ruilope 2011). Meanwhile, progressive renal disease can exacerbate uncontrolled hypertension due to volume expansion and increased systemic vascular resistance. Multiple guidelines discuss the importance of lowering BP to slow the progression of renal disease and reduce cardiovascular morbidity and mortality (National Kidney Foundation 2002; Chobanian et al. 2003; American Diabetes Association 2012). However, in order to achieve and maintain adequate BP control, most patients with CKD require combinations of antihypertensive agents; often up to three or four medication classes may need to be employed (Bakris et al. 2000).

12.5 NUTRITION IN CHRONIC KIDNEY DISEASE AND END-STAGE RENAL DISEASE

Patients with CKD, and particularly those with advanced or stage 5 CKD, have protein wasting with sarcopenia, resulting in fatigue and weakness. Moreover, due to aggravation of metabolic and hormonal parameters, protein wasting in these individuals is associated with increased morbidity and mortality (Kalantar-Zadeh et al. 2005; Menon et al. 2005; Muntner et al. 2005; Weiner et al. 2008). It has not been established whether protein depletion itself or secondary comorbidities, including cardiovascular risk factors such as elevated triglycerides, and inflammatory cytokines that often accompany renal failure, may be the cause of protein depletion (Kopple 1997; Kopple et al. 1999; Kalantar-Zadeh and Kopple 2001). Protein restriction is established as a standard component of the nutritional management of patients with advanced renal disease, since high-protein diets lead to the accumulation of potentially toxic metabolites of protein metabolism, as well as potassium, fat, and pro-inflammatory fatty acids. Thus, the balancing of protein intake is a complex undertaking, particularly as anorexia and other comorbid conditions often influence what patients can or will eat.

Numerous clinical studies of the effects of low-protein intake on the progression of CKD were carried out in the 1970s and 1980s. Subsequently, the National Institutes of Health supported the largest and most comprehensive multicenter trial of protein in renal disease ever conducted—the Modification of Diet in Renal Disease (MDRD) Study. This randomized prospective controlled trial was undertaken to test the effects of low-protein and low-phosphorus diets and strict BP control on the progression of renal disease (Klahr et al. 1994). The MDRD Study investigated the effects of three levels of dietary protein and phosphorus intakes and two BP goals on the progression of CKD. Eight hundred forty adults with various renal diseases, except for insulin-dependent diabetes mellitus, were studied.

MDRD Study A included 585 patients who had a GFR, measured by ^{125}I-iothalamate clearances, of 25–55 mL/minute/1.73 m^2. These persons were randomly assigned to 1.3 g of protein/kg of standard body weight/day and 16–20 mg of phosphorus/kg/day, or to 0.58 g of protein/kg/day and 5–10 mg of phosphorus/kg/day. They were also assigned to either a mean arterial BP goal of 107 mmHg (113 mmHg for those of 61 years of age or older) or 92 mmHg (98 mmHg for those of 61 years of age or older).

In MDRD Study B, 255 patients with a baseline GFR of 13–24 mL/minute/1.73 m^2 were randomly assigned to a 0.28 g of protein/kg/day and 4–9 mg of phosphorus/kg/day diet supplemented with 0.28 g/kg/day of keto acids and amino acids, or to 0.58 g of protein/kg/day with 5–10 mg of phosphorus/kg/day. They were also randomly assigned to either the above modest or strict BP control groups.

Progression of renal failure was measured periodically for an average of 2.2 years. There were no differences between the groups in the decline in GFR in Study A. In Study B, there was a borderline significantly greater rate of decline in GFR with the 0.58 g of protein/kg/day diet than with the very low-protein keto acid and amino acid diet ($p = 0.07$).

In the 12-year follow-up analysis of Study A, during the first 6 years after the initiation of dietary protein prescription, there was a significantly lower adjusted hazard ratio of reaching ESRD or a combination of ESRD and mortality in those assigned to the 0.58 g of protein/kg/day diet compared with those assigned to the 1.3 g of protein/kg/day diet (Levey et al. 2006).

In a long-term follow-up of the MDRD Study, assignment to a very low-protein diet did not delay progression to kidney failure, but appeared to increase the risk of death (Menon et al. 2009). It is important to appreciate that after an average of 2.2 years of follow-up, the patients were discharged to be followed up with their various primary care physicians, and therefore probably had little or no aggressive dietary therapy, and essentially no clinical follow-up data were available except for the times of onset of their dialysis therapy and mortality.

A large multicenter study proved that providing essential amino acids rather than a mixture of essential and nonessential amino acids during protein restriction does not affect the progression of renal disease (Menon et al. 2009). The principal goal of protein-restricted regimens is to decrease the accumulation of nitrogen waste products, hydrogen ions, phosphates, and inorganic ions while maintaining an adequate nutritional status to avoid secondary problems, such as metabolic acidosis, bone disease, and insulin resistance, as well as proteinuria and deterioration of renal function.

Probably the major safety issue concerning low-protein diets is the risk of protein–energy wasting. This concern is especially important when individuals are prescribed as little as 0.6 g of protein/kg/day. This concern is based on two related issues. The fact that the low-protein diet of 0.6 g/kg/day is close to the dietary requirement for clinically stable individuals who are normal or have CKD indicates that some people may be at increased risk for protein malnutrition. In contrast, rather extensive research indicates that such diets provide adequate daily protein for almost all clinically stable CKD patients (Eyre and Attman 2008).

The other issue is that with such restriction in protein intake, it often becomes more difficult to meet the average daily energy needs of the patient. This is particularly true because in order to provide adequate quantities of essential amino acids with these protein-restricted diets, a large proportion of the protein must be of high biological value, that is, animal protein. In contrast, it is often the foods higher in lower-quality protein that provide the most calories (e.g., bread, rolls, pasta, biscuits, and cakes). This is the case because high-calorie butter, jam, cream cheese, sauces, and so forth, can be readily added to these latter foods.

A solution to this dilemma is to frequently monitor the protein–energy status of the patient. If evidence for protein malnutrition emerges, the protein intake may be increased up to 0.80 g of protein/kg/day. Evidence for energy malnutrition may be treated with dietary counseling, by increasing the protein intake as above, as this will increase the availability of low-quality proteins that can be ingested with a consequent increase in energy intake, or with oral or parenteral high-energy supplements.

An analysis of 14 studies with a total of 666 subjects with CKD (GFR <20 mL/minute) who were prescribed a dietary protein intake from 0.3 g/kg/day (supplemented with keto acids and amino acids) to 0.5 g/kg/day of protein for more than 12 months found that in all but two studies, low-protein diets were not associated with deterioration in body composition (Fouque et al. 2000). Other recent studies have reported similar findings (Chauveau et al. 2003).

There is no clear evidence base on which to recommend a dietary protein intake for patients with stage 1 or 2 CKD. Published trials to a large extent have examined the effect of protein intake on the progression of renal failure in individuals with stages 3–5 CKD. Since the published data so far have not been definitive, consent should be obtained from the patient after a discussion of the evidence and the side effects of a low-protein diet, including possible loss of lean body mass. Then a diet providing 0.60–0.75 g of protein/kg/day can be prescribed. To ensure an adequate intake of essential amino acids, this diet should provide at least 50% of the protein as high biological value. This amount of protein intake normally will maintain a neutral or positive nitrogen balance (Kopple 1999).

For stages 4 and 5 CKD, the potential advantages of a low-protein and low-phosphorous diet at this degree of renal insufficiency are more compelling. The rationale for a low-protein diet at this stage is that toxic products of nitrogen metabolism begin to accumulate in significant amounts at these levels of renal insufficiency. A low-protein diet generates less nitrogenous and other compounds, including guanidines, organic acids, and minerals, which have been considered potentially toxic to the patient. Hence, a low-protein diet may reduce the risk of uremic symptoms.

Patients can suffer from anorexia and nausea. As a result, they may eat too little protein rather than too much. These patients are at increased risk for malnutrition. Encouragement and specific training to follow the prescribed diet may increase the likelihood that they do not ingest less than the recommended intake or other nutrients. To maintain a neutral or positive nitrogen balance, patients should be prescribed 0.60 g of protein/kg/day. For individuals who are unable to maintain adequate dietary energy intake with such a diet or will not accept this diet, an intake of up to 0.75 or 0.80 g of protein/kg/day may be recommended. This latter protein intake is easier for most people to adhere to and, as indicated above, frequently enables people to more readily ingest a higher dietary energy intake.

Nephrotic syndrome is a nonspecific disorder in which the kidneys are damaged, causing them to leak large amounts of protein. The prescribed protein intake in nephrotic patients is not increased unless their proteinuria exceeds 5.0 g/day. Above 5.0 g of proteinuria/day, the prescribed diet is increased by 1 g/day of high-biological-value protein for each additional gram per day of proteinuria. Proteinuria is monitored periodically; if urinary protein excretion changes the diet, protein intake can be modified accordingly. This approach is based on the adverse consequences observed in CKD patients who are protein wasted (Rambod et al. 2009).

Clinical practice guidelines for nutrition in CKD from the National Kidney Foundation recommend a protein intake of 1.2–1.3 g of protein/kg/day for clinically stable chronic peritoneal dialysis (CPD) patients (Clinical Practice Guidelines 2000). Dietary protein requirements in patients undergoing automated peritoneal dialysis appear to be similar. Patients undergoing hemodialysis lose protein in the dialysate. Nitrogen balance studies suggest that to maintain normal total body protein and protein balance, some maintenance hemodialysis patients require more than 1.0 g of protein/kg/day. Clinical practice guidelines (2000) on nutrition in CKD patients recommend 1.2 g of protein/kg of body weight/day for clinically stable patients; half of the dietary protein should be of high biological value.

During maintenance hemodialysis, monitoring nitrogen balance requires a consideration of total nitrogen appearance (TNA), which is defined as the sum of dialysate, urine, fecal nitrogen losses, and (in dialysis patients) the postdialysis increment in body urea nitrogen content (Westra et al. 2007).

As nitrogen is rather expensive to measure, and there are few commercial laboratories that measure nitrogen, urea is usually measured instead. Urea is the major nitrogenous product of protein and amino acid degradation, and unlike nitrogen, it can be both precisely and inexpensively measured. TNA usually can be estimated accurately by measuring urea nitrogen appearance (UNA).

UNA is the amount of urea nitrogen that appears or accumulates in body fluids and all outputs (most commonly, urine and dialysate).

Clinically stable people who are at zero nitrogen balance should theoretically have a total nitrogen output that is equal to nitrogen intake minus about 0.5 g of nitrogen/day from such unmeasured losses as sweat, blood drawing, growth of nails, and replacement of exfoliated skin. Nitrogen output therefore should closely correlate with nitrogen intake in these individuals and can be used to estimate dietary nitrogen output, and therefore dietary protein needs to maintain balance. In stable CKD patients, both TNA and UNA are in balance with dietary nitrogen and protein intake (Cook et al. 2007).

For the purpose of estimation, dietary proteins are assumed to have 6.25 g of nitrogen/g of protein. UNA is calculated as follows: UNA (g/day) = UUN + DUN + Change in Body UN (all in units of g/day), where Body UN is body urea nitrogen and DUN is the dialysate urea nitrogen. The change in body urea nitrogen (g/day) is different than blood urea nitrogen (BUN) and is calculated by subtracting the final BUN after dialysis from the initial BUN. Since BUN goes down during dialysis, this is expressed as BUN(final) minus BUN initial as a positive number. This difference is then multiplied by the body water volume estimated as 0.6 times body weight. You have now accounted for the change in BUN during dialysis from the point of view of BUN, but you also must correct for the change in body water that occurs as the result of dialysis. This is calculated by multiplying 0.6 times the difference between the final body weight and the initial body weight, and then multiplying this result by the final BUN in grams per liter. The final body weight will be greater than the initial body weight or body water, and by multiplying by the final BUN, you have accounted for this change during dialysis.

Mathematically, the formulas can be summarized as follows:

$$\text{UNA} = \text{UUN} + \text{DUN} + \Delta \text{ Body UN}$$

$$\Delta \text{ Body UN} = \left(\left[\text{BUN(final)} - \text{BUN(initial)}\right] \times 0.6 \text{ BW}\right) + \left(\left[\text{BW(final)} - \text{BW(initial)}\right] \times \text{BUN(final)}\right)$$

The calculation is made to reflect the time between dialysis intervals and then normalized to 24 hours. Body weight (BW) times 0.6 to estimate body water is valid for average body composition. In edematous or lean patients, the estimated proportion of body weight that is water is increased, and in the obese or the very young, it is decreased.

Although there are not yet any systematically collected data on which to recommend protein requirements in maintenance hemodialysis patients receiving more frequent dialysis treatments, this dietary intake is estimated to provide adequate protein nutrition.

Alterations in dietary protein intake have an important role in the prevention and management of CKD. Using soy protein instead of animal protein reduces the development of kidney disease in animals (Eknoyan and Agodoa 2002). Reducing protein intake preserves kidney function in persons with early diabetic kidney disease. These observations lead to the potential for substitution of soy protein for animal protein, to result in less hyperfiltration and glomerular hypertension, with resulting protection from diabetic nephropathy. Specific components of soy protein may lead to benefits for specific peptides, amino acids, and isoflavones. Substituting soy protein for animal protein usually decreases hyperfiltration in diabetic subjects and may reduce urine albumin excretion. Limited data are available on the effects of soy peptides, isoflavones, and other soy components on renal function in diabetes. Further studies are required to discern the specific benefits of soy protein and its components on renal function in diabetic subjects (Eknoyan and Agodoa 2002).

Studies clearly indicate that people prescribed special diets are much more likely to adhere to them if they are periodically monitored, educated, and encouraged to follow their dietary prescription. In order to maximize compliance, physicians and dietitians should schedule frequent, often monthly, visits with patients who have CKD stage 5 and often stage 4. Less frequent visits may be convened with patients who have stable and less severe renal insufficiency, as long as evidence indicates that they are adequately compliant.

12.6 SUMMARY

CKD is a global public health problem (Eknoyan and Agodoa 2002; Levey et al. 2007; Crowe et al. 2008), affecting 10–16% of the adult population on several continents (Chadban et al. 2003; Hallan et al. 2006a; Coresh et al. 2007; Wen et al. 2008) and increasing the risk of adverse outcomes (Chronic Kidney Disease Prognosis Consortium et al. 2010; Astor et al. 2011; Gansevoort et al. 2011; Levey et al. 2011; van der Velde et al. 2011). The definition and staging of CKD is based on the level of GFR and the presence of kidney damage, usually ascertained as albuminuria (Eknoyan and Agodoa 2002; Levey et al. 2011; Tonelli et al. 2011).

In international population cohorts, the crude prevalence of reduced eGFR (<60 mL/minute/1.73 m^2) in Asians, whites, and blacks was 5.1%, 15.8%, and 9.4%, respectively. The prevalence of elevated albuminuria (≥30 mg/g by albumin-to-creatinine ratio [ACR] or ≥1+ by urine dipstick) in these three racial groups was 2.8%, 9.7%, and 16.8%, respectively. The difference in prevalence of reduced eGFR and elevated albuminuria across racial groups was attenuated after age standardization, particularly for reduced eGFR.

The GFR thresholds for the definition and staging of CKD were first proposed in 2002, using data derived predominantly from a general U.S. population (Eknoyan and Agodoa 2002). In the last decade, these eGFR thresholds have been incorporated into clinical guidelines in other countries (Crowe et al. 2008; Levin et al. 2008; Japanese Society of Nephrology 2009). The recognition of albuminuria as an independent risk factor for adverse outcomes has now led to the incorporation of albuminuria categories into CKD staging, and this analysis has utilized the new recommendations for categories of albuminuria and eGFR (Kidney Disease 2013). The relationship of eGFR and albuminuria to overall CKD and CVD outcomes, irrespective of race, gives additional credence to their use in clinical detection of early CKD.

Aggressive screening of patients presenting with low eGFR and nutritional interventions designed to reduce BP, including the Dietary Approaches to Stop Hypertension (DASH) diet and increased fruit and vegetable intake, together with reasonable control of sodium intake in obese and hypertensive patients, should be standard practice in primary care. The emphasis in primary care education on hypertension treatment has traditionally been the use of various drugs, with only lip service paid to lifestyle and nutrition. This has been due to the recognized difficulties in dietary and lifestyle change, but prevention carried out by a multidisciplinary primary care team, including dietitians, using integrated methods of nutrition, lifestyle change, and appropriate individualized pharmacotherapy, should help reduce the morbidity and mortality of CKD.

Primary care providers need to be very attentive to the risks of progressive kidney disease and should screen patients, particularly those at increased risk—patients with hypertension, patients with diabetes mellitus, and patients with a family history of kidney disease—with blood tests for serum creatinine and urine testing to look for albuminuria, with a spot urine for calculation of an ACR. This is of particular importance among populations where there is an increased risk of CKD.

REFERENCES

ACCORD Study Group, H. C. Gerstein, M. E. Miller, S. Genuth, F. Ismail-Beigi, J. B. Buse, D. C. Goff Jr. et al. 2011. Long-term effects of intensive glucose lowering on cardiovascular outcomes. *N Engl J Med* 364 (9):818–828.

American Diabetes Association. 2012. Introduction: The American Diabetes Association's (ADA) evidence-based practice guidelines, standards, and related recommendations and documents for diabetes care. *Diabetes Care* 35 (Suppl 1):S1–S2.

Anon. 2000. Obesity: Preventing and managing the global epidemic. Report of a WHO consultation. *World Health Organ Tech Rep Ser* 894:i–xii, 1–253.

Aparicio, M., V. Bellizzi, P. Chauveau, A. Cupisti, T. Ecder, D. Fouque, L. Garneata et al. 2012. Protein-restricted diets plus keto/amino acids—A valid therapeutic approach for chronic kidney disease patients. *J Ren Nutr* 22 (2 Suppl):S1–S21.

Astor, B. C., K. Matsushita, R. T. Gansevoort, M. van der Velde, M. Woodward, A. S. Levey, P. E. Jong et al. 2011. Lower estimated glomerular filtration rate and higher albuminuria are associated with mortality and end-stage renal disease. A collaborative meta-analysis of kidney disease population cohorts. *Kidney Int* 79 (12):1331–1340.

Bakris, G. L., M. Williams, L. Dworkin, W. J. Elliott, M. Epstein, R. Toto, K. Tuttle, J. Douglas, W. Hsueh, and J. Sowers. 2000. Preserving renal function in adults with hypertension and diabetes: A consensus approach. National Kidney Foundation Hypertension and Diabetes Executive Committees Working Group. *Am J Kidney Dis* 36 (3):646–661.

Bosma, R. J., J. J. van der Heide, E. J. Oosterop, P. E. de Jong, and G. Navis. 2004. Body mass index is associated with altered renal hemodynamics in non-obese healthy subjects. *Kidney Int* 65 (1):259–265.

Botdorf, J., K. Chaudhary, and A. Whaley-Connell. 2011. Hypertension in cardiovascular and kidney disease. *Cardiorenal Med* 1 (3):183–192.

Bray, G. A., C. Bouchard, and W. P. T. James. 1998. *Handbook of Obesity*. New York: Marcel Dekker.

Brenner, B. M., M. E. Cooper, D. de Zeeuw, W. F. Keane, W. E. Mitch, H. H. Parving, G. Remuzzi, S. M. Snapinn, Z. Zhang, S. Shahinfar, and RENAAL Study Investigators. 2001. Effects of losartan on renal and cardiovascular outcomes in patients with type 2 diabetes and nephropathy. *N Engl J Med* 345 (12):861–869.

Burton, J. O., L. J. Gray, D. R. Webb, M. J. Davies, K. Khunti, W. Crasto, S. J. Carr, and N. J. Brunskill. 2012. Association of anthropometric obesity measures with chronic kidney disease risk in a non-diabetic patient population. *Nephrol Dial Transplant* 27 (5):1860–1866.

Calle, E. E., C. Rodriguez, K. Walker-Thurmond, and M. J. Thun. 2003. Overweight, obesity, and mortality from cancer in a prospectively studied cohort of U.S. adults. *N Engl J Med* 348 (17):1625–1638.

Centers for Disease Control and Prevention. 2012. Centers for Disease Control summary health statistics for U.S. adults: National Health Interview Survey, 2010. Atlanta, GA: Centers for Disease Control and Prevention.

Centers for Disease Control and Prevention. 2014. National chronic kidney disease fact sheet 2014. Atlanta, GA: Centers for Disease Control and Prevention. https://www.cdc.gov/diabetes/pubs/pdf/kidney_factsheet.pdf.

Chadban, S. J., E. M. Briganti, P. G. Kerr, D. W. Dunstan, T. A. Welborn, P. Z. Zimmet, and R. C. Atkins. 2003. Prevalence of kidney damage in Australian adults: The AusDiab kidney study. *J Am Soc Nephrol* 14 (7 Suppl 2):S131–S138.

Chagnac, A., M. Herman, B. Zingerman, A. Erman, B. Rozen-Zvi, J. Hirsh, and U. Gafter. 2008. Obesity-induced glomerular hyperfiltration: Its involvement in the pathogenesis of tubular sodium reabsorption. *Nephrol Dial Transplant* 23 (12):3946–3952.

Chalmers, L., F. J. Kaskel, and O. Bamgbola. 2006. The role of obesity and its bioclinical correlates in the progression of chronic kidney disease. *Adv Chronic Kidney Dis* 13 (4):352–364.

Chauveau, P., B. Vendrely, W. El Haggan, N. Barthe, V. Rigalleau, C. Combe, and M. Aparicio. 2003. Body composition of patients on a very low-protein diet: A two-year survey with DEXA. *J Ren Nutr* 13 (4):282–287.

Chobanian, A. V., G. L. Bakris, H. R. Black, W. C. Cushman, L. A. Green, J. L. Izzo Jr., D. W. Jones et al. 2003. The Seventh Report of the Joint National Committee on Prevention, Detection, Evaluation, and Treatment of High Blood Pressure: The JNC 7 report. *JAMA* 289 (19):2560–2572.

Chronic Kidney Disease Prognosis Consortium, K. Matsushita, M. van der Velde, B. C. Astor, M. Woodward, A. S. Levey, P. E. de Jong, J. Coresh, and R. T. Gansevoort. 2010. Association of estimated glomerular filtration rate and albuminuria with all-cause and cardiovascular mortality in general population cohorts: A collaborative meta-analysis. *Lancet* 375 (9731):2073–2081.

Clinical practice guidelines for nutrition in chronic renal failure. K/DOQI, National Kidney Foundation. 2000. *Am J Kidney Dis* 35 (6 Suppl 2):S1–S140.

Collins, A. J., R. N. Foley, B. Chavers, D. Gilbertson, C. Herzog, K. Johansen, B. Kasiske et al. 2012. United States Renal Data System 2011 annual data report: Atlas of chronic kidney disease & end-stage renal disease in the United States. *Am J Kidney Dis* 59 (1 Suppl 1):A7.e1–e420.

Cook, N. R., J. A. Cutler, E. Obarzanek, J. E. Buring, K. M. Rexrode, S. K. Kumanyika, L. J. Appel, and P. K. Whelton. 2007. Long term effects of dietary sodium reduction on cardiovascular disease outcomes: Observational follow-up of the trials of hypertension prevention (TOHP). *BMJ* 334 (7599):885–888.

Coresh, J., E. Selvin, L. A. Stevens, J. Manzi, J. W. Kusek, P. Eggers, F. Van Lente, and A. S. Levey. 2007. Prevalence of chronic kidney disease in the United States. *JAMA* 298 (17):2038–2047.

Crowe, E., D. Halpin, P. Stevens, and Guideline Development Group. 2008. Early identification and management of chronic kidney disease: Summary of NICE guidance. *BMJ* 337:a1530.

D'Agati, V. D., F. J. Kaskel, and R. J. Falk. 2011. Focal segmental glomerulosclerosis. *N Engl J Med* 365 (25):2398–2411.

Ejerblad, E., C. M. Fored, P. Lindblad, J. Fryzek, J. K. McLaughlin, and O. Nyren. 2006. Obesity and risk for chronic renal failure. *J Am Soc Nephrol* 17 (6):1695–1702.

Eknoyan, G., and L. Agodoa. 2002. On improving outcomes and quality of dialysis care, and more. *Am J Kidney Dis* 39 (4):889–891.

Erdmann, E. 2006. Worldwide spread of lifestyle diseases and its importance for cardiovascular events. *Drugs Today (Barc)* 42 (Suppl C):5–8.

Eyre, S., and P. O. Attman. 2008. Protein restriction and body composition in renal disease. *J Ren Nutr* 18 (2):167–186.

Fouque, D., P. Wang, M. Laville, and J. P. Boissel. 2000. Low protein diets delay end-stage renal disease in non diabetic adults with chronic renal failure. *Cochrane Database Syst Rev* (2):CD001892.

Fox, C. S., M. G. Larson, E. P. Leip, B. Culleton, P. W. Wilson, and D. Levy. 2004. Predictors of new-onset kidney disease in a community-based population. *JAMA* 291 (7):844–850.

Gansevoort, R. T., K. Matsushita, M. van der Velde, B. C. Astor, M. Woodward, A. S. Levey, P. E. de Jong, J. Coresh, and Chronic Kidney Disease Prognosis Consortium. 2011. Lower estimated GFR and higher albuminuria are associated with adverse kidney outcomes. A collaborative meta-analysis of general and high-risk population cohorts. *Kidney Int* 80 (1):93–104.

Garrison, R. J., W. B. Kannel, J. Stokes 3rd, and W. P. Castelli. 1987. Incidence and precursors of hypertension in young adults: The Framingham Offspring Study. *Prev Med* 16 (2):235–251.

Gomez, P., L. M. Ruilope, V. Barrios, J. Navarro, M. A. Prieto, O. Gonzalez, L. Guerrero, M. A. Zamorano, C. Filozof, and FATH Study Group. 2006. Prevalence of renal insufficiency in individuals with hypertension and obesity/overweight: The FATH study. *J Am Soc Nephrol* 17 (12 Suppl 3):S194–S200.

Hall, J. E., M. W. Brands, D. A. Hildebrandt, and H. L. Mizelle. 1992. Obesity-associated hypertension. Hyperinsulinemia and renal mechanisms. *Hypertension* 19 (1 Suppl):I45–I55.

Hall, J. E., E. D. Crook, D. W. Jones, M. R. Wofford, and P. M. Dubbert. 2002. Mechanisms of obesity-associated cardiovascular and renal disease. *Am J Med Sci* 324 (3):127–137.

Hall, J. E., J. R. Henegar, T. M. Dwyer, J. Liu, A. A. Da Silva, J. J. Kuo, and L. Tallam. 2004. Is obesity a major cause of chronic kidney disease? *Adv Ren Replace Ther* 11 (1):41–54.

Hallan, S. I., J. Coresh, B. C. Astor, A. Asberg, N. R. Powe, S. Romundstad, H. A. Hallan, S. Lydersen, and J. Holmen. 2006a. International comparison of the relationship of chronic kidney disease prevalence and ESRD risk. *J Am Soc Nephrol* 17 (8):2275–2284.

Hallan, S. I., K. Dahl, C. M. Oien, D. C. Grootendorst, A. Aasberg, J. Holmen, and F. W. Dekker. 2006b. Screening strategies for chronic kidney disease in the general population: Follow-up of cross sectional health survey. *BMJ* 333 (7577):1047.

Hashimoto, Y., M. Tanaka, H. Okada, T. Senmaru, M. Hamaguchi, M. Asano, M. Yamazaki et al. 2015. Metabolically healthy obesity and risk of incident CKD. *Clin J Am Soc Nephrol* 10 (4):578–583.

Heikkila, J., C. Holmberg, L. Kyllonen, R. Rintala, and S. Taskinen. 2011. Long-term risk of end stage renal disease in patients with posterior urethral valves. *J Urol* 186 (6):2392–2396.

Hsu, C. Y., C. E. McCulloch, C. Iribarren, J. Darbinian, and A. S. Go. 2006. Body mass index and risk for end-stage renal disease. *Ann Intern Med* 144 (1):21–28.

Iseki, K. 2006. Body mass index and the risk of chronic renal failure: The Asian experience. *Contrib Nephrol* 151:42–56.

Japanese Society of Nephrology. 2009. Evidence-based practice guideline for the treatment of CKD. *Clin Exp Nephrol* 13 (6):537–566.

Kalantar-Zadeh, K., R. D. Kilpatrick, N. Kuwae, C. J. McAllister, H. Alcorn Jr., J. D. Kopple, and S. Greenland. 2005. Revisiting mortality predictability of serum albumin in the dialysis population: Time dependency, longitudinal changes and population-attributable fraction. *Nephrol Dial Transplant* 20 (9):1880–1888.

Kalantar-Zadeh, K., and J. D. Kopple. 2001. Relative contributions of nutrition and inflammation to clinical outcome in dialysis patients. *Am J Kidney Dis* 38 (6):1343–1350.

Kambham, N., G. S. Markowitz, A. M. Valeri, J. Lin, and V. D. D'Agati. 2001. Obesity-related glomerulopathy: An emerging epidemic. *Kidney Int* 59 (4):1498–1509.

Keane, W. F., and G. Eknoyan. 1999. Proteinuria, albuminuria, risk, assessment, detection, elimination (PARADE): A position paper of the National Kidney Foundation. *Am J Kidney Dis* 33 (5):1004–1010.

Keller, U. 2006. From obesity to diabetes. *Int J Vitam Nutr Res* 76 (4):172–177.

Kidney Disease: Improving Global Outcomes (KDIGO) CKD Work Group. 2013. KDIGO 2012 clinical practice guideline for the evaluation and management of chronic kidney disease. *Kidney Int Suppl* 3:150.

Klahr, S., A. S. Levey, G. J. Beck, A. W. Caggiula, L. Hunsicker, J. W. Kusek, and G. Striker. 1994. The effects of dietary protein restriction and blood-pressure control on the progression of chronic renal disease. Modification of Diet in Renal Disease Study Group. *N Engl J Med* 330 (13):877–884.

Kopple, J. D. 1997. McCollum Award Lecture, 1996: Protein-energy malnutrition in maintenance dialysis patients. *Am J Clin Nutr* 65 (5):1544–1557.

Kopple, J. D. 1999. Pathophysiology of protein-energy wasting in chronic renal failure. *J Nutr* 129 (1S Suppl):247S–251S.

Kopple, J. D., X. Zhu, N. L. Lew, and E. G. Lowrie. 1999. Body weight-for-height relationships predict mortality in maintenance hemodialysis patients. *Kidney Int* 56 (3):1136–1148.

Kramer, H. 2006. Obesity and chronic kidney disease. *Contrib Nephrol* 151:1–18.

Levey, A. S., R. Atkins, J. Coresh, E. P. Cohen, A. J. Collins, K. U. Eckardt, M. E. Nahas et al. 2007. Chronic kidney disease as a global public health problem: Approaches and initiatives—A position statement from Kidney Disease Improving Global Outcomes. *Kidney Int* 72 (3):247–259.

Levey, A. S., P. E. de Jong, J. Coresh, M. El Nahas, B. C. Astor, K. Matsushita, R. T. Gansevoort, B. L. Kasiske, and K. U. Eckardt. 2011. The definition, classification, and prognosis of chronic kidney disease: A KDIGO controversies conference report. *Kidney Int* 80 (1):17–28.

Levey, A. S., T. Greene, M. J. Sarnak, X. Wang, G. J. Beck, J. W. Kusek, A. J. Collins, and J. D. Kopple. 2006. Effect of dietary protein restriction on the progression of kidney disease: Long-term follow-up of the Modification of Diet in Renal Disease (MDRD) Study. *Am J Kidney Dis* 48 (6):879–888.

Levin, A., B. Hemmelgarn, B. Culleton, S. Tobe, P. McFarlane, M. Ruzicka, K. Burns et al. 2008. Guidelines for the management of chronic kidney disease. *CMAJ* 179 (11):1154–1162.

Mallamaci, F., P. Ruggenenti, A. Perna, D. Leonardis, R. Tripepi, G. Tripepi, G. Remuzzi, C. Zoccali, and REIN Study Group. 2011. ACE inhibition is renoprotective among obese patients with proteinuria. *J Am Soc Nephrol* 22 (6):1122–1128.

Menon, V., T. Greene, X. Wang, A. A. Pereira, S. M. Marcovina, G. J. Beck, J. W. Kusek, A. J. Collins, A. S. Levey, and M. J. Sarnak. 2005. C-reactive protein and albumin as predictors of all-cause and cardiovascular mortality in chronic kidney disease. *Kidney Int* 68 (2):766–772.

Menon, V., J. D. Kopple, X. Wang, G. J. Beck, A. J. Collins, J. W. Kusek, T. Greene, A. S. Levey, and M. J. Sarnak. 2009. Effect of a very low-protein diet on outcomes: Long-term follow-up of the Modification of Diet in Renal Disease (MDRD) Study. *Am J Kidney Dis* 53 (2):208–217.

Morales, E., M. A. Valero, M. Leon, E. Hernandez, and M. Praga. 2003. Beneficial effects of weight loss in overweight patients with chronic proteinuric nephropathies. *Am J Kidney Dis* 41 (2):319–327.

Muntner, P., J. He, B. C. Astor, A. R. Folsom, and J. Coresh. 2005. Traditional and nontraditional risk factors predict coronary heart disease in chronic kidney disease: Results from the Atherosclerosis Risk in Communities study. *J Am Soc Nephrol* 16 (2):529–538.

Murphy, D., C. E. McCulloch, F. Lin, T. Banerjee, J. L. Bragg-Gresham, M. S. Eberhardt, H. Morgenstern et al. 2016. Trends in prevalence of chronic kidney disease in the United States. *Ann Intern Med* 165 (7):473–481.

National Institutes of Health. 2012. U.S. Renal Data System, 2012 annual data report: Atlas of chronic kidney disease and end-stage renal disease in the United States. Bethesda, MD: National Institutes of Health, National Institute of Diabetes and Digestive and Kidney Diseases. http://www.usrds.org/atlas12.aspx.

National Kidney Foundation. 2002. K/DOQI clinical practice guidelines for chronic kidney disease: Evaluation, classification, and stratification. *Am J Kidney Dis* 39 (2 Suppl 1):S1–S266.

Navaneethan, S. D., H. Yehnert, F. Moustarah, M. J. Schreiber, P. R. Schauer, and S. Beddhu. 2009. Weight loss interventions in chronic kidney disease: A systematic review and meta-analysis. *Clin J Am Soc Nephrol* 4 (10):1565–1574.

Nishiura, J. L., R. F. Neves, S. R. Eloi, S. M. Cintra, S. A. Ajzen, and I. P. Heilberg. 2009. Evaluation of nephrolithiasis in autosomal dominant polycystic kidney disease patients. *Clin J Am Soc Nephrol* 4 (4):838–844.

Parkin, D. M. 1998. The global burden of cancer. *Semin Cancer Biol* 8 (4):219–235.

Perneger, T. V., F. L. Brancati, P. K. Whelton, and M. J. Klag. 1995. Studying the causes of kidney disease in humans: A review of methodologic obstacles and possible solutions. *Am J Kidney Dis* 25 (5):722–731.

Praga, M., E. Hernandez, E. Morales, A. P. Campos, M. A. Valero, M. A. Martinez, and M. Leon. 2001. Clinical features and long-term outcome of obesity-associated focal segmental glomerulosclerosis. *Nephrol Dial Transplant* 16 (9):1790–1798.

Ram, R., D. N. Goswami, S. K. Bhattacharya, K. Bhattacharya, B. K. Saha, J. Saha, and B. Baur. 2006. An epidemiological study on risk factors of diabetes mellitus among patients attending a medical college hospital in Kolkata, West Bengal. *J Indian Med Assoc* 104 (8):428–430.

Rambod, M., R. Bross, J. Zitterkoph, D. Benner, J. Pithia, S. Colman, C. P. Kovesdy, J. D. Kopple, and K. Kalantar-Zadeh. 2009. Association of Malnutrition-Inflammation Score with quality of life and mortality in hemodialysis patients: A 5-year prospective cohort study. *Am J Kidney Dis* 53 (2):298–309.

Rao, M. V., Y. Qiu, C. Wang, and G. Bakris. 2008. Hypertension and CKD: Kidney Early Evaluation Program (KEEP) and National Health and Nutrition Examination Survey (NHANES), 1999–2004. *Am J Kidney Dis* 51 (4 Suppl 2):S30–S37.

Rashidi, A., A. R. Sehgal, M. Rahman, and A. S. O'Connor. 2008. The case for chronic kidney disease, diabetes mellitus, and myocardial infarction being equivalent risk factors for cardiovascular mortality in patients older than 65 years. *Am J Cardiol* 102 (12):1668–1673.

Ritz, E. 2006. Diabetic nephropathy. *Saudi J Kidney Dis Transpl* 17 (4):481–490.

Sarnak, M. J., A. S. Levey, A. C. Schoolwerth, J. Coresh, B. Culleton, L. L. Hamm, P. A. McCullough et al. 2003. Kidney disease as a risk factor for development of cardiovascular disease: A statement from the American Heart Association Councils on Kidney in Cardiovascular Disease, High Blood Pressure Research, Clinical Cardiology, and Epidemiology and Prevention. *Circulation* 108 (17):2154–2169.

Segura, J., and L. M. Ruilope. 2011. Hypertension in moderate-to-severe nondiabetic CKD patients. *Adv Chronic Kidney Dis* 18 (1):23–27.

Srivastava, T. 2006. Nondiabetic consequences of obesity on kidney. *Pediatr Nephrol* 21 (4):463–470.

Tchernof, A., and J. P. Despres. 2013. Pathophysiology of human visceral obesity: An update. *Physiol Rev* 93 (1):359–404.

Tonelli, M., P. Muntner, A. Lloyd, B. J. Manns, M. T. James, S. Klarenbach, R. R. Quinn, N. Wiebe, B. R. Hemmelgarn, and Alberta Kidney Disease Network. 2011. Using proteinuria and estimated glomerular filtration rate to classify risk in patients with chronic kidney disease: A cohort study. *Ann Intern Med* 154 (1):12–21.

Upadhyay, A., A. Earley, S. M. Haynes, and K. Uhlig. 2011. Systematic review: Blood pressure target in chronic kidney disease and proteinuria as an effect modifier. *Ann Intern Med* 154 (8):541–548.

U.S. Department of Health and Human Services. 2001. The surgeon general's call to action to prevent and decrease overweight and obesity. Rockville, MD: Office of the Surgeon General.

U.S. Department of Health and Human Services. 2013. Kidney disease statistics for the United States. NIH publication no. 12-3895. Bethesda, MD: U.S. Department of Health and Human Services, National Kidney and Urologic Diseases Clearinghouse. http://kidney.niddk.nih.gov/kudiseases/pubs/kustats/.

Vallon, V., and S. C. Thomson. 2012. Renal function in diabetic disease models: The tubular system in the pathophysiology of the diabetic kidney. *Annu Rev Physiol* 74:351–375.

van der Velde, M., K. Matsushita, J. Coresh, B. C. Astor, M. Woodward, A. Levey, P. de Jong et al. 2011. Lower estimated glomerular filtration rate and higher albuminuria are associated with all-cause and cardiovascular mortality. A collaborative meta-analysis of high-risk population cohorts. *Kidney Int* 79 (12):1341–1352.

Verberne, W. R., A. B. Geers, W. T. Jellema, H. H. Vincent, J. J. van Delden, and W. J. Bos. 2016. Comparative survival among older adults with advanced kidney disease managed conservatively versus with dialysis. *Clin J Am Soc Nephrol* 11 (4):633–640.

Wang, Y., X. Chen, M. J. Klag, and B. Caballero. 2006. Epidemic of childhood obesity: Implications for kidney disease. *Adv Chronic Kidney Dis* 13 (4):336–351.

Weiner, D. E., H. Tighiouart, E. F. Elsayed, J. L. Griffith, D. N. Salem, A. S. Levey, and M. J. Sarnak. 2008. The relationship between nontraditional risk factors and outcomes in individuals with stage 3 to 4 CKD. *Am J Kidney Dis* 51 (2):212–223.

Wen, C. P., T. Y. Cheng, M. K. Tsai, Y. C. Chang, H. T. Chan, S. P. Tsai, P. H. Chiang, C. C. Hsu, P. K. Sung, Y. H. Hsu, and S. F. Wen. 2008. All-cause mortality attributable to chronic kidney disease: A prospective cohort study based on 462 293 adults in Taiwan. *Lancet* 371 (9631):2173–2182.

Westra, W. M., J. D. Kopple, R. T. Krediet, M. Appell, and R. Mehrotra. 2007. Dietary protein requirements and dialysate protein losses in chronic peritoneal dialysis patients. *Perit Dial Int* 27 (2):192–195.

Yoshioka, T., H. G. Rennke, D. J. Salant, W. M. Deen, and I. Ichikawa. 1987. Role of abnormally high transmural pressure in the permselectivity defect of glomerular capillary wall: A study in early passive Heymann nephritis. *Circ Res* 61 (4):531–538.

Zandi-Nejad, K., and B. M. Brenner. 2005. Strategies to retard the progression of chronic kidney disease. *Med Clin North Am* 89 (3):489–509.

13 Nutrition and Heart Failure

13.1 INTRODUCTION

With increased aging of the world's population and increases in the comorbid diseases associated with cardiovascular disease, including metabolic syndrome, type 2 diabetes, and hypertension, the number of people globally affected by heart failure (HF) has increased over the last few decades both in the United States and around the world. Patients with HF can benefit from nutrition and lifestyle intervention, but the major emphasis for treating HF has been pharmacotherapy, as well as fluid and sodium restriction. Despite advances in drug treatment and mechanical assist devices, HF continues to be characterized by high morbidity and mortality comparable to common forms of advanced cancer (Curtis et al. 2008).

The economic impact associated with the very frequent hospitalization of patients with HF to treat acute HF decompensation has a significant public health impact (Writing Group Members et al. 2010). HF affects about 6 million individuals in the United States and 23 million worldwide. The direct costs of HF in the United States were $32 billion in 2013, and the cost is projected to increase threefold by 2030 (Heidenreich et al. 2013). The lifetime cost of HF per individual was estimated in 2011 to be $110,000/year, with more 75% of the cost consumed by "in-hospital care" (Dunlay et al. 2011). HF is a very serious disease with a 5-year mortality rate of approximately 50%, comparable to the mortality of some forms of advanced cancer (Askoxylakis et al. 2010). Among Medicare patients, 30-day, all-cause, risk-standardized readmission rates after hospital discharge are 20–25% (Ni and Xu 2015).

As noted, the prevalence of HF has markedly increased (Roger 2013), and it has been proposed that the increased number of aged individuals may be one of the reasons behind the increased prevalence of HF (Poole et al. 2012). Hospitalization due to acute decompensation of HF accounting for about 80% of HF-related hospital admissions can be caused by a number of factors, most commonly including nonadherence to medication, increased sodium intake, and uncontrolled hypertension. In addition, acute coronary syndrome, myocardial ischemia, arrhythmias, exacerbation of chronic pulmonary disease, alcohol intoxication, excess thyroid hormone, pregnancy, postoperative fluid overload, and administration of steroids or nonsteroidal anti-inflammatory drugs can all cause decompensation of a failing heart (Poole et al. 2012).

13.2 ETIOLOGY AND CLINICAL CLASSIFICATION OF HEART FAILURE

HF is caused by structural and functional defects in cardiac muscle, resulting in impairment of the ventricular filling or ventricular ejection fraction, the ratio of blood in the ventricle that is ejected during systole. The most common cause for HF is reduced left ventricular function due to prior myocardial function leaving behind nonfunctional heart muscle. However, disorders of the pericardium, endocardium, heart valves, or great vessels alone or in combination can also cause HF.

The heart is the only organ that provides its own blood supply, and it does so in proportion to oxygen demand for cardiac output in healthy hearts. Microvascular dysfunction and subsequent decrease in oxygen and nutrient delivery to the myocardium can be an important component of maintaining cardiac function in a failing heart. Therapeutic strategies to improve muscle microvascular nutritive and oxygen delivery functions via exercise training and anti-inflammatory and antioxidant agents have been proposed to be essential to provide better exercise tolerance and quality of life for patients with HF (Ohtani et al. 2012).

Low-output failure is the most common form of HF. Large myocardial infarctions and acute pulmonary emboli typically cause low-output failure. High-output HF is an uncommon condition in which a very rapid heart rate does not allow adequate time for optimal filling of the cardiac chambers, resulting in reduced effective organ perfusion and edema. High-output HF can be caused by severe anemia, large intracardiac flow shunts, hyperthyroidism, and vitamin B1 deficiency.

Clinically, there are two important subtypes of HF based on the function of the ventricles. HF with preserved ejection fraction is differentiated from HF with reduced ejection fraction. In patients with preserved ejection fraction of greater than 50%, the volume of the left ventricle is typically normal, but the left-ventricle wall is thick with reduced wall motion (Dassanayaka and Jones 2015). In HF with reduced ejection fraction, the left ventricle is typically enlarged and floppy. The size of heart muscle cells is smaller in HF with reduced ejection fraction than in HF with preserved ejection fraction (Dassanayaka and Jones 2015). These clinical subtypes are important because they influence the likelihood of treatment responses. Patients who have HF with reduced ejection fraction typically respond to pharmacotherapy, while patients who have HF with preserved ejection fraction respond to nitrates but not to the forms of pharmacotherapy meant to counteract activation of the renin–angiotensin axis. Patients with preserved ejection fraction also have a worse prognosis than patients with reduced ejection fraction (Glean et al. 2015; Zamani et al. 2015).

HF is also classified according to the functional capacity of patients. The New York Heart Association (NYHA) functional classification defines four functional classes as

- Class I: HF that does not cause limitations to physical activity. Ordinary physical activity does not cause symptoms.
- Class II: HF that causes slight limitations to physical activity. The patients are comfortable at rest, but ordinary physical activity results in HF symptoms.
- Class III: HF that causes marked limitations of physical activity. The patients are comfortable at rest, but less than ordinary activity causes symptoms of HF.
- Class IV: HF patients are unable to carry on any physical activity without HF symptoms or have symptoms when at rest.

The American College of Cardiology/American Heart Association (ACC/AHA) staging system is defined by four stages:

- Stage A: High risk of HF, but no structural heart disease or symptoms of HF
- Stage B: Structural heart disease, but no symptoms of HF
- Stage C: Structural heart disease and symptoms of HF
- Stage D: Refractory HF requiring specialized interventions

HF is a clinical diagnosis and can present with symptoms of shortness of breath, orthopnea, paroxysmal nocturnal dyspnea, fatigue, edema, distended abdomen, rales on auscultation, and pleural effusion (Watson et al. 2000; Yancy et al. 2013). Early stages of HF are more difficult to diagnose due to a lack of specific signs, as compensatory physiological mechanisms are activated.

13.3 DIAGNOSIS AND MEDICAL TREATMENT OF HEART FAILURE

13.3.1 Heart Failure with Preserved Ejection Fraction

Patients with HF are also classified based on ejection fraction in terms of either preserved or reduced ejection fraction. Systolic HF refers to HF with reduced ejection fraction, while diastolic HF refers to HF with preserved ejection fraction. Approximately 50% of the patients with HF have preserved ejection fraction, and they have higher morbidity and mortality rates than patients with reduced ejection fraction. HF with preserved ejection fraction is an emerging epidemic because of the rising prevalence in patients over the age of 65 and the lack of effective treatment for impaired myocardial energy availability (Oktay et al. 2013).

It has been proposed that increased production of radical oxygen species within the myocardium in response to activation of the renin–angiotensin–aldosterone system (RAAS) and sympathetic nervous system (SNS) leads to impairment of the mitochondrial bioenergetics with decreased adenosine triphosphate production (Munzel et al. 2015). Both of these factors are now believed to be major mechanisms for the development of HF with preserved ejection fraction (van Heerebeek et al. 2012b; Paulus and Tschope 2013; Andersen and Borlaug 2014). Research on mitochondrial bioenergetics in the myocardium and supplementation of antioxidants is being explored for this subtype of HF.

The principal symptoms of HF with preserved ejection fraction include exertional shortness of breath and fatigue (van Heerebeek et al. 2012a). The majority of patients are older women with a history of hypertension. In addition, these patients have many comorbidities, such as obesity, diabetes mellitus, dyslipidemia, and coronary artery disease (Owan et al. 2006; Lee et al. 2009). There are no pharmaceutical agents that have altered the clinical course of HF with preserved ejection fraction.

Studies have indicated that moderate walking exercise for these patients is associated with improved symptoms of fatigue and shortness of breath, and with weight loss and improved quality of life. However, exercise may not change the patient's systolic or diastolic function (Kitzman et al. 2013; Fleg et al. 2015; Pandey et al. 2015). Adjunctive therapy, such as omega-3 polyunsaturated fatty acids (PUFAs) (Macchia et al. 2005; Tavazzi et al. 2008), coenzyme Q10 (CoQ10) (Mortensen et al. 2014), and D-ribose (Bayram et al. 2015) supplementation, has been found useful for reducing the symptoms of HF with preserved ejection fraction, but more research is needed because the recommended management has not been effective in reversing the poor prognosis for these patients.

13.3.2 Pharmacotherapy of Heart Failure with Reduced Ejection Fraction

About half of all patients with HF have reduced ejection fraction, and the pharmacotherapy of this type of HF is based on using drugs that modify the RAAS and SNS responses to the reduction in cardiac output (Figure 13.1). The ACC and AHA jointly published updated clinical guidelines for

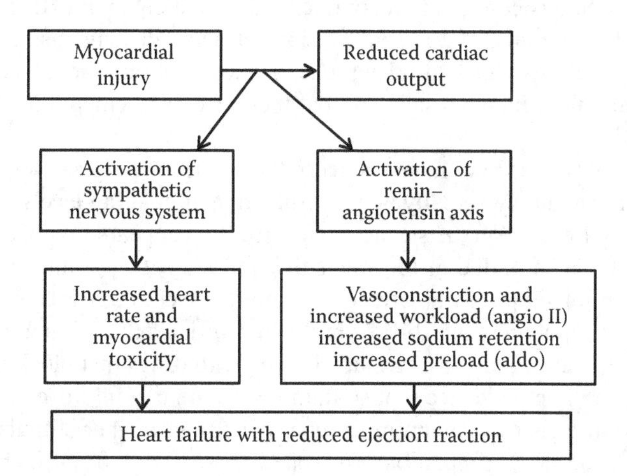

FIGURE 13.1 Pathophysiology of HF with reduced ejection fraction. Low blood pressure triggers carotid baroreceptors, which activate the SNS, leading to tachycardia and increased myocardial oxygen needs. Increases in epinephrine and norepinephrine lead to increased afterload via peripheral vasoconstriction. Reduced renal blood flow leads to activation of the renal–angiotensin axis, resulting in sodium and water retention. Angiotensin II (Angio II) also leads to vasoconstriction and increased afterload. Aldo, aldosterone.

the treatment of HF in May 2016, updating their 2013 guidelines (Yancy et al. 2016). These guidelines focus primarily on pharmacotherapy and follow a form that attempts to provide digestible blocks of information in response to specific issues, as suggested by the Institute of Medicine and formulated by the ACC/AHA (Greenfield and Steinberg 2011; Institute of Medicine 2011; Jacobs et al. 2013; Anderson et al. 2014; Arnett et al. 2014; Jacobs et al. 2014). However, beyond sodium and fluid restriction, dietary recommendations are general and encourage eating a "healthy diet."

The SNS and RAAS are activated as a physiological means to retain sodium and water, elevate heart rate, and increase peripheral vasoconstriction. Increased epinephrine and norepinephrine levels act to increase heart rate, contractility, and afterload via peripheral vasoconstriction. In the short term, this will work to increase cardiac output and relieve HF symptoms; however, chronically this has deleterious effects and causes further left ventricular systolic decline. β-Blockers are used to reduce SNS activation and angiotensin-converting enzyme (ACE). The activation of the RAAS has been demonstrated to contribute to negative remodeling of the heart, resulting in even worse overall cardiac function.

B-type natriuretic peptide and A-type natriuretic peptide have beneficial effects on blood flow during HF and represent another physiological mechanism activated to reverse changes secondary to low cardiac output. These peptides are released in the atrium as the elevated cardiac pressures stretch atrial myocytes. They act to vasodilate and cause sodium excretion, resulting in natriuresis.

Natriuretic peptide levels may be used to monitor diuretic therapy during hospitalizations for acute fluid overload and pulmonary edema (Berger et al. 2010; Januzzi 2012; Sanders-van Wijk et al. 2013). Diuretic therapy is only of secondary value, due to potential worsening of the underlying physiology, which is triggered by reduced blood pressure and so may worsen the underlying evolution of HF. On the other hand, fluid overload with edema secondary to HF remains the overwhelming reason for hospital admission, and diuretics remain the mainstay for treating volume overload. Detecting marked elevation or increased natriuretic peptide concentrations can facilitate more effective and prompt use of diuretics, leading to reduced hospital stays for congestion. Another benefit of monitoring with natriuretic peptides may be a reduction in needed doses of diuretics, lessening the risk of hypotension.

13.3.3 Sodium Restriction in Low-Output Heart Failure

Dietary sodium restriction is commonly recommended for patients with HF to prevent fluid retention, exacerbation of symptoms, and hospitalization for acute decompensated HF. However, evidence for effectiveness of this widely used approach is mostly observational. All current guidelines emphasize sodium and fluid intake restriction, but there is disagreement on whether strict sodium restriction is beneficial.

Results from several studies have raised concern that restricting dietary sodium to <2 g/day may not be beneficial in HF and may actually be harmful. High circulating levels of aldosterone lead to retention of sodium and water. On the surface, salt restriction appears to make physiological sense, given that interstitial edema is due to the water that follows salt into interstitial spaces. Clinical evidence suggests that for subjects who are not sodium deprived, high sodium intake may actually expand intravascular volume via fluid shift from the interstitial space without increasing total body water. Moreover, in the setting of HF pharmacotherapy with drugs that block the RAAS as well as diuretics, there is little direct evidence that sodium restriction can improve HF symptoms. In fact, increasing doses of diuretics can compromise renal perfusion, further stimulating the RAAS and increasing edema. In addition, stimulation of vasopressin secretion from the hypothalamus due to reduced perfusion can cause retention of free water and hyponatremia.

Controlled trials supporting the notion of less severe sodium restriction were carried out in which patients were randomized to either a 1.8 or 2.8 g sodium diet. Patients were also placed on a 1–2 L fluid restriction and high doses of diuretics. The earliest of these studies included a sample of 107 patients with severe HF followed for 7–36 months after discharge for the treatment of HF exacerbation. Survival in the 2.8 g sodium diet group was significantly better than in the 1.8 g sodium group (55% vs. 13%) (Licata et al. 2003). Similar results were reported in a larger study of 232 patients with less severe HF (NYHA class II) enrolled 30 days postdischarge from hospitalization for exacerbation of HF (Paterna et al. 2008). Over the 180-day study period, patients in the 1.8 g sodium intake group had a higher readmission rate. At 12 months, patients on the 1.8 g sodium diet had higher rates of combined end points of hospital admissions and death than patients on a 2.8 g diet (Parrinello et al. 2009). Additional clinical trials are underway to address the long-term effects of dietary sodium restriction on clinical outcomes in patients with HF (Butler et al. 2015; Colin-Ramirez et al. 2015).

13.3.4 Heart Failure Treatment: Medical Therapy

Educating patients in regards to the importance of medication compliance is crucial to prevent episodes of HF decompensation leading to hospitalization. There are many available pharmacotherapies for patients with low-output congestive HF. It is important to understand which therapies are the most important and reduce mortality versus those that are for symptom relief only.

13.3.4.1 ACE Inhibitors and Angiotensin Receptor Blockers

ACE inhibitors act primarily through blockade of the ACE, which converts angiotensin I to angiotensin II. Angiotensin II causes vasoconstriction, increasing afterload and systemic blood pressure. Angiotensin also contributes to the production of aldosterone, which leads to sodium and water retention.

Reducing the activity of the RAAS is crucial in HF, during which it is overactive and contributes to negative remodeling. ACE inhibitors can reduce the symptoms of HF and have been shown in multiple clinical trials to have a mortality benefit in systolic HF patients with reduced ejection fraction. Commonly used ACE inhibitors include lisinopril, captopril, Ramipril, and enalapril.

Angiotensin receptor blockers (ARBs) act by blocking the angiotensin receptor. Very similar effects on the RAAS are achieved when using ARBs compared with ACE inhibitors. ARBs are primarily used when a systolic HF patient is not able to tolerate an ACE inhibitor, frequently due to the side effect of coughing sometimes associated with ACE inhibitors.

ACE inhibitors reduce morbidity and mortality in HF with reduced ejection fraction. Randomized controlled trials (RCTs) clearly establish the benefits of ACE inhibition in patients with mild, moderate, or severe symptoms of HF and in patients with or without coronary artery disease (The CONSENSUS Trial Study Group 1987; The SOLVD Investigators 1991; Pfeffer et al. 1992; The Acute Infarction Ramipril Efficacy (AIRE) Study Investigators 1993; Kober et al. 1995; Packer et al. 1999).

ACE inhibitors can produce angioedema and should be given with caution to patients with low systemic blood pressures, renal insufficiency, or elevated serum potassium. ACE inhibitors also inhibit kininase and increase levels of bradykinin, which can induce cough, but also may contribute to their beneficial effect through vasodilation.

ARBs were developed with the rationale that angiotensin II production continues in the presence of ACE inhibition, driven through alternative enzyme pathways. ARBs do not inhibit kininase and are associated with a much lower incidence of cough and angioedema than ACE inhibitors, but like ACE inhibitors, ARBs should be given with caution to patients with low systemic blood pressure, renal insufficiency, or elevated serum potassium. Long-term therapy with ARBs produces hemodynamic, neurohormonal, and clinical effects consistent with those expected after interference with the renin–angiotensin system and have been shown in RCTs to reduce morbidity and mortality, especially in ACE inhibitor-intolerant patients (Cohn et al. 2001; Pfeffer et al. 2003a,b; Konstam et al. 2009).

13.3.4.2 β-Blockers

β-Blockers antagonize β-1 and β-2 receptors, which are the usual targets of the SNS, including epinephrine and norepinephrine. The overactive SNS has deleterious effects on long-term cardiac function, as described earlier.

β-Blockers improve outcomes in HF by lowering blood pressure, reducing left ventricular hypertrophy and diastolic dysfunction, slowing the heart rate, and reducing myocardial oxygen demand (Brophy et al. 2001; Klingbeil et al. 2003; Bergstrom et al. 2004; Lund et al. 2014). Three β-blockers are approved in the United States by the Food and Drug Administration (FDA) for the treatment of systolic congestive HF: metoprolol succinate, carvedilol, and bisoprolol. β-Blockers are contraindicated specifically in systolic HF when pulmonary edema is present, which can include signs of cardiogenic shock, severe bradycardia, hypotension, or wheezing related to asthma.

13.3.4.3 Aldosterone Antagonists

Aldosterone antagonists (spironolactone and eplerenone), also known as "potassium-sparing diuretics," block the action of aldosterone, inhibiting the reuptake of sodium and water. Normally, when sodium is reabsorbed, it is exchanged with potassium, which is then excreted. Since aldosterone inhibition decreases sodium reabsorption, it also decreases potassium excretion, resulting in higher serum potassium levels.

Spironolactone is indicated in systolic HF with recent or current NYHA functional class IV symptoms, preserved renal function, and a normal potassium concentration. Spironolactone was investigated in the Randomized Aldactone Evaluation Study (RALES) trial, and a mortality benefit was shown in NYHA functional class III and IV patients (Vardeny et al. 2014). However, significant hyperkalemia did contribute to sudden cardiac death.

13.3.4.4 Digoxin

Digoxin blocks the sodium-potassium ATPase pump. The mechanism by which this decreases atrioventricular conduction is not clear; however, it is perhaps due to increased vagal tone. Intracellular calcium within the cardiac myocytes is increased by digoxin, resulting in increased inotropy (contractility), and thus digoxin is frequently used when atrial fibrillation and left ventricular systolic dysfunction coexist.

While digoxin therapy is indicated for the treatment of symptomatic systolic congestive HF, the Digitalis Intervention Group (DIG) trial showed no mortality benefit; however, there was improvement in symptoms and fewer hospitalizations for HF (Abdul-Rahim et al. 2016). Digoxin toxicity is a concern, and the dose must be adjusted in the setting of renal failure.

13.3.4.5 Diuretics

The loop diuretics furosemide, bumetanide, and torsemide are utilized to help maintain euvolemia in HF patients. These drugs are for symptom relief only and have never been shown to have a mortality benefit. The dose frequently needs adjusting based on the patient's lifestyle, including fluid and salt intake.

13.3.4.6 ADH Antagonists

Tolvaptan is a vasopressin receptor antagonist. Vasopressin (aka antidiuretic hormone [ADH]) helps to regulate water retention by absorbing water in the collecting ducts of the nephron. Blocking this receptor will allow water to be excreted more readily. Many HF patients present with some degree of hyponatremia from water retention.

Tolvaptan has been shown in more than one clinical trial to raise sodium levels; however, mortality and rehospitalization were not improved (Felker et al. 2017). While tolvaptan is FDA approved for the treatment of euvolemic hyponatremia and hypervolemic hyponatremia, it has no place in the treatment of HF.

13.3.4.7 Nesiritide

Nesiritide is a recombinant form of B-type natriuretic peptide and is used for the treatment of acute decompensated HF. Nesiritide has potent vasodilatory properties and reduces pulmonary capillary wedge pressure effectively. This results in improvement of dyspnea.

One large trial (ASCEND-HF) randomized 7141 patients to nesiritide versus placebo. While nesiritide did improve the symptom of dyspnea better than placebo, there was no reduction in 30-day rehospitalization and no mortality benefit. Hypotension was significant in the nesiritide group.

Nesiritide is not recommended for routine use during decompensated HF. If patients with normal blood pressures are not responding well to typical management with loop diuretics, then nesiritide can be considered.

13.3.4.8 Hydralazine and Nitrates

Hydralazine is a direct arterial vasodilator that decreases afterload. Isosorbide mononitrate is a long-acting oral nitrate that decreases preload. The combination of these two drugs has an effect similar to that of an ACE inhibitor or ARB without reducing renal function or causing hyperkalemia. The combination of hydralazine and nitrates, however, does not have the neurohormonal blockade benefit of ACE inhibitors or ARBs, which is thought to play an important role. Despite this, a clear mortality benefit has been present with this combination when ACE inhibitors or ARBs are contraindicated, especially in the African American population (Sliwa et al. 2016).

13.3.5 Heart Failure Treatment: Mechanical, Revascularization, and Heart Transplant

The treatment of HF with therapies other than medications, such as the use of devices, is considered mechanical therapy. This includes biventricular pacing, implantable cardioverter defibrillators (ICDs), and left ventricular assist devices (LVADs). Revascularization with stenting and coronary bypass surgery are also implemented in some cases. Heart transplant is a last resort in treating HF. A discussion of these options is outside the scope of this chapter, which includes medical therapies, and sodium and fluid restriction simply to increase understanding of the physiology and potential impact of altering the responses to low-output HF.

13.4 BMI PARADOX IN HEART FAILURE

Despite evidence demonstrating the adverse effects of excess weight, the relationship between body mass index (BMI) and mortality in HF patients remains controversial. Because obesity and diabetes mellitus increase the risk of HF, it is attractive to hypothesize that weight loss would be beneficial to patients with HF and obesity, with or without diabetes mellitus. Paradoxically, several large cohort studies have shown that overweight and obese HF patients seem to have better survival than their healthy-weight counterparts (Horwich et al. 2001; Curtis et al. 2005; Lavie et al. 2005), which is inconsistent with our understanding of the negative effects associated with obesity and contradicts current recommendations to promote weight loss in the HF population.

There are a number of limitations in these studies that must be addressed before definitive conclusions can be drawn about the association between increased body fat and survival:

1. Many samples were composed primarily of men; thus, women have been underrepresented.
2. Many studies have been retrospective.
3. Few of the previous studies examined the impact of percent body fat on outcomes, while BMI may not be the right clinical indicator to assess excess body fat, especially in the presence of sarcopenia obesity.
4. None of the studies examined the effects of nutritional intake and nutritional status on outcomes.
5. None of the studies examined possible mechanisms that may be responsible for the positive effects of increased body fat on survival, so it is not possible to determine whether this relationship is causal.
6. None of the studies examined the effect of voluntary weight loss on outcomes.

7. Some of the findings reflect outcomes related to involuntary weight reduction that involves loss of lean tissue, muscle, and bone (cardiac cachexia), which is an independent predictor of increased mortality in advanced stages of HF (Kalantar-Zadeh et al. 2005).
8. None of the studies controlled for age, medication regimen, NYHA class, HF severity, or ejection fraction; thus, there are limited data to support the argument that weight loss may be detrimental to patients with HF, obesity, and diabetes mellitus.

Prospective studies that address limitations of past studies are needed before recommendations to change practice can be made.

Recently, in this advanced HF cohort, an unadjusted obesity survival paradox disappeared after adjustment for confounders. Overweight and obese males had higher adjusted mortality than normal-weight males, whereas a BMI in the overweight range was associated with a significant survival benefit in females (Vest et al. 2015). Another study involving 2527 subjects with diabetes conducted over 10 years demonstrated no benefit from the obesity paradox in congestive heart failure (Zamora et al. 2016).

13.5 MACRONUTRIENTS

13.5.1 Protein in Sarcopenia and Cardiac Cachexia

While the loss of body weight is a defining component of cachexia, sarcopenia is not necessarily associated with changes in body weight, because declining muscle mass can be masked by proportional increases in adipose tissue. Alternatively, high BMI may be associated with increased muscle mass, as already discussed in the previous section with regard to the BMI paradox. The failure to use body composition methods rather than simply body weight may hinder the clinical detection of sarcopenia and requires the use of imaging techniques for muscle mass, including dual-energy x-ray absorptiometry, computed tomography, or magnetic resonance imaging.

Clinically, it is virtually impossible to distinguish between sarcopenia and cachexia-related muscle wasting in advanced stages of HF. Yet, it should be noted that muscle mass is lost earlier than adipose tissue during the progression of HF. Older patients with HF may develop sarcopenia before becoming cachectic (von Haehling 2015). Although sarcopenia is primarily an age-dependent phenomenon, its course is accelerated by HF (Buford et al. 2010). Indeed, sarcopenia affects approximately 20% of older adults with HF, which exceeds the prevalence observed in individuals of the same age without HF (Fulster et al. 2013). Older patients with HF and sarcopenia show a lower exercise capacity than those with preserved muscle mass and function (Fulster et al. 2013). This finding suggests that the recognition of sarcopenia in the context of HF and the implementation of nutritional strategies to increase muscle mass, along with exercise, may help ameliorate functional capacity, before the wasting disorder enters its later stages.

HF treatment guidelines provide no recommendations regarding the intake of protein. It has recently been suggested that the amount and composition of dietary macronutrients may affect the symptoms and outcomes in HF patients (Chess and Stanley 2008). Specifically, it has been suggested that a high-protein diet might be beneficial in the advanced stages of HF. Current HF treatment guidelines provide no recommendations regarding the intake of protein, fat, and carbohydrate (Lindenfeld et al. 2010). An adequate energy–protein intake, when combined with amino acid supplementation, was shown to improve nutritional and metabolic status in most cardiac cachexia patients (Aquilani et al. 2008). A 12-week high-protein diet tested at the University of California, Los Angeles (UCLA) resulted in moderate weight loss and reduced adiposity in overweight and obese patients with HF and was associated with improvements in functional status, lipid profiles, glycemic control, and quality of life (Evangelista et al. 2009). It has been proposed that increasing protein and/or total energy intake in cachexic HF patients may prevent or reverse cachexia, but this remains to be definitively established (Rozentryt et al. 2010). High-protein intake might improve protein synthesis and cell function, and prevent deterioration in mitochondrial and left ventricular function.

13.5.2 Balancing Omega-3 and Omega-6 Fats in the Diet

Linoleic acid is a major constituent of diets in industrialized nations and increasingly in the developing world as processed foods are distributed globally. In the North American diet, this single fatty acid, at an intake of 16 g/day, accounts for approximately 7% of daily caloric intake and 20% of total dietary fatty acid intake (Blasbalg et al. 2011). This intake is more than threefold higher than the historic norm of 2%, owing mainly to the increased consumption of seed oils containing 20–54% of total fatty acids as linoleic acids (Blasbalg et al. 2011).

The mammalian liver can convert linoleic acid to longer-chain omega-6 PUFAs, particularly arachidonic acid, through elongation and desaturation reactions. Linoleic acid competes with α-linolenic acid for the same elongation and desaturation enzymes capable of converting α-linolenic acids to longer-chain omega-3 PUFAs, including eicosapentaenoic acid (EPA) and docosahexaenoic acid (DHA) (Bazinet et al. 2003; Domenichiello et al. 2014), which are associated with potential health benefits (Yurko-Mauro et al. 2010; Carter et al. 2013; Dalli et al. 2013). Linoleic acid and arachidonic acid are both n-6 fatty acids that are metabolized to pro-inflammatory bioactive oxidation products (Ramsden et al. 2012) and eicosanoids (Toborek et al. 1999). Increased levels of both fatty acids in the blood have been associated with conditions including nonalcoholic steatohepatitis, Alzheimer's disease, and asthma (Yoshida et al. 2009; Feldstein et al. 2010; Mabalirajan et al. 2013) in which inflammation plays a major pathogenic role. On the other hand, omega-3 EPA, docosapentaenoic acid (DPA), and DHA can be converted into anti-inflammatory and pro-resolving lipid mediators (Tjonahen et al. 2006; Bazan 2013; Dalli et al. 2013; Orr et al. 2013). This has been characterized as an imbalance of omega-6 and omega-3 fatty acids, which need to be balanced by both reducing omega-6 fat intake from processed foods and increasing omega-3 fat intake from ocean-caught fish and fish oil or algal oil supplements.

Data from the Atherosclerosis Risk in Communities (ARIC) study and the Physicians' Health Study have shown an inverse relationship between omega-3 PUFA intake and incident HF (Yamagishi et al. 2008; Wilk et al. 2012). Supplementation with omega-3 PUFAs has been of potential interest as a therapy for HF. Trials in primary and secondary prevention of coronary heart disease showed that omega-3 fatty acid supplementation results in a relative risk reduction of 10–20% in fatal and nonfatal cardiovascular events (Tavazzi et al. 2004). The Cardiovascular Health Study showed an inverse association in the intake of baked or broiled fish and incidence of congestive HF (Mozaffarian et al. 2005).

Further evidence on the benefit of omega-3 PUFA in HF was shown by the Gruppo Italiano per lo Studio della Sopravvivenza nell'Infarto Miocardico Heart Failure (GISSI-HF) investigators. Almost 7000 patients with NYHA class II through IV chronic HF were randomized to receive 1 g/day of omega-3 PUFAs or matching placebo (Tavazzi et al. 2008). Death from any cause was reduced from 29% with placebo to 27% in those treated with omega-3 fatty acids. The coprimary outcome of death or admission to hospital for a cardiovascular event was also reduced. In a follow-up study, 3-month treatment with omega-3 PUFA markedly enriched circulating EPA and DHA, independently of fish intake, and lowered pentraxin-3. Low EPA levels are inversely related to total mortality in patients with chronic HF (Masson et al. 2013).

Omega-3 PUFA supplementation may represent a novel therapeutic approach in late-stage HF characterized by cardiac cachexia (Mehra et al. 2006; Wang et al. 2006).

Further studies are needed to determine not only the optimal dose of omega-3 PUFA protection in different stages of HF, but also the underlying mechanism of action responsible for these benefits. It is clear that supplementation with omega-3 PUFA provides significant overall benefit with minimal risk (Fonarow 2008). Recent reviews have discussed the basic pathophysiological mechanisms and treatment effects in clinical trials (Endo and Arita 2016; Glück and Alter 2016). Integration of omega-3 into the microenvironment of cardiomyocyte ion channels led to allosteric changes and increased the electrical stability. Moreover, omega-3 also prevents the conversion of arachidonic acid into pro-inflammatory eicosanoids by serving as an alternative substrate for cyclooxygenase or lipoxygenase, resulting in the production of less potent products. In addition, a number of enzymatically oxygenated metabolites derived from omega-3 PUFAs were recently identified as anti-inflammatory mediators. These omega-3 metabolites may contribute to the beneficial effects against cardiovascular diseases that are attributed to omega-3. A better understanding of these interacting endogenous mechanisms appears to be required for interpreting the findings of recent experimental and clinical studies.

13.6 MICRONUTRIENTS

HF is now recognized as a systemic illness in which hormonal and neural activation results in the release of inflammatory cytokines, which cause oxidative stress in tissues and organs, including the heart. The role of micronutrients and minerals beyond sodium has been recognized in patients with HF. The vast majority of patients with HF follow a diet deficient in calcium, magnesium, and potassium (Lemon et al. 2010).

Micronutrient deficiencies, including calcium, magnesium, selenium, zinc, and vitamin D, may play a more important role than previously thought. Elevated levels of aldosterone and chronic use of diuretics increase urinary excretion of calcium and magnesium, leading to secondary hyperparathyroidism. Hyperparathyroidism depletes calcium from the bone and drives calcium into cells, increasing oxidative stress. Other micronutrients, including selenium, zinc, thiamine, and CoQ10, also appear to be reduced in patients with HF.

A combination of micronutrient supplements was administered to 30 elderly patients with stable systolic dysfunction and ejection fractions less than 35% due to ischemic heart disease, and the effects on left ventricular function and quality of life were determined (Witte et al. 2005). Patients were randomized to receive a combination of calcium; magnesium; zinc; copper; selenium; vitamins A, B6, B12, C, D, and E; thiamine; riboflavin; folate; and CoQ10 or placebo for 9 months. At the end of the study, the supplemented group had an increase of 5% in left ventricular ejection fraction ($p < 0.05$) and improved quality of life scores, while patients receiving placebo exhibited no changes. The sample size was small and included only elderly patients with HF due to ischemic heart disease and micronutrients at varying doses between 1/3 and 200 times the recommended dietary allowance (RDA). The study suggests the need for more research on which micronutrients are most important and whether these observations are extended to other types of HF and at which stages benefits are observed. In the balance of this chapter, the evidence available on selected micronutrients in HF is reviewed.

13.6.1 Coenzyme Q10 Supplementation

Mechanistically, the hallmarks of the failing heart include abnormal energy metabolism, increased production of reactive oxygen species (ROS), and defects in excitation–contraction coupling. HF is a highly dynamic pathological process, and observed alterations in cardiac metabolism and function depend on the disease progression (Akhmedov et al. 2015).

In the early stages, cardiac remodeling characterized by normal or slightly increased fatty acid oxidation plays a compensatory, cardioprotective role. However, upon progression of HF, fatty acid oxidation and mitochondrial oxidative activity are decreased, resulting in a significant drop in cardiac ATP levels. In HF, as a compensatory response to decreased oxidative metabolism, glucose uptake and glycolysis are upregulated, but this upregulation is not sufficient to compensate for a drop in ATP production.

Elevated mitochondrial ROS generation and ROS-mediated damage, when they overwhelm the cellular antioxidant defense system, induce heart injury and contribute to the progression of HF (Akhmedov et al. 2015). Mitochondrial uncoupling proteins (UCPs), which promote proton leak across the inner mitochondrial membrane, have emerged as essential regulators of mitochondrial membrane potential, respiratory activity, and ROS generation. Although the physiological role of UCP2 and UCP3, expressed in the heart, has not been clearly established, increasing evidence suggests that these proteins, by promoting mild uncoupling, could reduce mitochondrial ROS generation and cardiomyocyte apoptosis and thereby ameliorate myocardial function. Further investigation on the alterations in cardiac UCP activity and regulation will advance our understanding of their physiological roles in the healthy and diseased heart, and also may facilitate the development of novel and more efficient therapies.

CoQ10 (also called ubiquinone) is an antioxidant, the main function of which is the production of ATP through the electron transport chain. CoQ10 has been shown in all tissues and organs in the body, with highest concentrations in the heart. It has been postulated to improve functional status in congestive HF. Observational studies have reported that the plasma CoQ10 concentration was an independent predictor of mortality in patients with HF (Molyneux et al. 2008). Several RCTs have examined the effects of CoQ10 on congestive heart failure with inconclusive results. A meta-analysis in 2013 including 13 RCTs showed that supplementation with CoQ10 resulted in a net change of 3.67% in the EF and a significant decrease of the NYHA functional class (Fotino et al. 2013).

The effects of CoQ10 on morbidity and mortality in chronic HF were further studied in a 2-year prospective trial in patients with moderate to severe HF. A total of 420 patients were randomly assigned to either 100 mg of CoQ10 three times daily or placebo, in addition to standard therapy. Patients in the supplement group had improved symptoms and reduced major adverse cardiovascular events (Mortensen et al. 2014).

13.6.2 Thiamine

Thiamine, otherwise known as vitamin B1, serves as a key cofactor in carbohydrate metabolism. It is not synthesized in humans, and little thiamine is stored endogenously. As such, continual ingestion is required to prevent thiamine deficiency. Severe thiamine deficiency can result in severe vasodilatation and high-output HF, known as wet beriberi. This form of thiamine deficiency clearly warrants thiamine supplementation; however, wet beriberi is increasingly uncommon (Sole and Jeejeebhoy 2000). The benefit of thiamine supplementation in less severe forms of thiamine deficiency is still unclear. Thiamine deficiency in HF has typically been attributed to the use of loop diuretics, which promote the excretion of thiamine and other water-soluble B vitamins (Brady et al. 1995; Zenuk et al. 2002). However, poor dietary intake is likely a contributing factor in many patients (Brady et al. 1995). A series of studies have shown thiamine deficiency to be fairly common in the HF population, with prevalence ranging from 13% to 33% (Kwok et al. 1992; Hanninen et al. 2006). The prevalence may be even higher in hospitalized and elderly patients with HF (Kwok et al. 1992; Pfitzenmeyer et al. 1994). A number of small studies have shown improved markers of LV function after thiamine supplementation (Seligmann et al. 1991; Shimon et al. 1995). Other studies have shown mixed results from thiamine supplementation in HF (Pfitzenmeyer et al. 1994). Larger studies are necessary to examine the benefit of thiamine supplementation in HF, but it appears reasonable to supplement thiamine in chronic HF patients, especially those taking high-dose loop diuretics.

13.7 CONCLUSION

Despite significant progress in cardiovascular medicine, myocardial ischemia and infarction, progressing eventually to the final end-point of HF, remain the leading cause of morbidity and mortality in the United States. HF is a complex syndrome that results from any structural or functional impairment in ventricular filling or blood ejection. Ultimately, the heart's inability to supply the body's tissues with enough blood may lead to death.

There is no doubt that diet and exercise can have profound effects on age-related chronic diseases, including HF. Randomized trials have demonstrated the dramatic impact of combinations of diet and exercise on cardiovascular disease and diabetes. To extend these recommendations to HF, more evidence is needed on the effects of various components of diet, fluid restriction, and nutritional supplements. The high rates of hospital admissions, readmissions, and mortality associated with HF make such clinical research feasible. Considering the persistently high morbidity and costs associated with HF, it is time for primary care practices and researchers to optimize pharmacotherapy adherence and define the role of protein, lipid, antioxidant, and micronutrient supplementation in patients with stable and advancing HF. In the absence of well-developed clinical guidelines on nutrition, commonsense supplementation and nutritional support may benefit patients with HF.

REFERENCES

Abdul-Rahim, A. H., R. L. MacIsaac, P. S. Jhund, M. C. Petrie, K. R. Lees, and J. J. McMurray, on behalf of the VICCTA-Heart Failure Collaborators. 2016. Efficacy and safety of digoxin in patients with heart failure and reduced ejection fraction according to diabetes status: An analysis of the Digitalis Investigation Group (DIG) trial. *Int J Cardiol* 209:310–316.

The Acute Infarction Ramipril Efficacy (AIRE) Study Investigators. 1993. Effect of ramipril on mortality and morbidity of survivors of acute myocardial infarction with clinical evidence of heart failure. *Lancet* 342 (8875):821–828.

Akhmedov, A. T., V. Rybin, and J. Marin-Garcia. 2015. Mitochondrial oxidative metabolism and uncoupling proteins in the failing heart. *Heart Fail Rev* 20 (2):227–249.

Andersen, M. J., and B. A. Borlaug. 2014. Heart failure with preserved ejection fraction: Current understandings and challenges. *Curr Cardiol Rep* 16 (7):501.

Anderson, J. L., P. A. Heidenreich, P. G. Barnett, M. A. Creager, G. C. Fonarow, R. J. Gibbons, J. L. Halperin et al. 2014. ACC/AHA statement on cost/value methodology in clinical practice guidelines and performance measures: A report of the American College of Cardiology/American Heart Association Task Force on Performance Measures and Task Force on Practice Guidelines. *J Am Coll Cardiol* 63 (21):2304–2322.

Aquilani, R., C. Opasich, A. Gualco, M. Verri, A. Testa, E. Pasini, S. Viglio, P. Iadarola, O. Pastoris, and M. Dossena. 2008. Adequate energy-protein intake is not enough to improve nutritional and metabolic status in muscle-depleted patients with chronic heart failure. *Eur J Heart Fail* 10 (11):1127–1135.

Arnett, D. K., R. A. Goodman, J. L. Halperin, J. L. Anderson, A. K. Parekh, and W. A. Zoghbi. 2014. AHA/ACC/HHS strategies to enhance application of clinical practice guidelines in patients with cardiovascular disease and comorbid conditions: From the American Heart Association, American College of Cardiology, and U.S. Department of Health and Human Services. *J Am Coll Cardiol* 64 (17):1851–1856.

Askoxylakis, V., C. Thieke, S. T. Pleger, P. Most, J. Tanner, K. Lindel, H. A. Katus, J. Debus, and M. Bischof. 2010. Long-term survival of cancer patients compared to heart failure and stroke: A systematic review. *BMC Cancer* 10:105.

Bayram, M., J. A. St. Cyr, and W. T. Abraham. 2015. D-Ribose aids heart failure patients with preserved ejection fraction and diastolic dysfunction: A pilot study. *Ther Adv Cardiovasc Dis* 9 (3):56–65.

Bazan, N. G. 2013. The docosanoid neuroprotectin D1 induces homeostatic regulation of neuroinflammation and cell survival. *Prostaglandins Leukot Essent Fatty Acids* 88 (1):127–129.

Bazinet, R. P., H. Douglas, and S. C. Cunnane. 2003. Whole-body utilization of n-3 PUFA in n-6 PUFA-deficient rats. *Lipids* 38 (2):187–189.

Berger, R., D. Moertl, S. Peter, R. Ahmadi, M. Huelsmann, S. Yamuti, B. Wagner, and R. Pacher. 2010. N-terminal pro-B-type natriuretic peptide-guided, intensive patient management in addition to multidisciplinary care in chronic heart failure: A 3-arm, prospective, randomized pilot study. *J Am Coll Cardiol* 55 (7):645–653.

Bergstrom, A., B. Andersson, M. Edner, E. Nylander, H. Persson, and U. Dahlstrom. 2004. Effect of carvedilol on diastolic function in patients with diastolic heart failure and preserved systolic function. Results of the Swedish Doppler-echocardiographic study (SWEDIC). *Eur J Heart Fail* 6 (4):453–461.

Blasbalg, T. L., J. R. Hibbeln, C. E. Ramsden, S. F. Majchrzak, and R. R. Rawlings. 2011. Changes in consumption of omega-3 and omega-6 fatty acids in the United States during the 20th century. *Am J Clin Nutr* 93 (5):950–962.

Brady, J. A., C. L. Rock, and M. R. Horneffer. 1995. Thiamin status, diuretic medications, and the management of congestive heart failure. *J Am Diet Assoc* 95 (5):541–544.

Brophy, J. M., L. Joseph, and J. L. Rouleau. 2001. Beta-blockers in congestive heart failure. A Bayesian meta-analysis. *Ann Intern Med* 134 (7):550–560.

Buford, T. W., S. D. Anton, A. R. Judge, E. Marzetti, S. E. Wohlgemuth, C. S. Carter, C. Leeuwenburgh, M. Pahor, and T. M. Manini. 2010. Models of accelerated sarcopenia: Critical pieces for solving the puzzle of age-related muscle atrophy. *Ageing Res Rev* 9 (4):369–383.

Butler, J., L. Papadimitriou, V. Georgiopoulou, H. Skopicki, S. Dunbar, and A. Kalogeropoulos. 2015. Comparing sodium intake strategies in heart failure rationale and design of the Prevent Adverse Outcomes in Heart Failure by Limiting Sodium (PROHIBIT) Study. *Circ Heart Fail* 8 (3):636–645.

Carter, J. R., C. E. Schwartz, H. Yang, and M. J. Joyner. 2013. Fish oil and neurovascular reactivity to mental stress in humans. *Am J Physiol Regul Integr Comp Physiol* 304 (7):R523–R530.

Chess, D. J., and W. C. Stanley. 2008. Role of diet and fuel overabundance in the development and progression of heart failure. *Cardiovasc Res* 79 (2):269–278.

Cohn, J. N., G. Tognoni, and Valsartan Heart Failure Trial Investigators. 2001. A randomized trial of the angiotensin-receptor blocker valsartan in chronic heart failure. *N Engl J Med* 345 (23):1667–1675.

Colin-Ramirez, E., F. A. McAlister, Y. Zheng, S. Sharma, P. W. Armstrong, and J. A. Ezekowitz. 2015. The long-term effects of dietary sodium restriction on clinical outcomes in patients with heart failure. The SODIUM-HF (Study of Dietary Intervention under 100 mmol in Heart Failure): A pilot study. *Am Heart J* 169 (2):274–281.e1.

The CONSENSUS Trial Study Group. 1987. Effects of enalapril on mortality in severe congestive heart failure. Results of the Cooperative North Scandinavian Enalapril Survival Study (CONSENSUS). *N Engl J Med* 316 (23):1429–1435.

Curtis, J. P., J. G. Selter, Y. Wang, S. S. Rathore, I. S. Jovin, F. Jadbabaie, M. Kosiborod, E. L. Portnay, S. I. Sokol, and F. Bader. 2005. The obesity paradox: Body mass index and outcomes in patients with heart failure. *Arch Intern Med* 165 (1):55–61.

Curtis, L. H., M. A. Greiner, B. G. Hammill, J. M. Kramer, D. J. Whellan, K. A. Schulman, and A. F. Hernandez. 2008. Early and long-term outcomes of heart failure in elderly persons, 2001–2005. *Arch Intern Med* 168 (22):2481–2488.

Dalli, J., R. A. Colas, and C. N. Serhan. 2013. Novel n-3 immunoresolvents: Structures and actions. *Sci Rep* 3:1940.

Dassanayaka, S., and S. P. Jones. 2015. Recent developments in heart failure. *Circ Res* 117 (7):e58–e63.

Domenichiello, A. F., C. T. Chen, M. O. Trepanier, P. M. Stavro, and R. P. Bazinet. 2014. Whole body synthesis rates of DHA from alpha-linolenic acid are greater than brain DHA accretion and uptake rates in adult rats. *J Lipid Res* 55 (1):62–74.

Dunlay, S. M., N. D. Shah, Q. Shi, B. Morlan, H. VanHouten, K. H. Long, and V. L. Roger. 2011. Lifetime costs of medical care after heart failure diagnosis. *Circ Cardiovasc Qual Outcomes* 4 (1):68–75.

Endo, J., and M. Arita. 2016. Cardioprotective mechanism of omega-3 polyunsaturated fatty acids. *J Cardiol* 67 (1):22–27.

Evangelista, L. S., D. Heber, Z. Li, S. Bowerman, M. A. Hamilton, and G. C. Fonarow. 2009. Reduced body weight and adiposity with a high-protein diet improves functional status, lipid profiles, glycemic control, and quality of life in patients with heart failure: A feasibility study. *J Cardiovasc Nurs* 24 (3):207.

Feldstein, A. E., R. Lopez, T. A. Tamimi, L. Yerian, Y. M. Chung, M. Berk, R. Zhang, T. M. McIntyre, and S. L. Hazen. 2010. Mass spectrometric profiling of oxidized lipid products in human nonalcoholic fatty liver disease and nonalcoholic steatohepatitis. *J Lipid Res* 51 (10):3046–3054.

Felker, G. M., R. J. Mentz, R. Cole, K. F. Adams, G. F. Egnaczyk, M. Fiuzat, C. B. Patel et al. 2017. Efficacy and safety of tolvaptan in patients hospitalized with acute heart failure. *J Am Coll Cardiol* 69 (11):1399–1406.

Fleg, J. L., L. S. Cooper, B. A. Borlaug, M. J. Haykowsky, W. E. Kraus, B. D. Levine, M. A. Pfeffer et al. 2015. Exercise training as therapy for heart failure: Current status and future directions. *Circ Heart Fail* 8 (1):209–220.

Fonarow, G. C. 2008. Statins and n-3 fatty acid supplementation in heart failure. *Lancet* 372 (9645):1195–1196.

Fotino, A. D., A. M. Thompson-Paul, and L. A. Bazzano. 2013. Effect of coenzyme Q10 supplementation on heart failure: A meta-analysis. *Am J Clin Nutr* 97 (2):268–275.

Fulster, S., M. Tacke, A. Sandek, N. Ebner, C. Tschope, W. Doehner, S. D. Anker, and S. von Haehling. 2013. Muscle wasting in patients with chronic heart failure: Results from the studies investigating co-morbidities aggravating heart failure (SICA-HF). *Eur Heart J* 34 (7):512–519.

Glean, A. A., S. K. Ferguson, C. T. Holdsworth, T. D. Colburn, J. L. Wright, A. J. Fees, K. S. Hageman, D. C. Poole, and T. I. Musch. 2015. Effects of nitrite infusion on skeletal muscle vascular control during exercise in rats with chronic heart failure. *Am J Physiol Heart Circ Physiol* 309 (8):H1354–H1360.

Glück, T., and P. Alter. 2016. Marine omega-3 highly unsaturated fatty acids: From mechanisms to clinical implications in heart failure and arrhythmias. *Vasc Pharmacol* 82:11–19.

Greenfield, S., and E. Steinberg. 2011. *Clinical Practice Guidelines We Can Trust.* Washington, DC: National Academies Press.

Hanninen, S. A., P. B. Darling, M. J. Sole, A. Barr, and M. E. Keith. 2006. The prevalence of thiamin deficiency in hospitalized patients with congestive heart failure. *J Am Coll Cardiol* 47 (2):354–361.

Heidenreich, P. A., N. M. Albert, L. A. Allen, D. A. Bluemke, J. Butler, G. C. Fonarow, J. S. Ikonomidis et al. 2013. Forecasting the impact of heart failure in the United States: A policy statement from the American Heart Association. *Circ Heart Fail* 6 (3):606–619.

Horwich, T. B., G. C. Fonarow, M. A. Hamilton, W. R. MacLellan, M. A. Woo, and J. H. Tillisch. 2001. The relationship between obesity and mortality in patients with heart failure. *J Am Coll Cardiol* 38 (3):789–795.

Institute of Medicine. 2011. *Finding What Works in Health Care: Standards for Systematic Reviews*, ed. J. Eden, L. Levit, A. Berg, and S. Morton. Washington, DC: National Academies Press.

Jacobs, A. K., J. L. Anderson, and J. L. Halperin. 2014. The evolution and future of ACC/AHA clinical practice guidelines: A 30-year journey: A report of the American College of Cardiology/American Heart Association Task Force on Practice Guidelines. *J Am Coll Cardiol* 64 (13):1373–1384.

Jacobs, A. K., F. G. Kushner, S. M. Ettinger, R. A. Guyton, J. L. Anderson, E. M. Ohman, N. M. Albert et al. 2013. ACCF/AHA clinical practice guideline methodology summit report: A report of the American College of Cardiology Foundation/American Heart Association Task Force on Practice Guidelines. *J Am Coll Cardiol* 61 (2):213–265.

Januzzi, J. L., Jr. 2012. The role of natriuretic peptide testing in guiding chronic heart failure management: Review of available data and recommendations for use. *Arch Cardiovasc Dis* 105 (1):40–50.

Kalantar-Zadeh, K., S. D. Anker, A. J. S. Coats, T. B. Horwich, and G. C. Fonarow. 2005. Obesity paradox as a component of reverse epidemiology in heart failure. *Arch Intern Med* 165 (15):1797.

Kitzman, D. W., P. H. Brubaker, D. M. Herrington, T. M. Morgan, K. P. Stewart, W. G. Hundley, A. Abdelhamed, and M. J. Haykowsky. 2013. Effect of endurance exercise training on endothelial function and arterial stiffness in older patients with heart failure and preserved ejection fraction: A randomized, controlled, single-blind trial. *J Am Coll Cardiol* 62 (7):584–592.

Klingbeil, A. U., M. Schneider, P. Martus, F. H. Messerli, and R. E. Schmieder. 2003. A meta-analysis of the effects of treatment on left ventricular mass in essential hypertension. *Am J Med* 115 (1):41–46.

Kober, L., C. Torp-Pedersen, J. E. Carlsen, H. Bagger, P. Eliasen, K. Lyngborg, J. Videbaek, D. S. Cole, L. Auclert, and N. C. Pauly. 1995. A clinical trial of the angiotensin-converting-enzyme inhibitor trandolapril in patients with left ventricular dysfunction after myocardial infarction. Trandolapril Cardiac Evaluation (TRACE) Study Group. *N Engl J Med* 333 (25):1670–1676.

Konstam, M. A., J. D. Neaton, K. Dickstein, H. Drexler, M. Komajda, F. A. Martinez, G. A. Riegger et al. 2009. Effects of high-dose versus low-dose losartan on clinical outcomes in patients with heart failure (HEAAL study): A randomised, double-blind trial. *Lancet* 374 (9704):1840–1848.

Kwok, T., J. F. Falconer-Smith, J. F. Potter, and D. R. Ives. 1992. Thiamine status of elderly patients with cardiac failure. *Age Ageing* 21 (1):67–71.

Lavie, C. J., M. R. Mehra, and R. V. Milani. 2005. Obesity and heart failure prognosis: Paradox or reverse epidemiology? *Eur Heart J* 26 (1):5–7.

Lee, D. S., P. Gona, R. S. Vasan, M. G. Larson, E. J. Benjamin, T. J. Wang, J. V. Tu, and D. Levy. 2009. Relation of disease pathogenesis and risk factors to heart failure with preserved or reduced ejection fraction: Insights from the Framingham Heart Study of the National Heart, Lung, and Blood Institute. *Circulation* 119 (24):3070–3077.

Lemon, S. C., B. Olendzki, R. Magner, W. Li, A. L. Culver, I. Ockene, and R. J. Goldberg. 2010. The dietary quality of persons with heart failure in NHANES 1999–2006. *J Gen Intern Med* 25 (2):135–140.

Licata, G., P. Di Pasquale, G. Parrinello, A. Cardinale, A. Scandurra, G. Follone, C. Argano, A. Tuttolomondo, and S. Paterna. 2003. Effects of high-dose furosemide and small-volume hypertonic saline solution infusion in comparison with a high dose of furosemide as bolus in refractory congestive heart failure: Long-term effects. *Am Heart J* 145 (3):459–466.

Lindenfeld, J., N. M. Albert, J. P. Boehmer, S. P. Collins, J. A. Ezekowitz, M. M. Givertz, S. D. Katz, M. Klapholz, D. K. Moser, and J. G. Rogers. 2010. HFSA 2010 comprehensive heart failure practice guideline. *J Cardiac Fail* 16 (6):e1–e194.

Lund, L. H., L. Benson, U. Dahlstrom, M. Edner, and L. Friberg. 2014. Association between use of beta-blockers and outcomes in patients with heart failure and preserved ejection fraction. *JAMA* 312 (19):2008–2018.

Mabalirajan, U., R. Rehman, T. Ahmad, S. Kumar, S. Singh, G. D. Leishangthem, J. Aich et al. 2013. Linoleic acid metabolite drives severe asthma by causing airway epithelial injury. *Sci Rep* 3:1349.

Macchia, A., G. Levantesi, M. G. Franzosi, E. Geraci, A. P. Maggioni, R. Marfisi, G. L. Nicolosi et al. 2005. Left ventricular systolic dysfunction, total mortality, and sudden death in patients with myocardial infarction treated with n-3 polyunsaturated fatty acids. *Eur J Heart Fail* 7 (5):904–909.

Masson, S., R. Marchioli, D. Mozaffarian, R. Bernasconi, V. Milani, L. Dragani, M. Tacconi, R. M. Marfisi, L. Borgese, and V. Cirrincione. 2013. Plasma n-3 polyunsaturated fatty acids in chronic heart failure in the GISSI-Heart Failure Trial: Relation with fish intake, circulating biomarkers, and mortality. *Am Heart J* 165 (2):208–215.e4.

Mehra, M. R., C. J. Lavie, H. O. Ventura, and R. V. Milani. 2006. Fish oils produce anti-inflammatory effects and improve body weight in severe heart failure. *J Heart Lung Transplant* 25 (7):834–838.

Molyneux, S. L., C. M. Florkowski, P. M. George, A. P. Pilbrow, C. M. Frampton, M. Lever, and A. M. Richards. 2008. Coenzyme Q10: An independent predictor of mortality in chronic heart failure. *J Am Coll Cardiol* 52 (18):1435–1441.

Mortensen, S. A., F. Rosenfeldt, A. Kumar, P. Dolliner, K. J. Filipiak, D. Pella, U. Alehagen, G. Steurer, G. P. Littarru, and Q-SYMBIO Study Investigators. 2014. The effect of coenzyme Q10 on morbidity and mortality in chronic heart failure: Results from Q-SYMBIO: A randomized double-blind trial. *JACC Heart Fail* 2 (6):641–649.

Mozaffarian, D., C. L. Bryson, R. N. Lemaitre, G. L. Burke, and D. S. Siscovick. 2005. Fish intake and risk of incident heart failure. *J Am Coll Cardiol* 45 (12):2015–2021.

Munzel, T., T. Gori, J. F. Keaney Jr., C. Maack, and A. Daiber. 2015. Pathophysiological role of oxidative stress in systolic and diastolic heart failure and its therapeutic implications. *Eur Heart J* 36 (38):2555–2564.

Ni, H., and J. Xu. 2015. Recent trends in heart failure-related mortality: United States, 2000–2014. *NCHS Data Brief* (231):1–8.

Ohtani, T., S. F. Mohammed, K. Yamamoto, S. M. Dunlay, S. A. Weston, Y. Sakata, R. J. Rodeheffer, V. L. Roger, and M. M. Redfield. 2012. Diastolic stiffness as assessed by diastolic wall strain is associated with adverse remodelling and poor outcomes in heart failure with preserved ejection fraction. *Eur Heart J* 33 (14):1742–1749.

Oktay, A. A., J. D. Rich, and S. J. Shah. 2013. The emerging epidemic of heart failure with preserved ejection fraction. *Curr Heart Fail Rep* 10 (4):401–410.

Orr, S. K., S. Palumbo, F. Bosetti, H. T. Mount, J. X. Kang, C. E. Greenwood, D. W. Ma, C. N. Serhan, and R. P. Bazinet. 2013. Unesterified docosahexaenoic acid is protective in neuroinflammation. *J Neurochem* 127 (3):378–393.

Owan, T. E., D. O. Hodge, R. M. Herges, S. J. Jacobsen, V. L. Roger, and M. M. Redfield. 2006. Trends in prevalence and outcome of heart failure with preserved ejection fraction. *N Engl J Med* 355 (3):251–259.

Packer, M., P. A. Poole-Wilson, P. W. Armstrong, J. G. Cleland, J. D. Horowitz, B. M. Massie, L. Ryden, K. Thygesen, and B. F. Uretsky. 1999. Comparative effects of low and high doses of the angiotensin-converting enzyme inhibitor, lisinopril, on morbidity and mortality in chronic heart failure. ATLAS Study Group. *Circulation* 100 (23):2312–2318.

Pandey, A., A. Parashar, D. J. Kumbhani, S. Agarwal, J. Garg, D. Kitzman, B. D. Levine, M. Drazner, and J. D. Berry. 2015. Exercise training in patients with heart failure and preserved ejection fraction: Meta-analysis of randomized control trials. *Circ Heart Fail* 8 (1):33–40.

Parrinello, G., P. Di Pasquale, G. Licata, D. Torres, M. Giammanco, S. Fasullo, M. Mezzero, and S. Paterna. 2009. Long-term effects of dietary sodium intake on cytokines and neurohormonal activation in patients with recently compensated congestive heart failure. *J Cardiac Fail* 15 (10):864–873.

Paterna, S., P. Gaspare, S. Fasullo, F. M. Sarullo, and P. Di Pasquale. 2008. Normal-sodium diet compared with low-sodium diet in compensated congestive heart failure: Is sodium an old enemy or a new friend? *Clin Sci* 114 (3):221–230.

Paulus, W. J., and C. Tschope. 2013. A novel paradigm for heart failure with preserved ejection fraction: Comorbidities drive myocardial dysfunction and remodeling through coronary microvascular endothelial inflammation. *J Am Coll Cardiol* 62 (4):263–271.

Pfeffer, M. A., E. Braunwald, L. A. Moye, L. Basta, E. J. Brown Jr., T. E. Cuddy, B. R. Davis et al. 1992. Effect of captopril on mortality and morbidity in patients with left ventricular dysfunction after myocardial infarction. Results of the survival and ventricular enlargement trial. The SAVE Investigators. *N Engl J Med* 327 (10):669–677.

Pfeffer, M. A., J. J. McMurray, E. J. Velazquez, J. L. Rouleau, L. Kober, A. P. Maggioni, S. D. Solomon et al. 2003a. Valsartan, captopril, or both in myocardial infarction complicated by heart failure, left ventricular dysfunction, or both. *N Engl J Med* 349 (20):1893–1906.

Pfeffer, M. A., K. Swedberg, C. B. Granger, P. Held, J. J. McMurray, E. L. Michelson, B. Olofsson, J. Ostergren, S. Yusuf, S. Pocock, and CHARM Investigators and Committees. 2003b. Effects of candesartan on mortality and morbidity in patients with chronic heart failure: The CHARM-Overall programme. *Lancet* 362 (9386):759–766.

Pfitzenmeyer, P., J. C. Guilland, Ph. d'Athis, C. Petit-Marnier, and M. Gaudet. 1994. Thiamine status of elderly patients with cardiac failure including the effects of supplementation. *Int J Vitam Nutr Res* 64 (2):113–118.

Poole, D. C., D. M. Hirai, S. W. Copp, and T. I. Musch. 2012. Muscle oxygen transport and utilization in heart failure: Implications for exercise (in)tolerance. *Am J Physiol Heart Circ Physiol* 302 (5):H1050–H1063.

Ramsden, C. E., A. Ringel, A. E. Feldstein, A. Y. Taha, B. A. MacIntosh, J. R. Hibbeln, S. F. Majchrzak-Hong et al. 2012. Lowering dietary linoleic acid reduces bioactive oxidized linoleic acid metabolites in humans. *Prostaglandins Leukot Essent Fatty Acids* 87 (4–5):135–141.

Roger, V. L. 2013. Epidemiology of heart failure. *Circ Res* 113 (6):646–659.

Rozentryt, P., S. von Haehling, M. Lainscak, J. U. Nowak, K. Kalantar-Zadeh, L. Polonski, and S. D. Anker. 2010. The effects of a high-caloric protein-rich oral nutritional supplement in patients with chronic heart failure and cachexia on quality of life, body composition, and inflammation markers: A randomized, double-blind pilot study. *J Cachexia Sarcopenia Muscle* 1 (1):35–42.

Sanders-van Wijk, S., A. D. van Asselt, H. Rickli, W. Estlinbaum, P. Erne, P. Rickenbacher, A. Vuillomenet, M. Peter, M. E. Pfisterer, H. P. Brunner-La Rocca, and TIME-CHF Investigators. 2013. Cost-effectiveness of N-terminal pro-B-type natriuretic-guided therapy in elderly heart failure patients: Results from TIME-CHF (Trial of Intensified versus Standard Medical Therapy in Elderly Patients with Congestive Heart Failure). *JACC Heart Fail* 1 (1):64–71.

Seligmann, H., H. Halkin, S. Rauchfleisch, N. Kaufmann, R. Tal, M. Motro, Z. Vered, and D. Ezra. 1991. Thiamine deficiency in patients with congestive heart failure receiving long-term furosemide therapy: A pilot study. *Am J Med* 91 (2):151–155.

Shimon, H., S. Almog, Z. Vered, H. Seligmann, M. Shefi, E. Peleg, T. Rosenthal, M. Motro, H. Halkin, and D. Ezra. 1995. Improved left ventricular function after thiamine supplementation in patients with congestive heart failure receiving long-term furosemide therapy. *Am J Med* 98 (5):485–490.

Sliwa, K., A. Damasceno, B. A. Davison, B. M. Mayosi, M. U. Sani, O. Ogah, C. Mondo et al. 2016. Bi treatment with hydralazine/nitrates vs. placebo in Africans admitted with acute HEart Failure (BA-HEF). *Eur J Heart Fail* 18(10):1248–1258.

Sole, M. J., and K. N. Jeejeebhoy. 2000. Conditioned nutritional requirements and the pathogenesis and treatment of myocardial failure. *Curr Opin Clin Nutr Metab Care* 3 (6):417–424.

The SOLVD Investigators. 1991. Effect of enalapril on survival in patients with reduced left ventricular ejection fractions and congestive heart failure. *N Engl J Med* 325 (5):293–302.

Tavazzi, L., A. P. Maggioni, R. Marchioli, S. Barlera, M. G. Franzosi, R. Latini, D. Lucci, G. L. Nicolosi, M. Porcu, G. Tognoni, and GISSI-HF Investigators. 2008. Effect of n-3 polyunsaturated fatty acids in patients with chronic heart failure (the GISSI-HF trial): A randomised, double-blind, placebo-controlled trial. *Lancet* 372 (9645):1223–1230.

Tavazzi, L., G. Tognoni, M. G. Franzosi, R. Latini, A. P. Maggioni, R. Marchioli, G. L. Nicolosi, and M. Porcu. 2004. Rationale and design of the GISSI heart failure trial: A large trial to assess the effects of n-3 polyunsaturated fatty acids and rosuvastatin in symptomatic congestive heart failure. *Eur J Heart Fail* 6 (5):635–641.

Tjonahen, E., S. F. Oh, J. Siegelman, S. Elangovan, K. B. Percarpio, S. Hong, M. Arita, and C. N. Serhan. 2006. Resolvin E2: Identification and anti-inflammatory actions: Pivotal role of human 5-lipoxygenase in resolvin E series biosynthesis. *Chem Biol* 13 (11):1193–1202.

Toborek, M., A. Malecki, R. Garrido, M. P. Mattson, B. Hennig, and B. Young. 1999. Arachidonic acid-induced oxidative injury to cultured spinal cord neurons. *J Neurochem* 73 (2):684–692.

van Heerebeek, L., C. P. Franssen, N. Hamdani, F. W. Verheugt, G. A. Somsen, and W. J. Paulus. 2012a. Molecular and cellular basis for diastolic dysfunction. *Curr Heart Fail Rep* 9 (4):293–302.

van Heerebeek, L., N. Hamdani, I. Falcao-Pires, A. F. Leite-Moreira, M. P. Begieneman, J. G. Bronzwaer, J. van der Velden et al. 2012b. Low myocardial protein kinase G activity in heart failure with preserved ejection fraction. *Circulation* 126 (7):830–839.

Vardeny, O., B. Claggett, I. Anand, P. Rossignol, A. S. Desai, F. Zannad, B. Pitt, S. D. Solomon, and Randomized Aldactone Evaluation Study Investigators. 2014. Incidence, predictors, and outcomes related to hypo- and hyperkalemia in patients with severe heart failure treated with a mineralocorticoid receptor antagonist. *Circ Heart Fail* 7 (4):573–579.

Vest, A. R., Y. Wu, R. Hachamovitch, J. B. Young, and L. Cho. 2015. The heart failure overweight/obesity survival paradox: The missing sex link. *JACC Heart Fail* 3 (11):917–926.

von Haehling, S. 2015. The wasting continuum in heart failure: From sarcopenia to cachexia. *Proc Nutr Soc* 74 (4):367–377.

Wang, C., W. S. Harris, M. Chung, A. H. Lichtenstein, E. M. Balk, B. Kupelnick, H. S. Jordan, and J. Lau. 2006. n-3 fatty acids from fish or fish-oil supplements, but not α-linolenic acid, benefit cardiovascular disease outcomes in primary-and secondary-prevention studies: A systematic review. *Am J Clin Nutr* 84 (1):5–17.

Watson, R. D., C. R. Gibbs, and G. Y. Lip. 2000. ABC of heart failure. Clinical features and complications. *BMJ* 320 (7229):236–239.

Wilk, J. B., M. Y. Tsai, N. Q. Hanson, J. M. Gaziano, and L. Djoussé. 2012. Plasma and dietary omega-3 fatty acids, fish intake, and heart failure risk in the Physicians' Health Study. *Am J Clin Nutr* 96 (4):882–888.

Witte, K. K., N. P. Nikitin, A. C. Parker, S. von Haehling, H. D. Volk, S. D. Anker, A. L. Clark, and J. G. Cleland. 2005. The effect of micronutrient supplementation on quality-of-life and left ventricular function in elderly patients with chronic heart failure. *Eur Heart J* 26 (21):2238–2244.

Writing Group Members, D. Lloyd-Jones, R. J. Adams, T. M. Brown, M. Carnethon, S. Dai, G. De Simone et al. 2010. Heart disease and stroke statistics—2010 update: A report from the American Heart Association. *Circulation* 121 (7):e46–e215.

Yamagishi, K., J. A. Nettleton, A. R. Folsom, and ARIC Study Investigators. 2008. Plasma fatty acid composition and incident heart failure in middle-aged adults: The Atherosclerosis Risk in Communities (ARIC) Study. *Am Heart J* 156 (5):965–974.

Yancy, C. W., M. Jessup, B. Bozkurt, J. Butler, D. E. Casey Jr., M. M. Colvin, M. H. Drazner et al. 2016. 2016 ACC/AHA/HFSA focused update on new pharmacological therapy for heart failure: An update of the 2013 ACCF/AHA guideline for the management of heart failure: A report of the American College of Cardiology/American Heart Association Task Force on Clinical Practice Guidelines and the Heart Failure Society of America. *J Am Coll Cardiol* 68 (13):1476–1488.

Yancy, C. W., M. Jessup, B. Bozkurt, J. Butler, D. E. Casey Jr., M. H. Drazner, G. C. Fonarow et al. 2013. 2013 ACCF/AHA guideline for the management of heart failure: A report of the American College of Cardiology Foundation/American Heart Association Task Force on Practice Guidelines. *J Am Coll Cardiol* 62 (16):e147–e239.

Yoshida, Y., A. Yoshikawa, T. Kinumi, Y. Ogawa, Y. Saito, K. Ohara, H. Yamamoto, Y. Imai, and E. Niki. 2009. Hydroxyoctadecadienoic acid and oxidatively modified peroxiredoxins in the blood of Alzheimer's disease patients and their potential as biomarkers. *Neurobiol Aging* 30 (2):174–185.

Yurko-Mauro, K., D. McCarthy, D. Rom, E. B. Nelson, A. S. Ryan, A. Blackwell, N. Salem Jr., M. Stedman, and MIDAS Investigators. 2010. Beneficial effects of docosahexaenoic acid on cognition in age-related cognitive decline. *Alzheimers Dement* 6 (6):456–464.

Zamani, P., D. Rawat, P. Shiva-Kumar, S. Geraci, R. Bhuva, P. Konda, P. T. Doulias et al. 2015. Effect of inorganic nitrate on exercise capacity in heart failure with preserved ejection fraction. *Circulation* 131 (4):371–380; discussion 380.

Zamora, E., J. Lupón, C. Enjuanes, D. Pascual-Figal, M. de Antonio, M. Domingo, J. Comín-Colet et al. 2016. No benefit from the obesity paradox for diabetic patients with heart failure. *Eur J Heart Fail* 18 (7):851–858.

Zenuk, C., J. Healey, J. Donnelly, R. Vaillancourt, Y. Almalki, and S. Smith. 2002. Thiamine deficiency in congestive heart failure patients receiving long term furosemide therapy. *Can J Clin Pharmacol* 10 (4):184–188.

14 Pulmonary Function, Asthma, and Obesity

14.1 INTRODUCTION

Obesity significantly interferes with pulmonary function by decreasing lung volumes, particularly the expiratory reserve volume (ERV) and functional residual capacity (FRC). Strength and resistance may be reduced as the result of muscle weakness, especially in those with sarcopenic obesity associated with aging. These mechanical limitations lead to inspiratory overload, which increases respiratory effort, oxygen consumption, and respiratory energy expenditure. Body fat distribution significantly influences the function of the respiratory system, likely via the direct mechanical effect of fat accumulation in the chest and abdominal regions, as well as the systemic cytokines released by visceral fat. Asthma and obstructive sleep apnea (OSA) are obesity-associated diseases that involve interactions among environmental, genetic, and behavioral factors.

Approximately 60% of obese individuals have metabolic syndrome (Beltran-Sanchez et al. 2013). In this context, an association between metabolic syndrome and pulmonary disease has been investigated in recent years (Samson and Garber 2014; Baffi et al. 2016). Metabolic syndrome has been identified as an independent risk factor for worsening respiratory symptoms, impairment of lung function, asthma, and pulmonary hypertension. Several possible mechanisms have been proposed to explain these associations, including exposure to high insulin levels during fetal maturation (which induces alterations in airway smooth muscle), the effects of abdominal adiposity, deregulation of adipokine metabolism, and inflammation induced by ectopic fat in the lungs (Lee et al. 2014). Inflammation also impacts asthma in children and adults, and the roles of oxidative stress and elevated adipokines are still being evaluated relative to other causative factors, such as allergies and air pollution.

Therefore, obesity and metabolic syndrome both combine to impair lung function in the overweight and obese patient. A strong correlation exists between lung function and body fat distribution, with greater impairment when fat accumulates in the chest and abdomen. In combination with reflux esophagitis and anatomic changes with obesity, OSA leads to sleep disturbances, which create a vicious circle of increased calorie intake and poor sleep. The concomitant use of continuous positive airway pressure (CPAP) devices, together with a diet and lifestyle plan to reduce excess body fat and build lean body mass, including diaphragmatic strength through respiratory therapy, promises to reduce the morbidity associated with obesity and reduced pulmonary function.

14.2 PULMONARY FUNCTION IN OBESITY

Normal pulmonary function depends on the operation of the structures that compose the respiratory system. In obese individuals, structural changes of the thoracic–abdominal region lead to limited diaphragm mobility and rib movement, both essential for appropriate ventilatory mechanics. Additionally, the adipose tissue is an endocrine and paracrine organ that produces a large number of cytokines and bioactive mediators, thus generating in obese individuals a pro-inflammatory state that is associated with allergic reactions, bronchial responsiveness, and increased risk of asthma.

In order to maintain pulmonary homeostasis, the structures of the respiratory and cardiovascular systems need to work in equilibrium; that is, the lungs should be ventilated and the gases should diffuse through the alveolar–capillary barrier in a balanced fashion. It is practical in primary care practice to evaluate lung function by determining lung volumes. The most accurate techniques for determining lung volumes are spirometry and plethysmography. In normal breathing, the diaphragm contracts, pushing the abdominal content downward and forward, and at the same time, contraction of the external intercostal muscles tractions the ribs upward and forward. In obese individuals, this mechanism is hindered, since the excess adiposity that covers the thorax and the abdomen encumbers the breathing muscles. Any interference in the chest bellows or in chest mobility, generating a decrease in lung volume, can be considered a restrictive illness. In the obese, excess fat in the abdominal cavity and chest limits the two primary inspiratory movements: diaphragm contraction propelling the abdominal content downward and forward, and increased chest diameter by means of rib movement.

Evaluation of static lung volumes in overweight and obese patients reveals a reduction in the ERV, FRC, and total lung capacity (TLC). Reductions in FRC and ERV are detectable even at a modest increase in weight. This results from a shift in the balance of inflationary and deflationary pressures on the lung due to the mass load of adipose tissue around the rib cage and abdomen (Salome et al. 2010). Elevated intra-abdominal pressure can be transmitted to the chest. This dramatically reduces the FRC and ERV and requires patients to breathe in a less efficient part of their pressure–volume curve, which in turn increases the work of breathing (Steier et al. 2014). Marked reductions in ERV may lead to abnormalities in ventilation distribution, with closure of airways in the dependent zones of the lung and inequalities in the ventilation–perfusion ratio (Salome et al. 2010).

Spirometry measurements of lung function in morbidly obese subjects reveal a proportional reduction in forced vital capacity (FVC) and forced expiratory volume in 1 second (FEV1), suggesting the occurrence of restrictive lung disease (Carpio et al. 2014; Melo et al. 2014). The FEV1/FVC ratio is generally well preserved or elevated even in morbidly obese individuals, indicating that FEV1 and FVC are affected at the same rate (Wells et al. 1995; Thyagarajan et al. 2008). A reduction in expiratory flows in an obese individual is unlikely to indicate bronchial obstruction unless the flow measurements have been normalized for the reduction in FVC (Salome et al. 2010). In the supine position, the weight of the abdomen in obese individuals causes the diaphragm to ascend into the chest, resulting in the closure of small airways at the base of the lung, and thereby generating an intrinsic positive end-expiratory pressure that results in increased ventilatory work and consequent respiratory muscle impairment (Chlif et al. 2009; Arena and Cahalin 2014).

Most obese individuals present an arterial partial pressure of oxygen (PaO_2) within the normal range. However, among morbidly obese subjects, the alveolar–arterial oxygen gradient ($P(A\text{-}a)O_2$) is slightly widened because of the presence of areas of atelectasis and maldistribution of ventilation (Rivas et al. 2015), which can cause a major ventilation–perfusion imbalance. In these individuals, the lower parts of the lungs are relatively poorly ventilated and perfused, possibly due to the closure of small airways, whereas the upper regions of the lungs exhibit enhanced ventilation (Brazzale et al. 2015).

14.3 ASTHMA AND OBESITY

Obesity is also associated with a higher incidence, prevalence, and severity of asthma. Asthma in obese patients is characterized by poor treatment response and greater morbidity (Torchio et al. 2009; Boulet et al. 2012; Dixon et al. 2015; Lu et al. 2015; Pakhale et al. 2015; Ulrik 2016). The incidence of asthma is almost one and a half times higher in obese individuals than in nonobese individuals, and a three-unit increase in body mass index (BMI) is associated with a 35% increase in the risk of asthma (Hjellvik et al. 2010; Brumpton et al. 2013). Decreases in FRC and tidal volume, in addition to sedentary lifestyle and limited ability to perform physical activities, may worsen asthma symptoms among obese patients (Hjellvik et al. 2010; Yawn et al. 2015; Ulrik 2016). In a cohort study of more than 25,000 children and adults with asthma, a higher BMI was associated with worsened asthma control and an increased risk of asthma exacerbations (Schatz et al. 2015).

Obesity and metabolic syndrome are associated with a state of chronic systemic inflammation that is driven predominantly by the action of substances released by adipose tissue. Chronic inflammation is caused by activation of the innate immune system, which promotes a pro-inflammatory state and oxidative stress and a consequent systemic acute-phase response Increased levels of leptin, tumor necrosis factor α (TNF-α), transforming growth factor β (TGF-β), C-reactive protein (CRP), and eotaxin may interact with asthma-associated inflammation from atopic reactions to exacerbate cytokine effects on the contractility of the bronchial airway smooth muscles (Torchio et al. 2009; de Lima Azambuja et al. 2015).

Different obesity-associated asthma phenotypes are now recognized (Bates 2016). An early-onset allergic form that is complicated by obesity and a late-onset nonallergic form that occurs only in the setting of obesity have been identified. Late-onset obese asthmatics have more compliant airways, while early-onset obese asthmatics demonstrate inflammatory thickening of the airways. These two phenotypes are characterized by different pathological findings, but more research is needed on the interactions of allergens, dietary pattern, and asthma in obesity.

14.4 OBSTRUCTIVE SLEEP APNEA AND HYPOVENTILATION SYNDROME

Obesity is associated with both hypoventilation and OSA. Obesity is the most common known risk factor for the development of OSA (Duarte and Magalhaes-da-Silveira 2015). The prevalence of OSA associated with high rates of morbidity and mortality increases with age; the peak incidence occurs at approximately age 55, and the condition is more prevalent in males than in females by a ratio of 2:1 (Pinto et al. 2016).

OSA is a systemic disease that causes an increase in TNF-α, IL-6, insulin resistance, and glucose intolerance; these inflammatory cytokines have also been implicated in the immunological mechanisms of obesity (Aurora and Punjabi 2013). Central obesity and increased neck circumference are predisposing factors for OSA (Blomster et al. 2015; Ren et al. 2015). The resulting reduction or interruption of airflow, which occurs despite inspiratory effort, causes poor alveolar ventilation and oxyhemoglobin desaturation and, in cases of prolonged events, a progressive increase in the arterial partial pressure of carbon dioxide (Pierce and Brown 2015). There is a strong association between OSA and metabolic syndrome as a whole or with its individual components (Baffi et al. 2016).

The prevalence of metabolic syndrome in patients with OSA is 60%, which is significantly higher than in the general population (Gil et al. 2013). This association is partially explained by the fact that patients with OSA are more likely to have high visceral adiposity, as well as abnormal glucose metabolism (Baffi et al. 2016; Bozkurt et al. 2016). There is ample evidence suggesting that OSA may exacerbate or induce the majority of the components of metabolic syndrome.

Some of these effects can be improved with the use of CPAP. However, the modest and inconsistent benefits obtained with this technique suggest that factors other than intermittent hypoxia or the apnea–hypopnea index may play an important role (Baffi et al. 2016). Some obese individuals develop obesity hypoventilation syndrome (OHS), which is defined by the triad of obesity. Hypoventilation during the day and sleep-disordered breathing represent hypoventilation that occurs in the absence of a neuromuscular, mechanical, or metabolic cause (Chau et al. 2012). The prevalence of OHS is estimated to be 8.5% in patients with OSA and 19–31% in obese subjects (BaHammam 2015; Shetty and Parthasarathy 2015). OHS is more prevalent in women than in men, and postmenopausal women with OSA have a higher prevalence of OHS. This has been attributed to hormonal influences, particularly to the role of progesterone as a respiratory stimulant prior to menopause (Jehan et al. 2015; BaHammam et al. 2016). Compared with eucapnic obese patients, patients with OHS have severe upper airway obstruction, restrictive pulmonary damage, a decreased central respiratory drive, an increased incidence of pulmonary hypertension, and increased mortality (Chau et al. 2012).

Among the possible mechanisms involved in the pathogenesis of OHS, some studies have reported damage to respiratory mechanics caused by obesity, leptin resistance leading to central hypoventilation, respiratory sleep disorders, and impaired compensatory responses to acute hypercapnia (Chau et al. 2012; Pierce and Brown 2015; Shetty and Parthasarathy 2015). With respect to pulmonary function, patients with OHS present a reduction in chest wall compliance compared with patients with eucapnic obesity, as well as increased pulmonary resistance that is likely secondary to the reduction in FRC (Chau et al. 2012).

14.5 EFFECTS OF POOR-QUALITY SLEEP IN OBESITY

Poor-quality sleep is characterized by a decrease in sleep duration and disruptions in sleep patterns and increased wake after sleep onset (Ohayon et al. 2004). A good night's sleep is dependent on a sufficient amount of deep sleep and a sleep efficiency, that is, total sleep time divided by time in bed, of greater than 85% (Akerstedt et al. 1994). In both obese and nonobese individuals, the quality of sleep declines with age, with a major reduction in the duration of slow-wave sleep and increased sleep fragmentation (Van Cauter et al. 2000).

Adequate sleep quality and quantity are important for the normal functioning of daily metabolic and hormonal processes, and appetite regulation (Van Cauter et al. 2008). These factors may contribute to energy dysregulation that leads to weight gain and obesity. Several epidemiological studies have demonstrated an association between sleep duration and obesity (Marshall et al. 2008; Nielsen et al. 2011).

While many obese individuals presenting with daytime sleepiness or somnolence will be diagnosed with OSA, a significant proportion of such patients will continue to have somnolence after weight loss. Clinical studies demonstrate that obesity without sleep apnea is also associated with a higher prevalence of somnolence, and that bariatric surgery can markedly improve somnolence before resolution of OSA. Patients with OSA and excessive daytime sleepiness who undergo bariatric surgery experience a dramatic improvement in subjective sleepiness (Dixon et al. 2005; Fritscher et al. 2007; Holty et al. 2011). In a study of severely obese patients with OSA who underwent gastric bypass, the Epworth sleepiness score for the group fell from 14 (severe sleepiness) preoperatively to 5 (normal) at 1 month after surgery, a time when weight loss was expected to be just 10–12 pounds (Varela et al. 2007).

Short-term sleep restriction in young healthy adults also promotes insulin resistance, impaired glucose tolerance, and obesity (Spiegel et al. 1999, 2005). Insufficient sleep, in combination with physical inactivity, has been shown to impede weight loss in overweight individuals matched for caloric intake (Nedeltcheva et al. 2010).

Regular consumption of high-fat foods and excessive calories predicts excessive daytime sleepiness and poor quality of nocturnal sleep (Craig and Richardson 1989; Wells et al. 1995, 1998; Harnish et al. 1998). Food-induced sleepiness may be due to the acute hormonal and neuroendocrine effects of a high-fat meal. High-fat content and excessive nutrients ingested on a regular basis could then cause regularly occurring symptoms of excessive sleepiness. For years, people attributed the sleepiness after a very large Thanksgiving meal to the tryptophan in the turkey typically served at this meal. The sleepiness is induced by both tryptophan and the effects of a high-glycemic-index meal, which increases tryptophan availability (Herrera et al. 2011).

While the mechanisms explaining sleepiness beyond obstructive apnea are not fully established, a number of hormonal studies have been carried out in lean and obese individuals. The most convincing of these studies demonstrate that sleep deprivation affects leptin and ghrelin levels and appetite. In two studies where leptin levels were measured at multiple time points throughout the day and food intake was controlled, several days of sleep deprivation or restriction to four hours per night in young healthy men resulted in increased appetite and decreased leptin levels, with flattening of circadian peaks in leptin (Mullington et al. 2003; Spiegel et al. 2004). In fact, shortening the sleep time by just 90 minutes per night for 2 weeks is sufficient to markedly increase appetite and caloric intake (Nedeltcheva et al. 2009). Interestingly, ghrelin increases in parallel with increased appetite (Schmid et al. 2008). Elevated ghrelin levels may predict food intake during sleep restriction, suggesting a potential mechanism by which sleep loss may lead to increased food intake and the development of weight gain.

14.6 PRIMARY CARE SLEEP HYGIENE RECOMMENDATIONS

Sleep problems are prevalent among patients seen in primary care practice beyond those with OSA, or clinical sleep disorders related to obesity. In these patients, sleep problems may promote overeating and lead to the development of overweight and obesity. Sleep problems of this type refer generally to any combination of acute or chronic problems with prolonged sleep onset latency, excessive wake after sleep onset, short total sleep time, low sleep efficiency, or poor-sleep quality based on subjective and/or objective assessments.

More than half (56%) of Americans suffer from sleep problems, compared with 31% of western Europeans and 29% of Japanese (Leger et al. 2008). Although the majority of these individuals report functional impairment as a result of their sleep problems, most (61–79%) do not meet clinical diagnostic criteria for insomnia based on self-reported symptoms (Leger et al. 2008).

Sleep problems are of growing concern, because poor sleep is associated with impairments in motivation, emotion, and cognitive functioning, as well as increased risk for serious medical conditions, including diabetes, cardiovascular disease, cancer, and all-cause mortality, even when the symptoms are below the threshold for clinical sleep disorders (Banks and Dinges 2007; Walker 2009; Zaharna and Guilleminault 2010).

Despite the potential widespread benefit for sleep promotion, established behavioral treatments such as cognitive behavioral therapy for insomnia are largely limited to practices directed by sleep medicine professionals rather than primary care teams. Patients with intermittent or less severe sleep impairments or those for whom specialized sleep treatments are unavailable or inaccessible are more likely to seek assistance from primary care providers or self-help materials to manage their sleep problems, and as a result will likely be exposed to sleep hygiene recommendations that are widely used in medical settings (Zarcone 2000; Stepanski and Wyatt 2003) and are easily accessible on the Internet.

It may be useful to establish a practical set of evidence-based behavioral recommendations regarding caffeine use, nicotine, exercise, and stress for patients in primary care reporting sleep problems but who do not have evidence from sleep studies of sleep apnea.

Current sleep hygiene recommendations on caffeine intake for such patients vary widely, ranging from complete abstinence to avoiding caffeine only in the afternoon or evening (Stepanski and Wyatt 2003). Few studies have actually tested the impact of morning caffeine consumption on subsequent nighttime sleep, but 400 mg of caffeine consumed in the late afternoon and evening within the half-life of caffeine has been demonstrated to impair sleep onset and quality. It was found that even doses ingested up to 6 hours before bedtime were associated with disturbances in both subjectively and objectively assessed sleep (Drake et al. 2013). The participants in these studies were often not regular consumers of caffeine, and therefore may differ in their response to caffeine from the general population of caffeine users (Roehrs and Roth 2008). Nonetheless, it is reasonable to conclude that consuming large quantities of caffeine near bedtime is likely to disrupt sleep, but less is known about the clinical significance of low to moderate amounts of caffeine.

Nicotine promotes arousal and wakefulness, primarily through stimulation of cholinergic neurons in the basal forebrain (Boutrel and Koob 2004). Sleep hygiene recommendations suggest avoidance of nicotine use to promote better sleep. Nicotine, whether from cigarette smoking or administration via pill or patch, is associated with impaired sleep (Jaehne et al. 2009). Whereas caffeine tolerance results in a lesser impact on sleep disturbance, data suggest that even after years of smoking, smokers experience significantly worse sleep than nonsmokers (Jaehne et al. 2009). In the early stages of smoking cessation, sleep complaints are very common. This is likely due to nicotine withdrawal, which results in heightened arousal and cravings. Symptoms of withdrawal peak a few days after cessation and last for 3–4 weeks (Hughes 2007).

Regular exercise is a common sleep hygiene recommendation, with the caveat that exercise should be avoided close to bedtime (Stepanski and Wyatt 2003). Exercise may improve sleep through its effects on body temperature, arousal, and/or adenosine levels (Youngstedt 2005).

In general, recommending regular exercise as part of a healthy active lifestyle will also contribute to improved sleep.

Although stress is not traditionally a core component of sleep hygiene, several recommendations have emerged over the years encouraging individuals to reduce worry or engage in relaxing activities, particularly right before bedtime (Stepanski and Wyatt 2003). Stress typified by an event or events that lead to acute or chronic physiological stresses, including increased heart rate and blood pressure, and psychological anxiety responses can precipitate cognitive arousal and physiological arousal, which can cause problems with sleep initiation and maintenance. Techniques known to reduce stress and arousal, such as relaxation and mindfulness-based stress reduction, have been examined in relation to sleep and have provided some preliminary support for stress management as an effective recommendation to promote sleep (Dijk and Czeisler 1995; Lichstein et al. 2001; Dijk and Lockley 2002).

Sleep hygiene recommendations often encourage regular bedtimes and wake times in order to maximize the synchrony between physiological sleep drive, circadian rhythms, and the nocturnal sleep episode. Homeostatic sleep drive and the circadian hormonal systems work together to promote stable patterns of sleep and wakefulness (Dijk and Czeisler 1995). Sleep duration and continuity are worsened with changes in sleep patterns associated with jet lag or rotating shift work (Dijk and Lockley 2002).

None of the above recommendations are backed by strong science, but are meant to provide some guidance for primary care practices dealing with sleep problems both as an initial presentation and as residual complaints in patients with obesity treated for either OSA or daytime sleepiness.

14.7 SUMMARY

Obesity is associated with abnormal pulmonary function based on the physical effects of excess body fat on respiratory muscle function, inflammation from adipokines, and the superimposition of allergies common in the general population, such as cat allergy, which affects one in three individuals.

OSA can be documented with sleep studies. A simple screening questionnaire can be used to detect those suitable for study. Beyond that, recommendations for weight management need to also include recommendations on sleep hygiene, as the evidence strongly suggests that sleep problems promote obesity and overweight.

REFERENCES

Akerstedt, T., K. Hume, D. Minors, and J. Waterhouse. 1994. The subjective meaning of good sleep, an intraindividual approach using the Karolinska Sleep Diary. *Percept Mot Skills* 79 (1 Pt 1):287–296.

Arena, R., and L. P. Cahalin. 2014. Evaluation of cardiorespiratory fitness and respiratory muscle function in the obese population. *Prog Cardiovasc Dis* 56 (4):457–464.

Aurora, R. N., and N. M. Punjabi. 2013. Obstructive sleep apnoea and type 2 diabetes mellitus: A bidirectional association. *Lancet Respir Med* 1 (4):329–338.

Baffi, C. W., L. Wood, D. Winnica, P. J. Strollo Jr., M. T. Gladwin, L. G. Que, and F. Holguin. 2016. Metabolic syndrome and the lung. *Chest* 149 (6):1525–1534.

BaHammam, A. S. 2015. Prevalence, clinical characteristics, and predictors of obesity hypoventilation syndrome in a large sample of Saudi patients with obstructive sleep apnea. *Saudi Med J* 36 (2):181–189.

BaHammam, A. S., S. R. Pandi-Perumal, A. Piper, S. A. Bahammam, A. S. Almeneessier, A. H. Olaish, and S. Javaheri. 2016. Gender differences in patients with obesity hypoventilation syndrome. *J Sleep Res* 25 (4):445–453.

Banks, S., and D. F. Dinges. 2007. Behavioral and physiological consequences of sleep restriction. *J Clin Sleep Med* 3 (5):519–528.

Bates, J. H. 2016. Physiological mechanisms of airway hyperresponsiveness in obese asthma. *Am J Respir Cell Mol Biol* 54 (5):618–623.

Beltran-Sanchez, H., M. O. Harhay, M. M. Harhay, and S. McElligott. 2013. Prevalence and trends of metabolic syndrome in the adult U.S. population, 1999–2010. *J Am Coll Cardiol* 62 (8):697–703.

Blomster, H., T. P. Laitinen, J. E. Hartikainen, T. M. Laitinen, E. Vanninen, H. Gylling, J. Sahlman, J. Kokkarinen, J. Randell, J. Seppa, and H. Tuomilehto. 2015. Mild obstructive sleep apnea does not modulate baroreflex sensitivity in adult patients. *Nat Sci Sleep* 7:73–80.

Boulet, L. P., H. Turcotte, J. Martin, and P. Poirier. 2012. Effect of bariatric surgery on airway response and lung function in obese subjects with asthma. *Respir Med* 106 (5):651–660.

Boutrel, B., and G. F. Koob. 2004. What keeps us awake: The neuropharmacology of stimulants and wakefulness-promoting medications. *Sleep* 27 (6):1181–1194.

Bozkurt, N. C., S. Beysel, B. Karbek, I. O. Unsal, E. Cakir, and T. Delibasi. 2016. Visceral obesity mediates the association between metabolic syndrome and obstructive sleep apnea syndrome. *Metab Syndr Relat Disord* 14 (4):217–221.

Brazzale, D. J., J. J. Pretto, and L. M. Schachter. 2015. Optimizing respiratory function assessments to elucidate the impact of obesity on respiratory health. *Respirology* 20 (5):715–721.

Brumpton, B. M., L. Leivseth, P. R. Romundstad, A. Langhammer, Y. Chen, C. A. Camargo Jr., and X. M. Mai. 2013. The joint association of anxiety, depression and obesity with incident asthma in adults: The HUNT study. *Int J Epidemiol* 42 (5):1455–1463.

Carpio, C., A. Santiago, A. Garcia de Lorenzo, and R. Alvarez-Sala. 2014. Changes in lung function testing associated with obesity [in Spanish]. *Nutr Hosp* 30 (5):1054–1062.

Chau, E. H., D. Lam, J. Wong, B. Mokhlesi, and F. Chung. 2012. Obesity hypoventilation syndrome: A review of epidemiology, pathophysiology, and perioperative considerations. *Anesthesiology* 117 (1):188–205.

Chlif, M., D. Keochkerian, D. Choquet, A. Vaidie, and S. Ahmaidi. 2009. Effects of obesity on breathing pattern, ventilatory neural drive and mechanics. *Respir Physiol Neurobiol* 168 (3):198–202.

Craig, A., and E. Richardson. 1989. Effects of experimental and habitual lunch-size on performance, arousal, hunger and mood. *Int Arch Occup Environ Health* 61 (5):313–319.

de Lima Azambuja, R., L. S. da Costa Santos Azambuja, C. Costa, and R. Rufino. 2015. Adiponectin in asthma and obesity: Protective agent or risk factor for more severe disease? *Lung* 193 (5):749–755.

Dijk, D. J., and C. A. Czeisler. 1995. Contribution of the circadian pacemaker and the sleep homeostat to sleep propensity, sleep structure, electroencephalographic slow waves, and sleep spindle activity in humans. *J Neurosci* 15 (5 Pt 1):3526–3538.

Dijk, D. J., and S. W. Lockley. 2002. Integration of human sleep-wake regulation and circadian rhythmicity. *J Appl Physiol (1985)* 92 (2):852–862.

Dixon, A. E., M. Subramanian, M. DeSarno, K. Black, L. Lane, and F. Holguin. 2015. A pilot randomized controlled trial of pioglitazone for the treatment of poorly controlled asthma in obesity. *Respir Res* 16:143.

Dixon, J. B., L. M. Schachter, and P. E. O'Brien. 2005. Polysomnography before and after weight loss in obese patients with severe sleep apnea. *Int J Obes (Lond)* 29 (9):1048–1054.

Drake, C., T. Roehrs, J. Shambroom, and T. Roth. 2013. Caffeine effects on sleep taken 0, 3, or 6 hours before going to bed. *J Clin Sleep Med* 9 (11):1195–1200.

Duarte, R. L., and F. J. Magalhaes-da-Silveira. 2015. Factors predictive of obstructive sleep apnea in patients undergoing pre-operative evaluation for bariatric surgery and referred to a sleep laboratory for polysomnography. *J Bras Pneumol* 41 (5):440–448.

Fritscher, L. G., C. C. Mottin, S. Canani, and J. M. Chatkin. 2007. Obesity and obstructive sleep apnea-hypopnea syndrome: The impact of bariatric surgery. *Obes Surg* 17 (1):95–99.

Gil, J. S., L. F. Drager, G. M. Guerra-Riccio, C. Mostarda, M. C. Irigoyen, V. Costa-Hong, L. A. Bortolotto, B. M. Egan, and H. F. Lopes. 2013. The impact of metabolic syndrome on metabolic, pro-inflammatory and prothrombotic markers according to the presence of high blood pressure criterion. *Clinics (Sao Paulo)* 68 (12):1495–1501.

Harnish, M. J., S. R. Greenleaf, and W. C. Orr. 1998. A comparison of feeding to cephalic stimulation on postprandial sleepiness. *Physiol Behav* 64 (1):93–96.

Herrera, C. P., K. Smith, F. Atkinson, P. Ruell, C. M. Chow, H. O'Connor, and J. Brand-Miller. 2011. High-glycaemic index and -glycaemic load meals increase the availability of tryptophan in healthy volunteers. *Br J Nutr* 105 (11):1601–1606.

Hjellvik, V., A. Tverdal, and K. Furu. 2010. Body mass index as predictor for asthma: A cohort study of 118,723 males and females. *Eur Respir J* 35 (6):1235–1242.

Holty, J. E., N. Parimi, M. Ballesteros, T. Blackwell, P. T. Cirangle, G. H. Jossart, N. D. Kimbrough, J. M. Rose, K. L. Stone, and D. M. Bravata. 2011. Does surgically induced weight loss improve daytime sleepiness? *Obes Surg* 21 (10):1535–1545.

Hughes, J. R. 2007. Effects of abstinence from tobacco: Valid symptoms and time course. *Nicotine Tob Res* 9 (3):315–327.

Jaehne, A., B. Loessl, Z. Barkai, D. Riemann, and M. Hornyak. 2009. Effects of nicotine on sleep during consumption, withdrawal and replacement therapy. *Sleep Med Rev* 13 (5):363–377.

Jehan, S., A. Masters-Isarilov, I. Salifu, F. Zizi, G. Jean-Louis, S. R. Pandi-Perumal, R. Gupta, A. Brzezinski, and S. I. McFarlane. 2015. Sleep disorders in postmenopausal women. *J Sleep Disord Ther* 4 (5):1000212.

Lee, H., S. R. Kim, Y. Oh, S. H. Cho, R. P. Schleimer, and Y. C. Lee. 2014. Targeting insulin-like growth factor-I and insulin-like growth factor-binding protein-3 signaling pathways. A novel therapeutic approach for asthma. *Am J Respir Cell Mol Biol* 50 (4):667–677.

Leger, D., B. Poursain, D. Neubauer, and M. Uchiyama. 2008. An international survey of sleeping problems in the general population. *Curr Med Res Opin* 24 (1):307–317.

Lichstein, K. L., B. W. Riedel, N. M. Wilson, K. W. Lester, and R. N. Aguillard. 2001. Relaxation and sleep compression for late-life insomnia: A placebo-controlled trial. *J Consult Clin Psychol* 69 (2):227–239.

Lu, Y., H. P. Van Bever, T. K. Lim, W. S. Kuan, D. Y. Goh, M. Mahadevan, T. B. Sim, R. Ho, A. Larbi, and T. P. Ng. 2015. Obesity, asthma prevalence and IL-4: Roles of inflammatory cytokines, adiponectin and neuropeptide Y. *Pediatr Allergy Immunol* 26 (6):530–536.

Marshall, N. S., N. Glozier, and R. R. Grunstein. 2008. Is sleep duration related to obesity? A critical review of the epidemiological evidence. *Sleep Med Rev* 12 (4):289–298.

Melo, L. C., M. A. Silva, and A. C. Calles. 2014. Obesity and lung function: A systematic review. *Einstein (Sao Paulo)* 12 (1):120–125.

Mullington, J. M., J. L. Chan, H. P. Van Dongen, M. P. Szuba, J. Samaras, N. J. Price, H. K. Meier-Ewert, D. F. Dinges, and C. S. Mantzoros. 2003. Sleep loss reduces diurnal rhythm amplitude of leptin in healthy men. *J Neuroendocrinol* 15 (9):851–854.

Nedeltcheva, A. V., J. M. Kilkus, J. Imperial, K. Kasza, D. A. Schoeller, and P. D. Penev. 2009. Sleep curtailment is accompanied by increased intake of calories from snacks. *Am J Clin Nutr* 89 (1):126–133.

Nedeltcheva, A. V., J. M. Kilkus, J. Imperial, D. A. Schoeller, and P. D. Penev. 2010. Insufficient sleep undermines dietary efforts to reduce adiposity. *Ann Intern Med* 153 (7):435–441.

Nielsen, L. S., K. V. Danielsen, and T. I. Sorensen. 2011. Short sleep duration as a possible cause of obesity: Critical analysis of the epidemiological evidence. *Obes Rev* 12 (2):78–92.

Ohayon, M. M., M. A. Carskadon, C. Guilleminault, and M. V. Vitiello. 2004. Meta-analysis of quantitative sleep parameters from childhood to old age in healthy individuals: Developing normative sleep values across the human lifespan. *Sleep* 27 (7):1255–1273.

Pakhale, S., J. Baron, R. Dent, K. Vandemheen, and S. D. Aaron. 2015. Effects of weight loss on airway responsiveness in obese adults with asthma: Does weight loss lead to reversibility of asthma? *Chest* 147 (6):1582–1590.

Pierce, A. M., and L. K. Brown. 2015. Obesity hypoventilation syndrome: Current theories of pathogenesis. *Curr Opin Pulm Med* 21 (6):557–562.

Pinto, J. A., D. K. Ribeiro, A. F. Cavallini, C. Duarte, and G. S. Freitas. 2016. Comorbidities associated with obstructive sleep apnea: A retrospective study. *Int Arch Otorhinolaryngol* 20 (2):145–150.

Ren, S. L., Y. R. Li, J. X. Wu, J. Y. Ye, and R. Jen. 2015. Effects of altered intra-abdominal pressure on the upper airway collapsibility in a porcine model. *Chin Med J (Engl)* 128 (23):3204–3210.

Rivas, E., E. Arismendi, A. Agusti, M. Sanchez, S. Delgado, C. Gistau, P. D. Wagner, and R. Rodriguez-Roisin. 2015. Ventilation/perfusion distribution abnormalities in morbidly obese subjects before and after bariatric surgery. *Chest* 147 (4):1127–1134.

Roehrs, T., and T. Roth. 2008. Caffeine: Sleep and daytime sleepiness. *Sleep Med Rev* 12 (2):153–162.

Salome, C. M., G. G. King, and N. Berend. 2010. Physiology of obesity and effects on lung function. *J Appl Physiol (1985)* 108 (1):206–211.

Samson, S. L., and A. J. Garber. 2014. Metabolic syndrome. *Endocrinol Metab Clin North Am* 43 (1):1–23.

Schatz, M., R. S. Zeiger, S. J. Yang, W. Chen, S. Sajjan, F. Allen-Ramey, and C. A. Camargo Jr. 2015. Prospective study on the relationship of obesity to asthma impairment and risk. *J Allergy Clin Immunol Pract* 3 (4):560–565.e1.

Schmid, S. M., M. Hallschmid, K. Jauch-Chara, J. Born, and B. Schultes. 2008. A single night of sleep deprivation increases ghrelin levels and feelings of hunger in normal-weight healthy men. *J Sleep Res* 17 (3):331–334.

Shetty, S., and S. Parthasarathy. 2015. Obesity hypoventilation syndrome. *Curr Pulmonol Rep* 4 (1):42–55.

Spiegel, K., K. Knutson, R. Leproult, E. Tasali, and E. Van Cauter. 2005. Sleep loss: A novel risk factor for insulin resistance and type 2 diabetes. *J Appl Physiol (1985)* 99 (5):2008–2019.

Spiegel, K., R. Leproult, and E. Van Cauter. 1999. Impact of sleep debt on metabolic and endocrine function. *Lancet* 354 (9188):1435–1439.

Spiegel, K., E. Tasali, P. Penev, and E. Van Cauter. 2004. Brief communication: Sleep curtailment in healthy young men is associated with decreased leptin levels, elevated ghrelin levels, and increased hunger and appetite. *Ann Intern Med* 141 (11):846–850.

Steier, J., A. Lunt, N. Hart, M. I. Polkey, and J. Moxham. 2014. Observational study of the effect of obesity on lung volumes. *Thorax* 69 (8):752–759.

Stepanski, E. J., and J. K. Wyatt. 2003. Use of sleep hygiene in the treatment of insomnia. *Sleep Med Rev* 7 (3):215–225.

Thyagarajan, B., D. R. Jacobs Jr., G. G. Apostol, L. J. Smith, R. L. Jensen, R. O. Crapo, R. G. Barr, C. E. Lewis, and O. D. Williams. 2008. Longitudinal association of body mass index with lung function: The CARDIA study. *Respir Res* 9:31.

Torchio, R., A. Gobbi, C. Gulotta, R. Dellaca, M. Tinivella, R. E. Hyatt, V. Brusasco, and R. Pellegrino. 2009. Mechanical effects of obesity on airway responsiveness in otherwise healthy humans. *J Appl Physiol (1985)* 107 (2):408–416.

Ulrik, C. S. 2016. Asthma symptoms in obese adults: The challenge of achieving asthma control. *Expert Rev Clin Pharmacol* 9 (1):5–8.

Van Cauter, E., R. Leproult, and L. Plat. 2000. Age-related changes in slow wave sleep and REM sleep and relationship with growth hormone and cortisol levels in healthy men. *JAMA* 284 (7):861–868.

Van Cauter, E., K. Spiegel, E. Tasali, and R. Leproult. 2008. Metabolic consequences of sleep and sleep loss. *Sleep Med* 9 (Suppl 1):S23–S28.

Varela, J. E., M. W. Hinojosa, and N. T. Nguyen. 2007. Resolution of obstructive sleep apnea after laparoscopic gastric bypass. *Obes Surg* 17 (10):1279–1282.

Walker, M. P. 2009. The role of sleep in cognition and emotion. *Ann NY Acad Sci* 1156:168–197.

Wells, A. S., N. W. Read, and A. Craig. 1995. Influences of dietary and intraduodenal lipid on alertness, mood, and sustained concentration. *Br J Nutr* 74 (1):115–123.

Wells, A. S., N. W. Read, C. Idzikowski, and J. Jones. 1998. Effects of meals on objective and subjective measures of daytime sleepiness. *J Appl Physiol (1985)* 84 (2):507–515.

Yawn, B. P., M. A. Rank, S. L. Bertram, and P. C. Wollan. 2015. Obesity, low levels of physical activity and smoking present opportunities for primary care asthma interventions: An analysis of baseline data from the Asthma Tools Study. *NPJ Prim Care Respir Med* 25:15058.

Youngstedt, S. D. 2005. Effects of exercise on sleep. *Clin Sports Med* 24 (2):355–365, xi.

Zaharna, M., and C. Guilleminault. 2010. Sleep, noise and health: Review. *Noise Health* 12 (47):64–69.

Zarcone, V. P. 2000. Sleep hygiene. In *Principles and Practice of Sleep Medicine*, ed. M. H. Kryger, T. Roth, and W. C. Demend. 3rd ed., 657–661. Philadelphia: W.B. Saunders.

15 Frailty, Nutrition, and the Elderly

15.1 INTRODUCTION

The term *frailty* describes elderly patients who have multiple chronic diseases, limited activities of daily living, and increased risk of disability and loss of independence. Frailty is a geriatric syndrome that compromises the ability to maintain organismal functioning and is associated with an increased risk for multiple adverse health-related outcomes, including falls, fractures, disability, institutionalization, and death. The components of frailty consist of weight loss, fatigue, slow gait speed, weakness, and low activity levels. According to this model, those individuals with one or two of these conditions would be considered "prefrail," just as we have classifications for prediabetes, prehypertension, and early stages of renal failure. The idea inherent in defining a state of prefrailty is to promote efforts to prevent the progression of this condition to frailty, which is defined as three or more of the above conditions of weight loss, fatigue, slow gait speed, weakness, and low activity levels (Fried et al. 2001). Once frailty develops, there are steps toward rehabilitation using physical therapy and nutrition, which will be discussed.

Loss of skeletal muscle mass is central to the development of frailty in older people. Sarcopenia is common with advancing age, and the rate of progression of sarcopenia is responsive to nutritional status, particularly dietary protein. Along with sarcopenia, increased fat mass and decreased bone mass combine with environmental factors to increase the risk of frailty.

Healthy older people consuming the current U.S. recommended dietary allowance (RDA) for protein are at risk of losing skeletal muscle at an accelerated rate and developing frailty. Therefore, increased dietary protein will preserve or increase muscle mass and function when combined with strength training. Just to be clear, as discussed in Chapter 2, we recommend a higher protein intake than the U.S. RDA for everyone, but it is critical in the elderly. Periods of extreme inactivity. such as prolonged bed rest during hospitalization. promote sarcopenia. Changes in taste and the ability to digest foods, as well as behavioral issues around eating and the quality of institutional foods, are additional factors promoting sarcopenia.

Another common feature of aging is an increase in body fatness, as the elderly often select sweet low-protein and high-fat snack foods to the exclusion of balanced meals. Body fat is an independent predictor of disability and poor functional status; however, caloric restriction intended to produce weight loss can result in substantial loss of muscle mass. Bone density is often decreased in combination with sarcopenia due to reduced physical activity and inadequate gravitational or exercise-induced stress across weight-bearing bones.

Sarcopenic obesity is the combination of excess body fat and decreased muscle mass. This clinical presentation presents a challenge, since resting metabolic rates are directly related to lean body mass. Therefore, usual caloric restriction for weight loss will be less effective and can be harmful in the absence of adequate attention to protein intake and muscle rehabilitation. Strategies for weight loss for older people should include exercise to help preserve lean mass and a shift in macronutrient intake toward a lower-fat and higher-protein and higher-carbohydrate intake to maintain nutritional status.

15.2 NATURE OF AGING

Biological aging varies in its rate of progression among individuals based on genetic and nutritional factors. Biologic aging is different than chronological aging, which is your age or the simple passing of time. Nonetheless, none of us are getting out of this alive, and aging inevitably leads to progressive deterioration in both the structure and function of various molecular, cellular, and tissue components. Research efforts and clinical interventions can influence the rate of progression of age-related changes, and some gerontologists view aging as a chronic disease process that can be influenced by a combination of pharmacological, nutritional, and lifestyle factors, so that we can achieve a theoretical maximum of 120 years or so of life. In fact, advances in medicine, sanitation, and nutrition have advanced the life span from 50 years at the beginning of the twentieth century to about 85 years currently, and it is predicted that individuals born today may live to over 100 years. Researchers are studying centenarians, who are a small but rapidly growing group of elders. The other effort that is important, beyond extending life span, is the extension of health span, and that critically depends on preventing age-related chronic diseases and the physical disability related to the development of frailty.

A number of basic theories have been proposed to explain aging mechanisms, including the shortening and/or loss of telomeres, the accumulation of damaged DNA in cells, and dysfunction of important cellular organelles, such as the endoplasmic reticulum (ER) and mitochondria. Mitochondria in muscle are not the little circular organelles inside cells as depicted in high school biology texts, but are long structures that can increase or decrease in size and modulate their activity in oxidative phosphorylation as needed to provide energy to the muscle fibers. Part of the age-related loss of muscle function involves a degradation of mitochondria and the muscle fibers adjacent to them.

Age-associated accumulation of senescent cells in various tissues and organs causes functional disruption of tissue structure, partly through the appearance and accumulation of senescent-associated secretory proteins (Coppe et al. 2008; Rodier and Campisi 2011). Organismal aging proceeds with a gradual decline in cell proliferation of the somatic cells. The macroscopic outcome is evidenced by the appearance of dysfunctional and "worn out" tissues that degrade continuously, finally resulting in structural instability and death of the organism.

Our bodies are composed of a combination of somatic and progenitor cells that have a range of capacities for cell division, and pluripotent stem cells with a high capacity for division. In addition to stem cells, there are immortal germ cells in the spermatogenic tubules of the male testis and at the base of the small intestinal epithelial crypts that divide rapidly. The latter two cell types have telomerase, which restores the ends of DNA lost with each cell division. The emergence of a cancer cell with telomerase occurs through neoplastic transformation and acquisition of cellular immortality, but at the expense of having corrupted genetic and epigenetic states that confer potentially lethal behavior. On the other hand, emergence of an aged cell occurs through the induction of cellular senescence.

Cellular senescence differs from loss of proliferation or quiescent states by the occurrence of altered gene expression and metabolic activity, as well as accumulated insults that lead to irreversible arrest. Senescent cells are resistant to apoptosis (Moiseeva et al. 2006). Another property of senescent cells is a secretory phenotype. Senescent cells convert into pro-inflammatory counterparts and promote pathology, including sarcopenia.

The immune system of older people declines in reliability and efficiency with age, resulting in greater susceptibility to pathology as a consequence of inflammation, for example, cardiovascular disease, Alzheimer's disease, autoreactivity, and vaccine failure, as well as an increased vulnerability to infectious disease (Pawelec 1999; Targonski et al. 2007; Weiskopf et al. 2009). These changes are further compounded by reduced responsiveness and impaired communication between all cells of the immune system. The overall change to the immune system with age is termed immunosenescence and has a multifactorial etiology, a consequence of the complexity of the immune system, as well as of multiple genetic and environmental influences (Weiskopf et al. 2009). Immunosenescence of the innate immune system is primarily characterized by reduced cellular superoxide production and capability for phagocytosis. Involution of the thymus and reduced responsiveness to a new antigen load, owing to a reduced naïve–memory cell ratio and expansion of mature cell clones, characterize immunosenescence of the acquired immune system.

The term *inflammaging* was developed to describe an upregulation of the inflammatory response that occurs with age, resulting in a low-grade chronic systemic pro-inflammatory state that plays a role in progressing aging (Franceschi et al. 2000; Vasto et al. 2007). In this sense, aging resembles age-related chronic diseases, and while aging cannot be reversed (you cannot stop time), the ravages of aging can be reduced through healthy diet and lifestyle. Inflammaging is characterized by raised levels of inflammatory cytokines, including interleukin 1 (IL-1), IL-6, and tumor necrosis factor α (TNF-α). These cytokines have been shown to rise with age (De Martinis et al. 2006) and be involved in the pathogenesis of most age-related chronic diseases (De Martinis et al. 2006). C-reactive protein (CRP), also known as high-sensitivity CRP (hsCRP), is an acute-phase protein produced by the liver in response to inflammation. It is also a useful marker of inflammation associated with aging and chronic diseases when the highly sensitive assay for it is used. hsCRP in the upper quartile of the normal range is used clinically as a predictor of the risk for cardiovascular and other age-related chronic diseases (Buckley et al. 2009; Ansar and Ghosh 2013). In practice, it is elevated well above the normal range by mild upper respiratory viral infections and other common infections, limiting its usefulness in screening and follow-up.

The physiological response to inflammation is an increase in circulating cortisol levels (Giunta 2008). Cortisol is a part of most stress responses, but it is also immunosuppressive. Cortisol secretion from the adrenal gland is stimulated by the hypothalamic corticotrophin-releasing hormone and pituitary adrenocorticotropic hormone (ACTH), which together are called the hypothalamic–pituitary–adrenal (HPA) axis (Phillips et al. 2010). Neuronal cells within the HPA axis contain multiple cytokine receptors, particularly for IL-1, IL-6, and TNF (Turnbull and Rivier 1999), and it has been demonstrated in human beings *in vivo that* injection of IL-6 or TNF induces a marked change in HPA axis activity (Straub et al. 2000).

While the anti-inflammaging response attempts to counter the inflammaging process, it may also have negative implications via catabolic effects of cortisol on several tissue types, such as liver (gluconeogenesis), muscle (protein catabolism), and bone (resorption) (Giunta 2008), which promote the development of frailty.

15.3 EPIDEMIOLOGY OF FRAILTY

Muscle mass and strength decline with aging, due to a combination of α-motor neuron loss and inherent reductions in the number and size of muscle fibers (Evans and Campbell 1993; Evans 1995; Rosenberg 1997). Consequently, strength decreases with age, and muscle weakness can compromise well-being and activities of daily living. Sarcopenia is estimated to affect up to 30% of adults over the age of 70 years (Rosenberg 1997; Baumgartner et al. 1998; Morley 2001). Health care costs attributed to sarcopenia amount to tens of billions of dollars per year (Morley et al. 2005).

There are many causes of sarcopenia, including disuse atrophy, endocrine disorders such as Cushing's disease or glucocorticoid overuse, chronic disease conditions, inflammation, insulin resistance, and nutritional deficiencies. While advanced malnutrition or cachexia may be a component of sarcopenia, these conditions are not the same. Sarcopenia can occur at normal or even increased body weights.

The diagnosis of sarcopenia should be considered in all older patients who present with observed declines in physical function, strength, or overall health. Sarcopenia should specifically be considered in patients who are bedridden, cannot independently rise from a chair, or have a measured gait speed of less than 3 feet/second. Patients who meet these criteria should further undergo body composition assessment using bioelectrical impedance and dual-energy x-ray absorptiometry (DEXA), with sarcopenia being defined using currently validated definitions.

A diagnosis of sarcopenia is consistent with a reduced gait speed and an objectively measured low muscle mass. Sarcopenia is a highly prevalent condition in older persons that leads to disability, hospitalization, and death.

Sarcopenia is correlated with functional decline and disability (Baumgartner et al. 1998; Melton et al. 2000; Janssen et al. 2002; Lauretani et al. 2003; Delmonico et al. 2007). Findings are often stronger in men than in women, depending on the indexing method used. Sarcopenia has also been associated with increased mortality (Metter et al. 2002), although (Newman et al. 2006) weakness has been demonstrated to be a more powerful predictor of mortality in elderly people than muscle mass. In the longitudinal Rancho Bernardo study, sarcopenia was shown to be predictive of falls (Castillo et al. 2003).

The term *sarcopenic obesity* was first used by our group at the University of California, Los Angeles (UCLA) in 1996 (Heber et al. 1996) and describes persons with reduced body mass out of proportion to their adipose mass. Sarcopenic obesity is associated with disability, gait problems, and falls to a greater extent than persons with sarcopenia without increased body fat (Baumgartner et al. 2004). In longitudinal studies over 8 years, sarcopenic obesity was a better predictor of physical disabilities, abnormalities in gait or balance, and falls in the prior year than either sarcopenia or obesity alone.

These observations were confirmed in the Framingham and National Health and Nutrition Examination Survey (NHANES) studies, demonstrating that elderly people with high body fat and low muscle mass had the highest rate of disabilities (Davison et al. 2002). These data point to the fact that the development of disability and impaired mobility in older people has multiple etiologies, not just loss of muscle.

Muscle mass is an important, but not the only, predictor of muscle strength or physical function. Fat has several adverse effects on muscle function. Higher body fatness and older age have been associated with greater intramuscular lipid and reduced muscle quality, defined as reduced strength or cross-sectional area (Kelley et al. 1999; Goodpaster et al. 2006). It is also possible that higher body fatness decreases the capacity to generate power (force × speed), and muscle power is more closely related to functional capacity than muscle strength (Bassey et al. 1992). Several indices of sarcopenia that account for muscle and fat mass have been examined in relationship to function. These studies illustrate the complexity in defining sarcopenia in relationship to fat mass (Newman et al. 2003). When fat mass is considered, the role of lean mass per se is apparently small.

In addition to muscle loss and fat gain, there is a loss of bone mineral density with aging and an increase in fracture risk. Epidemiological studies have now clearly established that in both women and men, bone loss begins as early as the early part of the third decade—immediately after peak bone mass and long before any change in sex steroid production (Looker et al. 1998). Supporting these epidemiological data, volumetric bone mineral density analysis at the tibia and spine, in a large age- and sex-stratified population sample using quantitative computed tomography, demonstrated substantial trabecular bone loss in both sexes even when sex steroids were sufficient (Riggs et al. 2008). In women, the loss of trabecular bone in the spine accelerates substantially after menopause, as does the rate of fractures at the wrist, spine, and hip (Khosla and Riggs 2005), attesting to the adverse role of estrogen deficiency on skeletal homeostasis and its contribution to the acceleration of the age-associated bone loss. Cortical bone loss begins to decline after the age of 50 in both sexes, albeit at a faster rate in women than men.

Osteoporosis, determined as decreased bone mass per unit volume of anatomical bone, is only one of the factors responsible for the compromised bone strength that predisposes to an increased risk of fracture in the frailty syndrome. Aging contributes to fracture risk independent of bone mass (Hui et al. 1988). At the same bone mineral density, a 20-year increase in age is accompanied by a fourfold increase in fracture risk. Increased propensity to falls due to age-related decline in neuromuscular function is without doubt a factor for the age-related increase in fracture risk. However, there are also age-related changes in the bone itself, which contribute to the increase in fracture risk at the same mineral density due to an increase in age-related changes in the bone (Hui et al. 1988). For example, type I collagen is structurally complex and can deteriorate as it ages, with changes such as loss of cross-linking between the component chains (Bailey and Knott 1999). Collagen can also be damaged by accumulation of advanced glycation end products (Vashishth et al. 2001), another general feature of the aging process. Such changes could account for the age-related decline in cortical bone tensile strength (Wall et al. 1979). Defective collagen cannot be repaired, so the bone containing it must be replaced by remodeling.

15.4 SARCOPENIA

Aging is associated with a reduction in myofibrillar (Welle et al. 1993; Balagopal et al. 1997; Proctor et al. 1998) and mitochondrial (Rooyackers et al. 1996) protein synthetic rates and partially attributed to a reduction in growth factors such as insulin-like growth factor 1 (IGF-1) (Proctor et al. 1998). An acute bout of resistance exercise increases the muscle protein fractional synthetic rate and the absolute magnitude to a degree similar to that seen for young adults (Yarasheski et al. 1993; Hasten et al. 2000). Muscle cells hypertrophy when stretched in an eccentric movement. They then attract and merge with satellite cells, resulting in a thickened and stronger muscle fiber. This process is targeted to the muscle fibers activated in the movement that induced the stretch and attraction of satellite cells (Figure 15.1). There appears to be less activation of satellite cells in older adults in response to a single bout of resistance exercise (Dreyer et al. 2006). Therefore, nutrition and training exercises that enhance satellite cell recruitment (Olsen et al. 2006; Mackey et al. 2007) may be particularly effective in treating the sarcopenia of aging.

There is also a decrease in mitochondrial enzyme activity and mitochondrial transcriptome pattern and an increase in oxidative stress associated with aging (Evans and Campbell 1993;

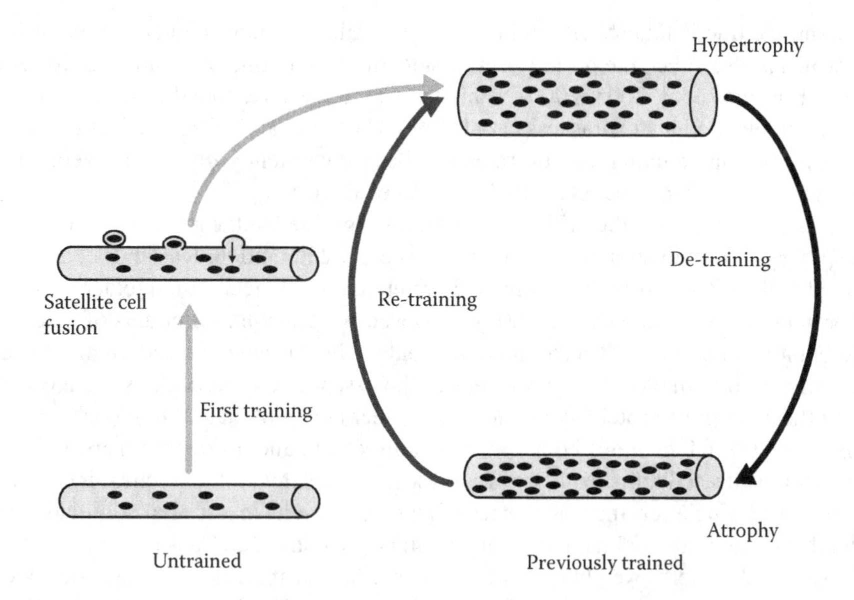

FIGURE 15.1 **(See color insert.)** Model for the connection between muscle size and number of myonuclei. In this model, myonuclei are permanent. Previously untrained muscles acquire newly formed nuclei by fusion of satellite cells preceding the hypertrophy. Subsequent detraining leads to atrophy but no loss of myonuclei. The elevated number of nuclei in muscle fibers that had experienced a hypertrophic episode would provide a mechanism for muscle memory, explaining the long-lasting effects of training and the ease with which previously trained individuals are more easily retrained. (Reprinted from Egner, I. M. et al., *Development*, 143(16), 2898–2906, 2016.)

Evans 1995; Baumgartner et al. 1998; Parise et al. 2005a,b; Melov et al. 2007). These two processes may be linked in that oxidative stress per se can lead to DNA, lipid, and protein damage that can disrupt the structure and replicative capacity of mitochondria.

Disuse atrophy results in an increase in reactive oxygen species (ROS) production in skeletal muscle. There is also a decreased expression of mitochondrial proteins and decreased mitochondrial oxidative phosphorylation for ATP production. Increased ROS production alters redox signaling in muscle fibers that can increase proteolysis and decrease protein synthesis. To further compound these effects, disuse muscle atrophy is associated with an overall decrease in skeletal antioxidant capacity due to a decreased antioxidant scavenging ability.

Endurance exercise increases oxidative stress in skeletal muscle. The short-term increase in ROS production with exercise has been demonstrated to be a powerful signaling molecule in activating signaling pathways. The transient oxidative stress that occurs with exercise is likely required for skeletal muscle adaptation to occur.

The key difference between exercise-induced oxidative stress and oxidative stress associated with disuse atrophy is the duration of the exposure. Oxidative stress following exercise is transient in nature, while disuse atrophy results in chronic exposure to elevated ROS.

A reduction in the metabolic capacity of mitochondria to carry out oxidative phosphorylation to form ATP (Evans and Campbell 1993; Evans 1995; Parise et al. 2005a,b) and decreases in muscle blood flow during exercise (Morley 2001) contribute to the observed reduction of VO_2max that occurs with aging. Although VO_2max does decline with aging, there is no question that older trained athletes can have VO_2max values equivalent to those of sedentary young individuals and definitely higher than those of sedentary older adults, despite an inevitable loss of aerobic capacity with aging (Coggan et al. 1990; Rogers et al. 1990; Morley et al. 2005; Delmonico et al. 2007).

15.5 MUSCLE PROTEIN SYNTHESIS

The mixed muscle fractional protein synthetic rate is similar in younger and older adults in the fasting state, which is also called the postabsorptive state in the scientific literature (Paddon-Jones et al. 2004, 2006; Katsanos et al. 2005, 2006). While a few studies have found lower rates of fractional synthetic rate in older adults (Yarasheski et al. 1993; Hasten et al. 2000), a reduction in mitochondrial and myofibrillar protein synthetic rates has been consistently observed (Welle et al. 1993; Yarasheski et al. 1993; Balagopal et al. 1997; Hasten et al. 2000).

The data show that it is not the difference in the fasting state but the response to feeding that differentiates younger from older adults (Paddon-Jones et al. 2004, 2006; Katsanos et al. 2005, 2006; Symons et al. 2007). There is higher amino acid retention in younger than in older muscle at lower levels of protein intake (Symons et al. 2007). However, with adequate amounts of essential amino acids, this blunting of amino acid accumulation in older adults is not observed (Symons et al. 2007). It appears, in fact, that the leucine component of the essential amino acids is the most important in restoring the absorptive protein synthetic rate in older adults to that seen in younger individuals (Katsanos et al. 2006). Leucine is both a nutrient amino acid and a signal to increase protein synthesis via specific intracellular signals known as the mTOR pathway. Of practical interest, however, is the finding that a single serving of 4 ounces of lean beef results in a similar stimulation of muscle protein synthetic rate in both older and younger adults (Symons et al. 2007).

In response to short-term weight training, there is a similar increase in myosin heavy chain and mixed muscle protein synthetic rates of about 150% in both older and younger adults (Hasten et al. 2000). The consumption of carbohydrate plus protein plus leucine after 30 minutes of activities of daily living exercises leads to a significant increase in muscle fractional protein synthetic rate and a net positive balance, compared with a carbohydrate feeding alone, in both younger and older adults (Koopman et al. 2006). Greater myofibrillar proteolysis in skeletal muscle in older than in younger adults has been observed (Trappe et al. 2004). Consequently, strategies to reduce proteolysis and increase synthesis could be important countermeasures to sarcopenia. Overall, older adults retain the ability to stimulate muscle and myofibrillar protein synthesis following a bout of resistance exercise, and this effect is enhanced with carbohydrate and protein nutrition to a greater extent than carbohydrate alone. Furthermore, older adult muscle appears to be less responsive to acute feeding if protein intake is quite low; however, with adequate amounts of high-quality protein, the diet-induced stimulation appears to be similar to that seen in younger adults.

15.6 PROTEIN REQUIREMENTS

There is generally accepted science that the elderly require more protein to attain a positive nitrogen balance, and that clinical recommendations of 1.0–1.2 g/kg of body weight are generally accepted and recognized as being well above the RDA of 0.8 g/kg of body weight. We will not repeat here the argument that body weight independent of body composition is not an appropriate way to recommend protein intake, but this is discussed in detail in Chapter 2 and is an important principle in understanding research done on protein requirements in the elderly and attempts to prevent or delay the development of sarcopenia.

Protein requirements in resistance-trained older adults have been extensively investigated (Campbell et al. 1999a,b; Haub et al. 2002; Campbell 2007; Campbell and Leidy 2007). When dietary protein intake was between 1.03 and 1.17 g/kg/day, resistance training induced gains in muscle mass and strength to a similar extent in the groups consuming a beef-containing diet and those on the lacto-ovo vegetarian regimen (Haub et al. 2002). At the molecular level, it has been clearly shown that when older adults consume suboptimal levels of protein (0.5 g/kg/day), rather than an adequate amount (1.2 g/kg/day), there are alterations in mRNA transcript abundance, which is directionally supportive of adverse metabolic, functional, and structural components that would favor sarcopenia (Thalacker-Mercer et al. 2007). Taken together, these data suggest that older adults completing resistance-type exercise should ensure that their dietary protein intake is more than 0.8 g/kg/day (more appropriately between 1.0 and 1.2 g/kg/day), and that their sources of protein include those with high biological value (e.g., egg whites, milk, beef, and fish).

Studies have found that skeletal muscle with strength training has a net positive protein balance only with feeding, particularly with amino acids (Biolo et al. 1995a,b, 1997). Net protein balance is also more positive following resistance exercise in postmenopausal women receiving protein and carbohydrate than placebo (Holm et al. 2005). From a practical perspective, the provision of a supplement containing 10 g of protein, 7 g of carbohydrate, and 3 g of fat immediately after exercise, compared with 2 hours after exercise, resulted in greater muscle mass and strength gains in older adults following a 12-week resistance exercise training program three times per week (Esmarck et al. 2001). Such findings highlight the importance of the early provision of proteins with essential amino acids, including leucine and some carbohydrate, to promote an insulin response following exercise. This regimen takes advantage of the intracellular milieu of muscle cells at the time when the greatest increase in net protein retention can occur.

15.7 SMELL AND TASTE CHANGES WITH AGING

Loss of smell and taste with aging has been linked to inadequate nutritional intake, reduced social pleasure, and decreased psychological well-being. It may even be life threatening, impairing the detection of smoke in a fire or the ability to identify spoiled food.

The sense of smell is mediated through stimulation of the olfactory receptor cells by volatile chemicals. To stimulate the olfactory receptors, airborne molecules must pass through the nasal cavity with relatively turbulent air currents and contact the receptors. Odorants can also be perceived by entering the nose posteriorly through the nasopharynx to reach the olfactory receptor via retronasal olfaction. Each olfactory receptor cell is a primary sensory bipolar neuron. The average nasal cavity contains more than 100 million such neurons. There are more than 900 genes encoding these receptors. The olfactory neurons are unique because they are generated throughout life by the underlying basal cells. New receptor cells are generated approximately every 30–60 days.

Sense of smell decreases with age, and it has been shown that the number of fibers in the olfactory bulb decreases throughout one's lifetime. In one study (Bhatnagar et al. 1987), the average loss in human mitral cells was 520 cells/year, with a reduction in bulb volume of 0.19 mm^3 (Bhatnagar et al. 1987). These olfactory bulb losses may be secondary to sensory cell loss in the olfactory mucosa and/or general decline in the regenerative process from stem cells in the subventricular zone.

Various neuropsychiatric disorders (e.g., depression, schizophrenia, and seasonal affective disorder) have been linked to hyposmia. It has been shown that patients with acute major depressive disorder have reduced olfactory sensitivity and reduced olfactory bulb volumes (Negoias et al. 2010). Schizophrenia patients have also been shown to have decreased olfactory bulb volume and impaired odor detection abilities (Nguyen et al. 2011).

The toxicity of systemic and inhaled aminoglycosides, formaldehyde, and other drugs can contribute to olfactory dysfunction. Many other medications and compounds may alter smell sensitivity, including alcohol, nicotine, organic solvents, and direct application of zinc salts (Tuccori et al. 2011).

Much of what is perceived as a taste defect is truly a primary defect in detecting smells. The components that comprise the sensation of flavor include the food's smell, taste, texture, and temperature. Each of these sensory modalities is stimulated independently to produce a distinct flavor when food enters the mouth.

Ongoing research has identified odor and taste receptors in surprising places, including skeletal muscle, brain, respiratory tract, and gastrointestinal tract. Taste receptors are present from the stomach to the colon and function in nutrient sensing (Depoortere 2014).

Oral cavity and mucosal disorders, including oral infections, inflammation, and radiation-induced mucositis, can impair taste sensation. The site of injury with radiotherapy is probably the microvilli of the taste buds rather than the taste buds themselves, which are resistant to radiation damage.

Aging causes taste loss due to changes in taste cell membranes involving altered function of ion channels and receptors rather than taste bud loss (Boesveldt et al. 2011; Wylie and Nebauer 2011). Nutritional deficiencies, which can be associated with aging, are also involved in taste aberrations. For example, decreased zinc, copper, and nickel levels are associated with taste alterations. These and other nutritional deficiencies may be caused by changes in eating behaviors, anorexia, malabsorption, and/or increased urinary losses.

Smell and taste disorders traditionally have been overlooked in most aspects of medical practice because these specialized senses often are not considered critical to life. However, they affect enjoyment of food, and they impair detection of the potentially dangerous smells of smoke or spoiled food.

Anxiety and depression, as well as anorexia and nutritional deficiencies, may result from taste and smell disorders. Many causes of smell and taste disorders exist, and the modalities of treatment begin with treating the specific deficit, if possible.

15.8 PREVENTION AND TREATMENT OF FRAILTY

Nutritional support of the elderly with prefrailty and frailty is established practice, but is not comprehensive enough to make a difference for the frail elderly. Like the can of nutritional formula that sits on the bed table without being consumed, nutrition support alone does not consider all elements of the frailty state in the elderly. Nutrition intervention for frailty refers not only to nutritional improvement but also to associated efforts to strengthen or rehabilitate the elderly with functional disability through exercise and physical therapy (Wakabayashi 2010; Minnella et al. 2016). Nutrition intervention of the prevention and treatment of frailty is similar to sports nutrition in including nutrition, exercise, and behavioral components. The key aims are to assess the following: (1) the presence and cause of malnutrition, (2) the presence and cause of sarcopenia, (3) the presence and cause of dysphagia, (4) the adequacy of nutrition care management with prediction of future nutritional status, and (5) whether functional improvement, such as resistance training and endurance training, can be conducted (Minnella et al. 2016).

Following a stroke, hip fracture, major surgery, or any number of medical conditions requiring extended stays in bed, there is an associated deconditioning that leads to muscle loss, fat gain, and decreases in bone mineralization, which are hallmarks of unhealthy aging via poor nutrition and inactivity. The prevalence of malnutrition in those settings, such as hospitals and nursing homes where patients are sent for rehabilitation, is high. In elderly patients hospitalized for rehabilitation, the prevalence of compromised nutrition status is between 49% and 67% (Strakowski et al. 2002). In Australia, up to 51.5% of patients admitted to rehabilitation hospitals were classified as malnourished and at nutritional risk (Charlton et al. 2010). One study found that the prevalence of malnutrition in elderly people was highest in rehabilitation settings at 50.5%, in comparison with a prevalence of 38.7% in acute care hospitals (Kaiser et al. 2010). A study using the Mini Nutritional Assessment—Short Form (MNA-SF) revealed a 40.8% prevalence of malnutrition in rehabilitation settings (Kaiser et al. 2011).

A systematic review found that malnutrition in older adults admitted to rehabilitation units negatively affected functional recovery and quality of life following discharge to the community (Marshall et al. 2014). Furthermore, rehabilitation outcome has been shown to be poor in malnourished patients with stroke (Davis et al. 2004), hip fracture (Anker et al. 2006), hospital-associated deconditioning (Wakabayashi and Sashika 2011, 2014), and a variety of other diseases.

It is not surprising that sarcopenia is a frequent occurrence in the hospital and rehabilitation center settings. Sarcopenia affects between 10% and 30% of community-dwelling elderly (Fielding et al. 2011). In a study of patients who were 60 years and older in an ambulatory rehabilitation facility, it was found that about 40% of individuals had sarcopenia (Yaxley et al. 2012). It has been demonstrated that 46.5% patients admitted to a subacute geriatric care unit who underwent a rehabilitation intervention met the diagnostic criteria for sarcopenia (Sanchez-Rodriguez et al. 2014).

Sarcopenia can be classified into primary age-related sarcopenia and sarcopenia secondary to reduced activity, comorbid diseases, and nutrition-related sarcopenia (Cruz-Jentoft et al. 2010). Assessment of the multifactorial causes of primary and secondary sarcopenia is critical in determining therapeutic strategies for sarcopenia.

Age-related sarcopenia can be treated with resistance training, protein and amino acid supplementation, smoking cessation, and some pharmacological approaches, including androgens and anabolic agents (Wakabayashi and Sakuma 2013, 2014). Pharmaceutical therapy with androgens and anabolic drugs is adjunctive in the therapy of sarcopenia (Sakuma and Yamaguchi 2012; Sakuma et al. 2015), but nutrition and exercise are the foundation of treatment. Exercise, protein supplementation, and avoiding bed rest are important for preventing and treating activity-related sarcopenia. Treatment of disease-related sarcopenia also includes therapies for advanced organ failure, inflammation, malignancy, and endocrine disorders, in addition to appropriate nutrition supplementation to increase muscle mass. In the United States, the six most common conditions receiving inpatient rehabilitation are stroke, lower extremity fracture, lower extremity joint replacement, debility, neurologic disorders, and brain dysfunction (Ottenbacher et al. 2014).

Difficulty swallowing or dysphagia can be due to sarcopenia of generalized skeletal muscles and swallowing muscles (Kuroda and Kuroda 2012; Wakabayashi 2014). Age-related loss of the tongue and geniohyoid muscle mass has been demonstrated in the elderly and is termed sarcopenic dysphagia (Tamura et al. 2012; Feng et al. 2013). Sarcopenic dysphagia is an important public health issue, because it is common in the elderly and can lead to aspiration pneumonia, which is more common with the global aging of society (Wakabayashi 2014).

Hip fractures are associated with a greater degree of disability, more health care costs, and higher mortality than all other osteoporotic fractures combined (Ensrud 2013). In 2005, hip fractures in the United States accounted for only 14% of total fractures but 72% of total fracture-related health care costs (Ensrud 2013). Global trends are for an increased number of hip fractures in many countries. The number of hip fractures worldwide is expected to rise from 1.6 million documented in 2000 to an estimated 6.3 million in 2050 (Ensrud 2013). Hip fracture is the most common condition requiring geriatric musculoskeletal rehabilitation. Malnutrition has been demonstrated in hip fracture patients using a variety of methods. In a typical study, 11.6% of hip fracture patients were malnourished, 44.2% were at risk of malnutrition, and 44.2% were well nourished (Koren-Hakim et al. 2012). The presence of malnutrition predicted gait status and mortality 6 months after hip fracture (Gumieiro et al. 2013). Serum albumin level and weight loss, as documented by body mass index (BMI), significantly influenced mortality after hip fracture (Miyanishi et al. 2010). Malnutrition and being at risk for malnutrition are common in patients with hip fracture, and malnutrition clearly affects outcome.

Stroke is the most common cause of disability in the West and in East Asian countries. More than 60% of patients remain disabled after a stroke. About 50% of patients suffer from hemiparesis, and 30% remain unable to walk without assistance (Kelly-Hayes et al. 2003). Rehabilitation, including nutrition and physical therapy, plays a critical role in functional recovery after stroke (Scherbakov and Doehner 2011; Scherbakov et al. 2013).

Both malnutrition and obesity are nutritional problems in stroke, and both impair recovery of function. Malnutrition and dysphagia respectively occur in up to 53% of patients after a stroke (Foley et al. 2009). Stroke-induced sarcopenia is difficult to assess. In a review of loss of skeletal muscle mass after stroke (English et al. 2010), lean tissue mass was significantly less in the paralyzed than the unaffected lower limb and upper limb, as might be expected based on denervation atrophy. Thigh muscle area was significantly less in stroke patients 6 months after the event. The pathogenic mechanisms of muscle wasting in stroke-related sarcopenia include disuse atrophy, spasticity, inflammation, denervation, reinnervation, impaired feeding, and intestinal absorption (Scherbakov et al. 2013). More research is needed to diagnose and treat stroke-induced sarcopenia.

15.9 SUMMARY

The prevention of prefrailty and frailty in the elderly is possible by increasing protein intake as recommended in Chapter 2 of this book in proportion to lean body mass, while also advising patients in targeted resistance exercises to balance muscle function through the major muscle groups controlling posture and walking. As walking speed and falls both correlate with morbidity and mortality, targeting these two functions in an aggressive preventive manner will help to reduce health care costs. The primary care practice can serve as the central triage for the various specialties that need to be engaged in the process of prevention and treatment of frailty in the middle-aged and elderly.

REFERENCES

Anker, S. D., M. John, P. U. Pedersen, C. Raguso, M. Cicoira, E. Dardai, A. Laviano et al. 2006. ESPEN Guidelines on Enteral Nutrition: Cardiology and pulmonology. *Clin Nutr* 25 (2):311–318.

Ansar, W., and S. Ghosh. 2013. C-reactive protein and the biology of disease. *Immunol Res* 56 (1):131–142.

Bailey, A. J., and L. Knott. 1999. Molecular changes in bone collagen in osteoporosis and osteoarthritis in the elderly. *Exp Gerontol* 34 (3):337–351.

Balagopal, P., O. E. Rooyackers, D. B. Adey, P. A. Ades, and K. S. Nair. 1997. Effects of aging on in vivo synthesis of skeletal muscle myosin heavy-chain and sarcoplasmic protein in humans. *Am J Physiol* 273 (4 Pt 1):E790–E800.

Bassey, E. J., M. A. Fiatarone, E. F. O'Neill, M. Kelly, W. J. Evans, and L. A. Lipsitz. 1992. Leg extensor power and functional performance in very old men and women. *Clin Sci (Lond)* 82 (3):321–327.

Baumgartner, R. N., K. M. Koehler, D. Gallagher, L. Romero, S. B. Heymsfield, R. R. Ross, P. J. Garry, and R. D. Lindeman. 1998. Epidemiology of sarcopenia among the elderly in New Mexico. *Am J Epidemiol* 147 (8):755–763.

Baumgartner, R. N., S. J. Wayne, D. L. Waters, I. Janssen, D. Gallagher, and J. E. Morley. 2004. Sarcopenic obesity predicts instrumental activities of daily living disability in the elderly. *Obes Res* 12 (12):1995–2004.

Bhatnagar, K. P., R. C. Kennedy, G. Baron, and R. A. Greenberg. 1987. Number of mitral cells and the bulb volume in the aging human olfactory bulb: A quantitative morphological study. *Anat Rec* 218 (1):73–87.

Biolo, G., R. Y. Declan Fleming, and R. R. Wolfe. 1995a. Physiologic hyperinsulinemia stimulates protein synthesis and enhances transport of selected amino acids in human skeletal muscle. *J Clin Invest* 95 (2):811–819.

Biolo, G., S. P. Maggi, B. D. Williams, K. D. Tipton, and R. R. Wolfe. 1995b. Increased rates of muscle protein turnover and amino acid transport after resistance exercise in humans. *Am J Physiol* 268 (3 Pt 1):E514–E520.

Biolo, G., K. D. Tipton, S. Klein, and R. R. Wolfe. 1997. An abundant supply of amino acids enhances the metabolic effect of exercise on muscle protein. *Am J Physiol* 273 (1 Pt 1):E122–E129.

Boesveldt, S., S. T. Lindau, M. K. McClintock, T. Hummel, and J. N. Lundstrom. 2011. Gustatory and olfactory dysfunction in older adults: A national probability study. *Rhinology* 49 (3):324–330.

Buckley, D. I., R. Fu, M. Freeman, K. Rogers, and M. Helfand. 2009. C-reactive protein as a risk factor for coronary heart disease: A systematic review and meta-analyses for the U.S. Preventive Services Task Force. *Ann Intern Med* 151 (7):483–495.

Campbell, W. W. 2007. Synergistic use of higher-protein diets or nutritional supplements with resistance training to counter sarcopenia. *Nutr Rev* 65 (9):416–422.

Campbell, W. W., M. L. Barton Jr., D. Cyr-Campbell, S. L. Davey, J. L. Beard, G. Parise, and W. J. Evans. 1999a. Effects of an omnivorous diet compared with a lactoovovegetarian diet on resistance-training-induced changes in body composition and skeletal muscle in older men. *Am J Clin Nutr* 70 (6):1032–1039.

Campbell, W. W., L. J. Joseph, S. L. Davey, D. Cyr-Campbell, R. A. Anderson, and W. J. Evans. 1999b. Effects of resistance training and chromium picolinate on body composition and skeletal muscle in older men. *J Appl Physiol (1985)* 86 (1):29–39.

Campbell, W. W., and H. J. Leidy. 2007. Dietary protein and resistance training effects on muscle and body composition in older persons. *J Am Coll Nutr* 26 (6):696S–703S.

Castillo, E. M., D. Goodman-Gruen, D. Kritz-Silverstein, D. J. Morton, D. L. Wingard, and E. Barrett-Connor. 2003. Sarcopenia in elderly men and women: The Rancho Bernardo study. *Am J Prev Med* 25 (3):226–231.

Charlton, K. E., C. Nichols, S. Bowden, K. Lambert, L. Barone, M. Mason, and M. Milosavljevic. 2010. Older rehabilitation patients are at high risk of malnutrition: Evidence from a large Australian database. *J Nutr Health Aging* 14 (8):622–628.

Coggan, A. R., R. J. Spina, M. A. Rogers, D. S. King, M. Brown, P. M. Nemeth, and J. O. Holloszy. 1990. Histochemical and enzymatic characteristics of skeletal muscle in master athletes. *J Appl Physiol (1985)* 68 (5):1896–1901.

Coppe, J. P., C. K. Patil, F. Rodier, Y. Sun, D. P. Munoz, J. Goldstein, P. S. Nelson, P. Y. Desprez, and J. Campisi. 2008. Senescence-associated secretory phenotypes reveal cell-nonautonomous functions of oncogenic RAS and the p53 tumor suppressor. *PLoS Biol* 6 (12):2853–2868.

Cruz-Jentoft, A. J., J. P. Baeyens, J. M. Bauer, Y. Boirie, T. Cederholm, F. Landi, F. C. Martin et al. 2010. Sarcopenia: European consensus on definition and diagnosis: Report of the European Working Group on Sarcopenia in Older People. *Age Ageing* 39 (4):412–423.

Davis, J. P., A. A. Wong, P. J. Schluter, R. D. Henderson, J. D. O'Sullivan, and S. J. Read. 2004. Impact of premorbid undernutrition on outcome in stroke patients. *Stroke* 35 (8):1930–1934.

Davison, K. K., E. S. Ford, M. E. Cogswell, and W. H. Dietz. 2002. Percentage of body fat and body mass index are associated with mobility limitations in people aged 70 and older from NHANES III. *J Am Geriatr Soc* 50 (11):1802–1809.

Delmonico, M. J., T. B. Harris, J. S. Lee, M. Visser, M. Nevitt, S. B. Kritchevsky, F. A. Tylavsky, A. B. Newman, and Health, Aging and Body Composition Study. 2007. Alternative definitions of sarcopenia, lower extremity performance, and functional impairment with aging in older men and women. *J Am Geriatr Soc* 55 (5):769–774.

De Martinis, M., C. Franceschi, D. Monti, and L. Ginaldi. 2006. Inflammation markers predicting frailty and mortality in the elderly. *Exp Mol Pathol* 80 (3):219–227.

Depoortere, I. 2014. Taste receptors of the gut: Emerging roles in health and disease. *Gut* 63 (1):179–190.

Dreyer, H. C., C. E. Blanco, F. R. Sattler, E. T. Schroeder, and R. A. Wiswell. 2006. Satellite cell numbers in young and older men 24 hours after eccentric exercise. *Muscle Nerve* 33 (2):242–253.

Egner, I. M., J. C. Bruusgaard, and K. Gundersen. 2016. Satellite cell depletion prevents fiber hypertrophy in skeletal muscle. *Development* 143 (16):2898–2906.

English, C., H. McLennan, K. Thoirs, A. Coates, and J. Bernhardt. 2010. Loss of skeletal muscle mass after stroke: A systematic review. *Int J Stroke* 5 (5):395–402.

Ensrud, K. E. 2013. Epidemiology of fracture risk with advancing age. *J Gerontol A Biol Sci Med Sci* 68 (10):1236–1242.

Esmarck, B., J. L. Andersen, S. Olsen, E. A. Richter, M. Mizuno, and M. Kjaer. 2001. Timing of postexercise protein intake is important for muscle hypertrophy with resistance training in elderly humans. *J Physiol* 535 (Pt 1):301–311.

Evans, W. J. 1995. What is sarcopenia? *J Gerontol A Biol Sci Med Sci* 50 (Special issue):5–8.

Evans, W. J., and W. W. Campbell. 1993. Sarcopenia and age-related changes in body composition and functional capacity. *J Nutr* 123 (2 Suppl):465–468.

Feng, X., T. Todd, C. R. Lintzenich, J. Ding, J. J. Carr, Y. Ge, J. D. Browne, S. B. Kritchevsky, and S. G. Butler. 2013. Aging-related geniohyoid muscle atrophy is related to aspiration status in healthy older adults. *J Gerontol A Biol Sci Med Sci* 68 (7):853–860.

Fielding, R. A., B. Vellas, W. J. Evans, S. Bhasin, J. E. Morley, A. B. Newman, G. Abellan van Kan et al. 2011. Sarcopenia: An undiagnosed condition in older adults. Current consensus definition: Prevalence, etiology, and consequences. International Working Group on Sarcopenia. *J Am Med Dir Assoc* 12 (4):249–256.

Foley, N. C., R. E. Martin, K. L. Salter, and R. W. Teasell. 2009. A review of the relationship between dysphagia and malnutrition following stroke. *J Rehabil Med* 41 (9):707–713.

Franceschi, C., M. Bonafe, S. Valensin, F. Olivieri, M. De Luca, E. Ottaviani, and G. De Benedictis. 2000. Inflamm-aging. An evolutionary perspective on immunosenescence. *Ann NY Acad Sci* 908:244–254.

Fried, L. P., C. M. Tangen, J. Walston, A. B. Newman, C. Hirsch, J. Gottdiener, T. Seeman et al. 2001. Frailty in older adults: Evidence for a phenotype. *J Gerontol A Biol Sci Med Sci* 56 (3):M146–M156.

Giunta, S. 2008. Exploring the complex relations between inflammation and aging (inflamm-aging): Anti-inflamm-aging remodelling of inflamm-aging, from robustness to frailty. *Inflamm Res* 57 (12):558–563.

Goodpaster, B. H., S. W. Park, T. B. Harris, S. B. Kritchevsky, M. Nevitt, A. V. Schwartz, E. M. Simonsick, F. A. Tylavsky, M. Visser, and A. B. Newman. 2006. The loss of skeletal muscle strength, mass, and quality in older adults: The health, aging and body composition study. *J Gerontol A Biol Sci Med Sci* 61 (10):1059–1064.

Gumieiro, D. N., B. P. Rafacho, A. F. Goncalves, S. E. Tanni, P. S. Azevedo, D. T. Sakane, C. A. Carneiro et al. 2013. Mini Nutritional Assessment predicts gait status and mortality 6 months after hip fracture. *Br J Nutr* 109 (9):1657–1661.

Hasten, D. L., J. Pak-Loduca, K. A. Obert, and K. E. Yarasheski. 2000. Resistance exercise acutely increases MHC and mixed muscle protein synthesis rates in 78–84 and 23–32 yr olds. *Am J Physiol Endocrinol Metab* 278 (4):E620–E626.

Haub, M. D., A. M. Wells, M. A. Tarnopolsky, and W. W. Campbell. 2002. Effect of protein source on resistive-training-induced changes in body composition and muscle size in older men. *Am J Clin Nutr* 76 (3):511–517.

Heber, D., S. Ingles, J. M. Ashley, M. H. Maxwell, R. F. Lyons, and R. M. Elashoff. 1996. Clinical detection of sarcopenic obesity by bioelectrical impedance analysis. *Am J Clin Nutr* 64 (3 Suppl):472S–477S.

Holm, L., B. Esmarck, C. Suetta, K. Matsumoto, T. Doi, M. Mizuno, B. F. Miller, and M. Kjaer. 2005. Postexercise nutrient intake enhances leg protein balance in early postmenopausal women. *J Gerontol A Biol Sci Med Sci* 60 (9):1212–1218.

Hui, S. L., C. W. Slemenda, and C. C. Johnston Jr. 1988. Age and bone mass as predictors of fracture in a prospective study. *J Clin Invest* 81 (6):1804–1809.

Janssen, I., S. B. Heymsfield, and R. Ross. 2002. Low relative skeletal muscle mass (sarcopenia) in older persons is associated with functional impairment and physical disability. *J Am Geriatr Soc* 50 (5):889–896.

Kaiser, M. J., J. M. Bauer, C. Ramsch, W. Uter, Y. Guigoz, T. Cederholm, D. R. Thomas et al. 2010. Frequency of malnutrition in older adults: A multinational perspective using the Mini Nutritional Assessment. *J Am Geriatr Soc* 58 (9):1734–1738.

Kaiser, M. J., J. M. Bauer, W. Uter, L. M. Donini, I. Stange, D. Volkert, R. Diekmann et al. 2011. Prospective validation of the modified Mini Nutritional Assessment short-forms in the community, nursing home, and rehabilitation setting. *J Am Geriatr Soc* 59 (11):2124–2128.

Katsanos, C. S., H. Kobayashi, M. Sheffield-Moore, A. Aarsland, and R. R. Wolfe. 2005. Aging is associated with diminished accretion of muscle proteins after the ingestion of a small bolus of essential amino acids. *Am J Clin Nutr* 82 (5):1065–1073.

Katsanos, C. S., H. Kobayashi, M. Sheffield-Moore, A. Aarsland, and R. R. Wolfe. 2006. A high proportion of leucine is required for optimal stimulation of the rate of muscle protein synthesis by essential amino acids in the elderly. *Am J Physiol Endocrinol Metab* 291 (2):E381–E387.

Kelley, D. E., B. Goodpaster, R. R. Wing, and J. A. Simoneau. 1999. Skeletal muscle fatty acid metabolism in association with insulin resistance, obesity, and weight loss. *Am J Physiol* 277 (6 Pt 1):E1130–E1141.

Kelly-Hayes, M., A. Beiser, C. S. Kase, A. Scaramucci, R. B. D'Agostino, and P. A. Wolf. 2003. The influence of gender and age on disability following ischemic stroke: The Framingham study. *J Stroke Cerebrovasc Dis* 12 (3):119–126.

Khosla, S., and B. L. Riggs. 2005. Pathophysiology of age-related bone loss and osteoporosis. *Endocrinol Metab Clin North Am* 34 (4):1015–1030, xi.

Koopman, R., L. Verdijk, R. J. Manders, A. P. Gijsen, M. Gorselink, E. Pijpers, A. J. Wagenmakers, and L. J. van Loon. 2006. Co-ingestion of protein and leucine stimulates muscle protein synthesis rates to the same extent in young and elderly lean men. *Am J Clin Nutr* 84 (3):623–632.

Koren-Hakim, T., A. Weiss, A. Hershkovitz, I. Otzrateni, B. Grosman, S. Frishman, M. Salai, and Y. Beloosesky. 2012. The relationship between nutritional status of hip fracture operated elderly patients and their functioning, comorbidity and outcome. *Clin Nutr* 31 (6):917–921.

Kuroda, Y., and R. Kuroda. 2012. Relationship between thinness and swallowing function in Japanese older adults: Implications for sarcopenic dysphagia. *J Am Geriatr Soc* 60 (9):1785–1786.

Lauretani, F., C. R. Russo, S. Bandinelli, B. Bartali, C. Cavazzini, A. Di Iorio, A. M. Corsi, T. Rantanen, J. M. Guralnik, and L. Ferrucci. 2003. Age-associated changes in skeletal muscles and their effect on mobility: An operational diagnosis of sarcopenia. *J Appl Physiol (1985)* 95 (5):1851–1860.

Looker, A. C., H. W. Wahner, W. L. Dunn, M. S. Calvo, T. B. Harris, S. P. Heyse, C. C. Johnston Jr., and R. Lindsay. 1998. Updated data on proximal femur bone mineral levels of US adults. *Osteoporos Int* 8 (5):468–489.

Mackey, A. L., B. Esmarck, F. Kadi, S. O. Koskinen, M. Kongsgaard, A. Sylvestersen, J. J. Hansen, G. Larsen, and M. Kjaer. 2007. Enhanced satellite cell proliferation with resistance training in elderly men and women. *Scand J Med Sci Sports* 17 (1):34–42.

Marshall, S., J. Bauer, and E. Isenring. 2014. The consequences of malnutrition following discharge from rehabilitation to the community: A systematic review of current evidence in older adults. *J Hum Nutr Diet* 27 (2):133–141.

Melov, S., M. A. Tarnopolsky, K. Beckman, K. Felkey, and A. Hubbard. 2007. Resistance exercise reverses aging in human skeletal muscle. *PLoS One* 2 (5):e465.

Melton, L. J., 3rd, S. Khosla, C. S. Crowson, M. K. O'Connor, W. M. O'Fallon, and B. L. Riggs. 2000. Epidemiology of sarcopenia. *J Am Geriatr Soc* 48 (6):625–630.

Metter, E. J., L. A. Talbot, M. Schrager, and R. Conwit. 2002. Skeletal muscle strength as a predictor of all-cause mortality in healthy men. *J Gerontol A Biol Sci Med Sci* 57 (10):B359–B365.

Minnella, E. M., R. Awasthi, C. Gillis, J. F. Fiore Jr., A. S. Liberman, P. Charlebois, B. Stein, G. Bousquet-Dion, L. S. Feldman, and F. Carli. 2016. Patients with poor baseline walking capacity are most likely to improve their functional status with multimodal prehabilitation. *Surgery* 160 (4):1070–1079.

Miyanishi, K., S. Jingushi, and T. Torisu. 2010. Mortality after hip fracture in Japan: The role of nutritional status. *J Orthop Surg (Hong Kong)* 18 (3):265–270.

Moiseeva, O., F. A. Mallette, U. K. Mukhopadhyay, A. Moores, and G. Ferbeyre. 2006. DNA damage signaling and p53-dependent senescence after prolonged beta-interferon stimulation. *Mol Biol Cell* 17 (4):1583–1592.

Morley, J. E. 2001. Anorexia, sarcopenia, and aging. *Nutrition* 17 (7–8):660–663.

Morley, J. E., M. J. Kim, M. T. Haren, R. Kevorkian, and W. A. Banks. 2005. Frailty and the aging male. *Aging Male* 8 (3–4):135–140.

Negoias, S., I. Croy, J. Gerber, S. Puschmann, K. Petrowski, P. Joraschky, and T. Hummel. 2010. Reduced olfactory bulb volume and olfactory sensitivity in patients with acute major depression. *Neuroscience* 169 (1):415–421.

Newman, A. B., V. Kupelian, M. Visser, E. Simonsick, B. Goodpaster, M. Nevitt, S. B. Kritchevsky, F. A. Tylavsky, S. M. Rubin, T. B. Harris, and Health ABC Study Investigators. 2003. Sarcopenia: Alternative definitions and associations with lower extremity function. *J Am Geriatr Soc* 51 (11):1602–1609.

Newman, A. B., V. Kupelian, M. Visser, E. M. Simonsick, B. H. Goodpaster, S. B. Kritchevsky, F. A. Tylavsky, S. M. Rubin, and T. B. Harris. 2006. Strength, but not muscle mass, is associated with mortality in the health, aging and body composition study cohort. *J Gerontol A Biol Sci Med Sci* 61 (1):72–77.

Nguyen, A. D., P. E. Pelavin, M. E. Shenton, P. Chilakamarri, R. W. McCarley, P. G. Nestor, and J. J. Levitt. 2011. Olfactory sulcal depth and olfactory bulb volume in patients with schizophrenia: An MRI study. *Brain Imaging Behav* 5 (4):252–261.

Olsen, S., P. Aagaard, F. Kadi, G. Tufekovic, J. Verney, J. L. Olesen, C. Suetta, and M. Kjaer. 2006. Creatine supplementation augments the increase in satellite cell and myonuclei number in human skeletal muscle induced by strength training. *J Physiol* 573 (Pt 2):525–534.

Ottenbacher, K. J., A. Karmarkar, J. E. Graham, Y. F. Kuo, A. Deutsch, T. A. Reistetter, S. Al Snih, and C. V. Granger. 2014. Thirty-day hospital readmission following discharge from postacute rehabilitation in fee-for-service Medicare patients. *JAMA* 311 (6):604–614.

Paddon-Jones, D., M. Sheffield-Moore, C. S. Katsanos, X. J. Zhang, and R. R. Wolfe. 2006. Differential stimulation of muscle protein synthesis in elderly humans following isocaloric ingestion of amino acids or whey protein. *Exp Gerontol* 41 (2):215–219.

Paddon-Jones, D., M. Sheffield-Moore, X. J. Zhang, E. Volpi, S. E. Wolf, A. Aarsland, A. A. Ferrando, and R. R. Wolfe. 2004. Amino acid ingestion improves muscle protein synthesis in the young and elderly. *Am J Physiol Endocrinol Metab* 286 (3):E321–E328.

Parise, G., A. N. Brose, and M. A. Tarnopolsky. 2005a. Resistance exercise training decreases oxidative damage to DNA and increases cytochrome oxidase activity in older adults. *Exp Gerontol* 40 (3):173–180.

Parise, G., S. M. Phillips, J. J. Kaczor, and M. A. Tarnopolsky. 2005b. Antioxidant enzyme activity is up-regulated after unilateral resistance exercise training in older adults. *Free Radic Biol Med* 39 (2):289–295.

Pawelec, G. 1999. Immunosenescence: Impact in the young as well as the old? *Mech Ageing Dev* 108 (1):1–7.

Phillips, A. C., D. Carroll, C. R. Gale, J. M. Lord, W. Arlt, and G. D. Batty. 2010. Cortisol, DHEA sulphate, their ratio, and all-cause and cause-specific mortality in the Vietnam Experience Study. *Eur J Endocrinol* 163 (2):285–292.

Proctor, D. N., P. Balagopal, and K. S. Nair. 1998. Age-related sarcopenia in humans is associated with reduced synthetic rates of specific muscle proteins. *J Nutr* 128 (2 Suppl):351S–355S.

Riggs, B. L., L. J. Melton, R. A. Robb, J. J. Camp, E. J. Atkinson, L. McDaniel, S. Amin, P. A. Rouleau, and S. Khosla. 2008. A population-based assessment of rates of bone loss at multiple skeletal sites: Evidence for substantial trabecular bone loss in young adult women and men. *J Bone Miner Res* 23 (2):205–214.

Rodier, F., and J. Campisi. 2011. Four faces of cellular senescence. *J Cell Biol* 192 (4):547–556.

Rogers, M. A., J. M. Hagberg, W. H. Martin 3rd, A. A. Ehsani, and J. O. Holloszy. 1990. Decline in VO2max with aging in master athletes and sedentary men. *J Appl Physiol (1985)* 68 (5):2195–2199.

Rooyackers, O. E., D. B. Adey, P. A. Ades, and K. S. Nair. 1996. Effect of age on in vivo rates of mitochondrial protein synthesis in human skeletal muscle. *Proc Natl Acad Sci USA* 93 (26):15364–15369.

Rosenberg, I. H. 1997. Sarcopenia: Origins and clinical relevance. *J Nutr* 127 (5 Suppl):990S–991S.

Sakuma, K., W. Aoi, and A. Yamaguchi. 2015. Current understanding of sarcopenia: Possible candidates modulating muscle mass. *Pflugers Arch* 467 (2):213–229.

Sakuma, K., and A. Yamaguchi. 2012. Sarcopenia and cachexia: The adaptations of negative regulators of skeletal muscle mass. *J Cachexia Sarcopenia Muscle* 3 (2):77–94.

Sanchez-Rodriguez, D., E. Marco, R. Miralles, M. Fayos, S. Mojal, M. Alvarado, O. Vazquez-Ibar, F. Escalada, and J. M. Muniesa. 2014. Sarcopenia, physical rehabilitation and functional outcomes of patients in a subacute geriatric care unit. *Arch Gerontol Geriatr* 59 (1):39–43.

Scherbakov, N., and W. Doehner. 2011. Sarcopenia in stroke-facts and numbers on muscle loss accounting for disability after stroke. *J Cachexia Sarcopenia Muscle* 2 (1):5–8.

Scherbakov, N., S. von Haehling, S. D. Anker, U. Dirnagl, and W. Doehner. 2013. Stroke induced sarcopenia: Muscle wasting and disability after stroke. *Int J Cardiol* 170 (2):89–94.

Strakowski, M. M., J. A. Strakowski, and M. C. Mitchell. 2002. Malnutrition in rehabilitation. *Am J Phys Med Rehabil* 81 (1):77–78.

Straub, R. H., L. E. Miller, J. Scholmerich, and B. Zietz. 2000. Cytokines and hormones as possible links between endocrinosenescence and immunosenescence. *J Neuroimmunol* 109 (1):10–15.

Symons, T. B., S. E. Schutzler, T. L. Cocke, D. L. Chinkes, R. R. Wolfe, and D. Paddon-Jones. 2007. Aging does not impair the anabolic response to a protein-rich meal. *Am J Clin Nutr* 86 (2):451–456.

Tamura, F., T. Kikutani, T. Tohara, M. Yoshida, and K. Yaegaki. 2012. Tongue thickness relates to nutritional status in the elderly. *Dysphagia* 27 (4):556–561.

Targonski, P. V., R. M. Jacobson, and G. A. Poland. 2007. Immunosenescence: Role and measurement in influenza vaccine response among the elderly. *Vaccine* 25 (16):3066–3069.

Thalacker-Mercer, A. E., J. C. Fleet, B. A. Craig, N. S. Carnell, and W. W. Campbell. 2007. Inadequate protein intake affects skeletal muscle transcript profiles in older humans. *Am J Clin Nutr* 85 (5):1344–1352.

Trappe, T., R. Williams, J. Carrithers, U. Raue, B. Esmarck, M. Kjaer, and R. Hickner. 2004. Influence of age and resistance exercise on human skeletal muscle proteolysis: A microdialysis approach. *J Physiol* 554 (Pt 3):803–813.

Tuccori, M., F. Lapi, A. Testi, E. Ruggiero, U. Moretti, A. Vannacci, R. Bonaiuti et al. 2011. Drug-induced taste and smell alterations: A case/non-case evaluation of an Italian database of spontaneous adverse drug reaction reporting. *Drug Saf* 34 (10):849–859.

Turnbull, A. V., and C. L. Rivier. 1999. Regulation of the hypothalamic-pituitary-adrenal axis by cytokines: Actions and mechanisms of action. *Physiol Rev* 79 (1):1–71.

Vashishth, D., G. J. Gibson, J. I. Khoury, M. B. Schaffler, J. Kimura, and D. P. Fyhrie. 2001. Influence of non-enzymatic glycation on biomechanical properties of cortical bone. *Bone* 28 (2):195–201.

Vasto, S., G. Candore, C. R. Balistreri, M. Caruso, G. Colonna-Romano, M. P. Grimaldi, F. Listi, D. Nuzzo, D. Lio, and C. Caruso. 2007. Inflammatory networks in ageing, age-related diseases and longevity. *Mech Ageing Dev* 128 (1):83–91.

Wakabayashi, H. 2010. Seamless community coordination of rehabilitation nutrition care management in patients with dysphagia [in Japanese]. *Gan To Kagaku Ryoho* 37 (Suppl 2):198–200.

Wakabayashi, H. 2014. Presbyphagia and sarcopenic dysphagia: Association between aging, sarcopenia, and deglutition disorders. *J Frailty Aging* 3 (2):97–103.

Wakabayashi, H., and K. Sakuma. 2013. Nutrition, exercise, and pharmaceutical therapies for sarcopenic obesity. *J Nutr Ther* 2 (2):11.

Wakabayashi, H., and K. Sakuma. 2014. Comprehensive approach to sarcopenia treatment. *Curr Clin Pharmacol* 9 (2):171–180.

Wakabayashi, H., and H. Sashika. 2011. Association of nutrition status and rehabilitation outcome in the disuse syndrome: A retrospective cohort study. *Gen Med* 12 (2):6.

Wakabayashi, H., and H. Sashika. 2014. Malnutrition is associated with poor rehabilitation outcome in elderly inpatients with hospital-associated deconditioning a prospective cohort study. *J Rehabil Med* 46 (3):277–282.

Wall, J. C., S. K. Chatterji, and J. W. Jeffery. 1979. Age-related changes in the density and tensile strength of human femoral cortical bone. *Calcif Tissue Int* 27 (2):105–108.

Weiskopf, D., B. Weinberger, and B. Grubeck-Loebenstein. 2009. The aging of the immune system. *Transpl Int* 22 (11):1041–1050.

Welle, S., C. Thornton, R. Jozefowicz, and M. Statt. 1993. Myofibrillar protein synthesis in young and old men. *Am J Physiol* 264 (5 Pt 1):E693–E698.

Wylie, K., and M. Nebauer. 2011. "The food here is tasteless!" Food taste or tasteless food? Chemosensory loss and the politics of under-nutrition. *Collegian* 18 (1):27–35.

Yarasheski, K. E., J. J. Zachwieja, and D. M. Bier. 1993. Acute effects of resistance exercise on muscle protein synthesis rate in young and elderly men and women. *Am J Physiol* 265 (2 Pt 1):E210–E214.

Yaxley, A., M. D. Miller, R. J. Fraser, L. Cobiac, and M. Crotty. 2012. The complexity of treating wasting in ambulatory rehabilitation: Is it starvation, sarcopenia, cachexia or a combination of these conditions? *Asia Pac J Clin Nutr* 21 (3):386–393.

16 Nutrition in Neurodegenerative Disorders and Cognitive Impairment

16.1 INTRODUCTION

Cognitive impairment and dementia are increasing globally, as the population of the world ages at a rapid rate. This aging of the world's population has been attributed to advances in nutrition and sanitation, as well as a declining birth rate in developed nations. Aging is the primary risk factor for Alzheimer's disease (AD), which is the most common form of dementia (Ballard et al. 2011). Aging is the only risk factor that is consistently identified after age 80. In that age group, more women than men have dementia, but this may be due to the longer life span in women. The high prevalence of inherited dementias among individuals under age 65, previously called presenile dementia, has led to the identification of causative genes and subsequent molecular pathology of direct relevance to the more common sporadic disease seen in older patients.

In this chapter, the differences among the major dementia diseases, including (1) AD, (2) vascular disease, (3) dementia with Lewy bodies, (4) frontotemporal lobar degeneration (FTLD), and (5) chronic traumatic encephalopathy (CTE), are briefly reviewed, and other causes of dementia are mentioned. Although patients who present with the mild but consistent cognitive decline that accompanies aging, such as forgetting first names or losing objects like mobile phones, should not be categorized as having dementia, it is increasingly important to make a specific early diagnosis of the cause of cognitive impairment when appropriate, particularly with the possibility of disease-modifying treatments becoming available in the future.

Over the past 40 years, a great deal of information on the connections between nutrition and brain health has been developed. This has led to an explosion of research on various dietary supplements, drugs, and the effects of reducing visceral fat through diet and exercise as approaches to prevention of AD. Most of this research has been done in individuals with mild cognitive impairment (MCI) or age-related memory deficits and in numerous animal and cellular models in the laboratory.

Although the impact of nutrition on normal brain development in utero and during childhood is well established, having driven public health recommendations for adequate folate intake during pregnancy, as well as adequate nutrition during pediatric care, more recently, attention has focused on brain health and nutrition throughout the life span, including adult medicine and geriatrics, as the impact of global aging and associated age-related chronic diseases, such as type 2 diabetes mellitus, has been recognized. Approaches that result in the reduction of visceral fat lead to decreased inflammation. A healthy lifestyle also has an impact on other aspects of brain health, helping to maintain normal mood, mental focus, motivation, and attention. This chapter highlights some of the scientific evidence indicating a relationship between nutrition and brain health, and summarizes some nutritional recommendations for maintaining cognitive health and mood stability in adults as they age.

16.2 EPIDEMIOLOGY

Increasing age is the strongest risk factor for dementia, and the only risk factor consistently identified after age 80. While prevalence is consistently higher among women, incidence is not; thus, the higher prevalence is largely thought to be a function of longer life spans in women. Lower educational levels have been found to be associated with higher prevalence. Within the United States, prevalence has been reported as elevated in African American and Latino populations; some authors have attributed these findings to lower education and higher cardiovascular morbidity in those populations. An estimated 35.6 million people worldwide were living with dementia in 2010, and this number is expected to increase to 115.4 million people by 2050 (Prince et al. 2013).

Several modifiable risk factors contribute to the possibility of developing AD. Diabetes, physical inactivity, and obesity are among the risk factors that share pathologic features, including dyslipidemia and insulin resistance. In addition, the strongest genetic risk factor for sporadic AD is the presence of the E4 isoform of the lipoprotein carrier apolipoprotein E (apoE). This isoform alters lipid physiology in the brain and periphery (Liu et al. 2013). As a result, several diet- and metabolism-based treatments to reduce dyslipidemia and visceral fat are being examined in AD patients.

AD is the most common type of dementia among Western countries, corresponding to about 60% of cases (Kalaria et al. 2008; Horton 2012), while vascular dementia (VaD) is the second, with about 20% of all cases. Due to the overlaps in symptomatology, pathophysiology, and risk factors, AD and VaD are not easily distinguished. In fact, VaD refers to a group of clinical syndromes, which include dementia, resulting from ischemic, hemorrhagic, anoxic, or hypoxic brain damage. Ischemic VaD may be due to macrovascular or microvascular cerebral disease or a combination of both types of lesions. The cause of hemorrhagic VaD may be hypertension, leading to cerebral amyloid angiopathy, the source of intralobar hemorrhages, or multiple petechial hemorrhages.

In AD, causes and progression are not well understood. The disease is associated with tangles and plaques in the brain, loss of connections, inflammation, and eventual death of brain cells, so it is classified as a neurodegenerative disorder. All these brain changes lead to memory loss and alterations in thinking and other brain functions. The disease usually progresses slowly and gradually gets worse as more brain cells die. The distribution of dementia around the world seems to vary according to cultural and socioeconomic differences among nations. Interestingly, the overall prevalence of dementia in general and AD in particular appears to be higher in developed countries than in developing ones (Rizzi et al. 2014).

Nonetheless, in a global survey performed in 2001, 60.1% of all people with dementia were living in developing countries. This is not inconsistent with the higher prevalence in developed countries since the population in developing countries is so much greater. Aging of the world's population is proceeding rapidly, especially in China, India, and Latin America, where dementia is rapidly becoming the major public health problem. Although epidemiological information about the prevalence of dementia and its subtypes remains scarce (Ferri et al. 2005; Liu et al. 2013), the Delphi Consensus Study found that the prevalence of dementia was high in the Americas and low in less developed regions of the world, such as Africa and the Middle East. The prevalence of dementia in Latin America will be similar to that encountered in North America by 2040 (Ferri et al. 2005). Among developed countries, Japan has the lowest prevalence of both dementia in general and AD in particular.

Modifiable risk factors that contribute to the risk of developing AD include diabetes, physical inactivity, and obesity (Lee 2011). Pathologic features shared among these risk factors include dyslipidemia and insulin resistance. In addition, the strongest genetic risk factor for sporadic AD is the presence of the E4 isoform of the lipoprotein carrier apoE. This isoform alters lipid physiology in the brain and periphery (Braak and Braak 1991; Liu et al. 2013). As a result, treatments that include dietary interventions to balance nutrition and a healthy active lifestyle in order to reduce insulin resistance and dyslipidemia are being examined in AD patients. These studies are examining the interactions among apoE, lipids, inflammation, amyloid β (Aβ) peptides, glucose, central nervous system (CNS) insulin, and peripheral insulin and seem increasingly important.

Cardiovascular risk factors, including hypertension, diabetes, obesity, and dyslipidemia, contribute to the high prevalence of mixed dementias, including both AD and VaD in developed countries. On the other hand, developing societies where hypertension is the major problem seem to have a proportionally higher prevalence of VaDs.

16.3 DIAGNOSIS OF DEMENTIA

Dementia includes symptoms of memory loss, changes in mood and behavior, and problems with communication, reasoning, and the ability to carry out daily activities. A diagnosis of dementia requires substantial impairment to be present in one or more cognitive domains. The impairment must be sufficient to interfere with independence in everyday activities. The diagnosis of mild neurocognitive disorder or MCI is made when there is modest impairment in one or more cognitive domains. The individual is still independent in everyday activities, albeit with greater effort. The impairment must represent a decline from a previously higher level and should be documented both by history and by objective assessment. Further, the cognitive deficits must not occur exclusively in the context of a delirium or be better explained by another mental disorder.

A full discussion of the differential diagnosis of dementias and MCI is beyond the scope of this chapter. However, primary care providers working with specialized memory clinics can diagnose the syndromes of dementia and MCI. The diagnosis is based on history, examination, and objective assessments, using standard criteria established by the American Psychiatric Association *Diagnostic and Statistical Manual of Mental Disorders* (DSM-5) (Table 16.1) (American Psychiatric Association 2013).

Dementia is associated with diseases causing structural and chemical changes in the brain. Dementia can lead to depression, psychosis, aggression, and wandering. There are many diseases that result in dementia. The most common types of dementia include (1) AD; (2) VaD; (3) mixed dementia, commonly AD and VaD together; (4) dementia with Lewy bodies; (5) frontotemporal dementia, also known as Pick's disease; and (6) CTE.

Alzheimer's dementia presents with difficulty remembering recent conversations, names, or events. This is often an early clinical symptom. Apathy and depression are also often early symptoms. Later symptoms include impaired communication, poor judgment, disorientation, confusion, behavior changes, and difficulty speaking, swallowing, and walking. Revised criteria and guidelines for diagnosing Alzheimer's were published in 2011 and affirmed in 2013 (American Psychiatric Association 2013), recommending that Alzheimer's be considered a slowly progressive brain disease that begins well before symptoms emerge. Abnormalities are deposits of the protein fragment β-amyloid, also known as plaques. Whether these are the key causative factor remains in question, since there are documented cases of amyloid deposits detected by Pittsburgh compound

TABLE 16.1
Functional Limitations Associated with Impairment in Different Cognitive Domains

Cognitive Domain	Examples of Changes in Everyday Activities
Complex attention	Normal tasks take longer, especially when there are competing stimuli; easily distracted; tasks need to be simplified; difficulty retaining the information needed over several minutes to do mental arithmetic or dial a phone number
Executive functioning	Difficulty with multistage tasks, planning, organizing, multitasking, following directions, keeping up with shifting conversations
Learning and memory	Difficulty recalling recent events; repeating self; misplacing objects; losing track of actions already performed; increasing reliance on lists, reminders
Language	Word-finding difficulty; use of general phrase or wrong words; grammatical errors; difficulty with comprehension of others' language or written material
Perceptual motor/ visuospatial function	Getting lost in familiar places; more use of notes and maps; difficulty using familiar tools and appliances
Social cognition	Disinhibition or apathy; loss of empathy; inappropriate behavior; loss of judgment

Source: Adapted from American Psychiatric Association, *Diagnostic and Statistical Manual of Mental Disorders*, 5th ed., American Psychiatric Association, Arlington, VA, 2013.

B (PiB)–positron emission tomography (PET) imaging in individuals with normal cognition (Snitz et al. 2015). There are also twisted strands of the protein tau, also called tau tangles, as well as evidence of nerve cell damage and death in the brain. These latter changes would be consistent with inflammation being the primary driver of AD, and this is consistent with what is known about the risk factors, including those that could be impacted by nutrition. A recent study suggested that greater amounts of amyloid at baseline in a prospective study were associated with more rapid progression of AD (Petersen et al. 2016). However, the jury is still out on whether amyloid is the key pathogenic factor or a bystander to an inflammatory process.

VaD presents with changes in cognition, suddenly following strokes that block major brain blood vessels (O'Brien and Thomas 2015). Problems in cognition and reasoning may begin as mild changes that worsen gradually as a result of multiple minor strokes or other conditions that affect smaller blood vessels, leading to cumulative damage. At earlier stages, the term *vascular cognitive impairment* (VCI) is used rather than VaD to indicate that changes can range from mild to severe. VaD is the second most common cause of dementia, after AD, accounting for 20–30% of cases, and it may be underdiagnosed.

Mixed dementia presents with dementia findings, including both vascular brain changes and changes linked to other types of dementia, including AD and dementia with Lewy bodies (Claus et al. 2015). Several studies have found that vascular changes and other brain abnormalities may interact in ways that increase the likelihood of a mixed dementia diagnosis.

Dementia with Lewy bodies often presents with memory loss and thinking problems common in Alzheimer's, but those diagnosed with it are more likely than people with Alzheimer's to have initial or early symptoms, such as sleep disturbances, well-formed visual hallucinations, and slowness, gait imbalance, or other parkinsonian movement features (Morra and Donovick 2014). Lewy bodies are abnormal aggregations (or clumps) of the protein α-synuclein. When they develop in a part of the brain called the cortex, dementia can result. α-Synuclein also aggregates in the brains of people with Parkinson's disease, but the aggregates may appear in a pattern that is different from dementia with Lewy bodies.

The brain changes of dementia with Lewy bodies alone can cause dementia, or they can be present at the same time as the brain changes of AD and/or VaD, with each abnormality contributing to the development of dementia. When these pathologies occur together, it is another form of mixed dementia.

Frontotemporal dementia (Galimberti et al. 2015) is characterized by nerve cell damage and loss of function in the frontal and temporal brain regions, which variably cause deterioration in behavior and personality, language disturbances, or alterations in muscle or motor functions. There are a number of different diseases that cause frontotemporal degenerations. The two most prominent are (1) a group of brain disorders involving the protein tau and (2) a group of brain disorders involving the protein called TDP43. The reason these localize to the frontal and temporal regions is not known. This condition is also called Pick's disease after Arnold Pick, a physician who in 1892 first described a patient with distinct symptoms affecting language.

CTE is a brain condition associated with repeated blows to the head (Galimberti et al. 2015). This form of dementia came into public consciousness with the suicide deaths of several National Football League players in the United States. They shot themselves in parts of their bodies such as the chest and abdomen purposely far from their heads in order to enable a study of their brain tissue postmortem. Potential signs of CTE are problems with thinking and memory, personality changes, and behavioral changes, including aggression and depression. People may not experience potential signs of CTE until years or decades after brain injuries occur. A definitive diagnosis of CTE can only be made after death, when an autopsy can reveal whether the known brain changes of CTE are present.

Other diseases can also lead to secondary dementia. These rarer causes include alcohol-related brain damage such as Wernicke–Korsakoff syndrome, due to irreversible damage from thiamin deficiency (Ilomaki et al. 2015), HIV (Brew and Chan 2014), and Creutzfeldt–Jakob disease (Sobreira et al. 2013), a slow prion disease first discovered in cannibals. Bovine spongioform encephalopathy

(Wells and Wilesmith 1995) is another prion disease that is contracted by eating meat from cows that were fed nerve parts or brains from other animals.

Working with neurologists who specialize in dementias and memory disorders, it is possible to diagnose the etiological subtypes of dementia syndromes using standard criteria for each of them. Brain imaging and biomarkers are used in the differential diagnoses among the different disorders. Treatments for the most part are still symptomatic. Therefore, the role of nutrition and lifestyle is best employed as early as possible for the prevention or slowing of progression. Many nutritional approaches in use currently are based on a combination of evidence from epidemiological studies, animal and cellular studies, and a very limited number of clinical intervention studies of short duration.

16.4 AGE-RELATED CHANGES IN THE BRAIN

A well-functioning brain has intact neurons and synapses that communicate messages to control basic bodily functions like breathing, heart rate, sensation, and movement, as well as such mental experiences as mood, thinking, reasoning, attention, and visual-spatial skills. Age-related alterations in the striatum are accompanied by spatial disorientation, as well as declines in motor function that lead to diminished muscle strength and loss of balance and coordination.

As the brain ages, it atrophies, its synaptic connections become less effective, and cells do not communicate as well as during youth.

A gradual deposition of abnormal protein deposits, including amyloid plaques and tau tangles, accumulate in brain regions controlling cognition, and these accumulations correlate with cognitive decline (Wansink and Linder 2003). PET scanning can measure the extent of brain plaques and tangles when a specific indicator is used (FDDNP) (Merrill et al. 2012). In a study of middle-aged and older nondemented adults with a median age of 64 years, increases in frontal, posterior cingulate, and global FDDNP binding at follow-up correlated with progression of memory decline ($r = -0.32$ to -0.37, $p = 0.03–0.01$) after 2 years. Moreover, it was found that higher baseline FDDNP binding was associated with future decline in most cognitive domains, including language, attention, executive, and visuospatial abilities ($r = -0.31$ to -0.56, $p = 0.05–0.002$). These regional plaque and tangle binding patterns are consistent with known neuropathological patterns of plaque and tangle brain accumulation, spreading from the medial temporal to other neocortical regions as cognitive decline progresses. These abnormal protein deposits have also been found to correlate with late-life major depression and symptoms of anxiety and depression in nondemented volunteers (Quinn et al. 2010; Danthiir et al. 2011).

In addition to plaque and tangle accumulation, numerous neurotransmitter systems decline with aging, particularly cholinergic cells in the basal forebrain that project to brain regions controlling cognitive skills (e.g., frontal, parietal, and medial temporal) (Holmes et al. 2005). Neurons in the hippocampus (a brain region critical to forming new memories) show decline (Kepe et al. 2006), and age-associated general and regional brain atrophy accelerates when people develop MCI and dementia (Burggren et al. 2011). Loss of such neurotransmitters as dopamine and muscarine leads to decreased sensitivity to stimulation.

Age-related decline in brain health is accompanied by decline in cognitive skills. Although earlier studies suggested that cognitive decline did not begin until age 60, recent research indicates that such decline can be observed as early as age 45 years. Singh-Manoux and coworkers (2012) observed 5198 men and 2192 women who ranged in age from 45 and 70. Their cognitive abilities were assessed three times over a 10-year period. The investigators found that cognitive scores declined in all areas except vocabulary. They reported a 3.6% decline in mental reasoning in those aged 45–49 years and a 9.6% decline in men and 7.4% in women in the age range 65–70 years.

These and other investigators point to the public health implications of such findings for preventing dementia: since these gradual declines in brain health and cognitive abilities precede the onset of dementia symptoms by decades, it might be possible to develop prevention treatments that delay the onset of those symptoms. Moreover, targeting individuals with risk factors for heart disease—obesity, hypertension, or high cholesterol—could protect them not only from future cardiac disease but also from cognitive decline and dementia.

16.5 INFLAMMATION, OXIDATIVE STRESS, AND THE BRAIN

As the brain ages, inflammation and oxidation appear to contribute to neurodegeneration, just as they do in heart disease, diabetes, cancer, and aging of other body organs (Akiyama et al. 2000; Romano et al. 2010). In fact, the amyloid plaques that accumulate in the brains of AD patients show evidence of inflammation, including cytokines (protein molecules that attack foreign material) and activated microglia (cells that clean out cellular waste, ridding the brain of damaged neurons, plaques, and infectious agents). A growing body of evidence also suggests that Parkinson's disease is associated with oxidative damage via iron accumulation in the substantia nigra, where neurons are destroyed. Many scientists theorize that chronic inflammation in the brain destroys neurons, and several investigations have suggested that certain medicines, foods, and healthy behaviors can reduce inflammation. Age-related oxidative stress also damages neurons. Omega-3 fats from nuts and fish and antioxidant fruits and vegetables may diminish age-related inflammatory and oxidative neuronal damage.

Nourishing our brains through a healthy diet appears to protect us from cognitive decline. A recent study (Gu et al. 2010) of more than 2000 people age 65 and older showed that research subjects who ate a greater amount of nuts, fish, tomatoes, poultry, vegetables, and fruits, and a lesser amount of high-fat dairy products, red meat, and butter, had a lower risk for AD. These kinds of findings point to proper nutrition as a way to bolster brain health as we age.

A diet rich in anti-inflammatory omega-3 fatty acids from ocean-caught fish and seafood is associated with a lower risk for developing AD (Cole et al. 2009). The most abundant omega-3 fatty acid in the brain, docosahexaenoic acid (DHA), protects brain neurons against the toxic events associated with amyloid plaques and tau tangles. The prevalence of dementia among Nigerians, who eat a diet low in animal fat, is low compared with that of African Americans, who eat a diet with a higher intake of omega-6 fatty acids (Ogunniyi et al. 2000).

16.6 HEALTHY LIFESTYLE AND THE BRAIN

Considerable scientific evidence points to lifestyle as key to protecting brain health as people age (Small et al. 2000; Kosashvili et al. 2010; Lee et al. 2010; Rolland et al. 2010; Sofi et al. 2010; Merrill and Small 2011). Nutrition, mental and physical exercise, stress reduction, and social engagement can improve cognitive performance and possibly delay the onset of dementia. Dr. Gary Small and colleagues at the University of California, Los Angeles (UCLA) (Miller et al. 2012) found that a 6-week healthy lifestyle program, including healthy nutrition, physical conditioning, memory training, and stress management, improved both encoding and recalling of new verbal information, as well as self-perception of memory ability in older adults residing in continuing care retirement communities. In another study, the same group found that a 2-week healthy lifestyle program combining mental and physical exercise, stress reduction, and healthy diet was associated with significant effects on cognitive function and brain metabolism (Small et al. 2006). The reduced resting activity in the left dorsolateral prefrontal cortex observed following the 2-week program may reflect greater cognitive efficiency of a brain region involved in working memory. Such evidence suggests that the impact of nutrition on brain health could be augmented when combined with several healthy lifestyle behaviors.

16.6.1 Exercise and Brain Health

Exercise training can influence brain morphology at older ages. Hippocampal and medial temporal lobe volumes are larger in highly fit adults, and physical activity training increases hippocampal perfusion. A 52-week randomized controlled trial with 120 older adults (aged 55–80 years) showed that aerobic exercise training increased the size of the anterior hippocampus, leading to improvements in spatial memory (Erickson et al. 2011). Exercise training increased hippocampal volume by 2%, effectively reversing age-related losses in volume by 1–2 years. Hippocampal volume declined in the control group. Caudate nucleus and thalamus volumes were unaffected by the intervention. These findings indicate that aerobic exercise training is effective at reversing hippocampal volume loss in older adults, which is accompanied by improved memory function.

Brain-derived neurotrophic factor (BDNF) plays an important role in neuronal survival and growth, serves as a neurotransmitter modulator, and participates in neuronal plasticity, which is essential for learning and memory. It is widely expressed in the CNS, gut, and other tissues. Decreased levels of BDNF are associated with neurodegenerative diseases with neuronal loss, such as Parkinson's disease, AD, multiple sclerosis, and Huntington's disease.

Studies investigating the effects of physical activity and acute exercise and/or training on the plasma concentrations of BDNF in humans (Gold et al. 2003; Knaepen et al. 2010) demonstrated that exercise increased BDNF release (Goekint et al. 2008, 2010a,b, 2011; Goekint 2011). After training for 8 weeks, baseline BDNF levels are lower, possibly due to a receptor adaptation, while detraining will abolish the exercise-induced effects (Goekint et al. 2010a). Little is known about the effect of resistance exercise on hippocampus-dependent memory, although this type of exercise is increasingly recommended to improve muscle strength and bone density and to prevent age-related disabilities. It was shown that resistance training does not significantly increase peripheral BDNF levels (Goekint et al. 2008); however, it seems that resistance exercise increases cognitive performance, especially in the elderly population (Cassilhas et al. 2007).

16.6.2 Omega-3 Fatty Acids and Fish Oils

Although many Americans seem to prefer animal fat in their diet, at least one study suggested that substituting other healthier fats can promote satiety and may help with weight.

Theoretically fish oil supplements rich in DHA should have similar effects to seafood in reducing inflammation in the brain. A meta-analysis of randomized controlled trials of fish oil supplements alone without lifestyle changes failed to demonstrate a benefit in the treatment of dementias (Burckhardt et al. 2016). This is not surprising, as supplementation in the absence of reducing omega-6 fatty acids is less effective in altering tissue levels of omega-3 fatty acids.

It may be that patients with an apoE-4 isoform would be more responsive to changes in dietary fat from omega-6 to omega-3. An interesting 26-week study of cognitively intact subjects age 65 years or older demonstrated that those subjects with the apoE-4 genetic risk for AD demonstrated better attention span from ingesting either a low daily dose (226 mg of eicosapentaenoic acid [EPA], 176 mg of DHA) or a high daily dose (1093 mg EPA, 847 mg DHA) of fish oil than a placebo group (van de Rest et al. 2008).

Better cognitive health in older adults has been associated with omega-3 polyunsaturated fatty acids (PUFAs). The omega-3 long-chain PUFAs EPA and DHA are necessary for normal brain development and function (Danthiir et al. 2011). Epidemiological studies have demonstrated a clear connection between cognitive performance and omega-3 fatty acids, but clinical trials of DHA supplementation have not been successful in slowing the rate of cognitive and functional decline in patients with mild to moderate Alzheimer disease compared with placebo (Quinn et al. 2010). Even though a treatment may not show benefit in patients with dementia, it still may be effective in people with milder forms of cognitive impairment. To this end, an 18-month randomized, double-blind, controlled trial of omega-3 fatty acids in cognitively healthy older adults is currently in progress (Danthiir et al. 2011).

Omega-3 fatty acids also may offer a benefit in alleviating symptoms of depression. An 8-week controlled trial of 1050 mg of EPA and 150 mg of DHA daily found improvement in mood in patients with a major depressive episode without comorbid anxiety (Lesperance et al. 2011). EPA appears to be the key omega-3 fatty acid component that is associated with efficacy in major depressive disorders.

16.6.3 Antioxidant-Rich Foods

Antioxidant-rich foods protect neurons from oxidative free radicals that damage DNA. Polyphenols are potent antioxidants that can be found in strawberries, blackberries, blueberries, and other colorful berries, as well as grapes, pears, plums, cherries, broccoli, cabbage, celery, onions, and parsley.

Several large-scale studies indicate a link between dietary antioxidant intake and better brain health, including the Rotterdam Study, which demonstrated an association between higher dietary intake of the antioxidant vitamin E and a lower risk for developing AD (Devore et al. 2010). Another large-scale European study in people age 65 and older showed an association between daily consumption of fruits and vegetables and a lower risk for all forms of dementia (Barberger-Gateau et al. 2007).

Although memory impairment is associated with low antioxidant blood levels, short-term memory has been found to improve in laboratory animals fed antioxidant-rich berry extracts (Goyarzu et al. 2004). Other research suggests that when study subjects drink fruit or vegetable juice at least three times a week, they have a lower probability of developing AD than those who drink these juices less than once a week (Dai et al. 2006).

Pomegranate juice is rich in antioxidant polyphenols, and recent studies suggest its brain health benefits. Our group at UCLA performed a preliminary, placebo-controlled, randomized trial of pomegranate juice in older subjects with age-associated memory complaints using memory testing and functional brain activation (fMRI) as outcome measures (Bookheimer et al. 2013). Thirty-two subjects were enrolled and 28 completed the study. Subjects were randomly assigned to drink 8 ounces of either pomegranate juice or a flavor-matched placebo drink for 4 weeks. Subjects received memory testing, fMRI scans during cognitive tasks, and blood draws for peripheral biomarkers before and after the intervention. Investigators and subjects were all blind to group membership. After 4 weeks, only the pomegranate group showed a significant improvement in the Buschke selective reminding test of verbal memory and a significant increase in plasma antioxidant capacity and urolithin A–glucuronide, a metabolite of pomegranate ellagitannins formed by the colonic microflora. Furthermore, compared with the placebo group, the pomegranate group had increased fMRI activity during verbal and visual memory tasks. While preliminary, these results suggest a role for pomegranate juice in augmenting memory function through task-related increases in functional brain activity.

Research suggests that cocoa flavanols improve memory and learning, possibly as a result of their anti-inflammatory and neuroprotective effects (Lamport et al. 2015). These effects may be mediated by increased cerebral blood flow, with subsequent stimulation of neuronal function cerebral blood flow was measured before and after consumption of a 330 mL drink containing low (23 mg) or high (494 mg) amounts of cocoa flavanols. The drinks were matched for caffeine, theobromine, taste, calories, and appearance. The study was conducted in 8 males and 10 females between the ages of 50 and 65 using a randomized, counterbalanced, crossover, double-blind design and measured the study subjects' abilities to retain information over several minutes for doing mental arithmetic or dialing a phone number. Significant increases in regional perfusion across the brain were observed following consumption of the high-flavanol drink relative to the low-flavanol drink, particularly in the anterior cingulate cortex and the central opercular cortex of the parietal lobe. Other randomized placebo-controlled trials indicate that daily consumption of flavanol-rich cocoa drinks over 8 weeks is associated with improved cognitive function in healthy older adults (Mastroiacovo et al. 2015) and in older adults with MCI (Desideri et al. 2012).

Green tea contains a family of antioxidant phytochemicals known as catechins, including epigallocatechin gallate (EGCG). These antioxidant substances have both antiamyloid and anti-inflammatory properties and are bioavailable (Kim et al. 2010).

Used for centuries as a treatment for inflammatory diseases, curcumin (diferuloylmethane) is a yellow pigment in the spice turmeric. Considerable research has demonstrated that curcumin mediates its anti-inflammatory effects through the downregulation of inflammatory transcription factors, enzymes, and cytokines (Aggarwal and Sung 2009). A study including more than 1000 volunteers aged 60–93 years (Ringman et al. 2005) showed that volunteers who ate curried foods more frequently had higher scores on the Mini-Mental State Examination. Although evidence suggests that the antiamyloid and anti-inflammatory effects of curcumin might protect brain health and improve cognitive functioning, a previous study in patients with Alzheimer's dementia did not show cognitive benefits (Eskelinen and Kivipelto 2010).

It is still possible that the potential anti-inflammatory and antiamyloid effects of curcumin may only be observed in people at risk for dementia. The mechanism of action for curcumin is not clear, and evidence thus far has not confirmed that it is brain protective when taken as a supplement, since the oils used to cook curried dishes may be necessary for it to benefit neuronal health. Moreover, it may not be necessary for curcumin to penetrate the blood–brain barrier for it to exert anti-inflammatory effects, which may be triggered by interactions with immune cells in the gastrointestinal tract.

Our research team at UCLA recently initiated a study of curcumin versus placebo in nondemented older adults. Both neuropsychological tests and PET scans of amyloid plaques and tau tangles will be used as outcome measures. Curcumin is one of many spices and herbs that are antioxidant and have potential to promote brain health. Others are cinnamon, oregano, vanilla, parsley, ginger, basil, pepper, and chili.

16.6.4 Coffee, Caffeine, and the Brain

Several epidemiological studies have demonstrated an association between drinking coffee and better brain health. For example, a large-scale Swedish investigation showed that drinking up to three cups of coffee a day was associated with a 65% lower risk for AD (Chen et al. 2010). Coffee consumption is also associated with a lower rate of developing Parkinson's disease and diabetes, both of which increase the risk for dementia (Ng et al. 2006).

Coffee and other caffeinated beverages also have short-term effects on the mental state. Positive effects include an increase in alertness and attention, as well as an elevated mood. Drinking coffee can improve learning and recall; however, excessive caffeine consumption may result in irritability, anxiety, and insomnia. Some people cannot tolerate the acidity of coffee, so they prefer to get caffeine by drinking tea. Chocolate is another source of caffeine: 6 ounces of brewed coffee contains 100 mg of caffeine, compared with 40 mg from a similar amount of tea, and 10 mg from a chocolate bar.

16.6.5 Alcohol and the Brain

Clearly, alcoholism, with its distortion of nutrient and B vitamin intake, is both a major health problem worldwide and a cause of dementia. However, alcohol use in moderation is associated with a lower risk for dementia. A recent study demonstrated that light drinkers had almost a 30% lower risk for developing dementia than did people who either abstain from alcohol or drink in excess (Anstey et al. 2009). Because this study was not a double-blind, placebo-controlled trial, it does not definitely prove a cause-and-effect relationship. It is possible that drinking in moderation is also associated with some other factor that protects brain health and lowers risk for dementia. For example, moderate drinkers may deal with other aspects of their lives in moderation, which could reflect a personality style associated with lower stress levels.

Precisely what defines light or moderate alcohol use varies among studies, but many experts agree that one glass of wine or spirits for women and two glasses for men per day is a reasonable definition. The male–female differences likely reflect the body weight and size differences between men and women. Red wine compounds, including resveratrol, have been touted for their brain health effects (Liu et al. 2015). While there are many studies *in vitro* and in animals, resveratrol has poor bioavailability. A growing body of evidence indicates that resveratrol plays an important role in reducing organ damage following ischemia- and hemorrhage-induced reperfusion injury. Such a protective phenomenon is reported to be implicated in decreasing the formation and reaction of reactive oxygen species and pro-inflammatory cytokines, as well as the mediation of a variety of intracellular signaling pathways, including the nitric oxide synthase, nicotinamide adenine dinucleotide phosphate oxidase, deacetylase sirtuin 1, mitogen-activated protein kinase, peroxisome proliferator-activated receptor λ coactivator 1 α, hemeoxygenase-1, and estrogen receptor-related pathways. If bioavailability issues can be solved, this polyphenol may have some potential benefit for brain health in the future.

16.6.6 Dietary Supplements and the Brain

An antioxidant vitamin and mineral supplementation regimen was studied in a double-blind, placebo-controlled, randomized trial. A total of 4447 French participants aged 45–60 years were randomized to receive a combination of vitamin C (120 mg), β-carotene (6 mg), vitamin E (30 mg), selenium (100 μg), and zinc (20 mg), or a placebo. Subjects receiving the active antioxidant supplementation had better episodic memory scores. Verbal memory also improved by antioxidant supplementation only in subjects who were nonsmokers or who had low serum vitamin C concentrations at baseline (Kesse-Guyot et al. 2011).

Epidemiological studies have connected dietary vitamin D to brain health and better cognitive abilities. These investigations have led to randomized clinical trials demonstrating cognitive benefits, but these effects may be limited to older adults. For example, a 6-week controlled trial of daily vitamin D (5000 IU of cholecalciferol) or placebo included 128 young adult participants (mean age 22 years) and showed no cognitive benefits (Dean et al. 2011).

A cross-sectional study of nutrient status and psychometric and imaging indices of brain health was performed in 104 dementia-free older adults, with an average age of 87 years (Bowman et al. 2012). The investigators reported two nutrient biomarker patterns to be associated with better cognitive performance and MRI measures: one high in plasma vitamins B (B1, B2, B6, folate, and B12), C, D, and E, and the other high in plasma marine omega-3 fatty acids. A third pattern that was high in hydrogenated fats was associated with less favorable cognitive function and less total brain volume.

16.7 DIABETES, VISCERAL FAT, INFLAMMATION, AND ALZHEIMER'S DISEASE

Diabetes mellitus type 2, or "diabesity," is the most common metabolic disorder worldwide, and its prevalence is increasing dramatically. It is estimated that 387 million people live with diabetes, of which nearly 50% are unaware they have the disease, mostly due to the fact that diabetes can remain asymptomatic or be misdiagnosed for several years. The underlying determinants of diabetes are the same all over the world. Economic development is associated with increasingly "obesogenic environments," characterized by increasing access to energy-rich diets and decreased physical activity.

Diabetes causes micro- and macrovascular diseases (American Diabetes Association 2013). In addition, increasing evidence has also demonstrated that type 2 diabetes results in complications in the CNS, with many brain structures being sensitive to changes in glucose and insulin. Diabetes-associated cognitive decline (also known as diabetic encephalopathy) results from a complex interplay between direct and indirect metabolic consequences of long-term hyperglycemia, insulin deficiency, and additional components, such as genetic and environmental factors (Stranahan 2015). Diabetes-associated cognitive decline has been linked to learning and memory deficits, which in turn increase the risk for dementia, AD, and affective disorders (Biessels et al. 1994; Yates et al. 2012). In this context, recent studies have shown that elevated body mass index, obesity, and insulin resistance are correlated with increased risk of dementia and cognitive impairment (Raji et al. 2010; Grillo et al. 2011). The mechanisms by which cognitive abilities are impaired in diabetes have not been clearly identified. Nevertheless, it has been shown that altered neurogenesis, electrophysiological deficits, and oxidative stress injury, inflammation, and apoptosis can induce structural changes and be involved in brain dysfunction during the course of diabetes (Wrighten et al. 2009; Stranahan 2015).

16.8 PRIMARY CARE PHYSICIAN AND CASE MANAGER COLLABORATION IN DEMENTIA PATIENTS

People with dementia need help with challenging changes in behavior, memory, physical disability, and mood (van der Roest et al. 2007). All the nutritional knowledge in this chapter is useless if there is no way to deliver the physical and nutritional care needed to the patient.

The main source of help is family caregivers, who often suffer from the burdens of caregiving and from depression and health problems themselves (Dupuis et al. 2004). Therefore, the entire family or key caregivers become your patients as well in cases of dementia, and they may require psychological support.

It has been shown that early intervention makes the greatest difference in management of symptoms. The World Health Organization states that it would be challenging to intervene without effective involvement of primary care (World Health Organization and Alzheimer's Disease International 2012). Dementia case management interventions are becoming a central component of primary health care organizations in North America and Europe (Morales-Asencio et al. 2008; Bergman 2009; Bamford et al. 2014; Iliffe et al. 2014).

According to the Case Management Society of America, *case management* is "a collaborative process of assessment, planning, facilitation, care coordination, evaluation, and advocacy for options and services to meet an individual's and family's comprehensive health needs through communication and available resources" (Case Management Society of America 2016).

Case managers are health care professionals who provide follow-up, coordinate individual care, and interact with other health care providers. They also work in collaboration with family physicians, primary care teams, and dementia specialists (Laurant et al. 2004; Callahan et al. 2006; Stevenson and Herschell 2006; Vickrey et al. 2006; Jedenius et al. 2008, 2011; Schoenmakers et al. 2010; Jansen et al. 2011; Fortinsky et al. 2014). It is clear that dietitians knowledgeable in nutrition support, as well as neurological limitations to nutritional intake, will be critical in this effort, bringing their knowledge to bear in terms of the nutrition and supplements that patients and family members obtain so that no harm is done as every effort is made to implement ideas drawn from cutting-edge research on nutrition and brain health.

16.9 SUMMARY

The proportion of people with dementia is growing dramatically. According to the U.S. Alzheimer's Association, by 2030, 50% of Americans aged 65 years and older will be diagnosed with dementia (Alzheimer's Association 2014). In Canada in 2011, 747,000 Canadians lived with cognitive impairment (Alzheimer Society of Canada 2015). Today, the combined costs are $33 billion per year (Alzheimer's Association 2014), and they are projected to increase to $872 billion by 2038 (Dudgeon 2010; Prince et al. 2015). Worldwide, dementia is the main contributor to disability-adjusted life years (11.2%), representing a greater burden than cerebral vascular accident (9.5%), heart disease (5.0%), or cancer (2.4%) (Mathers and Leonardi 2000).

The interaction between nutrition and brain health is complex. Several gastrointestinal hormones or peptides, such as leptin and glucagon-like peptide 1 (GLP-1), have an influence on emotions and cognitive processes (Li et al. 2002; Komori et al. 2006). Leptin is synthesized in adipose tissue and sends signals to the brain to reduce appetite (receptors in the hypothalamus, cortex, and hippocampus). Leptin also elevates brain BDNF, a protein that stimulates brain cell growth and synaptic connections, leading to a more efficient, sensitive, and adaptive brain. Both leptin and BDNF facilitate synaptic plasticity in the hippocampus. Genetically obese rodents with dysfunctional leptin receptors show impaired spatial learning (Li et al. 2002; Komori et al. 2006).

Pro-inflammatory cytokines present in the adipose tissue of central obesity trigger excess inflammation throughout the body, and a low-calorie diet can alter the expression of inflammatory genes in this adipose tissue. A healthy brain diet includes many foods that fight inflammation, including fruits, vegetables, fish, whole grains, legumes, spices, and herbs. Flavonoids, present in cocoa, citrus fruits, and green leafy vegetables, also have anti-inflammatory effects and have been found to benefit cognition in older subjects and laboratory animals (Gomez-Pinilla 2008).

A diet that emphasizes antioxidant fruits and vegetables; proteins from fish, poultry, or lean beef; and complex carbohydrates and whole grains, as well as avoids processed foods and high-glycemic-index carbohydrates, maintains ideal body weight, and includes omega-3 fatty acids, is likely to support brain health and lower the risk for age-related cognitive decline and mood disturbances throughout life. Scientists are continuing to tease out the specific components of brain healthy nutrition in order to develop more evidence-based recommendations for consumers.

REFERENCES

Aggarwal, B. B., and B. Sung. 2009. Pharmacological basis for the role of curcumin in chronic diseases: An age-old spice with modern targets. *Trends Pharmacol Sci* 30 (2):85–94.

Akiyama, H., S. Barger, S. Barnum, B. Bradt, J. Bauer, G. M. Cole, N. R. Cooper et al. 2000. Inflammation and Alzheimer's disease. *Neurobiol Aging* 21 (3):383–421.

Alzheimer's Association. 2014. Alzheimer's disease facts and figures. Chicago: Alzheimer's Association.

Alzheimer Society of Canada. 2015. http://www.alzheimer.ca (accessed September 7, 2015).

American Diabetes Association. 2013. Diagnosis and classification of diabetes mellitus. *Diabetes Care* 36 (Suppl 1):S67–S74.

American Psychiatric Association. 2013. *Diagnostic and Statistical Manual of Mental Disorders*. 5th ed. Arlington, VA: American Psychiatric Association.

Anstey, K. J., H. A. Mack, and N. Cherbuin. 2009. Alcohol consumption as a risk factor for dementia and cognitive decline: Meta-analysis of prospective studies. *Am J Geriatr Psychiatry* 17 (7):542–555.

Ballard, C., S. Gauthier, A. Corbett, C. Brayne, D. Aarsland, and E. Jones. 2011. Alzheimer's disease. *Lancet* 377 (9770):1019–1031.

Bamford, C., M. Poole, K. Brittain, C. Chew-Graham, C. Fox, S. Iliffe, J. Manthorpe, L. Robinson, and CAREDEM team. 2014. Understanding the challenges to implementing case management for people with dementia in primary care in England: A qualitative study using normalization process theory. *BMC Health Serv Res* 14:549.

Barberger-Gateau, P., C. Raffaitin, L. Letenneur, C. Berr, C. Tzourio, J. F. Dartigues, and A. Alperovitch. 2007. Dietary patterns and risk of dementia: The three-city cohort study. *Neurology* 69 (20):1921–1930.

Bergman, H. 2009. Report of the Committee of Experts for the Development of an Action Plan on Alzheimer's Disease and Related Disorders. Montreal: Alzheimer Society of Montreal.

Biessels, G. J., A. C. Kappelle, B. Bravenboer, D. W. Erkelens, and W. H. Gispen. 1994. Cerebral function in diabetes mellitus. *Diabetologia* 37 (7):643–650.

Bookheimer, S. Y., B. A. Renner, A. Ekstrom, Z. Li, S. M. Henning, J. A. Brown, M. Jones, T. Moody, and G. W. Small. 2013. Pomegranate juice augments memory and FMRI activity in middle-aged and older adults with mild memory complaints. *Evid Based Complement Alternat Med* 2013:946298.

Bowman, G. L., L. C. Silbert, D. Howieson, H. H. Dodge, M. G. Traber, B. Frei, J. A. Kaye, J. Shannon, and J. F. Quinn. 2012. Nutrient biomarker patterns, cognitive function, and MRI measures of brain aging. *Neurology* 78 (4):241–249.

Braak, H., and E. Braak. 1991. Neuropathological stageing of Alzheimer-related changes. *Acta Neuropathol* 82 (4):239–259.

Brew, B. J., and P. Chan. 2014. Update on HIV dementia and HIV-associated neurocognitive disorders. *Curr Neurol Neurosci Rep* 14 (8):468.

Burckhardt, M., M. Herke, T. Wustmann, S. Watzke, G. Langer, and A. Fink. 2016. Omega-3 fatty acids for the treatment of dementia. *Cochrane Database Syst Rev* 4:CD009002.

Burggren, A. C., B. Renner, M. Jones, M. Donix, N. A. Suthana, L. Martin-Harris, L. M. Ercoli, K. J. Miller, P. Siddarth, G. W. Small, and S. Y. Bookheimer. 2011. Thickness in entorhinal and subicular cortex predicts episodic memory decline in mild cognitive impairment. *Int J Alzheimers Dis* 2011:956053.

Callahan, C. M., M. A. Boustani, F. W. Unverzagt, M. G. Austrom, T. M. Damush, A. J. Perkins, B. A. Fultz, S. L. Hui, S. R. Counsell, and H. C. Hendrie. 2006. Effectiveness of collaborative care for older adults with Alzheimer disease in primary care: A randomized controlled trial. *JAMA* 295 (18):2148–2157.

Case Management Society of America. 2016. What is a case manager? http://www.cmsa.org/Home/CMSA/WhatisaCaseManager/tabid/224/Default.aspx.

Cassilhas, R. C., V. A. Viana, V. Grassmann, R. T. Santos, R. F. Santos, S. Tufik, and M. T. Mello. 2007. The impact of resistance exercise on the cognitive function of the elderly. *Med Sci Sports Exerc* 39 (8):1401–1407.

Chen, X., O. Ghribi, and J. D. Geiger. 2010. Caffeine protects against disruptions of the blood-brain barrier in animal models of Alzheimer's and Parkinson's diseases. *J Alzheimers Dis* 20 (Suppl 1):S127–S141.

Claus, J. J., S. S. Staekenborg, J. J. Roorda, M. Stevens, D. Herderschee, W. van Maarschalkerweerd, L. Schuurmans, C. E. Tielkes, P. Koster, C. Bavinck, and P. Scheltens. 2015. Low prevalence of mixed dementia in a cohort of 2,000 elderly patients in a memory clinic setting. *J Alzheimers Dis* 50 (3):797–806.

Cole, G. M., Q. L. Ma, and S. A. Frautschy. 2009. Omega-3 fatty acids and dementia. *Prostaglandins Leukot Essent Fatty Acids* 81 (2–3):213–221.

Dai, Q., A. R. Borenstein, Y. Wu, J. C. Jackson, and E. B. Larson. 2006. Fruit and vegetable juices and Alzheimer's disease: The Kame Project. *Am J Med* 119 (9):751–759.

Danthiir, V., N. R. Burns, T. Nettelbeck, C. Wilson, and G. Wittert. 2011. The older people, omega-3, and cognitive health (EPOCH) trial design and methodology: A randomised, double-blind, controlled trial investigating the effect of long-chain omega-3 fatty acids on cognitive ageing and wellbeing in cognitively healthy older adults. *Nutr J* 10:117.

Dean, A. J., M. A. Bellgrove, T. Hall, W. M. Phan, D. W. Eyles, D. Kvaskoff, and J. J. McGrath. 2011. Effects of vitamin D supplementation on cognitive and emotional functioning in young adults—A randomised controlled trial. *PLoS One* 6 (11):e25966.

Desideri, G., C. Kwik-Uribe, D. Grassi, S. Necozione, L. Ghiadoni, D. Mastroiacovo, A. Raffaele et al. 2012. Benefits in cognitive function, blood pressure, and insulin resistance through cocoa flavanol consumption in elderly subjects with mild cognitive impairment: The Cocoa, Cognition, and Aging (CoCoA) study. *Hypertension* 60 (3):794–801.

Devore, E. E., F. Grodstein, F. J. van Rooij, A. Hofman, M. J. Stampfer, J. C. Witteman, and M. M. Breteler. 2010. Dietary antioxidants and long-term risk of dementia. *Arch Neurol* 67 (7):819–825.

Dudgeon, S. 2010. Rising tide: The impact of dementia on Canadian Society. Toronto: Alzheimer Society of Canada.

Dupuis, S., T. Epp, and B. Smale. 2004. A literature review. Caregivers of persons with dementia: Roles, experiences, supports, and coping. University of Waterloo. https://uwaterloo.ca/murray-alzheimer-research-and-education-program/sites/ca.murray-alzheimer-research-and-education-program/files/uploads/files/InTheirOwnVoices-LiteratureReview.pdf.

Erickson, K. I., M. W. Voss, R. S. Prakash, C. Basak, A. Szabo, L. Chaddock, J. S. Kim et al. 2011. Exercise training increases size of hippocampus and improves memory. *Proc Natl Acad Sci USA* 108 (7):3017–3022.

Eskelinen, M. H., and M. Kivipelto. 2010. Caffeine as a protective factor in dementia and Alzheimer's disease. *J Alzheimers Dis* 20 (Suppl 1):S167–S174.

Ferri, C. P., M. Prince, C. Brayne, H. Brodaty, L. Fratiglioni, M. Ganguli, K. Hall et al. 2005. Global prevalence of dementia: A Delphi Consensus Study. *Lancet* 366 (9503):2112–2117.

Fortinsky, R. H., C. Delaney, O. Harel, K. Pasquale, E. Schjavland, J. Lynch, A. Kleppinger, and S. Crumb. 2014. Results and lessons learned from a nurse practitioner-guided dementia care intervention for primary care patients and their family caregivers. *Res Gerontol Nurs* 7 (3):126–137.

Galimberti, D., B. Dell'Osso, A. C. Altamura, and E. Scarpini. 2015. Psychiatric symptoms in frontotemporal dementia: Epidemiology, phenotypes, and differential diagnosis. *Biol Psychiatry* 78 (10):684–692.

Goekint, M. 2011. Exercise and brain-derived neurotrophic factor. Vrije Universiteit Brussel, Brussels.

Goekint, M., K. De Pauw, B. Roelands, R. Njemini, I. Bautmans, T. Mets, and R. Meeusen. 2010a. Strength training does not influence serum brain-derived neurotrophic factor. *Eur J Appl Physiol* 110 (2):285–293.

Goekint, M., E. Heyman, B. Roelands, R. Njemini, I. Bautmans, T. Mets, and R. Meeusen. 2008. No influence of noradrenaline manipulation on acute exercise-induced increase of brain-derived neurotrophic factor. *Med Sci Sports Exerc* 40 (11):1990–1996.

Goekint, M., B. Roelands, K. De Pauw, K. Knaepen, I. Bos, and R. Meeusen. 2010b. Does a period of detraining cause a decrease in serum brain-derived neurotrophic factor? *Neurosci Lett* 486 (3):146–149.

Goekint, M., B. Roelands, E. Heyman, R. Njemini, and R. Meeusen. 2011. Influence of citalopram and environmental temperature on exercise-induced changes in BDNF. *Neurosci Lett* 494 (2):150–154.

Gold, S. M., K. H. Schulz, S. Hartmann, M. Mladek, U. E. Lang, R. Hellweg, R. Reer, K. M. Braumann, and C. Heesen. 2003. Basal serum levels and reactivity of nerve growth factor and brain-derived neurotrophic factor to standardized acute exercise in multiple sclerosis and controls. *J Neuroimmunol* 138 (1–2):99–105.

Gomez-Pinilla, F. 2008. Brain foods: The effects of nutrients on brain function. *Nat Rev Neurosci* 9 (7):568–578.

Goyarzu, P., D. H. Malin, F. C. Lau, G. Taglialatela, W. D. Moon, R. Jennings, E. Moy, D. Moy, S. Lippold, B. Shukitt-Hale, and J. A. Joseph. 2004. Blueberry supplemented diet: Effects on object recognition memory and nuclear factor-kappa B levels in aged rats. *Nutr Neurosci* 7 (2):75–83.

Grillo, C. A., G. G. Piroli, L. Junor, S. P. Wilson, D. D. Mott, M. A. Wilson, and L. P. Reagan. 2011. Obesity/hyperleptinemic phenotype impairs structural and functional plasticity in the rat hippocampus. *Physiol Behav* 105 (1):138–144.

Gu, Y., J. W. Nieves, Y. Stern, J. A. Luchsinger, and N. Scarmeas. 2010. Food combination and Alzheimer disease risk: A protective diet. *Arch Neurol* 67 (6):699–706.

Holmes, C., C. Ballard, D. Lehmann, A. David Smith, H. Beaumont, I. N. Day, M. Nadeem et al. 2005. Rate of progression of cognitive decline in Alzheimer's disease: Effect of butyrylcholinesterase K gene variation. *J Neurol Neurosurg Psychiatry* 76 (5):640–643.

Horton, R. 2012. GBD 2010: Understanding disease, injury, and risk. *Lancet* 380 (9859):2053–2054.

Iliffe, S., L. Robinson, C. Bamford, A. Waugh, C. Fox, G. Livingston, J. Manthorpe et al. 2014. Introducing case management for people with dementia in primary care: A mixed-methods study. *Br J Gen Pract* 64 (628):e735–e741.

Ilomaki, J., N. Jokanovic, E. C. Tan, and E. Lonnroos. 2015. Alcohol consumption, dementia and cognitive decline: An overview of systematic reviews. *Curr Clin Pharmacol* 10 (3):204–212.

Jansen, A. P., H. P. van Hout, G. Nijpels, F. Rijmen, R. M. Droes, A. M. Pot, F. G. Schellevis, W. A. Stalman, and H. W. van Marwijk. 2011. Effectiveness of case management among older adults with early symptoms of dementia and their primary informal caregivers: A randomized clinical trial. *Int J Nurs Stud* 48 (8):933–943.

Jedenius, E., K. Johnell, J. Fastbom, J. Stromqvist, B. Winblad, and N. Andreasen. 2011. Dementia management programme in a community setting and the use of psychotropic drugs in the elderly population. *Scand J Prim Health Care* 29 (3):181–186.

Jedenius, E., A. Wimo, J. Stromqvist, and N. Andreasen. 2008. A Swedish programme for dementia diagnostics in primary healthcare. *Scand J Prim Health Care* 26 (4):235–240.

Kalaria, R. N., G. E. Maestre, R. Arizaga, R. P. Friedland, D. Galasko, K. Hall, J. A. Luchsinger et al. 2008. Alzheimer's disease and vascular dementia in developing countries: Prevalence, management, and risk factors. *Lancet Neurol* 7 (9):812–826.

Kepe, V., J. R. Barrio, S. C. Huang, L. Ercoli, P. Siddarth, K. Shoghi-Jadid, G. M. Cole, N. Satyamurthy, J. L. Cummings, G. W. Small, and M. E. Phelps. 2006. Serotonin 1A receptors in the living brain of Alzheimer's disease patients. *Proc Natl Acad Sci USA* 103 (3):702–707.

Kesse-Guyot, E., L. Fezeu, C. Jeandel, M. Ferry, V. Andreeva, H. Amieva, S. Hercberg, and P. Galan. 2011. French adults' cognitive performance after daily supplementation with antioxidant vitamins and minerals at nutritional doses: A post hoc analysis of the Supplementation in Vitamins and Mineral Antioxidants (SU.VI.MAX) trial. *Am J Clin Nutr* 94 (3):892–899.

Kim, J., H. J. Lee, and K. W. Lee. 2010. Naturally occurring phytochemicals for the prevention of Alzheimer's disease. *J Neurochem* 112 (6):1415–1430.

Knaepen, K., M. Goekint, E. M. Heyman, and R. Meeusen. 2010. Neuroplasticity—Exercise-induced response of peripheral brain-derived neurotrophic factor: A systematic review of experimental studies in human subjects. *Sports Med* 40 (9):765–801.

Komori, T., Y. Morikawa, K. Nanjo, and E. Senba. 2006. Induction of brain-derived neurotrophic factor by leptin in the ventromedial hypothalamus. *Neuroscience* 139 (3):1107–1115.

Kosashvili, Y., O. Safir, A. Gross, G. Morag, D. Lakstein, and D. Backstein. 2010. Distal femoral varus osteotomy for lateral osteoarthritis of the knee: A minimum ten-year follow-up. *Int Orthop* 34 (2):249–254.

Lamport, D. J., D. Pal, C. Moutsiana, D. T. Field, C. M. Williams, J. P. Spencer, and L. T. Butler. 2015. The effect of flavanol-rich cocoa on cerebral perfusion in healthy older adults during conscious resting state: A placebo controlled, crossover, acute trial. *Psychopharmacology (Berl)* 232 (17):3227–3234.

Laurant, M. G., R. P. Hermens, J. C. Braspenning, B. Sibbald, and R. P. Grol. 2004. Impact of nurse practitioners on workload of general practitioners: Randomised controlled trial. *BMJ* 328 (7445):927.

Lee, E. B. 2011. Obesity, leptin, and Alzheimer's disease. *Ann NY Acad Sci* 1243:15–29.

Lee, Y., J. H. Back, J. Kim, S. H. Kim, D. L. Na, H. K. Cheong, C. H. Hong, and Y. G. Kim. 2010. Systematic review of health behavioral risks and cognitive health in older adults. *Int Psychogeriatr* 22 (2):174–187.

Lesperance, F., N. Frasure-Smith, E. St.-Andre, G. Turecki, P. Lesperance, and S. R. Wisniewski. 2011. The efficacy of omega-3 supplementation for major depression: A randomized controlled trial. *J Clin Psychiatry* 72 (8):1054–1062.

Li, X. L., S. Aou, Y. Oomura, N. Hori, K. Fukunaga, and T. Hori. 2002. Impairment of long-term potentiation and spatial memory in leptin receptor-deficient rodents. *Neuroscience* 113 (3):607–615.

Liu, C. C., T. Kanekiyo, H. Xu, and G. Bu. 2013. Apolipoprotein E and Alzheimer disease: Risk, mechanisms and therapy. *Nat Rev Neurol* 9 (2):106–118.

Liu, F. C., H. I. Tsai, and H. P. Yu. 2015. Organ-protective effects of red wine extract, resveratrol, in oxidative stress-mediated reperfusion injury. *Oxid Med Cell Longev* 2015:568634.

Mastroiacovo, D., C. Kwik-Uribe, D. Grassi, S. Necozione, A. Raffaele, L. Pistacchio, R. Righetti et al. 2015. Cocoa flavanol consumption improves cognitive function, blood pressure control, and metabolic profile in elderly subjects: The Cocoa, Cognition, and Aging (CoCoA) Study—A randomized controlled trial. *Am J Clin Nutr* 101 (3):538–548.

Mathers, C., and M. Leonardi. 2000. Global burden of dementia in the year 2000: Summary of methods and data sources. Geneva: World Health Organization.

Merrill, D. A., P. Siddarth, N. Y. Saito, L. M. Ercoli, A. C. Burggren, V. Kepe, H. Lavretsky, K. J. Miller, J. Kim, S. C. Huang, S. Y. Bookheimer, J. R. Barrio, and G. W. Small. 2012. Self-reported memory impairment and brain PET of amyloid and tau in middle-aged and older adults without dementia. *Int Psychogeriatr* 24 (7):1076–1084.

Merrill, D. A., and G. W. Small. 2011. Prevention in psychiatry: Effects of healthy lifestyle on cognition. *Psychiatr Clin North Am* 34 (1):249–261.

Miller, K. J., P. Siddarth, J. M. Gaines, J. M. Parrish, L. M. Ercoli, K. Marx, J. Ronch et al. 2012. The memory fitness program: Cognitive effects of a healthy aging intervention. *Am J Geriatr Psychiatry* 20 (6):514–523.

Morales-Asencio, J. M., E. Gonzalo-Jimenez, F. J. Martin-Santos, J. C. Morilla-Herrera, M. Celdraan-Manas, A. M. Carrasco, J. J. Garcia-Arrabal, and I. Toral-Lopez. 2008. Effectiveness of a nurse-led case management home care model in primary health care. A quasi-experimental, controlled, multi-centre study. *BMC Health Serv Res* 8:193.

Morra, L. F., and P. J. Donovick. 2014. Clinical presentation and differential diagnosis of dementia with Lewy bodies: A review. *Int J Geriatr Psychiatry* 29 (6):569–576.

Ng, T. P., P. C. Chiam, T. Lee, H. C. Chua, L. Lim, and E. H. Kua. 2006. Curry consumption and cognitive function in the elderly. *Am J Epidemiol* 164 (9):898–906.

O'Brien, J. T., and A. Thomas. 2015. Vascular dementia. *Lancet* 386 (10004):1698–1706.

Ogunniyi, A., O. Baiyewu, O. Gureje, K. S. Hall, F. Unverzagt, S. H. Siu, S. Gao et al. 2000. Epidemiology of dementia in Nigeria: Results from the Indianapolis-Ibadan study. *Eur J Neurol* 7 (5):485–490.

Petersen, R. C., H. J. Wiste, S. D. Weigand, W. A. Rocca, R. O. Roberts, M. M. Mielke, V. J. Lowe et al. 2016. Association of elevated amyloid levels with cognition and biomarkers in cognitively normal people from the community. *JAMA Neurol* 73 (1):85–92.

Prince, M., R. Bryce, E. Albanese, A. Wimo, W. Ribeiro, and C. P. Ferri. 2013. The global prevalence of dementia: A systematic review and metaanalysis. *Alzheimers Dement* 9 (1):63–75.e2.

Prince, M., A. Wimo, M. Guerchet, G.-C. Ali, Y.-T. Wu, and M. Prina. 2015. A world Alzheimer report 2015. The global impact of dementia. An analysis of prevalence, incidence, cost and trends. London: Alzheimer's Disease International.

Quinn, J. F., R. Raman, R. G. Thomas, K. Yurko-Mauro, E. B. Nelson, C. Van Dyck, J. E. Galvin et al. 2010. Docosahexaenoic acid supplementation and cognitive decline in Alzheimer disease: A randomized trial. *JAMA* 304 (17):1903–1911.

Raji, C. A., A. J. Ho, N. N. Parikshak, J. T. Becker, O. L. Lopez, L. H. Kuller, X. Hua, A. D. Leow, A. W. Toga, and P. M. Thompson. 2010. Brain structure and obesity. *Hum Brain Mapp* 31 (3):353–364.

Ringman, J. M., S. A. Frautschy, G. M. Cole, D. L. Masterman, and J. L. Cummings. 2005. A potential role of the curry spice curcumin in Alzheimer's disease. *Curr Alzheimer Res* 2 (2):131–136.

Rizzi, L., I. Rosset, and M. Roriz-Cruz. 2014. Global epidemiology of dementia: Alzheimer's and vascular types. *Biomed Res Int* 2014:908915.

Rolland, Y., G. Abellan van Kan, and B. Vellas. 2010. Healthy brain aging: Role of exercise and physical activity. *Clin Geriatr Med* 26 (1):75–87.

Romano, A. D., G. Serviddio, A. de Matthaeis, F. Bellanti, and G. Vendemiale. 2010. Oxidative stress and aging. *J Nephrol* 23 (Suppl 15):S29–S36.

Schoenmakers, B., F. Buntinx, and J. Delepeleire. 2010. Supporting family carers of community-dwelling elder with cognitive decline: A randomized controlled trial. *Int J Family Med* 2010:184152.

Singh-Manoux, A., M. Kivimaki, M. M. Glymour, A. Elbaz, C. Berr, K. P. Ebmeier, J. E. Ferrie, and A. Dugravot. 2012. Timing of onset of cognitive decline: Results from Whitehall II prospective cohort study. *BMJ* 344:d7622.

Small, G. W., L. M. Ercoli, D. H. Silverman, S. C. Huang, S. Komo, S. Y. Bookheimer, H. Lavretsky et al. 2000. Cerebral metabolic and cognitive decline in persons at genetic risk for Alzheimer's disease. *Proc Natl Acad Sci USA* 97 (11):6037–6042.

Small, G. W., D. H. Silverman, P. Siddarth, L. M. Ercoli, K. J. Miller, H. Lavretsky, B. C. Wright, S. Y. Bookheimer, J. R. Barrio, and M. E. Phelps. 2006. Effects of a 14-day healthy longevity lifestyle program on cognition and brain function. *Am J Geriatr Psychiatry* 14 (6):538–545.

Snitz, B. E., L. A. Weissfeld, A. D. Cohen, O. L. Lopez, R. D. Nebes, H. J. Aizenstein, E. McDade, J. C. Price, C. A. Mathis, and W. E. Klunk. 2015. Subjective cognitive complaints, personality and brain amyloid-beta in cognitively normal older adults. *Am J Geriatr Psychiatry* 23 (9):985–993.

Sobreira, S., I. A. Mota, J. E. Gomes da Cunha, R. Mello, and J. R. Oliveira. 2013. How heterogeneous can the clinical presentation for Creutzfeldt-Jacob disease be? *J Neuropsychiatry Clin Neurosci* 25 (4):E44–E45.

Sofi, F., C. Macchi, R. Abbate, G. F. Gensini, and A. Casini. 2010. Effectiveness of the Mediterranean diet: Can it help delay or prevent Alzheimer's disease? *J Alzheimers Dis* 20 (3):795–801.

Stevenson, G., and J. D. K. Herschell. 2006. An enhanced assessment and support team (EAST) for dementing elders—Review of a Scottish regional initiative. *J Ment Health* 15(2):251–258.

Stranahan, A. M. 2015. Models and mechanisms for hippocampal dysfunction in obesity and diabetes. *Neuroscience* 309:125–139.

van de Rest, O., J. M. Geleijnse, F. J. Kok, W. A. van Staveren, C. Dullemeijer, M. G. Olderikkert, A. T. Beekman, and C. P. de Groot. 2008. Effect of fish oil on cognitive performance in older subjects: A randomized, controlled trial. *Neurology* 71 (6):430–438.

van der Roest, H. G., F. J. Meiland, R. Maroccini, H. C. Comijs, C. Jonker, and R. M. Droes. 2007. Subjective needs of people with dementia: A review of the literature. *Int Psychogeriatr* 19 (3):559–592.

Vickrey, B. G., B. S. Mittman, K. I. Connor, M. L. Pearson, R. D. Della Penna, T. G. Ganiats, R. W. Demonte Jr. et al. 2006. The effect of a disease management intervention on quality and outcomes of dementia care: A randomized, controlled trial. *Ann Intern Med* 145 (10):713–726.

Wansink, B., and L. R. Linder. 2003. Interactions between forms of fat consumption and restaurant bread consumption. *Int J Obes Relat Metab Disord* 27 (7):866–868.

Wells, G. A., and J. W. Wilesmith. 1995. The neuropathology and epidemiology of bovine spongiform encephalopathy. *Brain Pathol* 5 (1):91–103.

World Health Organization and Alzheimer's Disease International. 2012. Dementia: A public health priority. Geneva: World Health Organization.

Wrighten, S. A., G. G. Piroli, C. A. Grillo, and L. P. Reagan. 2009. A look inside the diabetic brain: Contributors to diabetes-induced brain aging. *Biochim Biophys Acta* 1792 (5):444–453.

Yates, K. F., V. Sweat, P. L. Yau, M. M. Turchiano, and A. Convit. 2012. Impact of metabolic syndrome on cognition and brain: A selected review of the literature. *Arterioscler Thromb Vasc Biol* 32 (9):2060–2067.

17 Gene–Nutrient Interaction

17.1 INTRODUCTION

The interaction of nutrition with the human genome and the microbiome has attracted a great deal of attention in the last decade. The sequencing of the human genome was followed by the discovery that our bodies are covered with trillions of bacteria, and their genome outnumbers our own. Our understanding of the functioning of the genome has advanced far beyond the idea of a basic code for amino acids to an understanding of gene–gene, gene–nutrient, microRNA (miRNA), and epigenetic regulation of gene expression, with many of these processes influenced by nutrition. It is clear that gene sequencing is useful for the diagnosis of genetic diseases, but it is not ready for application in providing point-of-service personalization in diets to reduce age-related chronic diseases, as imagined by some commercial promoters who offered analysis of common genetic polymorphisms based on a sputum sample, followed by dietary recommendations. However, it is clear that what we already know about gene–nutrient interaction underscores the importance of an integrated approach to diet and lifestyle change in primary care practice.

Gene–nutrient interactions serve to moderate the certainty with which we provide some nutritional recommendations. We cannot assume that one size fits all for all nutrients, but genetics does not invalidate most commonsense nutrition recommendations. It is more likely from what we know that everyone benefits from balanced nutrition and a healthy active lifestyle, but some may benefit even more based on a genetic predisposition to inflammation and age-related chronic diseases.

Most age-related chronic diseases are still about 70% dependent on diet and lifestyle and only 30% on genetics. Identical twin studies examining the correlations among twins of common diseases tend to overestimate the impact of genetics on obesity and chronic diseases. However, identical twin studies have been used effectively to show the impact of microbiome changes on the risk of obesity. In these studies, identical twins who were different in that one twin was obese and other was lean were studied. Stool microflora from the obese twin and the normal twin were transplanted into germ-free mice, and on the same diet, the mouse with the microflora from the lean twin remained lean, while the mouse with the microflora from the obese twin gained weight.

Another important demonstration of the impact of nutrients on gene expression is the epigenetics, which occurs in utero. A yellow mouse called the agouti mouse has a heterozygous agouti gene mutation. This mutation confers a yellow coat color to the mice, obesity, and an increased risk of cancer. If a pregnant yellow agouti heterozygote mother is treated with methyl donor vitamins, including folic acid, then she gives birth to normal brown mice with no obesity or increased risk of cancer. The folic acid and other methyl donors prevent the expression of the agouti gene by methylation of CpG islands in the promoter region of the gene in utero. There are many other examples of epigenetic influences on gene expression based on in utero effects, and this phenomenon has been called nutrition programming.

While genetic diagnosis of rare inherited metabolic diseases is taught in medical schools, the emphasis is largely on those genes that can be targeted by drugs or used to diagnose an intolerance for certain nutrients, such as the amino acid phenylalanine in phenylketonuria (PKU). The search for small-molecule drugs that can treat cancers and other metabolic diseases, such as cystic fibrosis, has added to the general impression in medical school and primary care education that nutrition is less important than pharmacology.

In fact, nature's first pharmacy was the plant world, and prehuman mammals evolved with a plant-based diet for millions of years. The consumption of land-based mammals that were grass fed and ocean-caught fish and other seafood maintained the links to the plant world, since all these animals concentrated substances from their plant-based environment. Modern agriculture and animal husbandry is a relatively recent phenomenon in our human evolutionary history and has resulted in a number of gene–nutrient imbalances expressed through an increased risk of age-related chronic diseases. When first introducing the topic of gene–nutrient interaction in 1996 at the University of California, Los Angeles (UCLA) Center for Human Nutrition, with the dedication of the Dennis A. Tito Gene-Nutrient Interaction Laboratory, a great deal of skepticism was expressed by oncologists at UCLA about what exactly was meant by the term. This prejudice remains active, but the emphasis in this chapter and ongoing research on plant-based supplements and phytonutrient extracts aim to modify gene expression by restoring the balance of genes and nutrients through a diet rich in colorful phytonutrient-rich fruits, vegetables, and spices.

17.2 HUMAN NUTRITION AND GENE–NUTRIENT INTERACTION

The understanding of human nutrition has evolved throughout history in parallel to the development of key sciences, including chemistry, biochemistry, physiology, and most recently, genetics, with the sequencing of the human genome in the first decade of the twenty-first century.

During the "naturalistic era" (400 BC–1750 AD), Hippocrates (Karagiannis 2014) hypothesized that the body had "innate heat" and coined his famous phrase "Let food be your medicine and medicine be your food." During the next 500 years, little happened in the development of either scientific knowledge or nutrition science. However, the level of knowledge that could be gleaned from careful clinical observation of the effects of foods on physiological function was remarkable, as typified in the writings of Maimonides in the eleventh century AD. This medieval rabbi, physician, and philosopher was ahead of his time in applying Aristotelian understanding to the common ailments that could be modified by eating prescribed foods and carrying out simple hygienic practices that were not routine for many centuries after his death (Gesundheit 2011).

The late 1700s ushered in the "chemical-analytical era" (1750–1900), highlighted by Lavoisier's calorimetry studies (Severinghaus 2016). He discovered how food is metabolized by oxidation to carbon dioxide, water, and heat. He also invented the calorimeter, crucial to further understanding of heat energy. In the nineteenth century, Liebig (Usselman 2003) recognized that carbohydrates, proteins, and fats are oxidized by the body and calculated energy values for each. While chemists were examining the composition of foods and metabolism, physicians were studying the mechanisms and process of digestion, the means by which food is converted to useful intermediates that ultimately yield energy.

The "biological era" (1900–present) was founded on advances in chemistry, biochemistry, and understanding of metabolic pathways. In the early twentieth century, considerable research had been done on energy exchange and on the nature of foodstuffs. Once an understanding of macronutrients and better tools were developed, nutrition scientists turned their attention to the understanding of micronutrients, discovering the essential fatty acids and vitamins (McCollum 1967; Spector and Kim 2015).

The "cellular era" of the late twentieth century, beginning after the Second World War, focused on understanding functions of essential nutrients and the roles of micronutrients (vitamins and minerals) as cofactors for enzymes and hormones, and their subsequent roles in metabolic pathways. The roles of carbohydrates and fats in diseases such as diabetes and atherosclerosis were discovered, and underlying mechanisms were uncovered (Kritchevsky 1998).

Today, we are still in the era of cellular nutrition, but the "molecular and cellular" era is developing in the twenty-first century. It has been spurred on by the sequencing of the human genome, but it is not yet ready for application. Here is a glimpse of the future of nutritional science and personalized medicine.

17.3 NUTRIGENETICS

Observations of health and disease in the twentieth century raised some new questions. Why can some individuals consume high-fat diets and yet show no evidence of atherosclerotic disease?

Individual genetic differences in response to dietary components have been evident for years: lactose intolerance, alcohol dehydrogenase deficiency, and individual and population differences in blood lipid profiles and health outcomes after consumption of high-fat diets.

Genetic differences certainly were suspected, but elucidating and proving cellular, molecular, and ultimately genetic-level mechanisms in both healthy and unhealthy individuals proved to be a challenge. With the continuing developments in tools that enable molecular-level exploration of cause–effect phenomena, scientists have begun to develop hypotheses and conduct experiments to lay the foundation for a deeper level of understanding of gene–nutrient interactions. Today, an emerging field of nutritional research focuses on identifying and understanding molecular-level interaction between nutrients and other dietary bioactives with the human genome during transcription, translation, and expression, the processes during which proteins encoded by the genome are produced and expressed. The field of nutrition is likely to be the greatest beneficiary of the emerging trends in research on chronic diseases of aging, including cancer, heart disease, and mental dysfunction.

Nutrigenetics examines the individuality of response to nutrients based on genetics, while nutrigenomics examines the impact of nutrition on gene expression and disease risk. These definitions are often interchanged or confused even by scientists in the field, so you will see both terms.

The goal of nutrigenetics is to elucidate the effect of genetic variation on the interaction between diet and disease. Nutrigenetics has been used for decades in certain rare monogenic diseases such as PKU. In this disease, individuals must avoid phenylalanine-containing foods, or they risk development of serious mental dysfunction. More than 950 phenylalanine hydroxylase (PAH) gene variants have been identified in people with PKU. These vary in their consequences for the residual level of PAH activity, from having little or no effect to abolishing PAH activity completely (Blau 2016). A warning on diet soft drinks that use aspartame is specific to PKU. Advances in genotyping technology and the availability of locus-specific and genotype databases have greatly expanded the understanding of the correlations between individual gene variants, residual PAH enzymatic activity, and the clinical PKU phenotype.

Nutrigenetics in the general population has been proposed to have the potential to provide a basis for personalized dietary recommendations based on the individual's genetic makeup in order to prevent common multifactorial disorders decades before their clinical manifestation. A number of metabolic differences in metabolic pathways occur among individuals. Some of these affect the risk of certain cancers, such as lung and colon cancer.

One example of very common variants in nutrient metabolism that affect chronic disease risk is related to the metabolism of glucosinolates from cruciferous vegetables such as broccoli. The chemoprotective effect of cruciferous vegetables is due to their high glucosinolate content and the capacity of glucosinolate metabolites, such as isothiocyanates (ITCs) and indoles, to modulate biotransformation enzyme systems (e.g., cytochrome P450 and conjugating enzymes). Data from molecular epidemiologic studies suggest that genetic and associated functional variations in biotransformation enzymes, particularly glutathione S-transferase (GST) M1 and GSTT1, which metabolize ITCs, alter cancer risk in response to cruciferous vegetable exposure. Moreover, genetic polymorphisms in receptors and transcription factors that interact with these compounds may further contribute to variation in response to cruciferous vegetable intake.

Biotransformation enzymes, also referred to as xenobiotic- or drug-metabolizing enzymes, play a major role in regulating the toxic, mutagenic, and neoplastic effects of chemical carcinogens, as well as metabolizing other xenobiotics (e.g., phytochemicals and therapeutic drugs) and endogenous compounds (e.g., steroid hormones). Phytochemicals in plant foods modulate biotransformation enzyme activities, one mechanism by which fruits and vegetables, and cruciferous vegetables in particular, may contribute to reduced cancer risk.

There are two main groups of biotransformation enzymes. Phase I enzymes (cytochrome P450 and flavin-dependent monooxygenases) convert hydrophobic compounds to reactive electrophiles by oxidation, hydroxylation, and reduction reactions to prepare them for reaction with water-soluble moieties. Phase II enzymes (e.g., GST, UDP-glucuronosyltransferases [UGTs], sulfotransferases, and N-acetyltransferases) primarily catalyze conjugation reactions. Genetic polymorphisms in these enzyme systems can influence cancer susceptibility when coupled with the relevant carcinogen exposures. The understanding of how genetic differences in components of the biotransformation pathways alter response to chemopreventive foods such as cruciferous vegetables has only been discovered in the last few decades.

Null genotypes for *GSTM1* and *GSTT1* occur commonly and result in the absence of the respective enzymes. Both of these enzymes are involved in the metabolism of environmental carcinogens and reactive oxygen species. Thus, until recently, the primary hypothesis has been that individuals with the *GST* null genotypes are at higher risk for cancer because of reduced capacity to dispose of activated carcinogens. Numerous epidemiologic studies have focused on interactions between these polymorphisms and carcinogen exposure. Now, researchers are also studying relationships between *GST* polymorphisms and exposure to preventive agents (i.e., ITCs), with the hypothesis being that because ITCs are metabolized by GST, polymorphisms associated with reduced GST activity will result in longer circulating half-lives of ITCs and potentially greater chemoprotective effects of cruciferous vegetables (Lampe et al. 2000).

A null genotype has a modest effect on increasing the risk of cancer, but the individual with a null genotype has a greater opportunity to reduce the risk by eating cruciferous vegetables, which induce protective GST enzyme activity more briskly than is found in the wild-type GST individual. Therefore, a null mutation increases the risk of cancer modestly but provides that individual with an increased opportunity to benefit from nutrients beyond that of individuals who do not have the null mutation.

17.4 NUTRIGENOMICS: EFFECTS OF NUTRIENTS ON GENE EXPRESSION

Nutrigenomics explores the effects of nutrients on the genome, proteome (all of an organism's proteins), and metabolome (all the metabolites of a cell or organism). Nutrients previously thought to be simply sources of calories, such as lipids, can modulate gene expression—as can many phytochemicals derived from fruits, vegetables, and spices that were simply thought to be antioxidants.

Although epigenetic aberrations frequently occur in aging and cancer and form a core component of these conditions, perhaps the most useful aspect of epigenetic processes is that they are readily reversible. Unlike genetic effects that also play a role in cancer and aging, epigenetic aberrations can be relatively easily corrected. One of the most widespread approaches to the epigenetic alterations in cancer and aging is dietary control. This can be achieved not only through the quality of the diet, but also through the quantity of calories that are consumed. Many phytochemicals, such as sulforaphane (SFN) from cruciferous vegetables and green tea, have anticancer epigenetic effects and are also efficacious for preventing or treating the epigenetic aberrations of age-associated diseases besides cancer. Likewise, the quantity of calories that are consumed has proven to be advantageous in preventing cancer and extending the life span through control of epigenetic mediators.

17.5 EPIGENETICS AND DIET

Epigenetic processes involve changes that are heritable but are not encoded with the DNA sequence itself. There are numerous types of epigenetic mechanisms, but the three most important in humans include changes in DNA methylation, histone modifications, and noncoding RNAs.

DNA methylation is the most studied of the epigenetic processes and is based on the addition of a methyl group enzymatically from S-adenosylmethionine (SAM) to the 5-positon of cytosine, primarily occurring in CpG dinucleotides. This is carried out by three major methyltransferases

(DNMT1, DNMT3A, and DNMT3B). In general, the more methylated a gene regulatory region becomes, the less transcription will occur from the promoter, although there are notable exceptions to this dogma, as occurs with the gene that encodes human telomerase reverse transcriptase (hTERT), the key regulatory gene of telomerase (Poole et al. 2001; Daniel et al. 2012).

Epigenetic changes can also occur through modification of the histone proteins coating the chromosomes. Modification of the histones opens up the chromatin to allow transcription or, alternatively, to protect the DNA from inappropriate transcription. Although histone acetylation and methylation are the most studied of these modifications, others also occur, such as histone phosphorylation, ubiquitination, biotinylation, sumoylation, and ADP-ribosylation.

The number of enzymes that carry out histone modifications is large relative to those that mediate DNA methylation, and the two that often attract interest, especially with regard to cancer and aging, are the histone acetyltransferases (HATs) and the histone deactylases (HDACs) (Kouzarides 2007). In general, the more acetylated the histone amino tails become, the more likely it is that the gene promoter region that contains those histones will have increased transcriptional activity (Clayton et al. 2006).

Noncoding RNA, the third major type of epigenetic control in mammalian systems, is also important in gene expression. For example, miRNA consists of single-stranded noncoding RNAs that are usually about 21–23 nucleotides in length. These sequences suppress gene expression by altering the stability of gene transcripts and also by targeting the transcripts for degradation, although miRNA may also lead to an increase in gene transcription (Mathers et al. 2010). Many miRNAs have now been identified and can regulate a large number of varied genes that affect metabolism and oncogene expression (Esquela-Kerscher and Slack 2006).

Epigenetic alterations can also provide a format for long-term dietary programming of the genome, suggesting that nutritional supplementation may affect gene regulation in humans, and that well-adapted diets applied in utero and after birth may exert a fundamental and long-lasting positive impact. Some evidence shows that chronic diseases in adulthood are due to persistent influences from early-life nutrition.

Intrauterine growth restriction (IUGR) is a perinatal condition affecting fetal growth, with under the 10th percentile of the weight curve expected for gestational age, and it is more common among mothers with nutritional imbalances or malnutrition. This condition has been associated with higher cardiovascular and metabolic risk and postnatal obesity. There are also major changes in placental function, and particularly in a key molecule in this regulation, nitric oxide. The synthesis of nitric oxide has numerous control mechanisms and competition with arginase for their common substrate, the amino acid L-arginine. This competition is reflected in various vascular diseases, and particularly in the endothelium of the umbilical vessels of babies with IUGR. Along with this, there is regulation at the epigenetic level, where methylation in specific regions of some gene promoters, such as the nitric oxide synthase, regulates their expression (Casanello et al. 2016). The concept that a pregnant mother suffering nutritional insults has mechanisms in place for in utero epigenetic changes, preparing the newborn infant for an environment of nutritional deficiency, is being validated in numerous studies in both animals and humans.

Whereas many of the earlier studies had assumed that single-nucleotide polymorphisms (SNPs) were the main source of human genetic variability, an increasing body of evidence now suggests the importance of additional layers of variability, including copy number polymorphisms and epigenetic regulation, such as DNA methylation. Epigenetics is just beginning to reveal its possible implications in nutrition.

As diet is the most prominent lifelong environmental impact on human health and as, with prolonging life span and changing lifestyle in developed countries, chronic diseases become more prevalent, nutrigenomics and nutrigenetics are key scientific platforms to promote health and prevent disease through nutrition that better meets the requirements and constraints of consumer groups with specific health conditions and particular lifestyles, and in certain stages of life.

17.6 GENE–NUTRIENT INTERACTIONS IN CANCER AND AGING

Since aging is the primary risk factor for the development of cancer, it is worthwhile to examine the epigenetics of the regulation of cellular proliferation and cell death, as well as the epigenetics of aging, as common gene–nutrient interactions affect both processes. Nutrition can influence gene expression through epigenetics in cancer and aging. Over half of the gene defects that occur in cancer are due to epigenetic alterations rather than genetic mutations, and aging is associated with changes in methylation, as described below (Issa 1999). These acquired changes in gene expression can be influenced by changes in dietary intake, including both total calories and phytonutrients that have epigenetic effects.

General DNA hypomethylation has been described in cells, in addition to gene-specific hypermethylation, often leading the uncovering of gene expression leading to uncontrolled cell growth and neoplasia (Baylin et al. 1998). It is thought that these changes in DNA methylation play an early role in cancer genesis and lead to aberrations in cellular proliferation, as well as immortalization of previously normal cells.

Population studies demonstrate an association between green tea consumption and the inhibition of numerous cancers (Kim et al. 2010; Chen et al. 2011; Shanmugam et al. 2011). Among the antioxidants in green tea called catechins, the most widely studied is (–)-epigallocatechin-3-gallate (EGCG). Although EGCG has many effects on cells, it can inhibit DNA methyltransferase activity by directly interacting with the enzyme (Fang et al. 2003).

Another key dietary component that has epigenetic effects is SFN of cruciferous vegetables such as broccoli, cauliflower, brussels sprouts, cabbage, and kale. We have already discussed the role of glucosinolates in inducing metabolic enzymes in the liver and other tissues with detoxifying activities. In addition, SFN can inhibit DNMT (Meeran et al. 2010b), and can also inhibit HDAC activity (Myzak et al. 2007; Dashwood and Ho 2008; Schwab et al. 2008; Nian et al. 2009).

Curcumin (turmeric), resveratrol (grapes and red wine), and genistein (soybeans), as well as many other phytonutrients, have also been demonstrated to have epigenetic effects, suggesting that a general phenomenon of phytonutrients may be regulation of gene expression (Meeran et al. 2010a).

Changes in DNA methylation during aging likely contribute to a number of changes in the regulation of epigenetically controlled genes such as hTERT, which affects telomerase and can contribute to the aging process (Liu et al. 2003). Aging is associated with general hypomethylation of the genome, as well as regional or gene-specific hypermethylation (Issa 1999; Liu et al. 2003), which may be due to changes in the expression of the DNMTs (Lopatina et al. 2002; Casillas et al. 2003).

Histone modifications are also involved in the aging process. Sirtuin 1 (SIRT1) is a class II NAD+-dependent HDAC that has been demonstrated to increase the life span of a diverse range of animal models (Cohen et al. 2004; Kanfi et al. 2008). The SIRT1 enzyme appears to be an important nutrient sensor linked to metabolic rate. The redox potential, simplified as the NAD/NADH ratio, may be important in regulating SIRT1 activity, which is a key indicator for oxygen consumption and the respiratory chain. Although many other epigenetic changes occur during the aging process, the regulation of DNA methylation and histone modifications, as well as epigenetic control of hTERT and the role of SIRT1 in modulating aging biological processes, appear to be central to the nutrient modulation of the aging process.

Caloric restriction with constant protein intake in rodents has been shown to increase life span, and in multiple species, caloric restriction extends life span through multiple mechanisms, including epigenetic mechanisms (Weindruch et al. 1986; Sinclair 2005). In his original experiments at UCLA, working in the laboratory of Roy Walford, Richard Weindruch restricted calories at a set level below those of *ad libitum*-fed animals but kept protein constant (Weindruch et al. 1986). Protein restriction affects the lean body mass of rodents, including their tail, which is made of collagen. Therefore, Weindruch and coworkers wanted to control for differences in organ size in examining longevity. It turned out that the protein provided was a constant 30% of total energy intake (personal communication), which is very close to the 29% of resting energy expenditure in humans resulting from 1 g of protein/pound of lean body mass used in our obesity treatment regimens. The restriction of total calories by 25–60% relative to normally fed controls while providing essential nutrients and protein can lead to a 50% increase in life span (Holloszy and Fontana 2007; Colman et al. 2009; Cruzen and Colman 2009; Li and Tollefsbol 2011).

The life extension effects of sirtuins were originally discovered in yeast (Guarente and Picard 2005), and activation of SIRT1 is often observed in various tissues of animals subjected to caloric restriction, while inactivation of SIRT1 may lead to ablation of the life span-extending effects of caloric restriction. It is therefore apparent that epigenetic processes are not only central to the aging process, but also involved with key mediators of aging, such as DNA methylation and SIRT1.

17.7 GENOME-WIDE SCANNING AND DISEASE RISK

By scanning the genomes of thousands of people and comparing the sick with the healthy, markers for DNA sequences are being discovered that are believed to increase the risk of type 2 diabetes, cancer, heart disease, inflammatory bowel disease, and other common chronic diseases of aging. Genome-wide association studies derive their power from the Human Genome Project, which identified the complete genome of a few individuals. More recently, a haplotype map project has begun to catalog human genetic variation by grouping together those genetic variations that are associated in function across different ethnic groups. The research has been made possible by the much reduced cost of gene scanning and by efficient gene chip technologies, available only in the past few years.

In the past, geneticists focused only on single genes with marked effects on disease risk. They would examine a large family where a number of individuals have been afflicted with some rare disease. Typical examples include cystic fibrosis, Huntington's disease, and inherited forms of cancer. By tracking a small number of genetic markers that were linked to a rare disease in such families, researchers successfully isolated rare genes that caused disease.

For example, the gene variants BRCA1 and BRCA2 have been shown to increase breast cancer risk significantly. The lifetime risk of cancer associated with these rare variants is about 85–90%, leading women to elect to have a prophylactic mastectomy if they are found to have these genes. Other gene discoveries often led to insights into the pathway causing the disease, but had the drawback that only a small percent of common diseases, such as breast cancer, could be attributed to these rare gene defects. At most, inherited forms of colon, prostate, and breast cancer account for 10–15% of all cases. Family studies such as these lacked the power to pick up genetic variants that have a modest effect or that may interact with environmental exposures.

An alternative to traditional linkage studies is to search for "candidate genes" known to play a role in some biologic process, such as insulin production. Looking for associations between mutations in these candidates and common diseases has been going on for the past several decades. Hundreds of studies have reported such associations. But few have been reproduced more than once or twice.

Rather than work with a few thousand genomic markers, genome-wide association studies use gene chips that can scan an individual's DNA sample for anywhere from 100,000 to 500,000 or more single-base changes. Known as SNPs, these changes are selected to reflect patterns of common genetic diversity. Such high SNP density makes it much easier to detect potentially significant DNA changes. The studies can be done on tens of thousands of individuals as well, since the cost of using such chips has dropped in the past few years. By compiling the SNPs from every DNA sample in a database, and comparing the SNPs in heart attack patients with those in healthy people, it is possible to discern even subtle genetic signals that contribute to heart disease risk. However, the SNPs identified in these studies may not directly be involved in the cause of the disease, but are simply located in or near the problematic DNA.

With the exception of macular degeneration in Table 17.1, where the gene variant raises disease risk about two to three times in those with one copy, most of the genes found so far increase disease

TABLE 17.1
Selected Genome-Wide Scan Results

Disease	Publication Date	Sample Size	Gene or Variant	Approximate Risk
Macular degeneration	2005	1,700	1 new gene	400–600%
Inflammatory bowel disease	2006	4,500	1 new gene	120%
Prostate cancer	2007	17,500	2 variants in the same region (1 new)	123%
Obesity	2007	38,700	1 new gene	67%
Type 2 diabetes	2007	32,500	9 variants (3 new)	80%
Heart disease	2007	41,600	1 new variant	25–40%

Source: Couzin, J., and Kaiser, J., *Science*, 316, 820–822, 2007.

risk to a much lesser extent. Although a 50% increase may sound substantial, in absolute terms, it is modest. For example, assume that a 65-year-old man's prostate cancer risk is 3%. If he carries two copies of the most potent prostate cancer gene found to date, this makes him 1.23 times more likely to develop prostate cancer. In other words, his overall risk increases from 3% to about 3.7%.

17.8 THE MICROBIOME AND THE METAGENOME

Interest in the role of the microbiome in human health has burgeoned over the past decade, with the advent of new technologies for interrogating complex microbial communities. The large-scale dynamics of the microbiome can be described by many of the tools and observations used in the study of population ecology. Deciphering the metagenome and its aggregate genetic information can also be used to understand the functional properties of the microbial community. Both the microbiome and metagenome probably have important functions in health and disease; their exploration is a frontier in human genetics. However, at this point in the development of the research on the interactions of the microbiome, the immune system, and the expression of genes involved in chronic disease, there is too little information outside of gastrointestinal disorders to be of practical use in clinical applications.

17.9 CASE STUDY OF CLINICAL APPLICATION IN PRIMARY CARE OF GENE–NUTRIENT INTERACTIONS

There is no better example of the application and misapplication of medical genetics than familial hypercholesterolemia (FH), already discussed extensively in Chapter 9.

The FH phenotype can be divided into heterozygous and homozygous FH, with a prevalence of 1 in 300–500 and 1 in 1 million, respectively (Hopkins et al. 2011). The clinical syndrome of heterozygous FH is characterized by elevated plasma LDL cholesterol concentrations and premature coronary heart disease at ages 30–60. There is also a family history of heart disease and elevated cholesterol levels, along with tendon xanthomas. This presentation of FH is usually due to a single LDL receptor gene mutation; the very rare form of homozygous FH is caused by at least two *LDLR* mutations and presents with much higher cholesterol levels and much earlier presentation of heart disease, often in the twenties. LDL receptor mutations account for greater than 90% of the variants of the FH phenotype.

LDL particle size has also been associated with increased heart disease risk. Increased levels or percentage of small, dense LDL cholesterol has been correlated with increased future coronary heart disease events in the ARIC study (Hoogeveen et al. 2014). It is proposed that these smaller

LDL particles contribute to the pathogenesis of atherosclerosis due to a higher LDL particle number, or because smaller LDL circulating particles can penetrate the endothelium more easily. The finding of small, dense LDL has been related to increased markers of inflammation and the metabolic syndrome, and the development of adverse lipid profiles (Siri-Tarino et al. 2009).

Polygenic hypercholesterolemia is characterized by the FH phenotype, but none of the classic mutations that lead to heterozygous or homozygous FH. In a population study in the United Kingdom, it was demonstrated that 40% of those with the FH phenotype had no mutations in the described genes for LDL receptors, apolipoprotein B, or the enzyme PCSK9, which in the upregulated form degrades LDL receptors, increasing plasma cholesterol (Taylor et al. 2010; Santos and Maranhao 2014).

Given these findings, some have proposed the concept that less potent but more common gene variants across multiple genes may be playing a role in these cases (Teslovich et al. 2010). Based on genome-wide association studies that utilize high-throughput genotyping techniques, many SNPs have been found to have significant associations with elevated LDL cholesterol. It is thought that an individual may carry multiple variants that work together to produce an FH-like phenotype. Some investigators have proposed utilizing a polygenic or genotype score, which tallies SNPs from multiple LDL cholesterol-raising alleles, to use in risk assessment. In some studies, higher genotype scores have been associated with increased heart disease events (Kathiresan et al. 2008; Talmud et al. 2013; Santos and Maranhao 2014). Clearly, more research is needed to validate such genotype scores, especially when considered in the context of the classic risk factors for heart disease, including diabetes, hypertension, and visceral obesity.

Therefore, the genetics of hypercholesterolemia can be divided into two main groups. First is a classic clear pattern of Mendelian inheritance, which requires pharmacological intervention or liver transplantation for the homozygous condition. Second, and more commonly, there can be a presentation where an inheritance pattern is not easily found. In these patients, there may be a collection of gene variants that, together with traditional dietary and lifestyle factors, exert a compound effect similar to that of the classic gene mutations of FH. If index cases are found and are highly suggestive of FH on the basis of clinical criteria, genetic testing is not necessary to confirm a primary mutation, but it may still be done, and cascade screening of relatives is recommended. Some studies have shown the cost-effectiveness of the screening of relatives utilizing this approach (Marks et al. 2002; Ademi et al. 2014).

There is still controversy regarding universal screening of children for FH, with some believing that early identification can lead to early treatment and, as a result, reduction in total "cholesterol years." However, the long-term effects of statin therapy and the thresholds for initiation of treatment in young children are currently being debated. Groups such as the American Heart Association do not endorse universal screening, but they do state that cholesterol testing should be considered in children of parents with premature coronary heart disease and/or a history of elevated total cholesterol levels.

FH is an underdiagnosed condition worldwide, despite the fact that there are effective ways to treat it and prevent long-term damage. The National Lipid Association guidelines stressed the need, in the primary care setting, to identify FH on the basis of clinical criteria and cholesterol levels. These guidelines noted that a negative genetic test does not exclude FH, because up to 20% of patients will not be found to have a known mutation. Also, remember that the incidence of FH is 1 in 300–500 individuals, while the most common reason for elevated cholesterol levels is hypertriglyceridemia as part of the metabolic syndrome, occurring in about half of middle-aged populations. The lipids within very low-density lipoprotein particles, which carry triglycerides, are 20% cholesterol. Finally, beyond the effects of lifestyle change on cholesterol levels, normalization of excess body fat results can reverse the atherogenic lipid particle profile consisting of small, dense LDL particles.

17.10 SUMMARY

Personalized medicine based on gene–nutrient interaction is not ready for prime time. It is a futuristic concept promoted through the growing knowledge of genomics. Realistically, achieving this vision will require a personalized behavioral approach, as well as changes in foods that are eaten and exercises designed to maintain lean body mass. In the future, genomic information, including proteomics and genome-wide scanning, may be used to understand the basis of individual differences in response to dietary patterns, as well as the interaction of the human genome, the proteome, and the microbiome. The resulting nutrigenomic data have the potential to provide a sound basis for the development of safe and effective diet therapies for individuals or subgroups of the population. Another aspect of the future understanding of gene–nutrient interactions will be refined models of disease mechanisms based on understanding the genome. This understanding may provide new lines of research and possibly new diet and lifestyle interventions. The elaboration of physical and genetic linkage maps, combined with techniques to catalog massive databases of genetic information, may uncover new genes and gene interactions that, together with diet and lifestyle, may influence disease progression or even prevent common chronic diseases of aging and slow the aging process itself to maximize life span.

Who will do this? Public health officials will most likely continue to issue one-size-fits-all solutions and will necessarily need to run these through the funnel of special interests, which distort nutritional advice given to the public. The drug industry, while recognizing that nutrition may play a role, will minimize the role of diet and lifestyle and use only general government guidelines in patients given drugs to ameliorate conditions driven by diet and lifestyle, such as hypertension, hyperlipidemia, and diabetes. Food processors marketing mainstream products will wait a long time for the products to be created and the demand to be established. In the future, it will be primary care physicians and allied health care professionals, such as fitness instructors, dietitians, and psychologists armed with high-tech tools, who will catalyze lifestyle changes in those at risk of chronic diseases associated with aging, as well as the aging process itself.

REFERENCES

Ademi, Z., G. F. Watts, J. Pang, E. J. Sijbrands, F. M. van Bockxmeer, P. O'Leary, E. Geelhoed, and D. Liew. 2014. Cascade screening based on genetic testing is cost-effective: Evidence for the implementation of models of care for familial hypercholesterolemia. *J Clin Lipidol* 8 (4):390–400.

Baylin, S. B., J. G. Herman, J. R. Graff, P. M. Vertino, and J. P. Issa. 1998. Alterations in DNA methylation: A fundamental aspect of neoplasia. *Adv Cancer Res* 72:141–196.

Blau, N. 2016. Genetics of phenylketonuria: Then and now. *Hum Mutat* 37 (6):508–515.

Casanello, P., J. A. Castro-Rodriguez, R. Uauy, and B. J. Krause. 2016. Placental epigenetic programming in intrauterine growth restriction (IUGR) [in Spanish]. *Rev Chil Pediatr* 87 (3):154–161.

Casillas, M. A., Jr., N. Lopatina, L. G. Andrews, and T. O. Tollefsbol. 2003. Transcriptional control of the DNA methyltransferases is altered in aging and neoplastically-transformed human fibroblasts. *Mol Cell Biochem* 252 (1–2):33–43.

Chen, D., S. B. Wan, H. Yang, J. Yuan, T. H. Chan, and Q. P. Dou. 2011. EGCG, green tea polyphenols and their synthetic analogs and prodrugs for human cancer prevention and treatment. *Adv Clin Chem* 53:155–177.

Clayton, A. L., C. A. Hazzalin, and L. C. Mahadevan. 2006. Enhanced histone acetylation and transcription: A dynamic perspective. *Mol Cell* 23 (3):289–296.

Cohen, H. Y., C. Miller, K. J. Bitterman, N. R. Wall, B. Hekking, B. Kessler, K. T. Howitz, M. Gorospe, R. de Cabo, and D. A. Sinclair. 2004. Calorie restriction promotes mammalian cell survival by inducing the SIRT1 deacetylase. *Science* 305 (5682):390–392.

Colman, R. J., R. M. Anderson, S. C. Johnson, E. K. Kastman, K. J. Kosmatka, T. M. Beasley, D. B. Allison, C. Cruzen, H. A. Simmons, J. W. Kemnitz, and R. Weindruch. 2009. Caloric restriction delays disease onset and mortality in rhesus monkeys. *Science* 325 (5937):201–204.

Couzin, J., and J. Kaiser. 2007. Genome-wide association. Closing the net on common disease genes. *Science* 316 (5826):820–822.

Cruzen, C., and R. J. Colman. 2009. Effects of caloric restriction on cardiovascular aging in non-human primates and humans. *Clin Geriatr Med* 25 (4):733–743, ix–x.

Daniel, M., G. W. Peek, and T. O. Tollefsbol. 2012. Regulation of the human catalytic subunit of telomerase (hTERT). *Gene* 498 (2):135–146.

Dashwood, R. H., and E. Ho. 2008. Dietary agents as histone deacetylase inhibitors: Sulforaphane and structurally related isothiocyanates. *Nutr Rev* 66 (Suppl 1):S36–S38.

Esquela-Kerscher, A., and F. J. Slack. 2006. Oncomirs—microRNAs with a role in cancer. *Nat Rev Cancer* 6 (4):259–269.

Fang, M. Z., Y. Wang, N. Ai, Z. Hou, Y. Sun, H. Lu, W. Welsh, and C. S. Yang. 2003. Tea polyphenol (–)-epigallocatechin-3-gallate inhibits DNA methyltransferase and reactivates methylation-silenced genes in cancer cell lines. *Cancer Res* 63 (22):7563–7570.

Gesundheit, B. 2011. Maimonides' appreciation for medicine. *Rambam Maimonides Med J* 2 (1):e0018.

Guarente, L., and F. Picard. 2005. Calorie restriction—The SIR2 connection. *Cell* 120 (4):473–482.

Holloszy, J. O., and L. Fontana. 2007. Caloric restriction in humans. *Exp Gerontol* 42 (8):709–712.

Hoogeveen, R. C., J. W. Gaubatz, W. Sun, R. C. Dodge, J. R. Crosby, J. Jiang, D. Couper, S. S. Virani, S. Kathiresan, E. Boerwinkle, and C. M. Ballantyne. 2014. Small dense low-density lipoprotein-cholesterol concentrations predict risk for coronary heart disease: The Atherosclerosis Risk in Communities (ARIC) study. *Arterioscler Thromb Vasc Biol* 34 (5):1069–1077.

Hopkins, P. N., P. P. Toth, C. M. Ballantyne, D. J. Rader, and National Lipid Association Expert Panel on Familial Hypercholesterolemia. 2011. Familial hypercholesterolemias: Prevalence, genetics, diagnosis and screening recommendations from the National Lipid Association Expert Panel on Familial Hypercholesterolemia. *J Clin Lipidol* 5 (3 Suppl):S9–S17.

Issa, J. P. 1999. Aging, DNA methylation and cancer. *Crit Rev Oncol Hematol* 32 (1):31–43.

Kanfi, Y., V. Peshti, Y. M. Gozlan, M. Rathaus, R. Gil, and H. Y. Cohen. 2008. Regulation of SIRT1 protein levels by nutrient availability. *FEBS Lett* 582 (16):2417–2423.

Karagiannis, T. C. 2014. The timeless influence of Hippocratic ideals on diet, salicytates and personalized medicine. *Hell J Nucl Med* 17 (1):2–6.

Kathiresan, S., O. Melander, D. Anevski, C. Guiducci, N. P. Burtt, C. Roos, J. N. Hirschhorn et al. 2008. Polymorphisms associated with cholesterol and risk of cardiovascular events. *N Engl J Med* 358 (12):1240–1249.

Kim, J. W., A. R. Amin, and D. M. Shin. 2010. Chemoprevention of head and neck cancer with green tea polyphenols. *Cancer Prev Res (Phila)* 3 (8):900–909.

Kouzarides, T. 2007. Chromatin modifications and their function. *Cell* 128 (4):693–705.

Kritchevsky, D. 1998. History of recommendations to the public about dietary fat. *J Nutr* 128 (2 Suppl): 449S–452S.

Lampe, J. W., C. Chen, S. Li, J. Prunty, M. T. Grate, D. E. Meehan, K. V. Barale, D. A. Dightman, Z. Feng, and J. D. Potter. 2000. Modulation of human glutathione S-transferases by botanically defined vegetable diets. *Cancer Epidemiol Biomarkers Prev* 9 (8):787–793.

Li, Y., and T. O. Tollefsbol. 2011. p16(INK4a) suppression by glucose restriction contributes to human cellular lifespan extension through SIRT1-mediated epigenetic and genetic mechanisms. *PLoS One* 6 (2):e17421.

Liu, L., R. C. Wylie, L. G. Andrews, and T. O. Tollefsbol. 2003. Aging, cancer and nutrition: The DNA methylation connection. *Mech Ageing Dev* 124 (10–12):989–998.

Lopatina, N., J. F. Haskell, L. G. Andrews, J. C. Poole, S. Saldanha, and T. Tollefsbol. 2002. Differential maintenance and de novo methylating activity by three DNA methyltransferases in aging and immortalized fibroblasts. *J Cell Biochem* 84 (2):324–334.

Marks, D., D. Wonderling, M. Thorogood, H. Lambert, S. E. Humphries, and H. A. Neil. 2002. Cost effectiveness analysis of different approaches of screening for familial hypercholesterolaemia. *BMJ* 324 (7349):1303.

Mathers, J. C., G. Strathdee, and C. L. Relton. 2010. Induction of epigenetic alterations by dietary and other environmental factors. *Adv Genet* 71:3–39.

McCollum, E. V. 1967. The paths to the discovery of vitamins A and D. *J Nutr* 91 (21 Suppl):11–16.

Meeran, S. M., A. Ahmed, and T. O. Tollefsbol. 2010a. Epigenetic targets of bioactive dietary components for cancer prevention and therapy. *Clin Epigenetics* 1 (3–4):101–116.

Meeran, S. M., S. N. Patel, and T. O. Tollefsbol. 2010b. Sulforaphane causes epigenetic repression of hTERT expression in human breast cancer cell lines. *PLoS One* 5 (7):e11457.

Myzak, M. C., P. Tong, W. M. Dashwood, R. H. Dashwood, and E. Ho. 2007. Sulforaphane retards the growth of human PC-3 xenografts and inhibits HDAC activity in human subjects. *Exp Biol Med (Maywood)* 232 (2):227–234.

Nian, H., B. Delage, E. Ho, and R. H. Dashwood. 2009. Modulation of histone deacetylase activity by dietary isothiocyanates and allyl sulfides: Studies with sulforaphane and garlic organosulfur compounds. *Environ Mol Mutagen* 50 (3):213–221.

Poole, J. C., L. G. Andrews, and T. O. Tollefsbol. 2001. Activity, function, and gene regulation of the catalytic subunit of telomerase (hTERT). *Gene* 269 (1–2):1–12.

Santos, R. D., and R. C. Maranhao. 2014. What is new in familial hypercholesterolemia? *Curr Opin Lipidol* 25 (3):183–188.

Schwab, M., V. Reynders, S. Loitsch, D. Steinhilber, O. Schroder, and J. Stein. 2008. The dietary histone deacetylase inhibitor sulforaphane induces human beta-defensin-2 in intestinal epithelial cells. *Immunology* 125 (2):241–251.

Severinghaus, J. W. 2016. Eight sages over five centuries share oxygen's discovery. *Adv Physiol Educ* 40 (3):370–376.

Shanmugam, M. K., R. Kannaiyan, and G. Sethi. 2011. Targeting cell signaling and apoptotic pathways by dietary agents: Role in the prevention and treatment of cancer. *Nutr Cancer* 63 (2):161–173.

Sinclair, D. A. 2005. Toward a unified theory of caloric restriction and longevity regulation. *Mech Ageing Dev* 126 (9):987–1002.

Siri-Tarino, P. W., P. T. Williams, H. S. Fernstrom, R. S. Rawlings, and R. M. Krauss. 2009. Reversal of small, dense LDL subclass phenotype by normalization of adiposity. *Obesity (Silver Spring)* 17 (9):1768–1775.

Spector, A. A., and H. Y. Kim. 2015. Discovery of essential fatty acids. *J Lipid Res* 56 (1):11–21.

Talmud, P. J., S. Shah, R. Whittall, M. Futema, P. Howard, J. A. Cooper, S. C. Harrison et al. 2013. Use of low-density lipoprotein cholesterol gene score to distinguish patients with polygenic and monogenic familial hypercholesterolaemia: A case-control study. *Lancet* 381 (9874):1293–1301.

Taylor, A., D. Wang, K. Patel, R. Whittall, G. Wood, M. Farrer, R. D. Neely et al. 2010. Mutation detection rate and spectrum in familial hypercholesterolaemia patients in the UK pilot cascade project. *Clin Genet* 77 (6):572–580.

Teslovich, T. M., K. Musunuru, A. V. Smith, A. C. Edmondson, I. M. Stylianou, M. Koseki, J. P. Pirruccello et al. 2010. Biological, clinical and population relevance of 95 loci for blood lipids. *Nature* 466 (7307):707–713.

Usselman, M. C. 2003. Liebig's alkaloid analyses: The uncertain route from content to molecular formulae. *Ambix* 50 (1):71–89.

Weindruch, R., R. L. Walford, S. Fligiel, and D. Guthrie. 1986. The retardation of aging in mice by dietary restriction: Longevity, cancer, immunity and lifetime energy intake. *J Nutr* 116 (4):641–654.

18 Nutrition and the Risk of Common Forms of Cancer

18.1 INTRODUCTION

While cancer is not the leading cause of death with aging, it is the most feared, with the possible exception of dementia, which is a living death (Witte and Allen 2000). The public yearns for a cure for cancer. However, cancer is not a single disease, and many different solutions to its many different forms are needed. Cancer sometimes seems like a random killer of innocent people, but there are established risk factors, such as smoking, diet, and lifestyle.

Smoking tobacco, which is now an accepted risk factor for lung cancer, was not recognized as such even as recently as 70 or 80 years ago. In the 1940s and 1950s (Gardner and Brandt 2006), doctors appeared in advertisements for cigarettes and even endorsed specific brands. In 1964, the surgeon general's warning on cigarettes and lung cancer emerged based on a combination of population studies demonstrating an association and the work of basic scientists defining the pathways of tobacco carcinogenesis, including animal studies where rodents smoked cigarettes (U.S. Public Health Service 1964). Nonetheless, cigarette smoke was still rising over the slide projectors at major scientific meetings, such as those held in Atlantic City by the Federation of Societies of Experimental Biology in the 1970s. These scientific meetings included the most prominent medical experts in the nation, including many who were aware of the cancer connection to tobacco. Nonetheless, an equilibrium existed between the large tobacco companies aided by lobbies and their own select scientists and the larger scientific community that advanced basic research to describe the mechanisms of tobacco carcinogenesis at a cellular level. Extensive public health advertising, beginning in California and combined with tobacco taxes, ultimately reduced smoking in California and in many parts of the country, as these practices were applied nationally (Hu et al. 1995). The annual U.S. per capita cigarette consumption among adults ≥18 years of age rose from virtually zero in the early 1900s to more than 4000 during the 1960s, before declining to nearly 1700 in 2006, a level not seen since 1935 (National Center for Chronic Disease Prevention and Health Promotion 2014). In concert with this, there has been a significant decrease in the prevalence of squamous and small-cell carcinoma since the 1990s, although less rapidly among females than males. Adenocarcinoma rates decreased among males only through 2005, after which they then rose during 2006–2010 among every racial, ethnic, and gender group (Lewis et al. 2014). Laws in many cities prohibit smoking in restaurants and places of business. In airports, smokers are confined to glass-enclosed ventilated rooms. Public health can work to decrease cancer risk at least for smoking. Despite this background, tobacco products continue to be promoted globally. However, a final rule issued by the U.S. Food and Drug Administration (FDA) in 2016 has made tobacco products subject to the Federal Food, Drug, and Cosmetic Act, as amended by the Family Smoking Prevention and Tobacco Control Act, so that there are finally restrictions on the sale and distribution of tobacco products and required warning statements for tobacco products (Food and Drug Administration 2016).

The challenge for relating nutrition to cancer risk is much greater than for tobacco, which has taken more than 80 years from scientific discovery to implementation of a rule by the FDA. Nutrition-related cancer risks are more complex and require more carefully designed research. It is easy do studies demonstrating a lack of effect of a single nutrient, such as fat, but it is difficult to carry out comprehensive studies of dietary patterns. While you can encourage the public to stop smoking, it is not possible to tell them to stop eating.

The idea that somehow diet and lifestyle could impact the collection of deadly diseases comprising cancer has for decades seemed unlikely to the oncology and general medical communities, which continue to this day to emphasize screening for prevention and early treatment as a sort of prevention. In common with the diabetes and cardiology communities, only minimal attention is given to primary prevention through lifestyle change. Until the 1980s, the only government guidelines on nutrition for cancer patients emphasized restoring lost body weight in patients with advanced cancer and weight loss by recommending high-calorie foods and intravenous nutrition. The idea of encouraging some cancer patients to lose weight was not even considered.

It was the rediscovery of the impact of obesity on cancer, which had first been identified in the 1930s, that spurned a renewal of research efforts on nutrition in animal models of breast cancer and other obesity-associated cancers (Kritchevsky 1997). The prevalent view that high-fat diets were the sole cause of obesity led to several large trials in breast cancer patients, including the Women's Health Initiative (Prentice et al. 2006) and the Women's Intervention Nutrition Study (Chlebowski et al. 1992), which concentrated on lowering dietary fat without addressing the other causes of obesity, including refined carbohydrates, hidden sugar, and sedentary lifestyles. When these studies were proposed, there was controversy on the use of federal funds for such "soft science" coming from the biochemical nutrition community (Palmer 1986). When these expensive clinical trials failed to show a benefit, a general cooling of interest in nutrition and cancer followed at the National Institutes of Health and the National Cancer Institute. It was only the efforts of the public through prominent donors and nonprofit foundations such as the Prostate Cancer Foundation that kept dietary risk factors in the public eye (Lohse et al. 2016).

Primary care practices are conscious of the relation of obesity to type 2 diabetes, hypertension, pulmonary diseases, and heart disease. However, there is still a lack of understanding among many of the impact of obesity, poor-quality diets, and sedentary lifestyle on the risk of common forms of cancer. In this chapter, we review those risk factors and their impact on cancer, emphasizing not only weight management but also the role of phytonutrients from colorful fruits and vegetables and spices, which are also part of the solution to the obesity epidemic.

18.2 NUTRITION AND PHYSICAL ACTIVITY AS RISK FACTORS

Nutrition and physical activity are the most modifiable risk factors for the prevention of common forms of cancer other than smoking cessation (Lohse et al. 2016). Around the world, an estimated 11 million people are diagnosed each year with cancer, and nearly 7 million people are recorded as dying from cancer. Projections for 2030 predict that these figures will double. Cancer is increasing at rates faster than the increase in global population, in part due to the aging of the world's population (DeSantis et al. 2014).

As a result of the export of Western dietary habits and urbanization, obesity and cancer are becoming more common in high-income but also in middle-income and low-income countries. The global epidemic of obesity and the nutritional changes and sedentary lifestyles that cause obesity are associated with dietary patterns that have characteristics likely to promote the development of common forms of cancer, such as breast cancer and prostate cancer. The World Health Organization noted some years ago that for the first time in human history, there are more overweight than underweight individuals in the world (Vandevijvere et al. 2015). As treatments for these cancers improved and screening caught prostate and breast cancers at an earlier curable stage, a growing population of cancer survivors developed. For those individuals where obesity was a risk factor for the development of their cancer, they often ultimately die not of the cancer, but of complications of diabetes and heart disease (Demark-Wahnefried et al. 2015).

Human diets have moved away from plant-based origins that dominated our food supply for tens of thousands of years to a diet based on processed foods with greater amounts of sugar, fat, and calories than ever consumed in human history, but also with a lack of antioxidant phytonutrients, vitamins, and minerals that may help to prevent common forms of cancer. Processed snack foods and soft drinks became ever present in American diets over the last 50 years through the efforts of the media and advertisers encouraging people to eat when they are not hungry. It is clear that some methods of food production, processing, preservation, and preparation influence the development of some cancers. The consumption of colorful antioxidant-rich fruits and vegetables, and spices is associated with a reduced incidence of cancer, and only recently have these habits received more attention from segments of the public. Nonetheless, 80% of Americans fail to eat the five to nine servings of fruits and vegetables recommended by the National Cancer Institute (Sangita et al. 2013).

Evidence has also been developed that physical activity and resulting changes in body composition can impact the risk of a number of cancers, suggesting that bioenergetics is another factor determining cancer risk and tumor development (Hoffman 2016). As far back as the 1970s, evidence began to develop that obesity and excess body fat through effects of hormones could increase the risk of common forms of cancer, most notably breast, prostate, and colon cancer (Lipsett 1975).

Since obesity measured by body mass index (BMI) is a surrogate for increased body fat, the impact of diet and lifestyle on body composition and fat distribution were linked to increased risks of cancer. In this regard, visceral fat emerged as the key element in mediating the increased risks associated with obesity through its association with the secretion of inflammatory cytokines called adipokines (Moran Pascual et al. 2016). Common forms of cancer are age-related chronic diseases that share some pathogenic mechanisms, including oxidant stress and inflammation with heart disease and diabetes. This realization was a departure from the view that cancer was strictly a disease of the genome that could only be affected by pharmacological intervention. The realization that nutrition affects gene expression through epigenetics and immune function through the microbiome has breathed new energy into nutrition and cancer research.

The evidence that diet and lifestyle are risk factors for common forms of cancer has developed over decades from a combination of observational studies in populations, extensive studies in experimental model systems including animals, and a limited number of human intervention studies. Due to the interactive effects of multiple components of the Western diet pattern, studies of nutrition and cancer prevention are more complex than studies examining smoking and cancer. From 1991 until 2006, our group at the University of California, Los Angeles (UCLA) was fortunate to be one of only two National Cancer Institute-funded clinical nutrition research units in the nation charged to promote interdisciplinary research, education, training, and public awareness of the relationships of nutrition to cancer development. This center grant fostered research on nutrition and common forms of cancer through government and private foundation funding that led to some of the earliest published research on nutrition intervention in prostate cancer (Li et al. 2008). The evolution of our understanding of the impact of obesity and phytonutrients was developed through many other studies in our laboratories and others, including some of the first studies of the effects of pomegranate juice polyphenols in prostate cancer in both animal models and humans (Pantuck et al. 2015).

18.3 RISK FACTORS VERSUS STATISTICAL BAD LUCK AND CANCER RISK

Many patients, medical oncologists, and primary care providers simply view cancer as "bad luck," which supposes that nutrition and physical activity have little relationship to cancer risk. If this were true, then eating as much of anything that tastes good, regardless of fat, sugar, or salt content, and remaining sedentary would be justified in terms of cancer risk reduction.

A controversial paper by two esteemed scientists in a high-impact, widely read, and credible scientific journal demonstrated a statistical correlation between the number of stem cell divisions in an organ and the lifetime cancer risk in that organ. They argued that diet and lifestyle played a lesser role in cancer than mutations to DNA in dividing stem cells (Tomasetti and Vogelstein 2015). Stem cells are renewing cells, and their number differs in different tissues. The idea that random mutations in the DNA of dividing stem cells is the cause of the majority of age-related cancers has been interpreted to indicate that environmental and hereditary factors combined explain only one-third of cancers and deserve less emphasis (Witte and Allen 2000). However, this argument is methodologically flawed and has been widely criticized on technical bases too esoteric to repeat here. In summary, these counterarguments point out that the pool of dividing stem cells is the substrate on which risk factors act, and so risk factors deserve attention. Risk factors and proliferation rates are not independent, but interact to increase cancer risk (Coleman et al. 2010; Gotay et al. 2015; O'Callaghan 2015; Potter and Prentice 2015; Song and Giovannucci 2015; Weinberg and Zaykin 2015; Wild et al. 2015).

The cancers illustrated to represent lifetime risk as the result of mutations in dividing stems cell are all susceptible to risk factors common in the United States, including obesity, physical inactivity, tobacco, alcohol, diet, and infectious agents. There is little evidence that a cancer would exceed a substantial rate, greater than a 1% lifetime risk, in the absence of an important risk factor. In organs with low stem cell divisions, the lifetime cancer risk will typically be very low. The major types and most abundant cancers arise from tissues that have relatively high stem cell division rates and a high prevalence of strong relevant risk factors. The exception to this rule is prostate cancer, which has a small stem cell population that divides slowly.

There are many known risk factors (Table 18.1) that can influence cancer incidence, including age, gender, overweight and obesity, ethnic origin, geographic location, susceptibility genes modified by diet and lifestyle, and exposure to carcinogens, including chemical, physical, and infectious viruses or bacteria. For breast cancer, age at menarche, parity, hormonal status, and lactation are important risk factors likely mediated through effects of reproductive hormones, but also significantly modified by nutrition and obesity.

At autopsy, approximately 40% of women between 40 and 49 years of age have occult breast cancers (Nielsen et al. 1987), yet breast cancer is diagnosed in only 2% of women of this age. Similarly, prostate cancer has been found in 24% of men age 60–70 years (Sanchez-Chapado et al. 2003) yet is diagnosed in only 8% of these men. By age 90, it is estimated that 80–90% of men will have pathologically detectable but clinically undetectable prostate cancer. At surgery for prostatectomy, 98% of prostate glands have evidence of inflammation pathologically, as well as the frequent occurrence of a precancerous pathology called proliferative inflammatory neoplasia (PIN). In women with breast cancer, the precancerous form is called ductal carcinoma in situ (DCIS). It is also estimated that microscopic thyroid cancers are present in 98% of individuals by the age of 70 years (Harach et al. 1985; Black and Welch 1993), yet these cancers become clinically significant in less than 0.5% of these individuals. Pathologists have renamed some indolent thyroid cancers as hyperproliferative conditions rather than cancer. These clinically indolent, microscopic foci of cancers are likely due to the inability of the tumor itself to trigger angiogenesis, tumor-promoting inflammation, and suppression of immune surveillance (Albini et al. 2012) within the tumor microenvironment (Albini and Sporn 2007; Hanahan and Weinberg 2011). It is often difficult to identify

TABLE 18.1
Risk Factors

Unmodifiable Risk Factors	Modifiable Risk Factors	Treatable Risk Factors
Age	Tobacco	Chronic inflammation
Genetics	Overweight and obesity	Viral infections
Hereditary and mutations	Diet quality	Bacterial infections
Gender	Physical activity	Diabetes
Ethnicity	Exposure to carcinogens	Irradiation
Family history	Alcohol	Hormonal status
Geographic location	Lactation	

Source: Adapted from Albini, A. et al., *J. Natl. Cancer Inst.*, 107(10), 2015.

patients with precancerous lesions in adequate numbers to perform nutrition intervention studies, and often such patients have surgery or other forms of therapy to rid themselves of such lesions and would not participate in nutrition trials in any case. Given these difficulties, much information on nutritional risk factors comes from epidemiology and basic research rather than clinical trials.

Tumorigenesis describes the process that occurs in the period between the original mutation of DNA and when a tumor is formed (Figure 18.1). A mutation of nuclear DNA that is acquired or inherited is the transformation of a normal cell into a precancerous cell. From there to the development of a clinically detectable tumor from these transformed cells requires growth promotion to a detectable size and the development of a blood supply to feed the tumor through the process of angiogenesis, which is stimulated by inflammation.

However, the tumor microenvironment is also an integral, essential part of tumorigenesis (Figure 18.2). In fact, the microenvironment often mediates and amplifies the influence of nutritional and

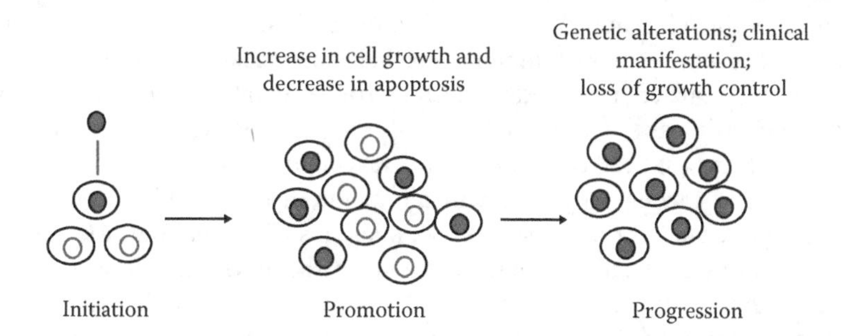

FIGURE 18.1 **(See color insert.)** Tumorigenesis is a multistep process initiated with mutation of genes that control cell cycle, cell differentiation, apoptosis, and DNA repair. Once the cancer stem cells are established, the tumor mass grows as angiogenesis provides the critical blood supply to the tumor. Once the tumor mass is clinically detected, the phase of progression leading to metastasis begins. The typical tumor develops over a window of 10–15 years, providing an opportunity for prevention prior to the formation of a clinically detectable tumor. Overexpression of oncogenes and failure of expression of tumor suppressor genes in tumor cells have been implicated in this process.

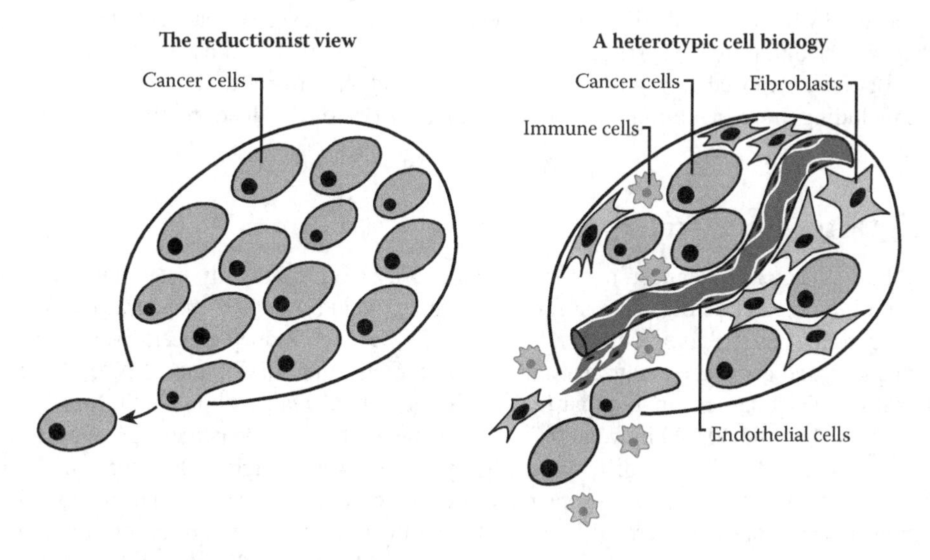

FIGURE 18.2 **(See color insert.)** Much research is done on isolated cancer cells in culture, but the tumor microenvironment is complex and may mediate effects of bioactive substances not found in pure cell culture. Nutrition may impact tumor growth by inhibiting angiogenesis or altering immune function. (Reprinted from Hanahan, D., and Weinberg, R. A., *Cell*, 100(1), 57–70, 2000.)

environmental risk factors. Therefore, it is necessary to consider not just the biology of the cancer cell but also the influence of the surrounding tumor microenvironment. The stromal, inflammatory, and endothelial cells have crucial roles in the developing tumor and might account for different tumor risk even in the presence of the same amount of dividing stem cells (Baker 2015). Chronic inflammation is linked to carcinogenesis (de Visser et al. 2006; Noonan et al. 2008). Immune, endothelial, and stromal cells in the microenvironment that normally maintain homeostasis can act to promote transformed cell survival and replication. The microenvironment can be a primary factor in determining whether stem cells after a transformation event will continue to grow and become a cancer or remain as a microhyperplasia or even be cleared by the immune system. Epigenetics, which defines changes due to methylation or histone acetylation affecting gene expression while the DNA base sequence remains constant, can be modified by nutritional factors. Epigenetics also appears to play a key role in permitting a mutated cell to become a tumor or remain in an indolent state (Burgio and Migliore 2015). Therefore, bad luck may be prevented by protecting the tumor microenvironment, curbing inflammation, or stimulating antitumor adaptive immune responses, as can be seen from the recent success of immune blockade anticancer drugs (Pardoll 2012).

The health impact of cancers is related to mortality rather than incidence, and the cancer survivor population is increasing as the result of improved screening, prevention, and treatment. Certain common tumors, such as basal cell carcinoma, have very high survival rates. Among 300,000 men diagnosed with prostate cancer, only 10% will die of the disease, while most will die of heart disease and other age-related chronic diseases. So, a key insight is that the risk factors promoting cancer need to be addressed even after diagnosis and treatment, as they may affect survival and, in some instances, tumor cell behavior and clinical recurrence. Proving the latter in clinical trials is a challenge that will require significant amounts of clinical research. Pancreatic carcinomas are diagnosed very late in their course and are often rapidly fatal, but there are some common risk factors for pancreatic cancer that have been identified that could be applied earlier as better surrogate biomarkers for prostate cancer are identified. Only 10–15% of cancers are due to inherited susceptibility genes by most estimates, suggesting that diet and environment influence clinical cancer, even though it is difficult to demonstrate that influence.

It is important to determine whether a cancer is present, but it is even more important to determine whether and when it will become clinically meaningful to the patient. Some individuals leading a healthy lifestyle will still be diagnosed with cancer because of bad luck, but on the average, they will be diagnosed less frequently with common cancers than those leading an unhealthy lifestyle or those exposed to known carcinogens. Therefore, efforts to address modifiable risk factors, including those involving diet and physical activity, are worth addressing in primary care practice.

18.3.1 Obesity and Cancer

Among the risk factors for cancer, overweight and obesity are prominently listed. Obesity is associated with increased risks of common forms of cancer, including postmenopausal breast cancer, advanced prostate cancer, colorectal cancer, endometrial cancer, kidney cancer, liver cancer, gallbladder cancer, and esophageal cancer. National Cancer Institute Surveillance, Epidemiology, and End Results (SEER) data estimated that in 2007 in the United States, about 34,000 new cases of cancer in men (4%) and 50,500 in women (7%) were due to obesity. The percentage of cases attributed to obesity varied widely for different cancer types, but was as high as 40% for some cancers, particularly endometrial cancer and esophageal adenocarcinoma. By 2030, assuming continuation of existing trends in obesity, there will be about 500,000 additional cases of cancer in the United States attributable to obesity. This analysis also found that if every adult reduced their BMI by 1%, which would be equivalent to a weight loss of roughly 1 kg, or 2.2 pounds, for an adult of average weight, this would prevent the increase in the number of cancer cases due to obesity and actually result in a reduction in cancer incidence of about 100,000 new cases per year. While these statistical estimates are only approximate and lifestyle changes should clearly result in more than a 1 kg weight loss, this calculation indicates the importance of weight management in cancer control.

The BMI associations with common forms of cancer may only be the tip of the iceberg for two reasons (IARC Working Group on the Evaluation of Carcinogenic Risks to Humans 2010). First, there are major ethnic differences in the correlation of BMI and visceral fat, especially among Asians and South Asians. In the normal BMI range of 20–25 kg/m^2, men and women in Asia have been found to have an increased risk of type 2 diabetes, which is related to increased visceral fat. Using MRI, studies in London found that 45% of women and 60% of men had excess visceral fat at normal BMI and normal waist circumference. Obesity in association with Western diets also has a number of other characteristics beyond simply excess energy. These include excess fat, sugar, and salt intake in processed foods, together with inadequate fiber intake and intakes of fruits and vegetables of only two to three servings per day, resulting in suboptimal consumption of antioxidant phytonutrients.

It is the multiple mechanisms integrated within a poor-quality diet and a sedentary lifestyle that combine to make obesity the nutritional risk factor most strongly associated with an increased risk of cancer, excluding nutritional toxins such as aflatoxin from moldy nuts and grains. Studies of individual nutrients, such as fat and sugar, studied in isolation have been disappointing. Human fat cells contain the enzyme aromatase, which converts adrenal androgens into estrogens. For postmenopausal women, the fat is the primary source of estrogen, and numerous studies have established that obese women have increased production of estrogen and increased blood levels of estrogens. Uterine cancer and breast cancer are known to be estrogen responsive, so increased estrogen from excess body fat is considered a risk factor for postmenopausal breast cancer. Excess body fat is also associated with increased levels of insulin and insulin-like growth factor 1 (IGF-1) due to insulin resistance. IGF-1 in experimental models increases the growth of a number of different cancers, including breast and prostate cancer. Fat cells also produce pro-inflammatory cytokines called adipokines that can stimulate tumor cell growth. Excess abdominal visceral fat causes a chronic low-level inflammation, which has been associated with increased cancer risk as well.

18.3.2 Alcohol

According to the National Institute on Alcohol Abuse and Alcoholism, an alcoholic drink in the United States contains 14 g of pure alcohol or ethanol. Generally, this amount of pure alcohol is found in 12 ounces of beer, 8 ounces of malt liquor, 5 ounces of wine, or 1.5 ounces of 80-proof liquor. The federal government's dietary guidelines define moderate alcohol drinking as up to one drink per day for women and up to two drinks per day for men. Heavy alcohol drinking is defined as having more than three drinks on any day or more than seven drinks per week for women, and more than four drinks on any day or more than 14 drinks per week for men. Alcohol is not calorie-free and contributes to obesity. A typical beer is 220 calories, and a light beer has about 110 calories/12 ounces. Wine has about 90 calories/5 ounce serving, and this is about the same number of calories as 1.5 ounces of hard liquor. In addition to the calories associated with alcohol, drinking excessive amounts of alcohol can lower the ability to control overall calorie intake at a meal.

Based on extensive research, there is a scientific consensus for a connection between alcohol consumption and several types of cancer (IARC Working Group on the Evaluation of Carcinogenic Risks to Humans 2010, 2012). The National Toxicology Program of the U.S. Department of Health and Human Services lists consumption of alcoholic beverages as a known human carcinogen. The research evidence indicates that both the amount of alcohol consumed and the number of years of regular alcohol consumption contribute to the risk of developing an alcohol-associated cancer. Based on data from 2009, an estimated 3.5% of all cancer deaths in the United States (about 19,500 deaths) were alcohol related (Nelson et al. 2013).

Clear patterns have emerged between alcohol consumption and a number of common forms of cancer. People who consume 50 g or more of alcohol per day, which is about 3½ or more drinks per day, have a two to three times greater risk of developing cancer of the head and neck, including the mouth, pharynx, and larynx, than nondrinkers (Baan et al. 2007). Moreover, the risks of these cancers are substantially higher among persons who consume this amount of alcohol and also use tobacco (Hashibe et al. 2009). Alcohol consumption is a major risk factor for esophageal squamous cell carcinoma (IARC Working Group on the Evaluation of Carcinogenic Risks to Humans 2012). In addition, people who inherit a deficiency in an enzyme that metabolizes alcohol have been found to have substantially increased risks of alcohol-related esophageal squamous cell carcinoma.

There are a number of other forms of cancer where alcohol consumption increases risk. Alcohol consumption is an independent risk factor for, and a primary cause of, liver cancer (Grewal and Viswanathen 2012). Population studies have demonstrated the association between alcohol consumption and the risk of breast cancer in women. These studies have consistently found increased risks of breast cancer associated with increasing alcohol intake. A meta-analysis of numerous studies, including 58,000 women with breast cancer, estimated that women who drank more than 45 g of alcohol/day, or about three drinks, had a 50% greater risk of developing breast cancer than nondrinkers (Hamajima et al. 2002). The Million Women Study in the United Kingdom, including more than 28,000 women with breast cancer, estimated that for every 10 g of alcohol consumed per day, there was a 12% increase in the risk of breast cancer (Allen et al. 2009). Alcohol consumption is associated with a modestly increased risk of colorectal cancer (Fedirko et al. 2011).

18.4 PHYTONUTRIENTS FROM FRUITS, VEGETABLES, AND SPICES

Phytonutrients are sometimes called phytochemicals, because some scientists focus on the potential toxicity of these compounds. In the amounts found in fruits, vegetables, and culinary spices, there are no toxic effects demonstrated. These compounds are aggressively metabolized by the same enzymes in the liver that detoxify drugs, and increased amounts in a reasonable range induce more enzyme activity for the metabolism and excretion of phytonutrients. These compounds are naturally found in fruits, vegetables, grains, and other plant products and are often responsible for distinct plant characteristics, such as color pigmentation and smell.

Basic studies have revealed that these compounds are able to affect cell proliferation and cell cycle regulation, and usually participate in multiple signaling pathways, which are often disrupted in tumor initiation, proliferation, and propagation (Surh 2003; Murakami 2009; Lee et al. 2011; Priyadarsini and Nagini 2012; Howes and Simmonds 2014). Although prior observations have resulted in many successful preclinical studies, only a limited number of clinical trials have been carried out (Surh 2003). Many of the investigators have attributed an inability to detect preventive effects to the variable bioavailability and distribution of compounds, and that the appreciable risk reduction may take several years to detect in large population studies. As global cancer incidence continues to rise, understanding the impact of these dietary modifications may fuel simple and inexpensive ways to improve health worldwide.

Clearly, eating more fruits and vegetables is an aspect of effective lifestyle modification for weight management while also providing phytonutrients and increasing the antioxidant and anti-inflammatory properties of the diet by comparison with diets not containing fruits, vegetables, and spices. One effective tool for educating patients on ways to enhance their intake of a variety of phytonutrients is to point out that the colors of fruits and vegetables represent families of phytonutrients (Heber and Bowerman 2001).

18.5 ANTIOXIDANT SUPPLEMENTS

Oxidative stress reflects an imbalance between the production of reactive oxygen species (ROS) and an adequate antioxidant defense. Due to the unchecked dramatic cell proliferation of cancer cells, higher amounts of ROS are produced with increased proliferation and a low level of intracellular oxidants have been shown to stimulate cancer cell proliferation (Palozza et al. 2010; Lee et al. 2011;

Ono et al. 2015; Tong et al. 2015). Numerous endogenous antioxidants are produced in the body to help neutralize ROS, and external sources of antioxidants from fruits, vegetables, and spices may also contribute to antioxidant defense, especially with aging, as endogenous oxidant stress is increased (Chlebowski et al. 1992; Tokarz and Blasiak 2014).

Since dietary interventions are more difficult and expensive, the first attempts to demonstrate the effects of antioxidant phytonutrients were carried out with dietary supplements. Lycopene; β-carotene; vitamins A, C, and E; selenium; and other purified micronutrients outside their normal food matrix have been broadly studied in humans for preventing common forms of cancer. Preclinical studies have shown that antioxidants are capable of preventing cellular damage induced by free ROS, suggesting that cancer development may be slowed in the setting of increased levels of dietary exogenous or endogenous antioxidant supplements (Glasauer and Chandel 2014; Key et al. 2015). However, these studies and the clinical trials on which they are based could not duplicate the food matrix and dietary patterns where these phytonutrients are found. Therefore, it is not surprising that many did not demonstrate preventive effects. The early so-called negative results of these studies have been used to minimize the impact of nutrition in cancer prevention, but there is much to be learned on how to conduct such studies in the future.

One of the most infamous early trials was the Carotene and Retinol Efficacy Trial (CARET), which examined the effects of daily supplementation with β-carotene and retinol on the incidence of lung cancer in smokers, and showed that both β-carotene (15 mg) and retinol (25,000 IU) daily supplementation was associated with increased lung cancer and increased overall mortality (Albanes et al. 1996; Ilic et al. 2011). Prior to the study, it was known that smoking affected the metabolism of β-carotene, and the dose selection was partly based on the ability of the chromatographs at that time to detect β-carotene. Furthermore, β-carotene in early population studies was often taken as the biomarker of overall antioxidant intake, which is clearly a flawed concept. The adverse effects in the CARET persisted up to 6 years after supplementation ended, as reported in an updated study, with the caveat that the higher risk of lung cancer and all-cause mortality was no longer statistically significant (Etminan et al. 2004; Goodman et al. 2004).

The Linxian trial showed that a combination of 15 mg of β-carotene, 30 mg of α-tocopherol, and 50 μg of selenium daily for 5 years initially showed a lower mortality risk from gastric cancer but not esophageal cancer. The study also concluded that polyphenols did not affect the risk of developing either gastric or esophageal cancer (Blot et al. 1993; Abdull Razis and Noor 2013). A new report 10 years later analyzing those who took this antioxidant supplementation compared with placebo failed to show a persistent reduced risk of mortality (Qiao et al. 2009; H. Wang et al. 2012).

Trials that have failed to show clinical significance of antioxidant therapy in cancer prevention have been performed in a variety of other models. β-Carotene and/or α-tocopherol has failed to show an effect on the incidence of lung cancer and other cancers, including urothelial, pancreatic, colorectal, and digestive tract cancers (The Alpha-Tocopherol, Beta Carotene Cancer Prevention Study Group 1994; Rautalahti et al. 1999; Virtamo et al. 2000; Wright et al. 2007; Mukherjee et al. 2008; Link et al. 2010; Mansuy 2011; X. Wang et al. 2012). Expanding this to other supplements has also yielded mixed results. Clinical studies of α-tocopherol (400 IU) and/or vitamin C (500 mg) in combination versus placebo did not reduce the incidence of prostate cancer or other cancers, including lymphoma, leukemia, melanoma, lung, bladder, pancreas, or colorectal cancers, in male U.S. physicians older than 50 years of age for a median of 7.6 years of follow-up (Gaziano et al. 2009; Wang et al. 2014). The authors also concluded after the trial that after a mean of 10.3 years of follow-up, α-tocopherol and vitamin C supplementation had no immediate or long-term detectable effects on the risk of total or site-specific cancers (Wang et al. 2014).

Differences in chemical composition of naturally occurring antioxidants in food compared with those purified into supplements may contribute to the failure to see positive impacts of antioxidant supplementation. Vitamin E is naturally found in eight different forms, called α-, β-, λ-, and δ-tocopherols and -tocotrienols, in nature but are usually studied in supplements only as α-tocopherol (Vance et al. 2013). In addition, studies in individuals without clinical cancer must be carried out over very long periods of time to show an effect and suffer from the same problem as antiaging studies in this regard.

18.5.1 Folic Acid

Preclinical studies have suggested that folate may have anticancer properties because of its role in DNA repair and its role in modulating S-adenosylmethionine, a universal methyl donor group for DNA methylation reactions. Therefore, several large-scale cross-sectional studies have shown that dietary folate intake may be associated with a lower risk of several cancers, including lung, breast, pancreatic, esophagus, stomach, and colorectal cancer (Lamprecht and Lipkin 2003; Tio et al. 2014). Results from large prospective studies have shown that there is a near 25% risk reduction in the risk of colorectal cancer in those with high folate intake compared with low intake. Recently, a meta-analysis of 16 prospective and 26 case-control studies demonstrated that women with higher daily dietary folate intake had a significant reduction in breast cancer risk compared with those with lower folate intake. Interestingly, despite this effect, there was no significant association between circulating folate levels and breast cancer risk (Chen et al. 2014).

18.5.2 Lycopene

Lycopene is a naturally occurring carotenoid found in many fruits and vegetables, with particularly high concentration in tomatoes and tomato-based products (Shi and Le Maguer 2000; Kaefer and Milner 2011). Lycopene localizes to the prostate gland and in preclinical studies lowers intracellular generation of ROS by augmenting proteins involved in antioxidant reactions, including superoxide dismutase-1 (SOD-1) and glutathione S-transferase Ω-1. Lycopene may also reduce oxidative stress by downregulating expression of ROS-generating proteins (Palozza et al. 2010; Rubio et al. 2013). Furthermore, lycopene has been shown to inhibit cell proliferation, induce apoptosis, and in prostate cancer models, attenuate the metastatic capacity of cancer cells (Palozza et al. 2010; Gupta et al. 2013; Rubio et al. 2013; Ono et al. 2015).

Consistent with the above experimental data, epidemiological and observational studies have linked increased consumption of lycopene-rich food with lower prostate cancer risks (Ilic et al. 2011; Butt et al. 2013; Chen et al. 2013; Fridlender et al. 2015; Key et al. 2015; Tyagi et al. 2015). In a meta-analysis of 21 observational studies, both moderate and high lycopene-rich diets were associated with lower prostate cancer incidence, 6% and 11%, respectively. Although the trend was not statistically significant, it highlighted that single interventional randomized trials are required to assess the true clinical effect (Etminan et al. 2004; Shehzad et al. 2010). A recent meta-analysis of eight randomized clinical trials showed a minor, insignificant decrease in the incidence of benign prostatic hyperplasia and prostate cancer patients compared with controls (Chen et al. 2013; Fridlender et al. 2015).

18.5.3 Glucosinolates from Cruciferous Vegetables

Glucosinolates are a group of sulfur-containing glycosides that occur in some 450 species of plants, but are primarily consumed from cruciferous vegetables such as broccoli, cabbage, brussels sprouts, and cauliflower. Many epidemiological and basic research studies have revealed that the consumption of cruciferous vegetables has substantial potential for the prevention of common forms of cancer (Abdull Razis and Noor 2013).

Glucosinolates and their derivatives, which include isothiocyanates, phenylethyl isothiocyanate, di-indolyl methane, and indole-3-carbinol, may modulate many relevant processes, such as the induction of metabolic enzymes in the liver; inhibition of inflammatory processes; modulation of cancer signaling pathways, including cellular proliferation; angiogenesis; the epithelial–mesenchymal transition; cancer stem cell self-renewal; and suppression of diverse oncogenic signaling pathways, including nuclear factor κB (NF-κB), hormone receptor, and the signal transducer and activator of transcription (Mukherjee et al. 2008; H. Wang et al. 2012; X. Wang et al. 2012). Glucosinolate derivatives have the potential to modulate epigenetic alterations, such as DNA methylation, histone modifications, noncoding microRNAs (miRNAs), regulation of polycomb group proteins, and epigenetic cofactor modifiers, all of which may contribute to carcinogenesis (Link et al. 2010; H. Wang et al. 2012).

Dietary glucosinolates are hydrolyzed by a plant enzyme called myrosinase when the vegetable is crushed, releasing the volatile metabolites, such as isothiocyanate. These compounds travel to the liver and induce phase 2 detoxifying enzymes, including glutathione S-transferases and UDP glucuronosyl transferases (UGTs). These enzymes in the liver catalyze conjugation reactions to inactivate or detoxify exogenous carcinogens and endogenous compounds, including sex steroid hormones related to cancer development (Mansuy 2011; Navarro et al. 2011; Boddupalli et al. 2012). Indole glucosinolate hydrolysis products, such as di-indolyl methane and indole-3-carbinol, also induce both phase 1 drug metabolic and phase 2 detoxifying enzymes by direct interaction with aryl-hydrocarbon receptor (AhR) or increasing the binding affinity of AhR to xenobiotic response elements (XREs) in target genes (Navarro et al. 2011).

Although there has been extensive research on dietary phytochemicals contributing to the overall understanding of glucosinolate derivatives in terms of their chemical and biological functions and beneficial effects in human health, clinical studies of human participants on the biological effects of dietary glucosinolate are lacking and limited to determining the effects of raw cruciferous vegetables or their extracts under some biological parameters (Singh and Singh 2012; Fujioka et al. 2014).

In a pilot study supported by the UCLA National Cancer Institute-funded clinical nutrition research unit in 1997, a case-control study was conducted of mainly asymptomatic subjects aged 50–74 years who underwent a screening sigmoidoscopy at either of two Southern California Kaiser Permanente medical centers during 1991–1993 (Lin et al. 1998). A total of 459 individuals had a first-time diagnosis of histologically confirmed adenomas detected by flexible sigmoidoscopy. Another 507 patients seen at the same clinics had no polyps detected. Subjects had a 45-minute in-person interview for information on various risk factors and basic demographic data and completed a 126-item food frequency questionnaire. Blood samples were used for glutathione S-transferase M1 (GSTM1) genotyping. In any normal population, approximately 50% of individuals have the null mutation, meaning that the GSTM1 enzyme is not functional.

Subjects with the highest quartile of broccoli intake (an average of 3.7 servings per week) had an odds ratio of 0.47 (95% confidence interval 0.30–0.73) for colorectal adenomas, compared with subjects who reportedly never ate broccoli. When stratified by GSTM1 genotype, a protective effect of broccoli was observed only among subjects with the GSTM1 null genotype (p for trend, 0.001; p for interaction, 0.01). The observed broccoli–GSTM1 interaction is compatible with the isothiocyanate mechanism described above. If a patient has a GSTM1 null mutation, meaning that the enzyme is inactive, they actually obtain a greater preventive benefit by eating broccoli than individuals with a functional enzyme. As the result of the absence of GSTM1 function, other glutathione S-transferases are upregulated to a greater extent, providing a greater preventive benefit of consuming glucosinolates. This mechanism was demonstrated in a metabolic ward study where cruciferous vegetables specifically upregulated a glutathione S-transferase in red blood cells (Lampe et al. 2000).

One clinical pearl is that many broccoli extracts are simply dried broccoli and have minimal levels of glucosinolate, and they cannot be cleaved to active metabolites due to the absence of myrosinase. Ongoing development of supplements with both glucosinolates and myrosinase is under evaluation currently.

18.5.4 Green Tea Polyphenols

The tea plant (*Camellia sinensis*) is cultivated in more than 30 countries. Green, black, and oolong teas are the most common varieties, all of which are derived from the leaves of the tea plant, but differ according to their manufacturing processes (Mukhtar and Ahmad 2000; Katiyar et al. 2007). Studies have shown that green tea possesses significant beneficial effects due to an abundance of monomeric catechins or epicatechins, which include (–)-epicatechin (EC), (–)-epicatechin-3-gallate (ECG), (–)-epigallocatechin (EGC), and (–)-epigallocatechin-3-gallate (EGCG) (Katiyar et al. 2007). Of these, EGCG is the major and most active ingredient of green tea polyphenols (GTPs) and is shown to have potent anticancer activities in both *in vitro* and *in vivo* models (Meeran and Katiyar 2008; Nandakumar et al. 2011). In particular, EGCG has been shown to inhibit cellular proliferation and to induce apoptosis in many cancer cell types through multiple mechanisms (Ahmad et al. 2000; Baliga et al. 2005; Meeran et al. 2006). Several elegant studies have addressed the modes of actions of various tea polyphenols, including EGCG, in cancers. Recent studies have suggested that the anticancer activity of EGCG is mediated, at least in part, through its epigenetic effects on DNA methylation and histone acetylation (Fang et al. 2003; Meeran et al. 2011; Nandakumar et al. 2011). EGCG is involved in direct inhibition of DNA methylating enzymes by forming hydrogen bonds to the active sites of the enzyme inhibiting substrate binding (Fang et al. 2003). Our group at UCLA has demonstrated that green tea but not black tea inhibited markers of oxidation and localized to the prostate gland when administered prior to prostatectomy (Henning et al. 2015). In preliminary studies, our group has also shown that the combination of quercetin and green tea extract leads to greater bioavailability of EGCG, as measured by plasma levels (P. Wang et al. 2012).

In a comprehensive study of many green teas, our group has found variations in the contents of catechins. In general, catechins are safe at doses consumed in green tea beverages (Henning et al. 2003). There have been rare reports in Europe of hepatotoxicity with highly concentrated extracts of green tea, where EGCG was concentrated far beyond the usual profile of catechins (Pillukat et al. 2014). In our research on prostate cancer patients prior to prostatectomy, we have used standardized brewed green tea (Henning et al. 2015).

If you are planning to use or recommend a green tea supplement, it is wise to use a standardized water- or alcohol-extracted green tea from a trusted supplement manufacturer or to drink tea with known amounts of catechins. As with many dietary supplements, there is no standardization required, as with drug preparations, which makes research on green tea in humans difficult.

18.6 SPICES

Spices have been consumed throughout the world as condiments for thousands of years because of their flavor, taste, and color. Spices were also used as food preservatives and as medicinal plants in folk medicine for the treatment of inflammation in various diseases. Some antioxidants from spices, such as curcumin (turmeric), eugenol (clove), and capsaicin (red pepper), have been shown in experimental model systems to control cellular oxidative stress due to their antioxidant properties and their capacity to block the production of ROS and interfere with signal transduction pathways (Kaefer and Milner 2011; Rubio et al. 2013). In addition, inflammatory mechanisms could be modulated by spice compounds such as curcumin (Gupta et al. 2013; Tyagi et al. 2015). Both epidemiological and experimental studies have demonstrated that certain spices could lower risks of some forms of cancer (Butt et al. 2013; Fridlender et al. 2015). Among spices, curcumin is one that has both basic and clinical research and will be reviewed below.

Curcumin, or turmeric (bis-α,β-unsaturated β-diketone), is a polyphenol derived from the roots of the perennial *Curcuma longa* plant, and is a gold-colored spice widely used in Indian cooking, textile dyes, and traditional Ayurvedic medicine (Shehzad et al. 2010). In recent decades, *in vitro* models have shown that curcumin inhibits the growth of a variety of cell lines by inducing cell cycle arrest and apoptosis, most importantly through pleiotropic modulation on several distinct cancer targets, including NF-κB, cyclooxygenase-2 (COX-2), tumor necrosis factor α (TNF-α), STAT-3, and cyclin D1 (Bar-Sela et al. 2010; Shehzad et al. 2010; Hasima and Aggarwal 2014; Bortel et al. 2015). Building on preclinical work, several phase 1 clinical trials have confirmed both the safety and pharmacokinetics of curcumin in patients with doses escalated up to 8 g/day, and these trials have shown measurable biological effects in patients with a variety of malignancies, including pancreatic cancer, multiple myeloma, and advanced colorectal cancer, refractory to standard chemotherapy (Sharma et al. 2001; Dhillon et al. 2008; Epelbaum et al. 2010; Yang et al. 2013).

Curcumin is preferentially distributed into the colonic mucosa compared with other tissues, leading many initial clinical studies to focus on identifying whether this compound may play a role in colorectal cancer models (Bar-Sela et al. 2010). This hypothesis was tested in patients with familial adenomatous polyposis (FAP), an inherited condition that leads to unregulated development of innumerable precancerous adenomatous growths throughout the colon, with eventual development of colorectal cancer at a young age. In one study, patients were given a combination of curcumin and quercetin (400/20 mg), a common flavonoid compound found in several supplements and foods. Compared with baseline colonoscopies performed prior to initiation of treatment, all five patients tested were found to have a decreased number of polyps and reduced polyp size after 6 months of treatment without other laboratory abnormalities and minimal adverse effects (Cruz-Correa et al. 2006). Although this study was limited and used a combination of both curcumin and quercetin, it raised awareness for future research testing the therapeutic potential of curcumin in precancerous models (Cruz-Correa et al. 2006).

18.7 MICROBIOTA METABOLISM OF PHYTONUTRIENTS AND IMMUNE FUNCTION

Polyphenols are metabolized by the gut microbiota into substances such as urolithin from pomegranate juice and phenolic acid from green tea catechins. These smaller metabolites of phytonutrients have anticancer properties *in vitro* and are an emerging area of research.

Pomegranate juice prepared by squeezing whole pomegranates contains a family of several high-molecular-weight hydrolyzable tannins, including punicalagin and punicalin, called ellagitannins, which have potential as nontoxic chemopreventive dietary agents for prostate cancer based on animal studies and some human observational studies in prostate cancer patients (Heber 2008). However, ellagitannins are not absorbed intact in the human gastrointestinal tract, but are hydrolyzed, generating different metabolites, including ellagic acid, which appears in the circulation between 30 minutes and 5 hours after consumption of pomegranate juice (Seeram et al. 2008). Through the action of human colonic microflora, ellagic acid is then partially converted into metabolites, including urolithin A. Both ellagic acid and urolithin A are absorbed, transported in the blood, conjugated in the liver, and excreted in glucuronidated form in the urine between 12 and 56 hours after pomegranate juice consumption (Cerda et al. 2005; Mertens-Talcott et al. 2006).

In vitro and mouse studies have demonstrated that pomegranate ellagitannins inhibit tumor angiogenesis (Sartippour et al. 2008), delay the transition from androgen-dependent to androgen-independent phenotype, and induce apoptosis through a NF-κB-dependent mechanism *in vitro* and in tumor tissue excised from castrated severe combined immunodeficiency mice with Los Angeles prostate cancer–human prostate cancer xenografts (Rettig et al. 2008). Previous *in vitro* studies have shown that pomegranate metabolites, ellagic acid and urolithin A, inhibit prostate cancer cell proliferation (Seeram et al. 2007; Malik et al. 2011) and affect multiple signaling pathways in several cell types (Li et al. 2005; Edderkaoui et al. 2008; Gonzalez-Sarrias et al. 2009). For instance, urolithin A decreased both activity and expression of tumor-specific cytochrome P450, CYP1B1, in a human prostate cancer cell line (Kasimsetty et al. 2009), while ellagic acid induced apoptosis via a caspase-dependent pathway (Malik et al. 2011) and cell cycle arrest involving cyclin-dependent kinase inhibitory protein p21 (Narayanan et al. 1999). Furthermore, ellagic acid showed a selective antiproliferative activity for cancer cell lines without affecting the viability of human nonneoplastic cells (Losso et al. 2004; Rocha et al. 2012).

The point of this detailed mechanistic discussion and proof of concept is simply to indicate that the gut microflora may play an active role in converting phytonutrients into smaller molecules that contribute to their cancer preventive effects. While this complicates research on phytonutrient effects, it also demonstrates the lasting effects of a single glass of pomegranate juice, since these conjugated metabolites persist for up to 48 hours after a single glass of juice (Seeram et al. 2006).

Moreover, in a study in human volunteers published in 2015, our group demonstrated that administration of pomegranate juice altered gut microbial populations and increased those producing urolithin A in individuals who were urolithin producers (Li et al. 2015). Based on urinary measurement of urolithin A, about 70% of normal subjects are producers and 30% are nonproducers. Some nonproducers can be induced to produce urolithin A through repeated administration of pomegranate juice daily for 28 days. Ongoing research is examining aspects of this phenomenon, but pomegranate polyphenols in common with green tea and cranberry juice appear to have polyphenols that change gut microbiota.

It is unlikely that the concept that metabolites are formed by microflora that have cancer preventive potential is unique to pomegranate, since we also found that consumption of green tea and black tea led to a rise in plasma and urine levels of phenolic acids as the result of microflora metabolism. These phenolic acids demonstrated antiproliferative effects on colon cancer cells (Henning et al. 2013). Emerging evidence from our lab indicates that green tea can also modify the microbiome. While prebiotics are typically fibers, there is now some consideration of classifying polyphenols as prebiotics as well.

18.8 SUMMARY

There is clearly a great deal of evidence on the impact of nutrition on the risk of common forms of cancer. The major factors are obesity, alcohol, and the lack of phytonutrients from fruits, vegetables, spices, and green tea. The modulation of immune function and inflammation by these dietary factors is mediated by the gut microflora, which metabolize phytonutrients and form recirculating substances such as phenolic acids and urolithins, which in turn are beginning to demonstrate some anticancer effects.

However, the complexity of nutritional patterns and the chemistry and biology of fruits and vegetables suggests that there is no single fruit, vegetable, or tea that would be a sole recommended cancer preventive food. Instead, a global dietary approach to achieve and maintain body composition through adequate protein and physical activity, five to nine servings of colorful fruits and vegetables, and the use of spices would be a reasonable recommendation for any patient concerned about reducing the risk of common forms of cancer. Dietary supplements should be taken with due consideration to all the factors already discussed in earlier chapters. Patients with fear of cancer are often targeted by charlatans, and the primary care practice can serve as a reasoned source for useful information on dietary supplements using the information provided in this text.

REFERENCES

Abdull Razis, A. F., and N. M. Noor. 2013. Cruciferous vegetables: Dietary phytochemicals for cancer prevention. *Asian Pac J Cancer Prev* 14 (3):1565–1570.

Ahmad, N., P. Cheng, and H. Mukhtar. 2000. Cell cycle dysregulation by green tea polyphenol epigallocatechin-3-gallate. *Biochem Biophys Res Commun* 275 (2):328–334.

Albanes, D., O. P. Heinonen, P. R. Taylor, J. Virtamo, B. K. Edwards, M. Rautalahti, A. M. Hartman et al. 1996. Alpha-tocopherol and beta-carotene supplements and lung cancer incidence in the alpha-tocopherol, beta-carotene cancer prevention study: Effects of base-line characteristics and study compliance. *J Natl Cancer Inst* 88 (21):1560–1570.

Albini, A., S. Cavuto, G. Apolone, and D. M. Noonan. 2015. Strategies to prevent "bad luck" in cancer. *J Natl Cancer Inst.* 107 (10):djv213.

Albini, A., and M. B. Sporn. 2007. The tumour microenvironment as a target for chemoprevention. *Nat Rev Cancer* 7 (2):139–147.

Albini, A., F. Tosetti, V. W. Li, D. M. Noonan, and W. W. Li. 2012. Cancer prevention by targeting angiogenesis. *Nat Rev Clin Oncol* 9 (9):498–509.

Allen, N. E., V. Beral, D. Casabonne, S. W. Kan, G. K. Reeves, A. Brown, J. Green, and Million Women Study Collaborators. 2009. Moderate alcohol intake and cancer incidence in women. *J Natl Cancer Inst* 101 (5):296–305.

The Alpha-Tocopherol, Beta Carotene Cancer Prevention Study Group. 1994. The effect of vitamin E and beta carotene on the incidence of lung cancer and other cancers in male smokers. *N Engl J Med* 330 (15):1029–1035.

Baan, R., K. Straif, Y. Grosse, B. Secretan, F. El Ghissassi, V. Bouvard, A. Altieri, V. Cogliano, and WHO International Agency for Research on Cancer Monograph Working Group. 2007. Carcinogenicity of alcoholic beverages. *Lancet Oncol* 8 (4):292–293.

Baker, S. G. 2015. A cancer theory kerfuffle can lead to new lines of research. *J Natl Cancer Inst* 107 (2):dju405.

Baliga, M. S., S. Meleth, and S. K. Katiyar. 2005. Growth inhibitory and antimetastatic effect of green tea polyphenols on metastasis-specific mouse mammary carcinoma 4T1 cells in vitro and in vivo systems. *Clin Cancer Res* 11 (5):1918–1927.

Bar-Sela, G., R. Epelbaum, and M. Schaffer. 2010. Curcumin as an anti-cancer agent: Review of the gap between basic and clinical applications. *Curr Med Chem* 17 (3):190–197.

Black, W. C., and H. G. Welch. 1993. Advances in diagnostic imaging and overestimations of disease prevalence and the benefits of therapy. *N Engl J Med* 328 (17):1237–1243.

Blot, W. J., J. Y. Li, P. R. Taylor, W. Guo, S. Dawsey, G. Q. Wang, C. S. Yang et al. 1993. Nutrition intervention trials in Linxian, China: Supplementation with specific vitamin/mineral combinations, cancer incidence, and disease-specific mortality in the general population. *J Natl Cancer Inst* 85 (18):1483–1492.

Boddupalli, S., J. R. Mein, S. Lakkanna, and D. R. James. 2012. Induction of phase 2 antioxidant enzymes by broccoli sulforaphane: Perspectives in maintaining the antioxidant activity of vitamins A, C, and E. *Front Genet* 3:7.

Bortel, N., S. Armeanu-Ebinger, E. Schmid, B. Kirchner, J. Frank, A. Kocher, C. Schiborr, S. Warmann, J. Fuchs, and V. Ellerkamp. 2015. Effects of curcumin in pediatric epithelial liver tumors: Inhibition of tumor growth and alpha-fetoprotein in vitro and in vivo involving the NFkappaB- and the beta-catenin pathways. *Oncotarget* 6 (38):40680–40691.

Burgio, E., and L. Migliore. 2015. Towards a systemic paradigm in carcinogenesis: Linking epigenetics and genetics. *Mol Biol Rep* 42 (4):777–790.

Butt, M. S., A. Naz, M. T. Sultan, and M. M. Qayyum. 2013. Anti-oncogenic perspectives of spices/herbs: A comprehensive review. *EXCLI J* 12:1043–1065.

Cerda, B., P. Periago, J. C. Espin, and F. A. Tomas-Barberan. 2005. Identification of urolithin a as a metabolite produced by human colon microflora from ellagic acid and related compounds. *J Agric Food Chem* 53 (14):5571–5576.

Chen, J., Y. Song, and L. Zhang. 2013. Lycopene/tomato consumption and the risk of prostate cancer: A systematic review and meta-analysis of prospective studies. *J Nutr Sci Vitaminol (Tokyo)* 59 (3):213–223.

Chen, P., C. Li, X. Li, J. Li, R. Chu, and H. Wang. 2014. Higher dietary folate intake reduces the breast cancer risk: A systematic review and meta-analysis. *Br J Cancer* 110 (9):2327–2338.

Chlebowski, R. T., D. Rose, I. M. Buzzard, G. L. Blackburn, W. Insull Jr., M. Grosvenor, R. Elashoff, and E. L. Wynder. 1992. Adjuvant dietary fat intake reduction in postmenopausal breast cancer patient management. The Women's Intervention Nutrition Study (WINS). *Breast Cancer Res Treat* 20 (2):73–84.

Coleman, H. A., J. P. Labrador, R. K. Chance, and G. J. Bashaw. 2010. The Adam family metalloprotease Kuzbanian regulates the cleavage of the roundabout receptor to control axon repulsion at the midline. *Development* 137 (14):2417–2426.

Cruz-Correa, M., D. A. Shoskes, P. Sanchez, R. Zhao, L. M. Hylind, S. D. Wexner, and F. M. Giardiello. 2006. Combination treatment with curcumin and quercetin of adenomas in familial adenomatous polyposis. *Clin Gastroenterol Hepatol* 4 (8):1035–1038.

Demark-Wahnefried, W., L. Q. Rogers, C. M. Alfano, C. A. Thomson, K. S. Courneya, J. A. Meyerhardt, N. L. Stout, E. Kvale, H. Ganzer, and J. A. Ligibel. 2015. Practical clinical interventions for diet, physical activity, and weight control in cancer survivors. *CA Cancer J Clin* 65 (3):167–189.

DeSantis, C. E., C. C. Lin, A. B. Mariotto, R. L. Siegel, K. D. Stein, J. L. Kramer, R. Alteri, A. S. Robbins, and A. Jemal. 2014. Cancer treatment and survivorship statistics, 2014. *CA Cancer J Clin* 64 (4):252–271.

de Visser, K. E., A. Eichten, and L. M. Coussens. 2006. Paradoxical roles of the immune system during cancer development. *Nat Rev Cancer* 6 (1):24–37.

Dhillon, N., B. B. Aggarwal, R. A. Newman, R. A. Wolff, A. B. Kunnumakkara, J. L. Abbruzzese, C. S. Ng, V. Badmaev, and R. Kurzrock. 2008. Phase II trial of curcumin in patients with advanced pancreatic cancer. *Clin Cancer Res* 14 (14):4491–4499.

Edderkaoui, M., I. Odinokova, I. Ohno, I. Gukovsky, V. L. Go, S. J. Pandol, and A. S. Gukovskaya. 2008. Ellagic acid induces apoptosis through inhibition of nuclear factor kappa B in pancreatic cancer cells. *World J Gastroenterol* 14 (23):3672–3680.

Epelbaum, R., M. Schaffer, B. Vizel, V. Badmaev, and G. Bar-Sela. 2010. Curcumin and gemcitabine in patients with advanced pancreatic cancer. *Nutr Cancer* 62 (8):1137–1141.

Etminan, M., B. Takkouche, and F. Caamano-Isorna. 2004. The role of tomato products and lycopene in the prevention of prostate cancer: A meta-analysis of observational studies. *Cancer Epidemiol Biomarkers Prev* 13 (3):340–345.

Fang, M. Z., Y. Wang, N. Ai, Z. Hou, Y. Sun, H. Lu, W. Welsh, and C. S. Yang. 2003. Tea polyphenol (–)-epigallocatechin-3-gallate inhibits DNA methyltransferase and reactivates methylation-silenced genes in cancer cell lines. *Cancer Res* 63 (22):7563–7570.

Fedirko, V., I. Tramacere, V. Bagnardi, M. Rota, L. Scotti, F. Islami, E. Negri et al. 2011. Alcohol drinking and colorectal cancer risk: An overall and dose-response meta-analysis of published studies. *Ann Oncol* 22 (9):1958–1972.

Food and Drug Administration, Department of Health and Human Services. 2016. Deeming tobacco products to be subject to the Federal Food, Drug, and Cosmetic Act, as amended by the Family Smoking Prevention and Tobacco Control Act; restrictions on the sale and distribution of tobacco products and required warning statements for tobacco products. Final rule. *Fed Regist* 81 (90):28973–29106.

Fridlender, M., Y. Kapulnik, and H. Koltai. 2015. Plant derived substances with anti-cancer activity: From folklore to practice. *Front Plant Sci* 6:799.

Fujioka, N., C. E. Ainslie-Waldman, P. Upadhyaya, S. G. Carmella, V. A. Fritz, C. Rohwer, Y. Fan, D. Rauch, C. Le, D. K. Hatsukami, and S. S. Hecht. 2014. Urinary 3,3′-diindolylmethane: A biomarker of glucobrassicin exposure and indole-3-carbinol uptake in humans. *Cancer Epidemiol Biomarkers Prev* 23 (2):282–287.

Gardner, M. N., and A. M. Brandt. 2006. "The doctors' choice is America's choice": The physician in US cigarette advertisements, 1930–1953. *Am J Public Health* 96 (2):222–232.

Gaziano, J. M., R. J. Glynn, W. G. Christen, T. Kurth, C. Belanger, J. MacFadyen, V. Bubes, J. E. Manson, H. D. Sesso, and J. E. Buring. 2009. Vitamins E and C in the prevention of prostate and total cancer in men: The Physicians' Health Study II randomized controlled trial. *JAMA* 301 (1):52–62.

Glasauer, A., and N. S. Chandel. 2014. Targeting antioxidants for cancer therapy. *Biochem Pharmacol* 92 (1):90–101.

Gonzalez-Sarrias, A., J. C. Espin, F. A. Tomas-Barberan, and M. T. Garcia-Conesa. 2009. Gene expression, cell cycle arrest and MAPK signalling regulation in Caco-2 cells exposed to ellagic acid and its metabolites, urolithins. *Mol Nutr Food Res* 53 (6):686–698.

Goodman, G. E., M. D. Thornquist, J. Balmes, M. R. Cullen, F. L. Meyskens Jr., G. S. Omenn, B. Valanis, and J. H. Williams Jr. 2004. The Beta-Carotene and Retinol Efficacy Trial: Incidence of lung cancer and cardiovascular disease mortality during 6-year follow-up after stopping beta-carotene and retinol supplements. *J Natl Cancer Inst* 96 (23):1743–1750.

Gotay, C., T. Dummer, and J. Spinelli. 2015. Cancer risk: Prevention is crucial. *Science* 347 (6223):728.

Grewal, P., and V. A. Viswanathen. 2012. Liver cancer and alcohol. *Clin Liver Dis* 16 (4):839–850.

Gupta, S. C., B. Sung, J. H. Kim, S. Prasad, S. Li, and B. B. Aggarwal. 2013. Multitargeting by turmeric, the golden spice: From kitchen to clinic. *Mol Nutr Food Res* 57 (9):1510–1528.

Hamajima, N., K. Hirose, K. Tajima, T. Rohan, E. E. Calle, C. W. Heath Jr., R. J. Coates et al. 2002. Alcohol, tobacco and breast cancer—Collaborative reanalysis of individual data from 53 epidemiological studies, including 58,515 women with breast cancer and 95,067 women without the disease. *Br J Cancer* 87 (11):1234–1245.

Hanahan, D., and R. A. Weinberg. 2000. The hallmarks of cancer. *Cell* 100 (1):57–70.

Hanahan, D., and R. A. Weinberg. 2011. Hallmarks of cancer: The next generation. *Cell* 144 (5):646–674.

Harach, H. R., K. O. Franssila, and V. M. Wasenius. 1985. Occult papillary carcinoma of the thyroid. A "normal" finding in Finland. A systematic autopsy study. *Cancer* 56 (3):531–538.

Hashibe, M., P. Brennan, S. C. Chuang, S. Boccia, X. Castellsague, C. Chen, M. P. Curado et al. 2009. Interaction between tobacco and alcohol use and the risk of head and neck cancer: Pooled analysis in the International Head and Neck Cancer Epidemiology Consortium. *Cancer Epidemiol Biomarkers Prev* 18 (2):541–550.

Hasima, N., and B. B. Aggarwal. 2014. Targeting proteasomal pathways by dietary curcumin for cancer prevention and treatment. *Curr Med Chem* 21 (14):1583–1594.

Heber, D. 2008. Multitargeted therapy of cancer by ellagitannins. *Cancer Lett* 269 (2):262–268.

Heber, D., and Bowerman, S. 2001. Applying science to changing dietary patterns. *J Nutr* 131:3078S–3081S.

Henning, S. M., C. Fajardo-Lira, H. W. Lee, A. A. Youssefian, V. L. Go, and D. Heber. 2003. Catechin content of 18 teas and a green tea extract supplement correlates with the antioxidant capacity. *Nutr Cancer* 45 (2):226–235.

Henning, S. M., P. Wang, N. Abgaryan, R. Vicinanza, D. M. de Oliveira, Y. Zhang, R. P. Lee, C. L. Carpenter, W. J. Aronson, and D. Heber. 2013. Phenolic acid concentrations in plasma and urine from men consuming green or black tea and potential chemopreventive properties for colon cancer. *Mol Nutr Food Res* 57 (3):483–493.

Henning, S. M., P. Wang, J. W. Said, M. Huang, T. Grogan, D. Elashoff, C. L. Carpenter, D. Heber, and W. J. Aronson. 2015. Randomized clinical trial of brewed green and black tea in men with prostate cancer prior to prostatectomy. *Prostate* 75 (5):550–559.

Hoffman, A. J. 2016. The impact of physical activity for cancer prevention: Implications for nurses. *Semin Oncol Nurs* 32 (3):255–272.

Howes, M. J., and M. S. Simmonds. 2014. The role of phytochemicals as micronutrients in health and disease. *Curr Opin Clin Nutr Metab Care* 17 (6):558–566.

Hu, T. W., H. Y. Sung, and T. E. Keeler. 1995. Reducing cigarette consumption in California: Tobacco taxes vs an anti-smoking media campaign. *Am J Public Health* 85 (9):1218–1222.

IARC Working Group on the Evaluation of Carcinogenic Risks to Humans. 2010. Alcohol consumption and ethyl carbamate. *IARC Monogr Eval Carcinog Risks Hum* 96:3–1383.

IARC Working Group on the Evaluation of Carcinogenic Risks to Humans. 2012. Personal habits and indoor combustions. A review of human carcinogens. *IARC Monogr Eval Carcinog Risks Hum* 100 (Pt E):1–538.

Ilic, D., K. M. Forbes, and C. Hassed. 2011. Lycopene for the prevention of prostate cancer. *Cochrane Database Syst Rev* (11):CD008007.

Kaefer, C. M., and J. A. Milner. 2011. Herbs and spices in cancer prevention and treatment. In *Herbal Medicine: Biomolecular and Clinical Aspects*, ed. I. F. F. Benzie and S. Wachtel-Galor, 361–383. Boca Raton, FL: CRC Press.

Kasimsetty, S. G., D. Bialonska, M. K. Reddy, C. Thornton, K. L. Willett, and D. Ferreira. 2009. Effects of pomegranate chemical constituents/intestinal microbial metabolites on CYP1B1 in 22Rv1 prostate cancer cells. *J Agric Food Chem* 57 (22):10636–10644.

Katiyar, S., C. A. Elmets, and S. K. Katiyar. 2007. Green tea and skin cancer: Photoimmunology, angiogenesis and DNA repair. *J Nutr Biochem* 18 (5):287–296.

Key, T. J., P. N. Appleby, R. C. Travis, D. Albanes, A. J. Alberg, A. Barricarte, A. Black et al. 2015. Carotenoids, retinol, tocopherols, and prostate cancer risk: Pooled analysis of 15 studies. *Am J Clin Nutr* 102 (5):1142–1157.

Kritchevsky, D. 1997. Caloric restriction and experimental mammary carcinogenesis. *Breast Cancer Res Treat* 46 (2–3):161–167.

Lampe, J. W., C. Chen, S. Li, J. Prunty, M. T. Grate, D. E. Meehan, K. V. Barale, D. A. Dightman, Z. Feng, and J. D. Potter. 2000. Modulation of human glutathione S-transferases by botanically defined vegetable diets. *Cancer Epidemiol Biomarkers Prev* 9 (8):787–793.

Lamprecht, S. A., and M. Lipkin. 2003. Chemoprevention of colon cancer by calcium, vitamin D and folate: Molecular mechanisms. *Nat Rev Cancer* 3 (8):601–614.

Lee, K. W., A. M. Bode, and Z. Dong. 2011. Molecular targets of phytochemicals for cancer prevention. *Nat Rev Cancer* 11 (3):211–218.

Lewis, D. R., D. P. Check, N. E. Caporaso, W. D. Travis, and S. S. Devesa. 2014. US lung cancer trends by histologic type. *Cancer* 120 (18):2883–2892.

Li, T. M., G. W. Chen, C. C. Su, J. G. Lin, C. C. Yeh, K. C. Cheng, and J. G. Chung. 2005. Ellagic acid induced p53/p21 expression, G1 arrest and apoptosis in human bladder cancer T24 cells. *Anticancer Res* 25 (2A):971–979.

Li, Z., W. J. Aronson, J. R. Arteaga, K. Hong, G. Thames, S. M. Henning, W. Liu, R. Elashoff, J. M. Ashley, and D. Heber. 2008. Feasibility of a low-fat/high-fiber diet intervention with soy supplementation in prostate cancer patients after prostatectomy. *Eur J Clin Nutr* 62 (4):526–536.

Li, Z., S. M. Henning, R. P. Lee, Q. Y. Lu, P. H. Summanen, G. Thames, K. Corbett, J. Downes, C. H. Tseng, S. M. Finegold, and D. Heber. 2015. Pomegranate extract induces ellagitannin metabolite formation and changes stool microbiota in healthy volunteers. *Food Funct* 6 (8):2487–2495.

Lin, H. J., N. M. Probst-Hensch, A. D. Louie, I. H. Kau, J. S. Witte, S. A. Ingles, H. D. Frankl, E. R. Lee, and R. W. Haile. 1998. Glutathione transferase null genotype, broccoli, and lower prevalence of colorectal adenomas. *Cancer Epidemiol Biomarkers Prev* 7 (8):647–652.

Link, A., F. Balaguer, and A. Goel. 2010. Cancer chemoprevention by dietary polyphenols: Promising role for epigenetics. *Biochem Pharmacol* 80 (12):1771–1792.
Lipsett, M. B. 1975. Hormones, nutrition, and cancer. *Cancer Res* 35 (11 Pt 2):3359–3361.
Lohse, T., D. Faeh, M. Bopp, S. Rohrmann, and Swiss National Cohort Study Group. 2016. Adherence to the cancer prevention recommendations of the World Cancer Research Fund/American Institute for Cancer Research and mortality: A census-linked cohort. *Am J Clin Nutr* 104 (3):678–685.
Losso, J. N., R. R. Bansode, A. Trappey 2nd, H. A. Bawadi, and R. Truax. 2004. In vitro anti-proliferative activities of ellagic acid. *J Nutr Biochem* 15 (11):672–678.
Malik, A., S. Afaq, M. Shahid, K. Akhtar, and A. Assiri. 2011. Influence of ellagic acid on prostate cancer cell proliferation: A caspase-dependent pathway. *Asian Pac J Trop Med* 4 (7):550–555.
Mansuy, D. 2011. Brief historical overview and recent progress on cytochromes P450: Adaptation of aerobic organisms to their chemical environment and new mechanisms of prodrug bioactivation. *Ann Pharm Fr* 69 (1):62–69.
Meeran, S. M., and S. K. Katiyar. 2008. Cell cycle control as a basis for cancer chemoprevention through dietary agents. *Front Biosci* 13:2191–2202.
Meeran, S. M., S. K. Mantena, C. A. Elmets, and S. K. Katiyar. 2006. (–)-Epigallocatechin-3-gallate prevents photocarcinogenesis in mice through interleukin-12-dependent DNA repair. *Cancer Res* 66 (10):5512–5520.
Meeran, S. M., S. N. Patel, T. H. Chan, and T. O. Tollefsbol. 2011. A novel prodrug of epigallocatechin-3-gallate: Differential epigenetic hTERT repression in human breast cancer cells. *Cancer Prev Res (Phila)* 4 (8):1243–1254.
Mertens-Talcott, S. U., P. Jilma-Stohlawetz, J. Rios, L. Hingorani, and H. Derendorf. 2006. Absorption, metabolism, and antioxidant effects of pomegranate (*Punica granatum* L.) polyphenols after ingestion of a standardized extract in healthy human volunteers. *J Agric Food Chem* 54 (23):8956–8961.
Moran Pascual, E., M. Martinez Sarmiento, A. Budia Alba, E. Broseta Rico, R. Camara Gomez, and F. Boronat Tormo. 2016. Central body fat mass measured by bioelectrical impedanciometry but not body mass index is a high-grade prostate cancer risk factor. *Urol Int* 98 (1):28–31.
Mukherjee, S., H. Gangopadhyay, and D. K. Das. 2008. Broccoli: A unique vegetable that protects mammalian hearts through the redox cycling of the thioredoxin superfamily. *J Agric Food Chem* 56 (2):609–617.
Mukhtar, H., and N. Ahmad. 2000. Tea polyphenols: Prevention of cancer and optimizing health. *Am J Clin Nutr* 71 (6 Suppl):1698S–1702S; discussion 1703S–1704S.
Murakami, A. 2009. Chemoprevention with phytochemicals targeting inducible nitric oxide synthase. *Forum Nutr* 61:193–203.
Nandakumar, V., M. Vaid, and S. K. Katiyar. 2011. (–)-Epigallocatechin-3-gallate reactivates silenced tumor suppressor genes, Cip1/p21 and p16INK4a, by reducing DNA methylation and increasing histones acetylation in human skin cancer cells. *Carcinogenesis* 32 (4):537–544.
Narayanan, B. A., O. Geoffroy, M. C. Willingham, G. G. Re, and D. W. Nixon. 1999. p53/p21(WAF1/CIP1) expression and its possible role in G1 arrest and apoptosis in ellagic acid treated cancer cells. *Cancer Lett* 136 (2):215–221.
National Center for Chronic Disease Prevention and Health Promotion, Office on Smoking and Health. 2014. The health consequences of smoking—50 years of progress: A report of the surgeon general. Atlanta, GA: Centers for Disease Control and Prevention.
Navarro, S. L., F. Li, and J. W. Lampe. 2011. Mechanisms of action of isothiocyanates in cancer chemoprevention: An update. *Food Funct* 2 (10):579–587.
Nelson, D. E., D. W. Jarman, J. Rehm, T. K. Greenfield, G. Rey, W. C. Kerr, P. Miller, K. D. Shield, Y. Ye, and T. S. Naimi. 2013. Alcohol-attributable cancer deaths and years of potential life lost in the United States. *Am J Public Health* 103 (4):641–648.
Nielsen, M., J. L. Thomsen, S. Primdahl, U. Dyreborg, and J. A. Andersen. 1987. Breast cancer and atypia among young and middle-aged women: A study of 110 medicolegal autopsies. *Br J Cancer* 56 (6):814–819.
Noonan, D. M., A. De Lerma Barbaro, N. Vannini, L. Mortara, and A. Albini. 2008. Inflammation, inflammatory cells and angiogenesis: Decisions and indecisions. *Cancer Metastasis Rev* 27 (1):31–40.
O'Callaghan, M. 2015. Cancer risk: Accuracy of literature. *Science* 347 (6223):729.
Ono, M., M. Takeshima, and S. Nakano. 2015. Mechanism of the anticancer effect of lycopene (tetraterpenoids). *Enzymes* 37:139–166.
Palmer, S. 1986. Dietary considerations for risk reduction. *Cancer* 58 (8 Suppl):1949–1953.
Palozza, P., N. Parrone, A. Catalano, and R. Simone. 2010. Tomato lycopene and inflammatory cascade: Basic interactions and clinical implications. *Curr Med Chem* 17 (23):2547–2563.

Pantuck, A. J., C. A. Pettaway, R. Dreicer, J. Corman, A. Katz, A. Ho, W. Aronson, W. Clark, G. Simmons, and D. Heber. 2015. A randomized, double-blind, placebo-controlled study of the effects of pomegranate extract on rising PSA levels in men following primary therapy for prostate cancer. *Prostate Cancer Prostatic Dis* 18 (3):242–248.

Pardoll, D. M. 2012. The blockade of immune checkpoints in cancer immunotherapy. *Nat Rev Cancer* 12 (4):252–264.

Pillukat, M. H., C. Bester, A. Hensel, M. Lechtenberg, F. Petereit, S. Beckebaum, K. M. Muller, and H. H. Schmidt. 2014. Concentrated green tea extract induces severe acute hepatitis in a 63-year-old woman—A case report with pharmaceutical analysis. *J Ethnopharmacol* 155 (1):165–170.

Potter, J. D., and R. L. Prentice. 2015. Cancer risk: Tumors excluded. *Science* 347 (6223):727.

Prentice, R. L., B. Caan, R. T. Chlebowski, R. Patterson, L. H. Kuller, J. K. Ockene, K. L. Margolis et al. 2006. Low-fat dietary pattern and risk of invasive breast cancer: The Women's Health Initiative Randomized Controlled Dietary Modification Trial. *JAMA* 295 (6):629–642.

Priyadarsini, R. V., and S. Nagini. 2012. Cancer chemoprevention by dietary phytochemicals: Promises and pitfalls. *Curr Pharm Biotechnol* 13 (1):125–136.

Qiao, Y. L., S. M. Dawsey, F. Kamangar, J. H. Fan, C. C. Abnet, X. D. Sun, L. L. Johnson et al. 2009. Total and cancer mortality after supplementation with vitamins and minerals: Follow-up of the Linxian General Population Nutrition Intervention Trial. *J Natl Cancer Inst* 101 (7):507–518.

Rautalahti, M. T., J. R. Virtamo, P. R. Taylor, O. P. Heinonen, D. Albanes, J. K. Haukka, B. K. Edwards, P. A. Karkkainen, R. Z. Stolzenberg-Solomon, and J. Huttunen. 1999. The effects of supplementation with alpha-tocopherol and beta-carotene on the incidence and mortality of carcinoma of the pancreas in a randomized, controlled trial. *Cancer* 86 (1):37–42.

Rettig, M. B., D. Heber, J. An, N. P. Seeram, J. Y. Rao, H. Liu, T. Klatte et al. 2008. Pomegranate extract inhibits androgen-independent prostate cancer growth through a nuclear factor-kappaB-dependent mechanism. *Mol Cancer Ther* 7 (9):2662–2671.

Rocha, A., L. Wang, M. Penichet, and M. Martins-Green. 2012. Pomegranate juice and specific components inhibit cell and molecular processes critical for metastasis of breast cancer. *Breast Cancer Res Treat* 136 (3):647–658.

Rubio, L., M. J. Motilva, and M. P. Romero. 2013. Recent advances in biologically active compounds in herbs and spices: A review of the most effective antioxidant and anti-inflammatory active principles. *Crit Rev Food Sci Nutr* 53 (9):943–953.

Sanchez-Chapado, M., G. Olmedilla, M. Cabeza, E. Donat, and A. Ruiz. 2003. Prevalence of prostate cancer and prostatic intraepithelial neoplasia in Caucasian Mediterranean males: An autopsy study. *Prostate* 54 (3):238–247.

Sangita, S., S. A. Vik, M. Pakseresht, and L. N. Kolonel. 2013. Adherence to recommendations for fruit and vegetable intake, ethnicity and ischemic heart disease mortality. *Nutr Metab Cardiovasc Dis* 23 (12):1247–1254.

Sartippour, M. R., N. P. Seeram, J. Y. Rao, A. Moro, D. M. Harris, S. M. Henning, A. Firouzi, M. B. Rettig, W. J. Aronson, A. J. Pantuck, and D. Heber. 2008. Ellagitannin-rich pomegranate extract inhibits angiogenesis in prostate cancer in vitro and in vivo. *Int J Oncol* 32 (2):475–480.

Seeram, N. P., W. J. Aronson, Y. Zhang, S. M. Henning, A. Moro, R. P. Lee, M. Sartippour et al. 2007. Pomegranate ellagitannin-derived metabolites inhibit prostate cancer growth and localize to the mouse prostate gland. *J Agric Food Chem* 55 (19):7732–7737.

Seeram, N. P., S. M. Henning, Y. Zhang, M. Suchard, Z. Li, and D. Heber. 2006. Pomegranate juice ellagitannin metabolites are present in human plasma and some persist in urine for up to 48 hours. *J Nutr* 136 (10):2481–2485.

Seeram, N. P., Y. Zhang, R. McKeever, S. M. Henning, R. P. Lee, M. A. Suchard, Z. Li et al. 2008. Pomegranate juice and extracts provide similar levels of plasma and urinary ellagitannin metabolites in human subjects. *J Med Food* 11 (2):390–394.

Sharma, R. A., H. R. McLelland, K. A. Hill, C. R. Ireson, S. A. Euden, M. M. Manson, M. Pirmohamed, L. J. Marnett, A. J. Gescher, and W. P. Steward. 2001. Pharmacodynamic and pharmacokinetic study of oral *Curcuma* extract in patients with colorectal cancer. *Clin Cancer Res* 7 (7):1894–1900.

Shehzad, A., F. Wahid, and Y. S. Lee. 2010. Curcumin in cancer chemoprevention: Molecular targets, pharmacokinetics, bioavailability, and clinical trials. *Arch Pharm (Weinheim)* 343 (9):489–499.

Shi, J., and M. Le Maguer. 2000. Lycopene in tomatoes: Chemical and physical properties affected by food processing. *Crit Rev Biotechnol* 20 (4):293–334.

Singh, S. V., and K. Singh. 2012. Cancer chemoprevention with dietary isothiocyanates mature for clinical translational research. *Carcinogenesis* 33 (10):1833–1842.

Song, M., and E. L. Giovannucci. 2015. Cancer risk: Many factors contribute. *Science* 347 (6223):728–729.
Surh, Y. J. 2003. Cancer chemoprevention with dietary phytochemicals. *Nat Rev Cancer* 3 (10):768–780.
Tio, M., J. Andrici, M. R. Cox, and G. D. Eslick. 2014. Folate intake and the risk of upper gastrointestinal cancers: A systematic review and meta-analysis. *J Gastroenterol Hepatol* 29 (2):250–258.
Tokarz, P., and J. Blasiak. 2014. Role of mitochondria in carcinogenesis. *Acta Biochim Pol* 61 (4):671–678.
Tomasetti, C., and B. Vogelstein. 2015. Cancer etiology. Variation in cancer risk among tissues can be explained by the number of stem cell divisions. *Science* 347 (6217):78–81.
Tong, L., C. C. Chuang, S. Wu, and L. Zuo. 2015. Reactive oxygen species in redox cancer therapy. *Cancer Lett* 367 (1):18–25.
Tyagi, A. K., S. Prasad, W. Yuan, S. Li, and B. B. Aggarwal. 2015. Identification of a novel compound (beta-sesquiphellandrene) from turmeric (*Curcuma longa*) with anticancer potential: Comparison with curcumin. *Invest New Drugs* 33 (6):1175–1186.
U.S. Public Health Service, Office of the Surgeon General. 1964. Smoking and health. Official report no. 1103. Washington, DC: U.S. Public Health Service, Office of the Surgeon General.
Vance, T. M., J. Su, E. T. Fontham, S. I. Koo, and O. K. Chun. 2013. Dietary antioxidants and prostate cancer: A review. *Nutr Cancer* 65 (6):793–801.
Vandevijvere, S., C. C. Chow, K. D. Hall, E. Umali, and B. A. Swinburn. 2015. Increased food energy supply as a major driver of the obesity epidemic: A global analysis. *Bull World Health Organ* 93 (7):446–456.
Virtamo, J., B. K. Edwards, M. Virtanen, P. R. Taylor, N. Malila, D. Albanes, J. K. Huttunen et al. 2000. Effects of supplemental alpha-tocopherol and beta-carotene on urinary tract cancer: Incidence and mortality in a controlled trial (Finland). *Cancer Causes Control* 11 (10):933–939.
Wang, H., T. O. Khor, L. Shu, Z. Y. Su, F. Fuentes, J. H. Lee, and A. N. Kong. 2012. Plants vs. cancer: A review on natural phytochemicals in preventing and treating cancers and their druggability. *Anticancer Agents Med Chem* 12 (10):1281–1305.
Wang, L., H. D. Sesso, R. J. Glynn, W. G. Christen, V. Bubes, J. E. Manson, J. E. Buring, and J. M. Gaziano. 2014. Vitamin E and C supplementation and risk of cancer in men: Posttrial follow-up in the Physicians' Health Study II randomized trial. *Am J Clin Nutr* 100 (3):915–923.
Wang, P., D. Heber, and S. M. Henning. 2012. Quercetin increased bioavailability and decreased methylation of green tea polyphenols in vitro and in vivo. *Food Funct* 3 (6):635–642.
Wang, X., J. P. de Rivero Vaccari, H. Wang, P. Diaz, R. German, A. E. Marcillo, and R. W. Keane. 2012. Activation of the nuclear factor E2-related factor 2/antioxidant response element pathway is neuroprotective after spinal cord injury. *J Neurotrauma* 29 (5):936–945.
Weinberg, C. R., and D. Zaykin. 2015. Is bad luck the main cause of cancer? *J Natl Cancer Inst* 107 (7):djv125.
Wild, C., P. Brennan, M. Plummer, F. Bray, K. Straif, and J. Zavadil. 2015. Cancer risk: Role of chance overstated. *Science* 347 (6223):728.
Witte, K., and M. Allen. 2000. A meta-analysis of fear appeals: Implications for effective public health campaigns. *Health Educ Behav* 27 (5):591–615.
Wright, M. E., J. Virtamo, A. M. Hartman, P. Pietinen, B. K. Edwards, P. R. Taylor, J. K. Huttunen, and D. Albanes. 2007. Effects of alpha-tocopherol and beta-carotene supplementation on upper aerodigestive tract cancers in a large, randomized controlled trial. *Cancer* 109 (5):891–898.
Yang, C., X. Su, A. Liu, L. Zhang, A. Yu, Y. Xi, and G. Zhai. 2013. Advances in clinical study of curcumin. *Curr Pharm Des* 19 (11):1966–1973.

19 Nutrition and the Cancer Patient

19.1 INTRODUCTION

Cancer screening and early detection of cancer are well established in primary care practice, and the follow-up care of cancer survivors is increasingly being triaged to primary care practices from oncology practices, as they are overburdened with the treatment of more cancer patients.

Primary care physicians and their multidisciplinary teams will be called on increasingly in the future to provide care to cancer patients while they are undergoing chronic treatment under the care of oncology specialists and during follow-up care. The increasing population of cancer survivors with concerns about the prevention of cancer recurrence with obesity and comorbid conditions will require lifestyle recommendations to reduce the risk of cancer recurrence.

Malnutrition in advanced cancer patients continues to be a vexing problem that contributes to morbidity and mortality. Nutrition support interventions have traditionally been used for patients with malnutrition secondary to cancer or cancer treatments. More recently, nutritional interventions including diet and lifestyle changes and dietary supplements have been studied and utilized in the primary and secondary prevention of common forms of cancer (Heber et al. 2006) and as part of the cancer treatment modality. As the number of cancer survivors who have successfully completed therapy increases, together with a growing population of patients with ongoing preventive pharmacology based on small-molecule cancer therapy (Hoelder et al. 2012), the need for nutrition counseling to decrease risk of cancer recurrence or for general health is becoming more recognized (Blanchard et al. 2008). During the emotional stress of dealing with a diagnosis, patients can derive increased quality of life and a sense of control over their lives as the result of receiving supportive advice on diet and lifestyle.

The evidence base for nutrition intervention in cancer patients is drawn from a combination of extensive epidemiological inference from association studies of the relationship of nutrition and physical activity to cancer and extensive animal studies demonstrating cellular and molecular mechanisms of the interaction. There are very limited nutrition intervention studies in humans. The general advice given for cancer prevention may also be beneficial to reduce risks of other common age-related chronic diseases, such as diabetes and heart disease. In the absence of proven benefits of nutrition intervention in this population, the interventions should be based on generally accepted macronutrient ranges according to the Institute of Medicine guidelines and be based on clinical trials that show a lack of adverse events when the nutrition interventions have been utilized. As is repeatedly emphasized here, the cancer patient is a vulnerable individual and easily subject to nutritional claims for curing cancer from unqualified and sometimes dangerous practitioners. Patient's families also read about the promise of nutrition for cancer in the popular press and must be educated as to its realistic and potential benefits, as well as limitations and potential harms, for each patient's situation.

19.2 PRIMARY CARE ONCOLOGY

The number of cancer patients presenting to primary care physicians is expected to increase, driven by the epidemic of obesity and the increased aging of the U.S. and world populations. The number of oncologists in practice over the coming decades will be inadequate to meet the demands for care by cancer patients. As cancer is converted in many cases to a chronic disease, and as the population of cancer survivors grows globally due to earlier detection and better treatments, primary care physicians and their multidisciplinary teams will be called on to deliver supportive care to cancer patients and to deliver healthy recommendations for secondary prevention to cancer survivors (Erikson et al. 2007; Warren et al. 2008).

A recent study estimated a 48% increase in the demand for oncology services, accompanied by a shortage of oncologists in the future (Warren et al. 2008). The greater involvement of primary care physicians in cancer care has been proposed as one means of addressing this shortfall (Warren et al. 2008), despite projections of a looming primary care physician shortage (Bodenheimer 2006).

While age is the primary risk factor for common forms of cancer, incidence rates, as already reviewed in Chapter 17, are influenced by diet and lifestyle. We are in the midst of a global epidemic of obesity and diabetes, which increases the risks of common forms of cancer, including prostate, breast, colon, uterine, gallbladder, liver, and pancreatic cancers. As the result of advances in screening, prevention, and treatment, there is a growing population of cancer survivors. This chapter written some 30 years ago would have concentrated solely on malnutrition in cancer. While nutrition support is still a vital need of patients with diagnosed cancer, it is also increasingly appreciated that cancer patients who have survived often contract common age-related chronic diseases. Some of the hormonal and inflammatory pathways that are important in diabetes and heart disease may also play a role in reducing tumor recurrence in survivors, but can also increase quality of life and reduce comorbid conditions.

Cancer care generally requires referral to medical oncologists, surgeons, and radiation oncologists for treatment. However, primary care practices are often the initial point of contact for patients in obtaining screening or evaluating symptoms. In addition, the primary care practice serves as the central contact point for cancer patients by making referrals, coordinating care with various specialists and support services, and managing both symptoms of cancer and its treatment, as well as preexisting medical conditions, such as diabetes, heart disease, or hypertension. Moreover, for cancer survivors, the primary care practice can be a central support service for lifestyle changes involving diet, exercise, and rational dietary supplementation.

Another important task for primary care practices is counseling cancer patients about treatment options and monitoring treatment progress and side effects (Williams 1994). Studies document the role that primary care physicians and practices can play in follow-up care for cancer survivors (Worster et al. 1995, 1996; Grunfeld et al. 2006; Keating et al. 2007; Snyder et al. 2008). The critical role of primary care practices in cancer screening and early detection is well established, and their role in the follow-up care of cancer survivors is emerging currently (Institute of Medicine 2006). Two general medical care roles are often assumed by primary care rather than by cancer specialists: (1) managing comorbid conditions and (2) evaluating and treating depression. Comorbid conditions and depression are common in cancer patients and survivors (Ko and Chaudhry 2002; Mao et al. 2007; Reich 2008). The management provided is important, as cancer patients with comorbid conditions such as diabetes experience worse outcomes (Ko and Chaudhry 2002; Smith et al. 2008; Lloyd-Williams et al. 2009). Oncologists often fail to identify depression in cancer patients experiencing moderate to severe depressive symptoms, and this is an area where primary care practices can provide important support for cancer patients and survivors (Passik et al. 1998).

The growth of the cancer patient and survivor populations in the United States, along with the anticipated shortages of oncologists, heightens the need for better information about participation of primary care physicians and their multidisciplinary teams in cancer care. Therefore, a greater knowledge of the nature of cancer and its treatment is an important background for primary care providers. Many of the nutritional principles of primary cancer prevention also apply to secondary prevention, such as increased intakes of fruits and vegetables and the achievement of optimal body composition.

19.3 CHANGING FACE OF CANCER

Due to advances in screening, early detection, and better treatment options, there has been an increase in overall 5-year survival rates among cancer patients. A total of 1,685,210 new cancer cases and 595,690 cancer deaths were projected to occur in the United States in 2016 (Siegel et al. 2016). Overall cancer incidence trends are stable in women, but declining by 3.1% per year in men from 2009 to 2012, much of which is because of recent rapid declines in prostate cancer diagnoses. The cancer death rate has dropped by 23% since 1991, translating to more than 1.7 million deaths averted through 2012. Despite this progress, death rates are increasing for cancers of the liver, pancreas, and uterine corpus, and cancer is now the leading cause of death in 21 states, primarily due to exceptionally large reductions in death from heart disease. Prostate, lung, and colorectal cancers account for 44% of all cases in men, with prostate cancer alone accounting for one in five new cases in the United States. For women, the three most commonly diagnosed cancers are breast, lung, and colorectal cancers, representing one-half of all cases. Breast cancer alone accounts for 29% of all new cancer diagnoses in American women.

19.4 CANCER SURVIVORS IN PRIMARY CARE

Patients presenting in primary care practice with a past medical history of cancer diagnosis and treatment are becoming much more common. As a result, more emphasis is being placed on recommendations to enhance overall health in this unique clinical population (Williams 1994). A recent report from the Institute of Medicine of the U.S. National Academy of Sciences specifically calls for lifestyle recommendations as part of implementing survivorship care planning in order to optimize health and quality of life after cancer treatment (Worster et al. 1995). Recommendations for cancer survivors are divided into three broad areas of weight management, physical activity, and diet quality.

The evidence supporting a weight management recommendation for cancer survivors is well established. A significant number of survivors of cancers where obesity and overweight are risk factors are overweight or obese when they are diagnosed with cancer and during follow-up. Survivors likely to be overweight or obese include postmenopausal breast cancer patients, as well as patients with cancers of the colon, endometrium, gastric cardia, kidney, pancreas, ovary, and gallbladder (Worster et al. 1996; Grunfeld et al. 2006; Keating et al. 2007). There is an increasing body of evidence suggesting that obesity may be contributing to recurrence and cancer-related mortality (Snyder et al. 2008).

Obesity and poor outcomes in cancer patients are most strongly linked in breast cancer, where numerous observational studies have evaluated the relation between body weight status at the time of cancer diagnosis and the risk of cancer recurrence and mortality. A recent meta-analysis of 82 studies that included 213,075 women with breast cancer demonstrated that for each 5 kg/m^2 increment in body mass index (BMI), there was a 14–29% increased risk of disease-specific mortality and an 8–17% increased risk of total mortality (Chan et al. 2014). Results of a similar magnitude were observed in a meta-analysis in prostate cancer; that analysis of 18,203 patients demonstrated that each 5 kg/m^2 increase in BMI was associated with a 21% increased risk of biochemical recurrence and a 20% higher risk of prostate cancer-specific mortality (Cao and Ma 2011). For colorectal cancer, a recent meta-analysis of 51,303 patients across 29 studies demonstrated slightly increased overall survival among obese individuals versus normal-weight individuals (Wu et al. 2014).

It should be noted that for breast cancer, the associations between body weight status and mortality are not linear, but instead indicate that the greatest risk is among women who are underweight (BMI <18.5 kg/m^2) or obese (BMI >29.9 kg/m^2) compared with those who are normal weight or overweight with a BMI between these extremes. For colorectal cancer, the lowest-risk patients appear to be those who are overweight, with higher risk observed among underweight and normal-weight patients (BMI <25 kg/m^2), as well as those who are obese (BMI ≥ 30 kg/m^2) (Cao and Ma 2011; Wu et al. 2014). Although meta-analyses have not been reported for other cancers, systematic reviews suggest that obesity is directly associated with recurrence and overall survival, although the data are less consistent (Parekh et al. 2012; Arem and Irwin 2013).

Obesity also can contribute to morbidity from cancer treatment and is a risk factor for poor wound healing, postoperative infections, and lymphedema, as well as for the development of comorbid illness (e.g., cardiovascular disease, cerebrovascular disease, and diabetes) and functional decline (Parekh et al. 2012; Arem and Irwin 2013). In addition, obesity places individuals at greater risk for developing second primary malignancies (Ligibel et al. 2014).

The associations between BMI and long-term outcomes and prognoses are weak in comparison with visceral obesity in cancer patients (Worster et al. 1995, 1996; Ko and Chaudhry 2002; Institute of Medicine 2006; Lee et al. 2008; Moon et al. 2008; Cecchini et al. 2011; Clark et al. 2013). In the nononcological setting, the waist circumference (WC) and waist-to-hip ratio (WHR) have been found to be better discriminators of diabetes and cardiovascular risks than BMI (Zimmet et al. 2005; Mao et al. 2007; Lee et al. 2008; Reich 2008). In the oncological setting, WC and WHR have been found to be associated with increased risk of endometrial, esophageal, colorectal, and breast cancers (Passik et al. 1998; Smith et al. 2008; Lloyd-Williams et al. 2009; Aune et al. 2015; Harding et al. 2015; Steffen et al. 2015). There is a suggestion that WC and WHR are associated with poor outcomes in colorectal cancer (Chan et al. 2014; Fedirko et al. 2014).

The combination of sarcopenia and obesity is classified as sarcopenic obesity (Heber et al. 1996). Several factors could increase the risk of sarcopenic obesity. Age-related body composition changes with progressive decline in muscle mass and/or strength are a significant risk factor. Hormonal changes, sedentary lifestyle, and malnutrition may also occur in the elderly, contributing to sarcopenic obesity. In addition, adipose tissue secretes pro-inflammatory cytokines and adipokines, promoting insulin resistance, and these pro-inflammatory markers can contribute toward low muscle mass and obesity (Roubenoff 2004; Schrager et al. 2007).

Studies have supported the clinical observation that the weight gain that breast cancer patients experience after treatment is different from the weight losses observed in other cancers, such as pancreatic cancer or lung cancer, since it occurs either in the absence of gains in lean tissue or in the presence of lean tissue losses (Cheney et al. 1997; Demark-Wahnefried et al. 1997; Aslani et al. 1998, 1999; Kutynec et al. 1999; Peterson et al. 2001).

It is clear that a combination of diet and exercise is necessary to correct sarcopenic obesity in cancer survivors. Preliminary data show some reversal of sarcopenia in premenopausal women undergoing adjuvant chemotherapy (Demark-Wahnefried et al. 2002). In a 12-week diet and exercise program in healthy but obese postmenopausal women, a diet and exercise regimen including resistance exercise led to improvements in body composition and exercise performance, including fat mass loss (14% average drop), improved VO_2max (+36% increase), and strength improvement (+26%) (Carpenter et al. 2012). Breast ductal fluid markers also declined from baseline, with estradiol showing a 24% reduction and interleukin 6 (IL-6) a 20% reduction. Reductions from baseline in hormones and cytokines were observed, including leptin (36% decline), estrone sulfate (10% decline), estradiol (25% decline), and IL-6 (33% decline) (Carpenter et al. 2012).

Based on this background, the American Cancer Society's practical recommendations for cancer survivors' weight management, physical activity, and diet quality (Demark-Wahnefried et al. 2015) are as follows:

1. Achieve and maintain a healthy weight. If overweight or obese, limit consumption of high-calorie foods and beverages and increase physical activity to promote weight loss.
2. Engage in regular physical activity.
3. Avoid inactivity and return to normal daily activities as soon as possible after diagnosis.
4. Aim to exercise at least 150 minutes/week, and include strength training exercises at least 2 days/week.
5. Achieve a dietary pattern that is high in vegetables, fruits, and whole grains.

In addition, limit consumption of processed meat and red meat and eat at least 2.5 cups of vegetables and fruits daily. Choose whole grains instead of refined grain products, and if you drink alcoholic beverages, limit consumption to no more than one drink daily for women or two drinks daily for men. This advice is reasonable and can be individualized to meet the needs of patients with comorbid conditions.

19.5 MALNUTRITION AND CANCER

Weight loss in cancer patients is due to depletion of both adipose tissue and skeletal muscle mass, while the nonmuscle protein compartment is relatively preserved, thus distinguishing cachexia from simple starvation (Fearon 1992). The loss of both adipose tissue and skeletal muscle mass can be extensive. Studies of the body composition of lung cancer patients showed that they lost 32% of their preillness stable weight, compared with a group of controls matched for age, sex, height, and preillness stable weight. Although the overall weight loss was 32%, the cachectic patients had lost 85% of their total body fat and 75% of their skeletal muscle, and there was also a significant decrease in mineral content, suggesting erosion of bone. This marked loss of skeletal muscle explains why patients with cachexia have a reduced mobility, and thus quality of life, together with a shorter life span, since loss of respiratory muscle function will lead to death from hypostatic pneumonia.

Death occurs with a 25–30% total body weight loss (Wigmore et al. 1997). A similar situation is found in patients with acquired immunodeficiency syndrome (AIDS), where death is imminent when they have lost 34% of their ideal body weight (Kotler et al. 1990). Respiratory failure has been found to be responsible for the death of 48% of cancer patients (Houten and Reilley 1980).

At the time of diagnosis, 80% of patients with upper gastrointestinal (GI) cancers and 60% of patients with lung cancer have significant weight loss (Bruera 1997; McMahon et al. 1998), defined as at least a 10% loss of body weight in the prior 6 months (Rivadeneira et al. 1998). In addition, malnutrition is a common complication of patients undergoing chemotherapy, radiation, or surgery for cancer.

This common problem in cancer patients has been recognized as a significant contributor to morbidity and mortality in cancer. Malnutrition is associated with a decreased quality of life in cancer patients, and significant weight loss is a biomarker of poor prognosis in cancer patients (McMahon et al. 1998). Nutrition intervention can help cancer patients maintain body weight and nutrition stores, offering relief from symptoms and improving their quality of life (American Cancer Society 2015). Poor nutrition practices, which can lead to undernutrition, can contribute to the incidence and severity of treatment side effects and increase the risk of infection and mortality in cancer patients (Vigano et al. 1994).

While weight loss is traditionally associated with cancer in the minds of professionals and the public, weight gain can occur as the result of chemotherapy treatment for early-stage cancers, possibly resulting from decreases in lean body mass and resting metabolism (Harvie et al. 2004). This is especially common in postmenopausal women with breast cancer who develop sarcopenic obesity after treatment. Sarcopenic obesity has been shown to be a risk factor for breast cancer progression (Prado et al. 2009). Obesity has also been associated with increased mortality in prostate cancer (Hsing et al. 2007). The nutrition of cancer patients should be assessed throughout the continuum of care to reflect changing objectives of nutrition intervention.

19.5.1 Protein–Energy Malnutrition

Protein–energy malnutrition (PEM) is the most common secondary diagnosis in individuals diagnosed with cancer. PEM leads to progressive wasting, weakness, and debilitation, as protein synthesis is reduced and lean body mass is lost, often leading to death (McMahon et al. 1998). PEM results most commonly from inadequate intake of macronutrients needed to meet energy requirements. In addition to reduced food intake, there are a number of associated abnormalities that can combine to worsen malnutrition, including reduced absorption of macronutrients secondary to changes in the GI tract. Cancer-induced metabolic abnormalities secondary to inflammation affect the metabolism of the major nutrients, including glucose and protein. Such abnormalities may include glucose intolerance and insulin resistance, increased lipolysis, and increased whole body protein turnover (Heber et al. 1986).

Increased turnover of liver and muscle proteins and gluconeogenesis from amino acids of muscle origin are thought to contribute to rapid muscle wasting seen in cancer-associated malnutrition (Mutlu and Mobarhan 2000; Nitenberg and Raynard 2000). Whole body protein breakdown is increased in lung cancer patients and has been shown to correlate with the degree of malnutrition, such that more malnourished patients have greater elevations of their whole body protein breakdown rates, expressed per kilogram of body weight. Muscle catabolism, measured by 3-methylhistidine excretion, was increased in lung cancer patients compared with that of healthy controls. Methylhistidine excretion rates did not correlate with weight loss, percentage of ideal body weight, or age in the lung cancer patients studied. Glucose production rates were markedly increased in lung cancer patients compared with healthy controls, and changes in glucose production rates in the cancer patients studied did not correlate with weight loss, percent of ideal body weight, or age.

Anorexia, the loss of appetite or desire to eat, is typically present in 15–25% of all cancer patients at diagnosis and may also occur as a side effect of treatments. Anorexia is an almost universal side effect in individuals with widely metastatic disease (Langstein and Norton 1991; Shills 1999), secondary to chemotherapy and radiation therapy side effects, which lead to taste and smell changes, nausea, and vomiting. Surgical treatments, such as esophagectomy and gastrectomy, may produce early satiety and lead to reduced food intake (Rivadeneira et al. 1998). Common psychological factors in cancer patients, including depression, loss of hope, anxiety, and morbid thoughts, may be enough to bring about anorexia and result in PEM (Bruera 1997). Evidence-based recommendations have been published describing various approaches to the problems of cancer-related fatigue, anorexia, depression, and dyspnea (Tisdale 1993). Other systemic or local effects of cancer or its treatment that may affect nutritional status include sepsis, malabsorption, maldigestion, and intestinal obstruction (Heber et al. 1986).

19.5.2 Carbohydrate Metabolism

Changes in carbohydrate metabolism, similar to those seen in type 2 diabetes, are common in patients with cancer-associated malnutrition. Although glucose turnover is increased, glucose is poorly utilized by peripheral tissues due to insulin resistance and glucose insensitivity (Rofe et al. 1994; Mutlu and Mobarhan 2000). Tumors have been demonstrated to increase the rate of glucose utilization in a number of tissues, acting as metabolic traps (Argiles and Azcon-Bieto 1988; Heber 1989). Since there are only 1200 kilocalories stored in the body as liver and muscle glycogen, blood glucose levels would be expected to fall. This does not occur since there is also an increase in hepatic glucose production in cachectic and anorectic tumor-bearing animals and humans. The regulation of protein metabolism is tightly linked to carbohydrate metabolism, since these processes are critical to the normal adaptation to starvation or underfeeding. During starvation, there is a decrease in glucose production, protein synthesis, and protein catabolism. The decrease in glucose production occurs as fat-derived fuels, primarily ketone bodies, are used for energy production. While there are 54,000 kilocalories of protein stored in the body cell mass, only about half of these are available for energy production. In fact, depletion below 50% of body protein stores is incompatible with life (Heber et al. 2006).

Early research demonstrated preferential metabolism of glucose through aerobic glycolysis, as opposed to oxidative phosphorylation (i.e., Warburg effect), for tumorigenesis. Most aggressive tumors exhibit a high rate of and dependence on glycolysis to meet their metabolic demands (Richtsmeier et al. 1987; Sandulache et al. 2011). It has therefore been reasoned that diets restricted in carbohydrates could target the altered metabolism of such glycolytic tumors (Seyfried and Shelton 2010; Seyfried et al. 2014). Those diets result in a state of systemic ketone body production and have thus been termed ketogenic diets. Indeed, there is some evidence that a ketogenic diet, a high-fat, low-carbohydrate (CHO) diet that leads to the elevation of circulating ketone bodies into the micromole range, may not only impair tumor cell metabolism and growth, but also fight cachexia and therapy-induced side effects (Holm and Kämmerer 2011; Klement and Kammerer 2011; Klement and Champ 2014). To date, ketogenic diets have been the most widely studied and rigorously explored, primarily in the management of medically refractory epilepsy, although studies are beginning to investigate their role in neurodegenerative conditions, migraine management, and oncology. Despite increasing interest and popularity, formal scientific studies of the majority of these interventions are lacking (Strowd and Grossman 2015).

19.5.3 Host–Tumor Interactions and Metabolic Abnormalities in the Cancer Patient

Based on autopsy studies performed in the 1920s (Terepka and Waterhouse 1956; Ogata et al. 2011) and animal studies done in the 1950s (Fenninger and Mider 1954), it was postulated that tumors acted to siphon off needed energy and protein from the host. In the 1970s and 1980s, specific abnormalities of intermediary metabolism were identified in cancer patients that could account for the common observation that such patients lost weight even in the face of apparently adequate nutrition. Studies conducted in a number of laboratories, including our own, have demonstrated that maladaptive metabolic abnormalities occur frequently in patients with cancer. In 1983, studies at the University of California, Los Angeles (UCLA) demonstrated that adequate calories and protein administered to six patients with active localized head and neck cancer via forced continuous enteral alimentation under metabolic ward conditions for 29 days failed to lead to significant weight gain (Heber et al. 1986). The observed failure of these patients to gain weight despite adequate caloric intake under metabolic ward conditions supports the concept that malnourished cancer patients are hypermetabolic.

If metabolic abnormalities promote the development of malnutrition or interfere with renutrition, then there should be some evidence of abnormally increased energy expenditure. A number of investigators have used indirect calorimetry and the abbreviated Weir formula to calculate energy expenditure at rest and then compared this with the basal energy expenditure (BEE) determined using the Harris–Benedict formulas. Studies have used this method to compare cancer patients to normal controls (Long et al. 1979). In one such study, 60% of a group of patients with advanced cancer had basal metabolic rates that were increased 20% above those predicted (Bozzetti et al. 1980). Among 173 malnourished GI cancer patients, 58% had abnormally increased resting energy expenditure (REE) by indirect calorimetry compared with BEE, but a greater number of patients were hypometabolic rather than hypermetabolic (36% vs. 22%) (Dempsey et al. 1984). In another study of 200 patients with a variety of cancers, abnormal energy metabolism was found in 59%, but this was more often hypometabolism than hypermetabolism (33% vs. 26%) (Knox et al. 1983). While standard formulas such as the Harris–Benedict can be used to estimate metabolic rate in normal individuals, the measured metabolic rates in patients with cancer have a much wider distribution. Controversy remains concerning the importance of REE in cancer-associated malnutrition; however, tumor resection has been shown to normalize REE in hypermetabolic cancer patients (Fredrix et al. 1997). Elevated REE and its role in the pathogenesis of cancer-associated malnutrition may depend on the individual patient and disease characteristics. When energy expenditure was studied in noncachectic patients with large localized sarcomas without prior treatment, weight loss, or history of decreased food intake, energy expenditure corrected for body cell mass determined by total body potassium counting or body surface area was significantly greater in sarcoma patients than in controls. This difference was due to both a decrease in body cell mass and an increase in REE in these patients before the onset of weight loss (Peacock et al. 1987).

Therefore, it is likely that lean body mass, rather than fat mass, correlates with the individual variations observed in measured REE. The hypothesis that the malnourished cancer patient may be hypermetabolic relative to the amount of lean body mass remaining is also likely based on the studies conducted in sarcoma patients.

One group of investigators have been studying short-term fasting as a means of enhancing the sensitivity of tumors to chemotherapy so as sensitize target tumor cells while having relatively low toxicity directed at normal cells and tissues (Safdie et al. 2009). This approach is still experimental and should only be considered within the context of a controlled clinical trial. However, the concept is novel and worthy of consideration. Longo and coworkers have proposed that changes in the levels of glucose, insulin-like growth factor 1 (IGF-1), insulin-like growth factor binding protein 1 (IGFBP-1), and other proteins caused by fasting have the potential to improve the efficacy of chemotherapy against tumors by protecting normal cells and tissues and possibly by diminishing multidrug resistance in malignant cells (Lee et al. 2012b). Starvation sensitized yeast cells (*Saccharomyces cerevisiae*) expressing the oncogene-like RAS2 (val19) to oxidative stress, and 15 of 17 mammalian cancer cell lines were sensitized to chemotherapeutic agents.

Short-term starvation (or fasting) protects normal cells and tumor-bearing mice from the harmful side effects of a variety of chemotherapy drugs. Cycles of starvation were as effective as chemotherapeutic agents in delaying progression of different tumors and increased the effectiveness of chemotherapy drugs against melanoma, glioma, and breast cancer cells. In mouse models of neuroblastoma, fasting cycles plus chemotherapy drugs—but not either treatment alone—resulted in long-term cancer-free survival. In 4T1 breast cancer cells, short-term starvation resulted in increased phosphorylation of the stress-sensitizing Akt and S6 kinases, increased oxidative stress, caspase 3 cleavage, DNA damage, and apoptosis. These studies suggest that multiple cycles of fasting promote differential stress sensitization in a wide range of tumors and could potentially replace or augment the efficacy of certain chemotherapy drugs in the treatment of various cancers, while reducing side effects of therapy in cancer patients. This counterintuitive idea of using short-term fasting prior to chemotherapy has yet to be tested and proven in humans (Lee et al. 2012a).

19.6 NUTRITION SCREENING

Nutrition intervention in cancer care embodies prevention of disease, treatment, cure, or supportive palliation. Prudence should always be exercised when considering alternative or unproven nutritional therapies for two reasons. First, these diets or supplements may prove harmful. Second, they may delay prudent and effective therapies, as was the case for Steve Jobs, who had a treatable tumor of the pancreas (insulinoma) that was not diagnosed promptly due to the use of ineffective herbal treatments for many months. Moreover, some physicians provide patients with anticancer dietary supplements while not emphasizing diet and lifestyle changes. Proactive nutritional care can prevent or reduce the complications typically associated with the treatment of cancer (Dewys et al. 1980).

Whether the goal of cancer treatment is cure or palliation, early detection of nutritional problems and prompt intervention are essential. Nutrition screening and nutrition assessment should be instituted by all members of the health care team caring for the cancer patient, including physicians, nurses, registered dietitians, social workers, and psychologists (Tchekmedyian et al. 1992). The Prognostic Nutrition Index (Dempsey and Mullen 1987; Dempsey et al. 1988) delayed hypersensitivity skin testing, institution-specific guidelines, and anthropometrics are all tools that can be used effectively to identify patients at nutritional risk. The selection of nutrition screening tools must be individualized and interpreted in light of clinical factors, as the various biomarkers can be affected by immune incompetence, inflammation, and hydration status (Sarhill et al. 2003).

The Patient-Generated Subjective Global Assessment (PG-SGA) is a simple and inexpensive approach to identifying individuals at nutritional risk and in triaging cancer patients for nutritional intervention (McMahon et al. 1998; Bauer et al. 2002). The PG-SGA is based on an earlier protocol called the Subjective Global Assessment (SGA) (Ottery 1994). With the PG-SGA, the individual and/or caretaker completes sections on weight history, food intake, symptoms, and function. Bioelectrical impedance analysis (BIA) is also used to assess nutritional status, as determined by body composition (Lukaski 1999). Single BIA measures show body cell mass, extracellular tissue, and fat as a percent of ideal, whereas sequential measurements can be used to show body composition changes over time. BIA is increasingly becoming available in ambulatory settings, and its use should be encouraged. With estimation of lean body mass, estimates of REE can be made by multiplying lean body mass by 14. This can guide nutritional interventions for weight gain or weight loss. The goals of nutrition intervention include

1. Preserving or increasing lean body mass
2. Reducing fatigue and improving quality of life
3. Correcting specific nutrition deficiencies
4. Improving tolerance of cancer therapy
5. Reducing side effects and complications related to nutrition
6. Enhancing immunity and decreasing the risk of infection
7. Promoting recovery and healing

19.7 SELECTING APPROPRIATE METHODS OF NUTRITION CARE

In patients with cancer, there is an association between poor nutritional parameters and worse overall morbidity and quality of life (Chlebowski et al. 1986). The benefits of initial and follow-up evaluations and counseling by a registered dietitian, preferably in the context of a team approach, can be enormous, although difficult to quantify (Ravasco et al. 2003). However, recent studies indicate improved nutritional intake and quality of life after individualized dietary counseling (Wickham et al. 1999; Ravasco et al. 2005). The main benefits relate to patient satisfaction, nutrition improvement or maintenance, compliance with team or institutional management protocols and guidelines, and a judicious use of risky and expensive treatments. The costs of nutritional counseling are modest when compared with other interventions.

Nutritional evaluation and counseling, usually undertaken by a registered dietitian, is a first and important step. Ideally, a dietitian should be an integral part of the cancer care team. Compliance with dietary advice can be promoted by regular contact between the health care provider and the patient, including regular nutritional assessments and advice (Parenteral and Enteral Nutrition Group 2004).

Dietitians typically obtain a 24- to 72-hour recall diet history either verbally or, preferably, as recorded at home. The diet record is then examined to assess the adequacy of calories and protein, utilizing food analysis tables, compared with estimated energy and protein needs. In addition to assessing current food and fluid intake, the dietitian should note any recent changes, along with food aversions, intolerances, or problems with feeding, such as taste changes. Alterations in protein metabolism are common in the course of cancer, including whole body protein turnover, increased protein synthesis and catabolism, and an increase in skeletal muscle breakdown. To account for the stress induced by the disease and treatment, protein requirements of cancer patients can be determined by adjusting the estimated requirement for healthy individuals to account for the stress induced by the disease and treatment.

19.7.1 Oral Nutrition Support

The first rule of nutrition intervention is to use the gut when it is available, and the preferred method of nutrition support is via the oral route using food. One goal of nutrition education and counseling is to have the patient increase consumption of nutrient-dense foods to correct nutritional imbalances and deficiencies in order to achieve and maintain a desirable weight. Calorically dense foods such as nuts and nut butters can be used to increase the efficiency of calorie conversion to body fat stores. One limitation of this approach is that malnourished cancer patients often are limited in their ability to absorb and digest fat due to the effects of malnutrition or enteritis as a result of radiation or chemotherapy. Therefore, overconsumption of high-fat foods can, in some cases, lead to GI distress.

Liquid supplements are the most common types of nutritional supplements, are readily available for patient consumption, and are effective when patients are unable to meet requirements with normal foods alone, despite dietary counseling (Ravasco et al. 2005). Patients may be anorectic due to illness or be affected by disabling factors, such as difficulty in chewing, inability to prepare foods for themselves, visual difficulties, decreased energy level, or poor access to foods. Nutritional supplements may be homemade and are usually milk based, or they are commercially prepared and packaged. Although somewhat expensive, commercial supplements provide balanced and fortified (vitamin- and mineral-enriched) nutrition that requires little or no preparation. Oral supplementation with liquid concentrated food supplements providing high-calorie, high-protein, low-volume nutrients is the simplest, most natural, and least invasive method of increasing nutrient intake. The benefits of oral supplementation include increased appetite and weight gain, decreased GI toxicity, and improved performance status (Nayel et al. 1992; Ovesen and Allingstrup 1992; Bell et al. 2003). These products are particularly helpful when patients cannot maintain an adequate intake through a regular diet but are able to swallow and have a relatively intact GI tract.

Dietitians can help patients select products based on tolerance and palatability. Commercially prepared supplements are available in a variety of flavors (including unflavored) and in a variety of nutrient compositions. Most commercially prepared supplements are available in ready-to-drink cans or boxes and are usually lactose-free, which for the patient is often more acceptable due to the increased incidence of perceived milk intolerance in this population. Vitamin- and mineral-fortified protein meal replacements designed to be mixed with milk provide an inexpensive and generally well-tolerated alternative for those who are not lactose intolerant. These supplements have vitamin, mineral, calorie, fat, carbohydrate, and protein contents similar to those of most commercially prepared supplements.

The success of supplementation depends on sufficient quantities being consumed over an extended period of time. The volume and choice of supplement is based on the patient's individual nutrient needs and preferences, and GI tolerance. Supplements with fiber, generally soy or oat fiber, are available and may be beneficial to the patient who has diarrhea or constipation. Nutritional supplements are generally well accepted and may offer relief to a patient who has difficulties eating solid food. Tolerability can be enhanced by starting with small quantities and by diluting the supplement with water or ice to decrease osmolality. A patient will usually accept one to three 8-ounce supplements per day, but there is great individual variability. Variety in supplements will help patients avoid taste fatigue, which is one main drawback to oral supplementation (Wargovich 1999). Patients who have alterations in taste or nausea may better tolerate an unflavored supplement.

Dietary modifications can be employed with the help of a registered dietitian to reduce the symptoms associated with cancer treatments. Appetite stimulants may be used to enhance the enjoyment of foods and to facilitate weight gain in the presence of significant anorexia (Seligman et al. 1998). Suggestions for appetite improvement are shown in Table 19.1 (Ottery 1995).

TABLE 19.1
Suggestions for Appetite Improvement

1	Establish a daily menu and record food intake.
2	Eat small, frequent, high-calorie meals.
3	Arrange for help in preparing meals.
4	Add extra protein and calories to food.
5	Prepare and store small portions of favorite foods.
6	Consume one-third of the daily protein and calorie requirements at breakfast.
7	Snack between meals with nuts or other healthy foods when possible.
8	Seek foods that appeal to the sense of smell.
9	Be creative with desserts.
10	Experiment with different foods.
11	Perform frequent mouth care to relieve symptoms and decrease unpleasant tastes.

19.7.2 Enteral Nutrition

Enteral nutrition is often needed in patients with cancers of the head and neck regions, esophagus, and stomach. Nasogastric tubes and tubes that extend into the duodenum or jejunum are best suited for short-term support (<2 weeks) (Heys et al. 1999). Enteral feeding into the jejunum is appropriate for patients at risk of aspiration. However, if the patient is at very high risk of aspirating, enteral nutritional support is contraindicated and parenteral nutrition should be considered. Moreover, patients with mucositis or esophagitis, and those who are immunocompromised and have herpetic, fungal, or candida lesions in the mouth or throat, may not be able to tolerate the presence of a nasogastric tube.

Percutaneous endoscopic gastrostomy (PEG) tubes and percutaneous endoscopic jejunostomy (PEJ) tubes are needed for long-term enteral feedings (for more than 2 weeks). Enteral nutrition can be delivered at different rates and durations. Bolus feedings that mimic meals are preferable because this method requires less time and equipment, offers greater flexibility to the patient, and enables normal physiological and hormonal mechanisms to operate (Heys et al. 1999). When administering bolus or intermittent enteral feeding, the steps in Table 19.2 should be followed.

Once the infusion method has been determined, a formula is selected. When a formula is being chosen, the institution nutrition formulary for available preparations, modular formulas, and additions such as glutamine or fiber should be considered. Consideration should also be given to the patient's medical condition, GI function, and financial resources. Enteral formulas, from elemental preparations of predigested nutrients to more complete and complex formulas that mimic oral nutrition intake, are available. More information on specific formulas and their ingredients and properties can be obtained from the manufacturers. There are also specialized formulas designed for specific disease conditions, including diabetes mellitus and compromised renal function, but the additional benefits of these formulas may not justify their cost, and the need for these should be carefully considered.

TABLE 19.2
Administering Bolus or Intermittent Enteral Feeding

1 Determine the calorie, nutrient, and free-water requirements in order to plan the feeding schedule. Dehydration will occur if adequate water is not included in the formulation, typically at 1 mL/calorie administered.
2 Administer bolus feedings three to six times per day. It is possible to give 250–500 cc over 10–15 minutes, as long as the patient tolerates these amounts without undue gastric distension.
3 Bolus feeding is only to be used when a nasogastric tube is in the stomach. Bolus feeding is contraindicated when feedings are delivered into the duodenum or jejunum, since gastric distention and dumping syndrome can occur.
4 Administer the bolus feeding using a gravity drip from a bag or syringe or a slow push with the syringe.
5 Change the amount of formula given at time 0, the type of formula, or added ingredients in the formula if diarrhea, a common side effect of this type of infusion, is encountered.

When instituting continuous or cyclic enteral feeding, the following steps should be followed:
1 Determine the calories per nutrient and free-water requirements in order to plan rate and timing recommendations, whether continuous or cyclic infusions.
2 Utilize a controlled enteral feeding pump that provides reliable, constant infusion rates in order to decrease the risk of gastric retention.
3 Initiate feeding into the stomach at rates of 25–30 mL/hour and start at 10 mL/hour into the jejunum (10 cc/hour), and then increase rates as tolerated every 4–6 hours until the rate needed to deliver the required caloric/nutrient needs is reached.
4 If continuous feed is used, it can be run at night to allow greater flexibility for the patient. In addition, night feeding can be combined with bolus feedings during the day to provide a more normal lifestyle for the patient.

19.7.3 Parenteral Nutrition

Parenteral nutrition is only required in patients who are unable to use the oral or enteral route. That is, if the gut is working, use it. Nutrients provided through the enteral route nourish the gut epithelium and provide better overall nutrition, as well as involving the gut peptides, which enhance insulin action. Patients with obstruction, intractable nausea and/or vomiting, short bowel syndrome, or ileus may require parenteral nutrition. Other indications to use total parenteral nutrition (TPN) in the cancer population include severe diarrhea or malabsorption, severe mucositis or esophagitis, high-output GI fistulas that cannot be bypassed by enteral intubation, and/or severe preoperative malnutrition (Heys et al. 1999). Despite some claims that TPN is a more aggressive form of nutrition, there are no advantages to using TPN over enteral nutrition for cancer care. The decision to utilize parenteral nutrition in patients with advanced cancer is difficult. The widespread use of TPN, as was done in the 1970s and 1980s, is not advised, since there is no evidence of improved survival in patients with advanced cancer (Chlebowski 1985; Bozzetti 1989). Most data point to the same conclusion: health care providers should not prescribe parenteral nutrition to patients with advanced, incurable cancer. A meta-analysis summarized findings from 15 clinical trials. Parenteral nutrition led to inferior survival, lower tumor response rates, and increased infection rates. The increased infection rate persisted even after catheter-related sepsis was excluded. This observation bolsters recommendations from recent guidelines that suggest parenteral nutrition may not be in the best interest of patients with advanced, incurable cancer (Jeffcoat and Kirkwood 1987).

19.8 DIET AND CANCER PREVENTION: THE ROLE OF COLORFUL FRUITS AND VEGETABLES

International studies of the food habits of a number of populations over the past 40 years have clearly documented the diversity of human dietary patterns and defined those associated with a lower risk of chronic diseases, including common forms of cancer (Glade 1999). In comparison with the diet of Americans, dietary patterns including a consistently higher intake of fruits, vegetables, whole grains, and plant proteins, such as soy, are associated with a markedly reduced risk of cancer. In the nutritional science and epidemiological literature, these dietary patterns have often been characterized as simply low-fat, high-fiber diets, or the intake of vegetables was quantitated as a single phytochemical, such as β-carotene (Garewal and Schantz 1995). Such simplified terminologies led to the concept that fiber or phytochemical supplementation could reproduce the benefits of the healthy dietary patterns they represented.

The idea that a dietary pattern conferred its benefits through a single component led to trials that purported to test one component of the diet in an American population, while all other variables were held constant. When research based on these flawed concepts was conducted, the expected benefits were not realized for fiber supplementation (Alberts et al. 2000) or β-carotene supplementation (The Alpha-Tocopherol, Beta Carotene Cancer Prevention Study Group 1994). This led to a series of publications resulting from intervention trials, which have been interpreted as evidence that nutrition simply does not work in cancer prevention. On the other hand, international studies suggest that for some cancers of the aerodigestive tract, a 50% reduction in risk is associated with intakes of 400–600 g/day of fruits and vegetables (Glade 1999). The challenge for nutrition scientists is to translate this scientific information into dietary guidelines that result in healthful changes in dietary patterns.

Over the past 200 years, a series of uniquely American foods have been developed through adaptation from other cultures: pizza made with oil added to the crust and large amounts of melted cheese, potato chips, corn chips, peanut butter, hot dogs, hamburgers made with beef fat flavoring, and profitable soft drinks made with corn sugar and artificial flavors (Schlosser 2001). Westernized Chinese food is among the highest-fat foods in America because it was adapted from low-fat Chinese versions to meet American tastes. Moreover, refried beans or frijoles have added lard or vegetable oil in the Mexican American adaptation of beans eaten in Mexico and South America without added fat. Special offers of larger portions delivering an extra 800 kilocalories for only an additional 39 cents have made fast-food restaurants especially popular with teenagers, low-income Americans, and the elderly. These foods have displaced the fruits, vegetables, and whole grains recommended in the U.S. dietary guidelines, and consumers have increasingly reduced their commitments to cooking healthy meals and eating as a family over the past few decades.

We are now separated from the system that enabled us to select foods according to color and taste. Humans and a few primate species have trichromatic color vision, so that they are able to distinguish red from green (Dominy and Lucas 2001). All other mammals have dichromatic vision and cannot distinguish between the two colors. One hypothesis for the evolution of this visual ability was that it conferred an advantage by enabling primates to distinguish red fruits from the green background of forest leaves. We could joke that today colors are still used to promote food choices, as most fast-food restaurants package their beige french fries in a red cardboard package. Contrasting colors have been shown to be one of the key factors in food selection by Drewnowski (1996). A new method for selecting fruits and vegetables based on colors keyed to the content of phytochemicals is described as a way of translating the science of phytochemical nutrition into dietary guidelines for the public. Most Americans eat only two to three servings of fruits and vegetables per day, without regard to the phytochemical contents of the foods being eaten. Certain phytochemicals give fruits and vegetables their colors and also indicate their unique physiological roles. All the colored phytochemicals that absorb light in the visible spectrum have antioxidant properties. In artificial membrane systems, it is possible to show synergistic interactions of lutein and lycopene in antioxidant capacity, and there are well-known antioxidant interactions of vitamins C and E based on their solubility in hydrophilic and hydrophobic compartments of cells.

However, many phytochemicals have other functions beyond acting as antioxidants. For example, lycopene stabilizes the connexin 43 gene product that is essential for gap junction communication (Stahl et al. 2000) while also interacting with vitamin D in the differentiation of HL-60 leukemia cells (Amir et al. 1999). In breast cancer cells, lycopene can interfere with IGF-1-stimulated tumor cell proliferation (Karas et al. 2000). Lycopene levels in the blood are associated with a reduced risk of prostate cancer (Gann et al. 1999), and lycopene administration may reduce proliferation and increase apoptosis in human prostate tissue where lycopene is the predominant carotenoid (Kucuk et al. 2001). Lutein is concentrated in the retina, where it may help prevent macular degeneration, the most common preventable form of age-related blindness (Mares-Perlman et al. 2001). Other studies have found that lycopene, α-carotene, and β-carotene are associated with a reduced risk of lung cancer (Heber 2000). On the basis of a recent review of functional properties of foods (Milner 2000) and research from our laboratories demonstrating that it is relatively simple to influence circulating levels of lycopene with the administration of only 177 mL (6 fluid ounces) of mixed vegetable juice daily (Heber et al. 2000), we developed a color code for a book aimed at helping consumers to change dietary patterns to include more fruits and vegetables by including one serving from each of seven color groups each day, selected on the basis of the family of phytochemicals they contain (Table 19.3) (Heber 2002).

TABLE 19.3
Color Code Relationship to Families of Phytochemicals

Color	Phytochemical	Fruits and Vegetables
Red	Lycopene	Tomatoes and tomato products, such as juice, soups, and pasta sauces
Red-purple	Anthocyanins and polyphenols	Grapes, blackberries, red wine, raspberries, blueberries
Orange	α- and β-carotene	Carrots, mangos, pumpkin
Orange-yellow	β-Cryptoxanthin and flavonoids	Cantaloupe, peaches, tangerines, papaya, oranges
Yellow-green	Lutein and zeaxanthin	Spinach, avocado, honeydew melon
Green	Glucosinolates and indoles	Broccoli, bok choi, kale
White-green	Allyl sulfides	Leeks, garlic, onion, chives

Although the color method is superior to the current system of simply encouraging increased fruit and vegetable intake, it does not account for actual phytochemical delivery to the consumer. Today, there is no labeling law that enables fruit and vegetable manufacturers to list the phytochemicals in their products. Fruits and vegetables are developed and grown less for their flavor and nutritional content and more to accommodate the need to transport these products over long distances and extend their shelf life once they get to the market. Finally, research in this area needs to continue on the >25,000 phytochemicals provided by fruits and vegetables, including those that do not have color, such as isoprenoids (Elson 1996). These important phytochemicals are widely distributed among different plant species, but the delivery of phytochemicals and their effects on biomarkers relevant to cancer prevention need to be documented.

19.9 COMPLEMENTARY AND ALTERNATIVE MEDICINES

Vitamin, mineral, and herbal supplement use is reported by nearly half of all breast cancer patients (DiGianni et al. 2002). There are two major concerns raised about the use of such supplements during chemotherapy. First, antioxidants can become pro-oxidants and so may influence the action of radiation or cytotoxic chemotherapy by enhancing or blocking oxidation in tumor cells (Sweet et al. 2016). This concern is theoretical and has never been demonstrated in clinical trials. Concentrated radiation delivered to tumor tissue is not going to be inhibited by vitamin E, which has been shown to reduce doxorubicin toxicity when provided pretreatment with nifedipine without impeding effectiveness (Lenzhofer et al. 1983). In most cases, antioxidant vitamins in a rational range will not affect chemotherapy or radiation, but may support the patient by reduction of side effects. Second, substances in botanicals may influence the pharmacodynamics of a chemotherapeutic regimen and thereby influence the effectiveness or safety of chemotherapy (Sweet et al. 2016). The most important CYP pathways for the metabolism of oncology pharmaceutical drugs are those involving the cytochrome P450 enzymes. The CYP cytochrome P450 3A4 isoform (commonly known as CYP3A4) is responsible for metabolizing greater than 50% of drugs that pass through the liver (Delgoda and Westlake 2004; Saxena et al. 2008). Several herbs and other CAM substances influence CYP3A4's function by either inducing or inhibiting the actions of these enzymes, and thus have the potential to influence the dose of a drug present in a patient's bloodstream (Delgoda and Westlake 2004; Saxena et al. 2008).

In working with oncologists and radiation therapists, you will find varying opinions about the use of supplements, ranging from recommending total abstinence to allowing multivitamins but not herbals or megadose vitamins. It is best to suggest to patients that they follow their oncologist's advice. In cases where a response is not achieved, it is often nutritional supplements or diets that are blamed by patients. If the patient follows the advice of oncologists even when the oncologist's views are contradicted by science, this is still the safest course of action for a primary care practitioner.

REFERENCES

Alberts, D. S., M. E. Martinez, D. J. Roe, J. M. Guillen-Rodriguez, J. R. Marshall, J. B. van Leeuwen, M. E. Reid et al. 2000. Lack of effect of a high-fiber cereal supplement on the recurrence of colorectal adenomas. Phoenix Colon Cancer Prevention Physicians' Network. *N Engl J Med* 342 (16):1156–1162.

The Alpha-Tocopherol, Beta Carotene Cancer Prevention Study Group. 1994. The effect of vitamin E and beta carotene on the incidence of lung cancer and other cancers in male smokers. *N Engl J Med* 330 (15):1029–1035.

American Cancer Society. 2015. Nutrition for the person with cancer: A guide for patients and families. Atlanta, GA: American Cancer Society.

Amir, H., M. Karas, J. Giat, M. Danilenko, R. Levy, T. Yermiahu, J. Levy, and Y. Sharoni. 1999. Lycopene and 1,25-dihydroxyvitamin D3 cooperate in the inhibition of cell cycle progression and induction of differentiation in HL-60 leukemic cells. *Nutr Cancer* 33 (1):105–112.

Arem, H., and M. L. Irwin. 2013. Obesity and endometrial cancer survival: A systematic review. *Int J Obes (Lond)* 37 (5):634–639.

Argiles, J. M., and J. Azcon-Bieto. 1988. The metabolic environment of cancer. *Mol Cell Biochem* 81 (1):3–17.

Aslani, A., R. C. Smith, B. J. Allen, and J. A. Levi. 1998. Changes in body composition during adjuvant chemotherapy for breast cancer. *Appl Radiat Isot* 49 (5–6):637–638.

Aslani, A., R. C. Smith, B. J. Allen, N. Pavlakis, and J. A. Levi. 1999. Changes in body composition during breast cancer chemotherapy with the CMF-regimen. *Breast Cancer Res Treat* 57 (3):285–290.

Aune, D., D. A. Navarro Rosenblatt, D. S. Chan, S. Vingeliene, L. Abar, A. R. Vieira, D. C. Greenwood, E. V. Bandera, and T. Norat. 2015. Anthropometric factors and endometrial cancer risk: A systematic review and dose-response meta-analysis of prospective studies. *Ann Oncol* 26 (8):1635–1648.

Bauer, J., S. Capra, and M. Ferguson. 2002. Use of the scored Patient-Generated Subjective Global Assessment (PG-SGA) as a nutrition assessment tool in patients with cancer. *Eur J Clin Nutr* 56 (8):779–785.

Bell, E. A., L. S. Roe, and B. J. Rolls. 2003. Sensory-specific satiety is affected more by volume than by energy content of a liquid food. *Physiol Behav* 78 (4–5):593–600.

Blanchard, C. M., K. S. Courneya, and K. Stein. 2008. Cancer survivors' adherence to lifestyle behavior recommendations and associations with health-related quality of life: Results from the American Cancer Society's SCS-II. *J Clin Oncol* 26 (13):2198–2204.

Bodenheimer, T. 2006. Primary care—Will it survive? *N Engl J Med* 355 (9):861–864.

Bozzetti, F. 1989. Effects of artificial nutrition on the nutritional status of cancer patients. *JPEN J Parenter Enteral Nutr* 13 (4):406–420.

Bozzetti, F., A. M. Pagnoni, and M. Del Vecchio. 1980. Excessive caloric expenditure as a cause of malnutrition in patients with cancer. *Surg Gynecol Obstet* 150 (2):229–234.

Bruera, E. 1997. ABC of palliative care. Anorexia, cachexia, and nutrition. *BMJ* 315 (7117):1219–1222.

Cao, Y., and J. Ma. 2011. Body mass index, prostate cancer-specific mortality, and biochemical recurrence: A systematic review and meta-analysis. *Cancer Prev Res (Phila)* 4 (4):486–501.

Carpenter, C. L., K. Duvall, P. Jardack, L. Li, S. M. Henning, Z. Li, and D. Heber. 2012. Weight loss reduces breast ductal fluid estrogens in obese postmenopausal women: A single arm intervention pilot study. *Nutr J* 11:102.

Cecchini, S., E. Cavazzini, F. Marchesi, L. Sarli, and L. Roncoroni. 2011. Computed tomography volumetric fat parameters versus body mass index for predicting short-term outcomes of colon surgery. *World J Surg* 35 (2):415–423.

Chan, D. S., A. R. Vieira, D. Aune, E. V. Bandera, D. C. Greenwood, A. McTiernan, D. Navarro Rosenblatt, I. Thune, R. Vieira, and T. Norat. 2014. Body mass index and survival in women with breast cancer—Systematic literature review and meta-analysis of 82 follow-up studies. *Ann Oncol* 25 (10):1901–1914.

Cheney, C. L., J. Mahloch, and P. Freeny. 1997. Computerized tomography assessment of women with weight changes associated with adjuvant treatment for breast cancer. *Am J Clin Nutr* 66 (1):141–146.

Chlebowski, R. T. 1985. Critical evaluation of the role of nutritional support with chemotherapy. *Cancer* 55 (1 Suppl):268–272.

Chlebowski, R. T., J. Herrold, I. Ali, E. Oktay, J. S. Chlebowski, A. T. Ponce, D. Heber, and J. B. Block. 1986. Influence of nandrolone decanoate on weight loss in advanced non-small cell lung cancer. *Cancer* 58 (1):183–186.

Clark, W., E. M. Siegel, Y. A. Chen, X. Zhao, C. M. Parsons, J. M. Hernandez, J. Weber, S. Thareja, J. Choi, and D. Shibata. 2013. Quantitative measures of visceral adiposity and body mass index in predicting rectal cancer outcomes after neoadjuvant chemoradiation. *J Am Coll Surg* 216 (6):1070–1081.

Delgoda, R., and A. C. Westlake. 2004. Herbal interactions involving cytochrome p450 enzymes: A mini review. *Toxicol Rev* 23 (4):239–249.

Demark-Wahnefried, W., V. Hars, M. R. Conaway, K. Havlin, B. K. Rimer, G. McElveen, and E. P. Winer. 1997. Reduced rates of metabolism and decreased physical activity in breast cancer patients receiving adjuvant chemotherapy. *Am J Clin Nutr* 65 (5):1495–1501.

Demark-Wahnefried, W., A. J. Kenyon, P. Eberle, A. Skye, and W. E. Kraus. 2002. Preventing sarcopenic obesity among breast cancer patients who receive adjuvant chemotherapy: Results of a feasibility study. *Clin Exerc Physiol* 4 (1):44–49.

Demark-Wahnefried, W., L. Q. Rogers, C. M. Alfano, C. A. Thomson, K. S. Courneya, J. A. Meyerhardt, N. L. Stout, E. Kvale, H. Ganzer, and J. A. Ligibel. 2015. Practical clinical interventions for diet, physical activity, and weight control in cancer survivors. *CA Cancer J Clin* 65 (3):167–189.

Dempsey, D. T., I. D. Feurer, L. S. Knox, L. O. Crosby, G. P. Buzby, and J. L. Mullen. 1984. Energy expenditure in malnourished gastrointestinal cancer patients. *Cancer* 53 (6):1265–1273.

Dempsey, D. T., and J. L. Mullen. 1987. Prognostic value of nutritional indices. *JPEN J Parenter Enteral Nutr* 11 (5 Suppl):109S–114S.

Dempsey, D. T., J. L. Mullen, and G. P. Buzby. 1988. The link between nutritional status and clinical outcome: Can nutritional intervention modify it? *Am J Clin Nutr* 47 (2 Suppl):352–356.

Dewys, W. D., C. Begg, P. T. Lavin, P. R. Band, J. M. Bennett, J. R. Bertino, M. H. Cohen et al. 1980. Prognostic effect of weight loss prior to chemotherapy in cancer patients. Eastern Cooperative Oncology Group. *Am J Med* 69 (4):491–497.

DiGianni, L. M., J. E. Garber, and E. P. Winer. 2002. Complementary and alternative medicine use among women with breast cancer. *J Clin Oncol* 20 (18 Suppl):34S–38S.

Dominy, N. J., and P. W. Lucas. 2001. Ecological importance of trichromatic vision to primates. *Nature* 410 (6826):363–366.

Drewnowski, A. 1996. From asparagus to zucchini: Mapping cognitive space for vegetable names. *J Am Coll Nutr* 15 (2):147–153.

Elson, C. E. 1996. Novel lipids and cancer. Isoprenoids and other phytochemicals. *Adv. Exp. Med. Biol* 399:71–86.

Erikson, C., E. Salsberg, G. Forte, S. Bruinooge, and M. Goldstein. 2007. Future supply and demand for oncologists: Challenges to assuring access to oncology services. *J Oncol Pract* 3 (2):79–86.

Fearon, K. C. 1992. The Sir David Cuthbertson Medal Lecture 1991. The mechanisms and treatment of weight loss in cancer. *Proc Nutr Soc* 51 (2):251–265.

Fedirko, V., I. Romieu, K. Aleksandrova, T. Pischon, D. Trichopoulos, P. H. Peeters, D. Romaguera-Bosch et al. 2014. Pre-diagnostic anthropometry and survival after colorectal cancer diagnosis in western European populations. *Int J Cancer* 135 (8):1949–1960.

Fenninger, L. D., and G. B. Mider. 1954. Energy and nitrogen metabolism in cancer. *Adv Cancer Res* 2:229–253.

Fredrix, E. W., A. J. Staal-van den Brekel, and E. F. Wouters. 1997. Energy balance in nonsmall cell lung carcinoma patients before and after surgical resection of their tumors. *Cancer* 79 (4):717–723.

Gann, P. H., J. Ma, E. Giovannucci, W. Willett, F. M. Sacks, C. H. Hennekens, and M. J. Stampfer. 1999. Lower prostate cancer risk in men with elevated plasma lycopene levels: Results of a prospective analysis. *Cancer Res* 59 (6):1225–1230.

Garewal, H. S., and S. Schantz. 1995. Emerging role of beta-carotene and antioxidant nutrients in prevention of oral cancer. *Arch Otolaryngol Head Neck Surg* 121 (2):141–144.

Glade, M. J. 1999. Food, nutrition, and the prevention of cancer: A global perspective. American Institute for Cancer Research/World Cancer Research Fund, American Institute for Cancer Research, 1997. *Nutrition* 15 (6):523–526.

Grunfeld, E., M. N. Levine, J. A. Julian, D. Coyle, B. Szechtman, D. Mirsky, S. Verma et al. 2006. Randomized trial of long-term follow-up for early-stage breast cancer: A comparison of family physician versus specialist care. *J Clin Oncol* 24 (6):848–855.

Harding, J. L., J. E. Shaw, K. J. Anstey, R. Adams, B. Balkau, S. L. Brennan-Olsen, T. Briffa et al. 2015. Comparison of anthropometric measures as predictors of cancer incidence: A pooled collaborative analysis of 11 Australian cohorts. *Int J Cancer* 137 (7):1699–1708.

Harvie, M. N., I. T. Campbell, A. Baildam, and A. Howell. 2004. Energy balance in early breast cancer patients receiving adjuvant chemotherapy. *Breast Cancer Res Treat* 83 (3):201–210.

Heber, D. 1989. Metabolic pathology of cancer malnutrition. *Nutrition* 5 (2):135–137.

Heber, D. 2000. Colorful cancer prevention: Alpha-carotene, lycopene, and lung cancer. *Am J Clin Nutr* 72 (4):901–902.

Heber, D. 2002. *What Color Is Your Diet?* New York: HarperCollins.

Heber, D., G. L. Blackburn, and J. Milner. 2006. *Nutritional Oncology.* 2nd ed. San Diego, CA: Academic Press.

Heber, D., L. O. Byerley, J. Chi, M. Grosvenor, R. N. Bergman, M. Coleman, and R. T. Chlebowski. 1986. Pathophysiology of malnutrition in the adult cancer patient. *Cancer* 58 (8 Suppl):1867–1873.

Heber, D., S. Ingles, J. M. Ashley, M. H. Maxwell, R. F. Lyons, and R. M. Elashoff. 1996. Clinical detection of sarcopenic obesity by bioelectrical impedance analysis. *Am J Clin Nutr* 64 (3 Suppl):472S–477S.

Heber, D., I. Yip, V. L. W. Go, W. Liu, R. M. Elashoff, and Q. Lu. 2000. Plasma carotenoids profiles in prostate cancer patients after dietary intervention. *FASEB J* 14:A719.

Heys, S. D., L. G. Walker, I. Smith, and O. Eremin. 1999. Enteral nutritional supplementation with key nutrients in patients with critical illness and cancer: A meta-analysis of randomized controlled clinical trials. *Ann Surg* 229 (4):467–477.

Hoelder, S., P. A. Clarke, and P. Workman. 2012. Discovery of small molecule cancer drugs: Successes, challenges and opportunities. *Mol Oncol* 6 (2):155–176.

Holm, E., and U. Kämmerer. 2011. Lipids and carbohydrates in nutritional concepts for tumor patients. *Aktuel Ernährungsmed* 36:13.
Houten, L., and A. A. Reilley. 1980. An investigation of the cause of death from cancer. *J Surg Oncol* 13 (2):111–116.
Hsing, A. W., L. C. Sakoda, and S. Chua Jr. 2007. Obesity, metabolic syndrome, and prostate cancer. *Am J Clin Nutr* 86 (3):s843–s857.
Institute of Medicine. 2006. *From Cancer Patient to Cancer Survivor: Lost in Transition.* Washington, DC: National Academies Press.
Jeffcoat, R., and S. Kirkwood. 1987. Implication of histidine at the active site of exo-beta-(1–3)-D-glucanase from *Basidiomycete* sp. QM 806. *J Biol Chem* 262 (3):1088–1091.
Karas, M., H. Amir, D. Fishman, M. Danilenko, S. Segal, A. Nahum, A. Koifmann, Y. Giat, J. Levy, and Y. Sharoni. 2000. Lycopene interferes with cell cycle progression and insulin-like growth factor I signaling in mammary cancer cells. *Nutr Cancer* 36 (1):101–111.
Keating, N. L., M. B. Landrum, E. Guadagnoli, E. P. Winer, and J. Z. Ayanian. 2007. Surveillance testing among survivors of early-stage breast cancer. *J Clin Oncol* 25 (9):1074–1081.
Klement, R. J., and C. E. Champ. 2014. Calories, carbohydrates, and cancer therapy with radiation: Exploiting the five R's through dietary manipulation. *Cancer Metastasis Rev* 33 (1):217–229.
Klement, R. J., and U. Kammerer. 2011. Is there a role for carbohydrate restriction in the treatment and prevention of cancer? *Nutr Metab (Lond)* 8:75.
Knox, L. S., L. O. Crosby, I. D. Feurer, G. P. Buzby, C. L. Miller, and J. L. Mullen. 1983. Energy expenditure in malnourished cancer patients. *Ann Surg* 197 (2):152–162.
Ko, C., and S. Chaudhry. 2002. The need for a multidisciplinary approach to cancer care. *J Surg Res* 105 (1):53–57.
Kotler, D. P., A. R. Tierney, J. A. Culpepper-Morgan, J. Wang, and R. N. Pierson Jr. 1990. Effect of home total parenteral nutrition on body composition in patients with acquired immunodeficiency syndrome. *JPEN J Parenter Enteral Nutr* 14 (5):454–458.
Kucuk, O., F. H. Sarkar, W. Sakr, Z. Djuric, M. N. Pollak, F. Khachik, Y. W. Li et al. 2001. Phase II randomized clinical trial of lycopene supplementation before radical prostatectomy. *Cancer Epidemiol Biomarkers Prev* 10 (8):861–868.
Kutynec, C. L., L. McCargar, S. I. Barr, and T. G. Hislop. 1999. Energy balance in women with breast cancer during adjuvant treatment. *J Am Diet Assoc* 99 (10):1222–1227.
Langstein, H. N., and J. A. Norton. 1991. Mechanisms of cancer cachexia. *Hematol Oncol Clin North Am* 5 (1):103–123.
Lee, C. M., R. R. Huxley, R. P. Wildman, and M. Woodward. 2008. Indices of abdominal obesity are better discriminators of cardiovascular risk factors than BMI: A meta-analysis. *J Clin Epidemiol* 61 (7):646–653.
Lee, C., L. Raffaghello, S. Brandhorst, F. M. Safdie, G. Bianchi, A. Martin-Montalvo, V. Pistoia et al. 2012a. Fasting cycles retard growth of tumors and sensitize a range of cancer cell types to chemotherapy. *Sci Transl Med* 4 (124):124ra27.
Lee, C., L. Raffaghello, and V. D. Longo. 2012b. Starvation, detoxification, and multidrug resistance in cancer therapy. *Drug Resist Updat* 15 (1–2):114–122.
Lenzhofer, R., U. Ganzinger, H. Rameis, and K. Moser. 1983. Acute cardiac toxicity in patients after doxorubicin treatment and the effect of combined tocopherol and nifedipine pretreatment. *J Cancer Res Clin Oncol* 106 (2):143–147.
Ligibel, J. A., C. M. Alfano, K. S. Courneya, W. Demark-Wahnefried, R. A. Burger, R. T. Chlebowski, C. J. Fabian et al. 2014. American Society of Clinical Oncology position statement on obesity and cancer. *J Clin Oncol* 32 (31):3568–3574.
Lloyd-Williams, M., C. Shiels, F. Taylor, and M. Dennis. 2009. Depression—An independent predictor of early death in patients with advanced cancer. *J Affect Disord* 113 (1–2):127–132.
Long, C. L., N. Schaffel, J. W. Geiger, W. R. Schiller, and W. S. Blakemore. 1979. Metabolic response to injury and illness: Estimation of energy and protein needs from indirect calorimetry and nitrogen balance. *JPEN J Parenter Enteral Nutr* 3 (6):452–456.
Lukaski, H. C. 1999. Requirements for clinical use of bioelectrical impedance analysis (BIA). *Ann NY Acad Sci* 873:72–76.
Mao, J. J., K. Armstrong, M. A. Bowman, S. X. Xie, R. Kadakia, and J. T. Farrar. 2007. Symptom burden among cancer survivors: Impact of age and comorbidity. *J Am Board Fam Med* 20 (5):434–443.
Mares-Perlman, J. A., A. I. Fisher, R. Klein, M. Palta, G. Block, A. E. Millen, and J. D. Wright. 2001. Lutein and zeaxanthin in the diet and serum and their relation to age-related maculopathy in the third National Health and Nutrition Examination Survey. *Am J Epidemiol* 153 (5):424–432.

McMahon, K., G. Decker, and F. D. Ottery. 1998. Integrating proactive nutritional assessment in clinical practices to prevent complications and cost. *Semin Oncol* 25 (2 Suppl 6):20–27.
Milner, J. A. 2000. Functional foods: The US perspective. *Am J Clin Nutr* 71 (6 Suppl):1654S–1659S.
Moon, H. G., Y. T. Ju, C. Y. Jeong, E. J. Jung, Y. J. Lee, S. C. Hong, W. S. Ha, S. T. Park, and S. K. Choi. 2008. Visceral obesity may affect oncologic outcome in patients with colorectal cancer. *Ann Surg Oncol* 15 (7):1918–1922.
Mutlu, E. A., and S. Mobarhan. 2000. Nutrition in the care of the cancer patient. *Nutr Clin Care* 3 (1):21.
Nayel, H., E. el-Ghoneimy, and S. el-Haddad. 1992. Impact of nutritional supplementation on treatment delay and morbidity in patients with head and neck tumors treated with irradiation. *Nutrition* 8 (1):13–18.
Nitenberg, G., and B. Raynard. 2000. Nutritional support of the cancer patient: Issues and dilemmas. *Crit Rev Oncol Hematol* 34 (3):137–168.
Ogata, R., Y. Tanio, J. Takashima, Y. Kato, T. Arizumi, R. Takada, Y. Tabata, K. Shimazu, and H. Fushimi. 2011. Retrospective analysis of immediate cause of death in lung cancer—Two case reports of lung cancer deaths due to bowel necrosis [in Japanese]. *Gan To Kagaku Ryoho* 38 (6):987–990.
Ottery, F. D. 1994. Rethinking nutritional support of the cancer patient: The new field of nutritional oncology. *Semin Oncol* 21 (6):770–778.
Ottery, F. D. 1995. Supportive nutrition to prevent cachexia and improve quality of life. *Semin Oncol* 22 (2 Suppl 3):98–111.
Ovesen, L., and L. Allingstrup. 1992. Different quantities of two commercial liquid diets consumed by weight-losing cancer patients. *JPEN J Parenter Enteral Nutr* 16 (3):275–278.
Parekh, N., U. Chandran, and E. V. Bandera. 2012. Obesity in cancer survival. *Annu Rev Nutr* 32:311–342.
Parenteral and Enteral Nutrition Group of the British Dietetic Association. 2004. *A Pocket Guide to Clinical Nutrition*. 3rd ed. Birmingham: British Dietetic Association.
Passik, S. D., W. Dugan, M. V. McDonald, B. Rosenfeld, D. E. Theobald, and S. Edgerton. 1998. Oncologists' recognition of depression in their patients with cancer. *J Clin Oncol* 16 (4):1594–1600.
Peacock, J. L., R. I. Inculet, R. Corsey, D. B. Ford, W. F. Rumble, D. Lawson, and J. A. Norton. 1987. Resting energy expenditure and body cell mass alterations in noncachectic patients with sarcomas. *Surgery* 102 (3):465–472.
Peterson, R. K., W. R. Shelton, and A. L. Bomboy. 2001. Allograft versus autograft patellar tendon anterior cruciate ligament reconstruction: A 5-year follow-up. *Arthroscopy* 17 (1):9–13.
Prado, C. M., V. E. Baracos, L. J. McCargar, T. Reiman, M. Mourtzakis, K. Tonkin, J. R. Mackey, S. Koski, E. Pituskin, and M. B. Sawyer. 2009. Sarcopenia as a determinant of chemotherapy toxicity and time to tumor progression in metastatic breast cancer patients receiving capecitabine treatment. *Clin Cancer Res* 15 (8):2920–2926.
Ravasco, P., I. Monteiro-Grillo, and M. E. Camilo. 2003. Does nutrition influence quality of life in cancer patients undergoing radiotherapy? *Radiother Oncol* 67 (2):213–220.
Ravasco, P., I. Monteiro-Grillo, P. M. Vidal, and M. E. Camilo. 2005. Dietary counseling improves patient outcomes: A prospective, randomized, controlled trial in colorectal cancer patients undergoing radiotherapy. *J Clin Oncol* 23 (7):1431–1438.
Reich, M. 2008. Depression and cancer: Recent data on clinical issues, research challenges and treatment approaches. *Curr Opin Oncol* 20 (4):353–359.
Richtsmeier, W. J., R. Dauchy, and L. A. Sauer. 1987. In vivo nutrient uptake by head and neck cancers. *Cancer Res* 47 (19):5230–5233.
Rivadeneira, D. E., D. Evoy, T. J. Fahey III, M. D. Lieberman, and J. M. Daly. 1998. Nutritional support of the cancer patient. *CA Cancer J. Clin* 48 (2):69–80.
Rofe, A. M., C. S. Bourgeois, P. Coyle, A. Taylor, and E. A. Abdi. 1994. Altered insulin response to glucose in weight-losing cancer patients. *Anticancer Res* 14 (2B):647–650.
Roubenoff, R. 2004. Sarcopenic obesity: The confluence of two epidemics. *Obes Res* 12 (6):887–888.
Safdie, F. M., T. Dorff, D. Quinn, L. Fontana, M. Wei, C. Lee, P. Cohen, and V. D. Longo. 2009. Fasting and cancer treatment in humans: A case series report. *Aging (Albany NY)* 1 (12):988–1007.
Sandulache, V. C., T. J. Ow, C. R. Pickering, M. J. Frederick, G. Zhou, I. Fokt, M. Davis-Malesevich, W. Priebe, and J. N. Myers. 2011. Glucose, not glutamine, is the dominant energy source required for proliferation and survival of head and neck squamous carcinoma cells. *Cancer* 117 (13):2926–2938.
Sarhill, N., F. A. Mahmoud, R. Christie, and A. Tahir. 2003. Assessment of nutritional status and fluid deficits in advanced cancer. *Am J Hosp Palliat Care* 20 (6):465–473.
Saxena, A., K. P. Tripathi, S. Roy, F. Khan, and A. Sharma. 2008. Pharmacovigilance: Effects of herbal components on human drugs interactions involving cytochrome P450. *Bioinformation* 3 (5):198–204.
Schlosser, E. 2001. *Fast Food Nation*. Boston, MA: Houghton Mifflin.

Schrager, M. A., E. J. Metter, E. Simonsick, A. Ble, S. Bandinelli, F. Lauretani, and L. Ferrucci. 2007. Sarcopenic obesity and inflammation in the InCHIANTI study. *J Appl Physiol (1985)* 102 (3):919–925.

Seligman, P. A., R. Fink, and E. J. Massey-Seligman. 1998. Approach to the seriously ill or terminal cancer patient who has a poor appetite. *Semin Oncol* 25 (2 Suppl 6):33–34.

Seyfried, T. N., R. E. Flores, A. M. Poff, and D. P. D'Agostino. 2014. Cancer as a metabolic disease: Implications for novel therapeutics. *Carcinogenesis* 35 (3):515–527.

Seyfried, T. N., and L. M. Shelton. 2010. Cancer as a metabolic disease. *Nutr Metab (Lond)* 7:7.

Shills, M. D. 1999. Nutrition and diet in cancer management. In *Modern Nutrition in Health and Disease*, 1317–1347. Baltimore, MD: Williams & Wilkins.

Siegel, R. L., K. D. Miller, and A. Jemal. 2016. Cancer statistics, 2016. *CA Cancer J Clin* 66 (1):7–30.

Smith, A. W., B. B. Reeve, K. M. Bellizzi, L. C. Harlan, C. N. Klabunde, M. Amsellem, A. S. Bierman, and R. D. Hays. 2008. Cancer, comorbidities, and health-related quality of life of older adults. *Health Care Financ Rev* 29 (4):41–56.

Snyder, C. F., C. C. Earle, R. J. Herbert, B. A. Neville, A. L. Blackford, and K. D. Frick. 2008. Trends in follow-up and preventive care for colorectal cancer survivors. *J Gen Intern Med* 23 (3):254–259.

Stahl, W., J. von Laar, H. D. Martin, T. Emmerich, and H. Sies. 2000. Stimulation of gap junctional communication: Comparison of acyclo-retinoic acid and lycopene. *Arch Biochem Biophys* 373 (1):271–274.

Steffen, A., J. M. Huerta, E. Weiderpass, H. B. Bueno-de-Mesquita, A. M. May, P. D. Siersema, R. Kaaks et al. 2015. General and abdominal obesity and risk of esophageal and gastric adenocarcinoma in the European Prospective Investigation into Cancer and Nutrition. *Int J Cancer* 137 (3):646–657.

Strowd, R. E., 3rd, and S. A. Grossman. 2015. The role of glucose modulation and dietary supplementation in patients with central nervous system tumors. *Curr Treat Options Oncol* 16 (8):36.

Sweet, E., F. Dowd, M. Zhou, L. J. Standish, and M. R. Andersen. 2016. The use of complementary and alternative medicine supplements of potential concern during breast cancer chemotherapy. *Evid Based Complement Alternat Med* 2016:4382687.

Tchekmedyian, N. S., C. Halpert, J. Ashley, and D. Heber. 1992. Nutrition in advanced cancer: Anorexia as an outcome variable and target of therapy. *JPEN J Parenter Enteral Nutr* 16 (6 Suppl):88S–92S.

Terepka, A. R., and C. Waterhouse. 1956. Metabolic observations during the forced feeding of patients with cancer. *Am J Med* 20 (2):225–238.

Tisdale, M. J. 1993. Cancer cachexia. *Anticancer Drugs* 4 (2):115–125.

Vigano, A., S. Watanabe, and E. Bruera. 1994. Anorexia and cachexia in advanced cancer patients. *Cancer Surv* 21:99–115.

Wargovich, M. J. 1999. Nutrition and cancer: The herbal revolution. *Curr Opin Gastroenterol* 15 (2):177–180.

Warren, J. L., A. B. Mariotto, A. Meekins, M. Topor, and M. L. Brown. 2008. Current and future utilization of services from medical oncologists. *J Clin Oncol* 26 (19):3242–3247.

Wickham, R. S., M. Rehwaldt, C. Kefer, S. Shott, K. Abbas, E. Glynn-Tucker, C. Potter, and C. Blendowski. 1999. Taste changes experienced by patients receiving chemotherapy. *Oncol Nurs Forum* 26 (4):697–706.

Wigmore, S. J., C. E. Plester, R. A. Richardson, and K. C. Fearon. 1997. Changes in nutritional status associated with unresectable pancreatic cancer. *Br J Cancer* 75 (1):106–109.

Williams, P. T. 1994. The role of family physicians in the management of cancer patients. *J Cancer Educ* 9 (2):67–72.

Worster, A., M. J. Bass, and M. L. Wood. 1996. Willingness to follow breast cancer. Survey of family physicians. *Can Fam Physician* 42:263–268.

Worster, A., M. L. Wood, I. R. McWhinney, and M. J. Bass. 1995. Who provides follow-up care for patients with early breast cancer? *Can Fam Physician* 41:1314–1320.

Wu, S., J. Liu, X. Wang, M. Li, Y. Gan, and Y. Tang. 2014. Association of obesity and overweight with overall survival in colorectal cancer patients: A meta-analysis of 29 studies. *Cancer Causes Control* 25 (11):1489–1502.

Zimmet, P., D. Magliano, Y. Matsuzawa, G. Alberti, and J. Shaw. 2005. The metabolic syndrome: A global public health problem and a new definition. *J Atheroscler Thromb* 12 (6):295–300.

20 Writing the Nutrition Prescription

20.1 INTRODUCTION

In this book, our goal has been to arm you with the necessary knowledge and tools to incorporate nutrition into your primary care practice. As a practical matter, this effort must be led by a dedicated primary care physician with the help of motivated registered dietitians, nurses, psychologists, physical therapists, and office staff, whether within your practice or by referral to the community. It is essential that the nutrition prescription provided by the physician be as efficient as possible. While many team members have superior knowledge in the areas of nutrition, exercise, and psychology, the doctor remains the focus of patient confidence in a therapy plan. Therefore, the endorsement of the plan, rather than the implementation of the plan, is the most important task of the physician. In this regard, we have provided detailed and referenced information on the role of nutrition in the most common conditions encountered in primary care practice. Much of this information was new and opposed to established teaching in American medical schools focused on drugs and surgery for the treatment of disease. Advanced technologies and drugs are effective for the treatment of acute disease, but many of the most common diseases, such as heart disease, diabetes, and cancer, are not preventable with drugs and surgery. While there is mention of prevention of heart disease, this largely relates to the use of statins, with some modest discussion of a healthy diet. Similarly, prevention of type 2 diabetes is the early introduction of metformin or intensive insulin therapy. We realize we are proposing a major change in attitude of primary health care providers in terms of the power of nutrition in the prevention and treatment of common disease.

20.2 NUTRITION PRESCRIPTIONS BY CHAPTER

This chapter provides the nutrition prescription relevant to each chapter, so that you will be able to initiate a plan within the difficult time constraints facing physicians today. As with prescriptions for drugs, long-term adherence is the challenge that must be faced after the nutrition prescription has been written. We will discuss how to engage your patients after they leave your office while maintaining a connection with your staff. The reach of the primary care practice can also be extended through commercial weight loss programs, Internet fitness and diet tools, and smartphone apps that are available to help patients improve their diet and lifestyle.

Chapter 1: Incorporating Nutrition into Your Practice

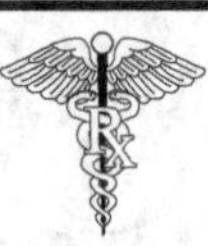

1. Survey your practice population's nutrition status and lifestyle.
2. Identify medical, nutritional, behavioral, and exercise resources available.
3. Obtain the equipment needed for primary care nutrition practice, including a bioimpedance scale with at least four contact points from a reliable manufacturer.
4. Review your office floor plan to accommodate obese patients in exam offices and provide space for group counseling and body composition at intake.
5. Train your staff to be empathetic and supportive in their interactions with the aged, the obese, and the nonadherent patients in your practice.
6. Modify routine practice steps to maintain efficient patient flow.
7. Provide Internet resources for self-monitoring and reporting progress to your practice.
8. Establish methods to obtain reimbursement for your services.

Chapter 2: Personalization of Nutrition Advice

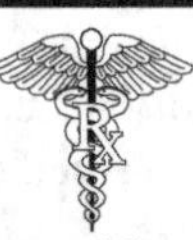

1. Measure lean body mass by bioimpedance and provide patients with protein recommendations and calorie recommendations for weight maintenance or weight loss to optimize body composition.
2. Evaluate fitness and provide an exercise prescription or referral to a physical therapist or certified trainer.
3. Through your registered dietitian, survey the diet and provide personalized food choices within the general guidelines based on the U.S. dietary guidelines for a healthy diet.
4. Optimize overall nutrition through diet and supplements.
5. Obtain information on botanical dietary supplements and provide advice.

Chapter 3: Nutrition and the Immune System

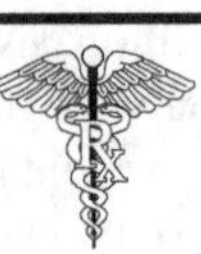

1. Determine if your patient has chronic inflammation complaints or frequent infections.
2. Optimize visceral fat measured by waist circumference through a combination of balanced diet and healthy active lifestyle.
3. Measure fatty acid profile and increase intake of omega-3 fatty acids from ocean-caught fish and seafood or fish oil or algae oil supplements. On a low-fat diet, about 2 g/day of eicosapentaenoic acid (EPA) and docosahexaenoic acid (DHA) should be optimum for most patients.
4. Determine whether patients are eating seven servings a day of colorful fruits and vegetables containing phytonutrients that optimize immune function.

Chapter 4: Nutrition and Gastrointestinal Disorders

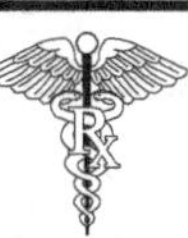

1. Determine if your patient has regular bowel movements or suffers from irritable bowel syndrome, including chronic constipation or diarrhea.
2. Determine whether food allergies or food intolerances are present. Ask about gluten sensitivity or enteropathy.
3. Assess whether there are any eating disorders or abnormal weight obsessions.
4. Optimize normal gastrointestinal function through hydration, fiber, and a regular biorhythm of eating and activity, including adequate sleep.
5. Ask your dietitian to determine sources of 25 g of dietary fiber per day from fruits, vegetables, and whole grains. Reduce intake of sugar and refined grains, as well as foods that cause bloating or other gastrointestinal symptoms.

Chapter 5: The Overweight and Obese Patient

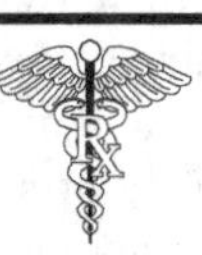

1. Determine the obesity phenotype.
2. Estimate energy expenditure and protein requirements.
3. Define a timescale for reaching the desirable weight range.
4. Provide structured diet programs that include the choice of using meal replacements and/or portion-controlled foods.
5. Prescribe leisure time physical activity and exercise.
6. Review behavioral strategies, including stress reduction, stimulus control, relapse prevention, social support, and self-monitoring.
7. Establish a plan for follow-up and social support individually or through groups.

Chapter 6: Nutrition and Evolution of Type 2 Diabetes

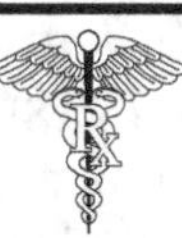

1. Determine the family history of type 2 diabetes and gestational diabetes to assess which patients require an intensive approach beyond the usual dietary guidelines.
2. Institute an intensive personalized diet, increased physical activity, educational sessions, and frequent follow-up patterned on the National Institutes of Health (NIH) Diabetes Prevention Program, but using the concepts outlined in Chapter 2 to optimize food and supplement intake.
3. In patients with excess body fat or metabolic syndrome, institute the program for weight management outlined in Chapter 5 and consider using meal replacements shown to be effective in the LOOK Ahead trial.
4. Reduce the consumption of sugar, especially from soft drinks and juices. Reduce high-glycemic-index foods and educate the patient on which foods to avoid.
5. Institute a personalized exercise program, including resistance exercises to build muscle, which will increase the uptake of glucose independent of insulin and reduce stress on the pancreatic β-cells.

Chapter 7: Managing Diabetes without Weight Gain

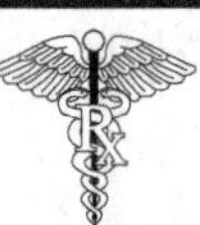

1. Determine the duration of type 2 diabetes mellitus and the likelihood that there are significant residual β-cell reserves of insulin. If necessary, conduct an oral glucose tolerance test measuring glucose, insulin, and C-peptide, the connecting peptide chain between the A and B chains of insulin and a validated measure of insulin reserves.
2. For patients with recent onset of diabetes or with significant insulin reserves, prescribe metformin according to the manufacturer's recommendations to spare pancreatic β-cell stress.
3. Emphasize weight management, since 95% of these patients are overweight or obese, over short-term tight glucose control.
4. When using insulin, incretins, or insulin secretagogue drugs to control blood sugar, use the minimum needed to maintain blood sugar at a level where there are no symptoms or immune impairment, but not to some tight control target that is theoretical. This is particularly dangerous in elderly patients or those with heart disease, where hypoglycemia causes a greater risk than mild hyperglycemia.
5. Avoid increasing insulin in patients not adherent to diet recommendations since this can result in a form of iatrogenic obesity due to high insulin levels promoting adipose tissue accumulation.
6. Utilize the principles in Chapters 5 and 6 to minimize weight gain through balanced diet and exercise prescriptions.
7. Institute a strong follow-up program, including exercise and food records, combined with blood glucose monitoring, so that patients can detect impacts of nonadherence to recommendations.

Chapter 8: Fatty Liver

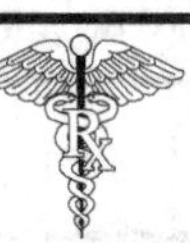

1. Assess liver function to determine the degree of suspicion for nonalcoholic steatohepatitis (NASH) disease. While fatty liver is very common, it is not sufficient for the diagnosis of NASH, which requires liver fat greater than 5% on MRI or, if clinically indicated, a liver biopsy, which should be performed by a liver specialist or gastroenterologist due to the significant risks of the procedure.
2. Assess whether metabolic syndrome or diabetes is present and utilize the steps in Chapters 6 and 7 if this is the case.
3. If there is no history of obesity, diabetes, or metabolic syndrome, consult a liver specialist to rule out other causes or contributors to the risk of liver failure or hepatocellular carcinoma.
4. Consider using 800 IU of vitamin E per day, milk thistle, and omega-3 fatty acid supplementation, together with the appropriate diet and exercise approaches emphasized. While not proven in clinical trials, shared decision making with patients is appropriate for these dietary supplements.
5. Institute a careful follow-up program to assess the impact of lifestyle changes on liver function tests (aspartate aminotransferase [AST], alanine aminotransferase [ALT], and gamma-glutamyltransferase [GGT]) and liver fat by MRI.

Chapter 9: Lipid Disorders and Management

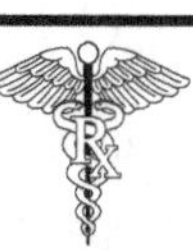

1. Determine whether the patient has dyslipidemia with elevated triglycerides and cholesterol or isolated hypercholesterolemia.
2. For isolated hypercholesterolemia, use statins or, in countries other than the United States, where legal, Chinese red yeast rice.
3. Add soluble fibers like guar or β-glucan supplements and phytosterol supplements to bind cholesterol in the intestine, which will reduce the size of the cholesterol pool and lower blood levels of LDL cholesterol.
4. In dyslipidemia, the most common lipid disorder, use fish oil supplements to lower triglycerides and β-glucan or phytosterols to lower cholesterol. Also, employ the same weight management strategies used to prevent type 2 diabetes mellitus or treat the metabolic syndrome, as these conditions often include hypertriglyceridemia.
5. In the diet, reduce excess sugar, refined carbohydrates, *trans* fats, and omega-6 fats to make the fish oils more effective in lowering triglyceride levels. Use monounsaturated fats from olive oil, avocados, and tree nuts to reduce inflammation, which promotes hypertriglyceridemia.

Chapter 10: Nutrition and Coronary Artery Disease

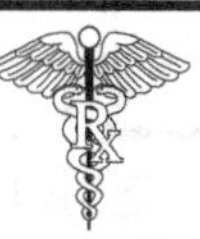

1. In patients with a prior cardiac event, institute statin therapy or, in countries other than the United States, Chinese red yeast rice. The statins and polyketides in Chinese red yeast rice have anti-inflammatory effects, in addition to lowering cholesterol levels.
2. Institute a diet consistent with the guidelines of the American Heart Association, but which incorporates a somewhat lower level of fat, in combination with restricted excess sugar and refined carbohydrates.
3. Fats should emphasize monounsaturated fats and limit hidden omega-6 and *trans* fats in processed foods. Fish oil from ocean-caught fish and fish oil supplements should be used to reduce inflammation. Prescribe aerobic exercise for cardiac rehabilitation, including behavior change strategies, such as meditation, combined with stress reduction and treatment of comorbid conditions, such as hypertension or type 2 diabetes mellitus.
4. Recommend seven servings per day of colorful fruits and vegetables. Evidence has been found for the benefits of lutein in stabilizing coronary arterial plaques, but other phytonutrients and antioxidants may also be of benefit.
5. Beetroot extract can be recommended to increase nitrite storage in myocardium, which is activated under conditions of hypoxia.

Chapter 11: Hypertension and Obesity

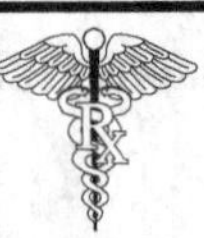

1. Diagnose and treat obesity—the most common cause of hypertension.
2. The Dietary Approaches to Stop Hypertension (DASH) diet, rich in nutrients from fruits, vegetables, and dairy, with modest levels of sodium and omega-3 and omega-6 fatty acids, has emerged as a balanced dietary strategy for the management of hypertension.
3. Soy protein rich in arginine can increase nitrite levels in the blood, as can beetroot extract rich in nitrate that is converted to nitrite by oral bacteria, absorbed in the blood as nitric oxide, and stored in the heart muscle and other organs as nitrite, which can be converted to nitric oxide under hypoxic conditions.
4. For sodium control, reduce the intake of processed foods with hidden sodium and increase potassium-rich fruits and vegetables. Excessive sodium restriction to levels of 1500 mg/day may be harmful and unattainable. Reasonable sodium intake controls, together with the DASH diet, are adequate to control blood pressure.
5. In obese patients not responsive to diet and sodium control, and in those with uncontrolled hypertension, adjunctive pharmacotherapy should be used, including agents targeting sympathetic activation, increased renal tubular sodium reabsorption, and overexpression of the renin–angiotensin–aldosterone system (RAAS) by the adipocyte.

Chapter 12: Nutrition and Renal Failure

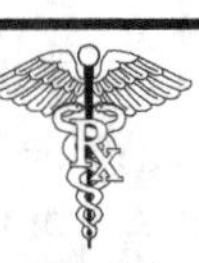

1. Review the estimated glomerular filtration rate (GFR) from the lab analysis based on serum creatinine, height, and weight. Check for proteinuria, microalbuminuria, and coexisting obesity or diabetes.
2. If it is borderline low in an individual with increased lean body mass, order a 24-hour urinary creatinine clearance test. If it is normal in an individual with a low lean body mass and a comorbid condition associated with sarcopenia, order a 24-hour urinary creatinine clearance.
3. If chronic kidney disease is found, concentrate on the treatment of hypertension, which is the one factor that can affect the rate of change in GFR.
4. Optimize the treatment of coexisting hyperlipidemia or diabetes.
5. Treat with an RAAS inhibitor in the obese diabetic patient with chronic kidney disease.
6. Address overweight and obesity with diet and exercise recommendations.

Chapter 13: Nutrition and Heart Failure

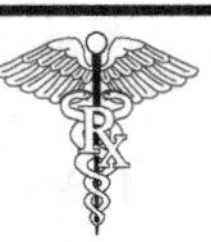

1. Educate patients on the importance of adhering to their medication regimen using inhibitors of the RAAS or sympathetic nervous system.
2. Use diuretics for symptomatic relief and minimize doses using B-natriuretic peptide monitoring.
3. Restrict sodium to 2.8 g/day and fluid intake to 1–2 L/day.
4. Patients should weigh themselves daily to detect fluid shifts and be taught that each quart or liter weighs about 2 pounds or 1 kg.
5. Supplement with omega-3 fatty acids and reduce omega-6 fats in the diet.
6. Supplement with coenzyme Q10 as ubiquinone or ubiquinol.
7. Supplement with a multivitamin or multimineral to compensate for vitamin and mineral losses through urine secondary to diuretic use.

Chapter 14: Pulmonary Function, Asthma, and Obesity

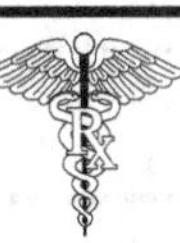

1. Ask obese patients about snoring and sleep quality. Conduct a formal sleep study if indicated. Poor sleep promotes overeating and obesity, which leads to poor sleep and sleep apnea.
2. Initiate weight management using the methods outlined in Chapter 5.
3. Initiate continuous positive airway pressure (CPAP) treatment at the same time, as they act together.
4. Initiate a sleep hygiene program to promote good-quality sleep.
5. Stress the avoidance of nicotine and caffeine as appropriate.
6. Initiate an exercise and stress reduction program for weight management and improvement of sleep quality.

Chapter 15: Frailty, Nutrition, and the Elderly

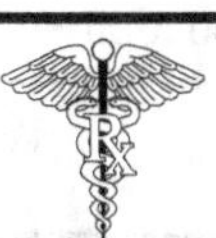

1. Increase protein intake to 1 g/pound of lean body mass and initiate a program of physical therapy and resistance training to combat sarcopenic obesity.
2. Increase fruit and vegetable intake, especially lutein-containing green vegetables, for the prevention of age-related macular degeneration and for brain health.
3. Initiate supplementation with a multivitamin or multimineral, 2000–5000 IU/day of vitamin D, and fish oils providing 2 g/day of EPA and DHA.
4. Survey taste changes and food preference changes to ensure that overall nutrition is adequate.
5. Prescribe daily walking and assess walking speed as a variable over time in response to physical therapy and resistance exercise, combined with protein supplementation.
6. Consider anabolic androgen treatment in advanced sarcopenia and assess the risks and benefits with each patient individually.

Chapter 16: Nutrition and Neurodegenerative Diseases

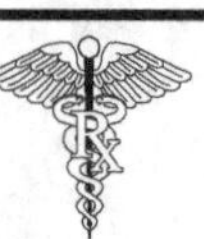

1. Assess cognitive function using questionnaires. If cognitive impairment is present, then initiate a program of mental and physical exercise, stress reduction, and social engagement.
2. Initiate a nutrition program to supplement protein, increase antioxidant intake, and reduce inflammation.
3. Initiate supplementation with a multivitamin or multimineral, 2000–5000 IU/day of vitamin D, and fish oils providing 2 g/day of EPA and DHA. Consider bioavailable forms of curcumin to ameliorate inflammation in the brain, even though clinical research is ongoing.
4. Increase intake of colorful fruits and vegetables, including cranberry, pomegranate, and cocoa flavonols. Consider beetroot extract to improve endothelial function.
5. If there are no contraindications, consider green tea extract, caffeine, and gingko biloba extract to improve concentration and attention.
6. Treat coexisting obesity and type 2 diabetes as indicated in Chapters 5 through 7.

Chapter 17: Gene–Nutrient Interactions

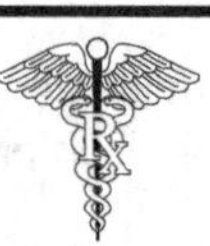

1. Recommend a multivitamin or multimineral supplement.
2. Measure homocysteine levels and supplement with folate, choline, and betaine as necessary to reduce levels of homocysteine.
3. Measure iron and iron-binding capacity to detect hemochromatosis. Genetic testing is not necessary to make the diagnosis.
4. Recommend cruciferous vegetable intake at three servings or more per week. Alternatively, recommend a broccoli sprout extract.
5. Consume seven servings per day of colorful fruits and vegetables.
6. Initiate supplementation with 5000 IU of vitamin D daily.
7. Do *not* recommend a commercial genetic test for the purpose of generating dietary recommendations.

Chapter 18: Nutrition and the Risks of Common Forms of Cancer

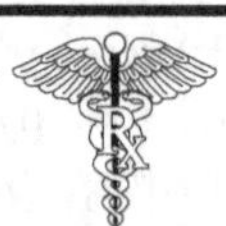

1. Assess family history of common forms of cancer. While usually sporadic, there are some families with a strong history of genetic forms of cancer.
2. Obtain the history of cancer treatment and site in cancer survivors.
3. In cancer survivors, initiate a preventive nutrition program to prevent recurrence, emphasizing achieving and maintaining a desirable body composition and weight, increased intake of fruits and vegetables, and judicious use of dietary supplements.

Chapter 19: Nutrition and the Cancer Patient 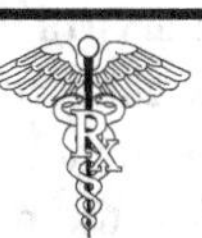

1. Assess nutrition status in patients with advanced cancer and support them with enteral nutrition supplementation after treatment. Work closely with oncologists on any dietary recommendations and potential nutritional side effects of cancer treatment.
2. In cancer patients, utilize nutrition intervention to preserve or increase lean body mass, reduce fatigue, improve quality of life, correct specific nutrition deficiencies, improve tolerance of cancer therapy, reduce side effects and complications related to nutrition, and enhance immunity and decrease the risk of infection.
3. In cancer cachexia, support the patient with enteral nutrition for basic needs and allow food intake for pleasure without concern as to calorie intake.
4. Initiate a program for appetite improvement, as outlined in the chapter.
5. Consider using appetite-enhancing drugs such as megestrol acetate and marijuana or cannabinoid extract supplements.

20.3 ENGAGING WITH PATIENTS USING WEARABLE DEVICES AND SOCIAL MEDIA

The Internet has had a major impact on the lives of primary care physicians. While word processing has been a feature of medical practice since the 1980s, it was mainly used for the production of physical letters sent to patients or insurers. Today, virtually all communications about patients are conducted electronically, including widespread use of electronic health records, which record all lab tests and visits. There are also patient-accessible services, allowing them to see their medical records and empowering them to see the changes that result from altering diet and lifestyle habits.

While there is no documentation yet, it is hoped that the use of electronic health records will enable better communication among health care providers, greater accountability for therapeutic decisions, and a greater ability to study the quality of care. In addition, the advent of PubMed, supported by the U.S. government, has made a major difference in the ability of physicians to access research and clinical information relevant to their daily challenges in a timely fashion. Just 40 years ago, it was necessary to go to the physical library and read or copy heavy bound books containing annual collections of medical or scientific journal articles. Textbooks were only available in libraries, and the general information that lives on Internet-accessible sites today was limited to physical books. All the above advances fall under the heading of the internal Internet designed for the benefit of the physician or primary care provider, with some benefit for the process of patient care. Most physicians have used private e-mail or patient communication systems linked to their institution, which patients can access independently to review lab tests or medical notes. The advent of these services has made it easier to meet privacy requirements mandated in the United States in the 1990s as the Health Insurance Portability and Accountability Act (HIPAA). Prior to the enactment of this law, insurance companies and individuals could access medical record information without the consent of the patient.

There is also an external-facing use of the Internet, including social media. Social media has exploded over the past decade, as Facebook, Instagram, What's App, and We Chat have become a part of the American culture. Recently, the founder of Facebook, Mark Zuckerberg, launched a multi-billion-dollar initiative to utilize social media in the battle for better health and new discoveries that solve the most pressing chronic diseases to improve quality of life and health span. Facebook now has the capability to host video and live TV shows, which enables primary care providers to create a virtual community in which patient education can be provided efficiently to large numbers of patients simultaneously using an interactive forum.

The power of big data to create information that can be mined by epidemiologists promises to provide new clues to the prevention and treatment of chronic disease, much as we have opened new avenues for primary care practices to use diet and exercise to reduce risk factors for disease in multiple organ systems. As diet and exercise interventions become more common in primary care practice, observations in clinical practice will form a new database for the evolution of controlled clinical trials, which will also be carried out using social media. Using Instagram, it is possible to take photographs of meals being eaten or supplements consumed, enabling better assessment of adherence to treatment and research study protocols.

A Facebook page for the primary care practice can also accomplish several other objectives, including providing patients with more information about their provider's human side, including interests and expertise. Primary care patient education can also be provided on a blog that is part of your primary care practice website. In all these places, you can provide your patients with links to controversial newspaper and magazine articles, with summaries and the doctor or primary care provider's opinions appended. This will start a conversation between patients and providers and lead to a meeting of the minds on a central philosophy that motivates both providers and patients as a mission for better nutrition.

Shared decision making has been emphasized for therapeutic decisions on pharmacotherapy but has not been emphasized in nutrition and exercise, where the default position is the government's dietary guidelines, which do not provide adequate personalization since they were designed for the average healthy population. As a result, more than 80% of the public do not meet either dietary guidelines or the guidelines designed to encourage physical activity. Through social media, it is possible for you to provide patients with special advice for different disease conditions, as discussed in this text.

This chapter reviews the range of these types of opportunities for enhanced interaction between patients, providers, and communities in order to enhance your ability to communicate your personal philosophy of nutrition and chronic disease to your patients.

20.3.1 Wearable Devices

A major reason that guidelines do not change behavior is that there is no provision for patient accountability to themselves or to the primary care practice. There is a coming revolution in wearable devices to monitor physical activity, blood pressure, blood glucose, sleep quality, and temperature throughout the day. From these measures, it will be possible to estimate total energy expenditure or calorie burning during the day. While the accuracy of these estimates can be questioned by scientists studying these physiological functions in detail, the inaccuracies of the methods are beside the point, as these devices are mainly intended to provide feedback to both patients and the primary care provider as changes occur that indicate adherence with recommended nutrition and exercise recommendations.

Wearable devices can be used to monitor the most basic aspect of physical activity passively. Counting steps per day and increasing them gradually to 10,000 per day is a first step in incorporating a healthy active lifestyle into one's daily routine. A walk after dinner can promote better digestion. A brisk morning walk can serve to activate the body and prepare it for targeted muscle-building exercises. There are a number of watches and other devices, including smartphones, that have internal accelerometers. These devices register movements and record them, from simply shaking up and down during walking to actually monitoring the movement involved in walking. While these devices do not record all physical activity, they do a good job of monitoring walking and running steps. They also often link to programs for monitoring food intake. The interesting aspect of recording food intake is that it is not only a monitoring method but also an intervention to change dietary patterns as a result of recording food intake.

All the above automated and interactive computer applications are wonderful, but they do not substitute for personal contact. Office visits can be supplemented by group intervention lectures involving up to 20 people. The interchange that results from a question-and-answer session can build strong relationships between patients and primary care providers. Volunteering for media opportunities on local television or speaking to local civic groups also enhances the prestige of a primary care practice.

20.3.2 Social Media

The greatest opportunity provided by social media is to humanize a primary care practice for patients. A Facebook page with photos of staff and physicians, along with some basic background information, can help patients get to know their doctors better, which is not always possible during a rushed office visit. Some of the posts can also be used to educate patients on health practices, nutrition, exercise, and prevention. In addition to basic information, it is helpful to promote a dialogue on controversial issues. This will engage patients and let them see how you make your decisions and the specifics of your nutrition philosophy. Patients should be discouraged from posting information on their own medical conditions, but should be encouraged to ask questions with regard to practice services.

When social media is used strictly as a marketing tool with a one-way lecture on information about a practice, it loses its appeal. Too much of a strong advertisement will defeat the community-building purpose of social media by lacking authenticity. The goal of social media should be to engage with patients and build trust. The marketing will flow naturally via word of mouth that your site is worth visiting. The various social media platforms can be used together. For example, you can promote a message on healthy lifestyles in a 60-second video. You can then incorporate it into your Facebook page or link it into a 140-character Twitter message. There are applications that allow you to post the same message on multiple platforms, including Facebook, Twitter, Google Plus, and LinkedIn. You can post messages that link to a blog on your practice website. You can share interesting information you may have read on various platforms. Patients may also follow your Twitter account with links to other social media where you appear.

Millennials use social media, and although many physicians are not familiar with various platforms, such as Instagram and Pinterest, these patients and their young families do use these services. An online presence is going to be a routine way for medical practices to be noticed in their communities, and it would be worthwhile to begin to get familiar with social media's potential.

20.4 MANAGING INFORMATION OVERLOAD TO KEEP UP WITH NUTRITION RESEARCH

Just 20 years ago, the typical busy practitioner would subscribe to several well-established medical journals. Between patients or at lunch, there would be time to read at least the abstract and then clip a few interesting articles to place in a file cabinet. Medical information management was so inefficient as to make physicians dependent on continuing education courses. These courses were often supported by the drug industry, and well-known authorities would cleverly transmit the messages that the drug industry needed to promote sales of their products. There was much less to know and far fewer controversies to handle.

Today, primary care providers are flooded with information and misinformation on nutrition, medicines, and putative cures for chronic diseases by social media, television news, e-mail, and print and online reports. In 2013, the Institute of Medicine acknowledged this problem, stating, "The ever-increasing volume of evidence makes it difficult for clinicians to maintain a working knowledge of new clinical information" (Mehta et al. 2016). The huge volume of information confronting primary care providers today has meant that rather than try to maintain a routine habit of professional reading, many primary care providers now seek information only when answers to specific clinical questions are needed for patient care. The advantage of this approach, which is reactive rather than proactive searching, is that it promotes the skills of problem-based learning.

The disadvantage is that it assumes that physicians and their associates are consciously aware of the need to search for new information. It is also time-consuming to constantly scan sources for new evidence in primary care practice nutrition to avoid the problem of knowing obsolete or contradicted concepts. Physicians are expected to practice so-called evidence-based medicine relying on meta-analyses of efficacy, which is often a valid approach for some forms of pharmacotherapy. In general, the approach of looking at the Cochrane Library or PubMed for meta-analyses will only be clear on well-established practices, but will be of less utility in nutrition. Nutrition does not easily lend itself to the types of randomized placebo-controlled trials typical of the evaluation of a new drug, Methods for assessing food intake in free-living populations are not yet adequate for this purpose, relying on self-report or supervised dietary recall. Similarly, methods for assessing physical activity are indirect, and outside the metabolic ward setting, they are difficult to quantitate.

20.5 INFORMATION MANAGEMENT STRATEGIES

A powerful information management strategy is a way to become aware of relevant new information in primary care nutrition practice or research by setting up feeds of information from reliable and authentic sources. These feeds can be browsed on any computer or smart mobile device. There are several ways to establish these feeds. One option is to subscribe to the table of contents of relevant journals via e-mail. Another option is a research site summary (RSS) feed reader. RSS is a standard for publishing summaries of frequently updated content on the World Wide Web, such as journal tables of contents and articles from medical journal news sites. Scientific societies such as the American Society for Nutrition also release article summaries from their journal. You can subscribe to these using feed reader software from Feedly (www.feedly.com) or Inoreader (www.inoreader.com), which can be used with any browser on a desktop or laptop. They are also available as apps for mobile devices such as smartphones and tablets. The feed reader periodically checks for new content and automatically downloads it to the device. Thus, you do not need to check multiple websites for updates. Instead, the content is delivered to your device for reading and scanning at your convenience.

Patients will often ask about a news feature that they heard only briefly and often take away incomplete or incorrect information. Surveys have found that up to one-third of local news is devoted to health stories, and these are often about nutrition and weight loss. The Internet is full of misinformation associated with the sale of products promoting ideas that have no basis in science. You do not have much control over these information streams, and so it is important to be able to determine the information that is most important and most relevant to you and your practice. Accessing, reading, organizing, storing, and retrieving useful medical information can both improve patient care and provide you with a feeling of greater control over this information.

It is possible to create a personalized stream of relevant information that can be scanned regularly and saved so that it is readily accessible. You simply have to dedicate some staff time up front to set up the topics. This does not substitute for an understanding of the subject, but it will keep you updated.

20.6 CONTINUING EDUCATION AND CERTIFICATION

If you have developed a strong interest in clinical nutrition, there are opportunities for you to obtain certification. Here, we provide just an overview of three examples.

20.6.1 American Board of Nutrition Physician Specialists

Originally founded as the American Board of Nutrition in 1948, Physician Nutrition Specialist (NBPNS) administers the comprehensive Certification Examination for Physician Nutrition

Specialists (PNSs). The diplomats generally have backgrounds in the specialties of internal medicine, pediatrics, family medicine, or general surgery, and sometimes in subspecialties such as adult or pediatric gastroenterology, endocrinology, critical care, nephrology, or cardiology.

To be eligible to take the NBPNS exam, a candidate must meet three requirements:

1. Current licensure to practice medicine in the United States, or the equivalent in other countries. All candidates for certification and recertification must be licensed to practice medicine in the country in which they reside.
2. American Board of Medical Specialties (ABMS) certification or the equivalent outside the United States.
3. Demonstrated expertise in nutrition defined by one or more of the following:
   a. Mentored training in clinical nutrition (requires letter of recommendation from mentor)
   b. Dedicated service on a hospital multidisciplinary nutrition team (requires letter of recommendation from hospital chief of staff or physician head of department)
   c. Performance of research with publications in nutrition (provide documentation on curriculum vitae)
   d. Teaching position involving nutrition at an academic medical center (requires letter of recommendation from department chairman)
   e. Committee membership and/or leadership role in a national nutrition society (provide documentation on curriculum vitae)
   f. Completion of a minimum of 150 hours of continuing medical education (CME) devoted to clinical nutrition (provide CME documentation)
   g. Regional peer-recognized leadership role in nutrition (requires letter of recommendation from peer in community)
4. Completion and filing of an application for the Certification Examination for Physician Nutrition Specialists, including copies of the candidate's current medical license and board certification.

Unlike less rigorous certifications, NBPNS accepts only physician applicants. To qualify for the exam, a physician must first be licensed in his or her state or jurisdiction and have boards in a primary specialty. Current diplomats hold primary specialty certification in either internal medicine, pediatrics, family medicine, or general surgery. Many of the internists and pediatricians are also subspecialists in either gastroenterology, endocrinology, or critical care. Many of the surgeons are subspecialists in critical care, trauma, or burns. They must then complete an approved fellowship in clinical nutrition, or a time-limited alternate pathway exists for demonstrating expertise in nutrition based on mentored training and self-learning.

Approved fellowships are currently available at the following 13 institutions: University of Alabama at Birmingham, Boston University, University of California at Los Angeles, University of Chicago, Children's Hospital of Philadelphia, Cleveland Clinic, University of Alberta, Canada, University of Colorado, Columbia University Medical Center, Geisinger Health System, Harvard/Massachusetts General Hospital, Memorial-Sloan Kettering Cancer Center, and Atlantic Health/Morristown Medical Center. Fellowships are 1–2 years in duration.

An applicant who passes the NBPNS exam receives a PNS certification that is valid for 10 years, after which the candidate must retake the certification examination or meet maintenance of certification (MOC) requirements.

NBPNS is a collaboration of the eight major nutrition professional societies. These include the American Society of Nutrition (ASN), American College of Nutrition (ACN), American Society of Parenteral and Enteral Nutrition (ASPEN), Canadian Nutrition Society (CNS), The Obesity Society (TOS), American Gastroenterological Association (AGA), American Association of Clinical Endocrinology (AACE), and Society for Critical Care Medicine (SCCM). Each stakeholder has a board seat.

Website: http://www.nutritioncare.org/NBPNS/

20.6.2 American Board of Obesity Medicine

The American Board of Obesity Medicine (ABOM) serves the public and the field of obesity medicine by maintaining standards for the assessment and credentialing of physicians. Certification as an ABOM diplomate signifies specialized knowledge in the practice of obesity medicine and distinguishes a physician as having achieved competency in obesity care.

To be eligible for the ABOM certification, a candidate must have three credentials:

1. Proof of an active medical license in the United States or Canada
2. Proof of completion of a residency in the United States or Canada
3. Active board certification in an ABMS member board or osteopathic medicine equivalent

A candidate must also have the required CME credit hours:

1. A minimum of 60 credit hours of CME recognized by the American Medical Association Physician Recognition Award (AMA PRA) Category 1 Credits on the topic of obesity are required for certification.
2. At least 30 credit hours must be obtained in person at a live meeting or conference.
3. The remaining 30 credit hours may be obtained by at-home CME activity.

All 60 CME credits must be earned within 36 months of the application deadline (e.g., from August 30, 2013 to August 30, 2016). All CME credits must be earned and documented at the time of application, except in the case of two specific meetings that take place each fall. CME credit hours from the Obesity Medicine Association's fall 2016 meeting and The Obesity Society's Obesity Week 2016 meeting will be valid for the 2016 ABOM exam with meeting registration documentation submitted with all other application requirements.

An applicant who passes the ABOM exam becomes a ABOM diplomate, and the certification is valid for 10 years, after which the candidate must meet the recertification requirements to be recertified.

Website: http://abom.org/

20.6.3 Specialist Certification of Obesity Professional Education

Specialist Certification of Obesity Professional Education (SCOPE) is a program supported by the World Obesity Federation and is the only internationally recognized certification in obesity management, endorsed by the National Health Service (NHS) and more than 50 national scientific obesity associations globally. It equips health professionals with up-to-date, evidence-based obesity management resources, to better treat their obese patients and excel in their careers. This certification is available not only to physicians but also to all professionals engaged in obesity treatment, including psychologists, nurses, dietitians, and exercise specialists.

To be eligible for the SCOPE certification, a candidate must meet the following criteria:

1. Evidence of 6 months of practical experience related to obesity management within a medical or allied health care professional setting.
2. At least 4 points from SCOPE e-learning modules.
3. Twelve points are required for certification. You may choose to accumulate the remaining 8 points through e-learning or combine e-learning with
   a. SCOPE schools (4 points)
   b. SCOPE-accredited instructor-led courses

SCOPE certification is renewable annually by completing two additional SCOPE modules and submitting a renewal fee.

Website: http://www.worldobesity.org/scope/

There are separate certifications for dietitians through the Academy of Nutrition and Dietetics. Beginning in 2017 Registered Dietitians will need to obtain a Masters' Degree in Nutrition. Fitness trainers can obtain certification through the American College of Sports Medicine. While certification is not necessary, it may serve to establish the expertise of your primary care practice. Finally, we hope you have enjoyed reading this text and will recommend it to your colleagues.

REFERENCE

Mehta, N. B., S. A. Martin, J. Maypole, and R. Andrews. 2016. Information management for clinicians. *Cleve Clin J Med* 83 (8):589–595.

Index

D

E

F

G

H

I

P

R

S

T

U

V

W

X